HISTOLOGY OF THE FETUS AND NEWBORN

Marie A. Valdés-Dapena, M.D.
Director, Section of Pediatric Pathology
Department of Pathology
University of Miami-Jackson Memorial
Medical Center
Professor of Pathology and Pediatrics
University of Miami School of Medicine
Miami, Florida

1979
W. B. SAUNDERS COMPANY
Philadelphia, London, Toronto

W. B. Saunders Company: West Washington Square
Philadelphia, PA 19105

1 St. Anne's Road
Eastbourne, East Sussex BN21 3UN, England

1 Goldthorne Avenue
Toronto, Ontario M8Z 5T9, Canada

Histology of the Fetus and Newborn   ISBN 0-7216-8948-5

© 1979 by the W. B. Saunders Company. Copyright under the International Copyright Union. All rights reserved. This book is protected by copyright. No part of it may be reproduced, stored in a retrieval system or transmitted in any form or by any means, electronic, mechanical, photocopying, recording, or otherwise, without written permission from the publisher. Made in the United States of America. Press of W. B. Saunders Company. Library of Congress catalog card number 78-64731.

Last digit is the print number: 9   8   7   6   5   4   3   2   1

Dedicated to

Antonio M. Valdés-Dapena, M.D., my husband,
who has enriched my life beyond measure,

Our children, Vicki, Debi, Cris, Andy, Teddy, Bob,
Mark, Dan, Patty, Caty and Peter Paul . . . and to

James B. Arey, M.D., my teacher and my friend.

Preface

Ever since I began working in the field of pathologic anatomy, as a first year resident, I have had difficulty knowing what comprises the normal histology of organs and tissues. The problem was magnified, or multiplied, whenever I dealt with the tissues of fetuses or newborns because, particularly in that age group, normal morphology changes so much from stage to stage of development.

It was that sense of inadequacy which impelled me to put together my first atlas on perinatal histology, published in 1957. I felt certain then that there must be others, particularly persons in training like me, who needed some kind of fixed and graded set of visual images against which to measure their perceptions of the sections they were examining. Because at the time the audience for such a work was correctly assumed by the publisher to be limited, the book itself was made of modest size; the market would not have supported anything more elaborate.

In the intervening twenty years, interest in pediatric pathology has burgeoned. Not only are many more physicians practicing the subspecialty now, but many more are devoting themselves to it exclusively and there are many more training programs in the field as well. Logically, then, the need to recognize what constitutes normal tissue has grown in parallel fashion. Thus it seemed reasonable to attempt once more to respond to that relative void in the realm of reference books, by constructing a second and more comprehensive compilation of illustrations, limited to tissues of infants as they are seen by light microscopy.

This book was created to answer the simple questions we all encounter daily: What does the normal lung of an infant of 36 weeks gestation look like under the microscope, in routine hematoxylin and eosin stained sections? — or the lung at 28 weeks? — or the spleen at 30 weeks?

This book makes no pretense at being anything other than a ready, work-a-day reference for the practitioner of pathology and the resident in anatomic pathology; it is presented because there is no other. It fills a void. It serves a common need.

MARIE VALDÉS-DAPENA, M.D.

Acknowledgments

I am deeply indebted to Mr. Otto Lehmann of the Department of Medical Communications at Temple University School of Medicine for his patience, diligence and expertise; it is he who produced most of the photomicrographs in this book. Special thanks are due Mr. Charles Bailey of the Department of Biomedical Communications at the University of Miami School of Medicine, who finished the job so well begun by Mr. Lehmann.

Four secretaries assisted in compilation of data and typing of the manuscript; I am grateful to them all—Mrs. Louise Rhodes, Miss Dorothy Ardente, Mrs. Jeanne Logue and Miss Anne O'Connor.

Microscopic sections, autopsy protocols and surgical pathology reports utilized in the creation of this collection were derived from the following institutions:

1. Temple University Health Sciences Center, Philadelphia, Pa. (1959–1976)
2. St. Christopher's Hospital for Children, Philadelphia, Pa. (1959–1976)
3. University of Miami–Jackson Memorial Medical Center, Miami, Fla. (1976–1978)
4. Fitzgerald-Mercy Hospital, Lansdowne, Pa. (1949–1951)
5. Women's Medical College Hospital, Philadelphia, Pa. (1951–1959)
6. Graduate Hospital of the University of Pennsylvania, Philadelphia, Pa. (1951–1959)

MARIE VALDÉS-DAPENA, M.D.

Contents

Part One: **CARDIOVASCULAR SYSTEM** 1
    1. Heart 3
    2. Blood Vessels 31

Part Two: **LYMPHOID TISSUE** 43
    3. Thymus 45
    4. Palatine Tonsils 59
    5. Lymph Nodes 65

Part Three: **SPLEEN** 79
    6. Spleen 81

Part Four: **ENDOCRINE GLANDS** 101
    7. Pituitary Gland 103
    8. Thyroid Gland 117
    9. Parathyroid Glands 126
   10. Adrenal Gland 131

Part Five: **SKIN** 155
   11. Skin 157

Part Six: **GASTROINTESTINAL TRACT** 167
   12. Tongue 168
   13. Salivary Glands 183
   14. Esophagus 193
   15. Stomach 207
   16. Small Intestine 223
   17. Large Intestine 233
   18. Liver and Gallbladder 245
   19. Pancreas 269

Part Seven: **RESPIRATORY SYSTEM** 285

    20. Upper Respiratory Tract 287
    21. Lower Respiratory Tract 309

Part Eight: **URINARY SYSTEM** 343

    22. Kidney 345
    23. Urinary Bladder and Urethra 383

Part Nine: **MALE REPRODUCTIVE SYSTEM** 395

    24. Testis 397
    25. Prostate 415

Part Ten: **FEMALE REPRODUCTIVE SYSTEM** 431

    26. Ovary 433
    27. Fallopian Tubes 469
    28. Uterus and Vagina 479

Part Eleven: **Breast** 501

    29. Breast 503

Part Twelve: **EYE** 513

    30. Eye 515

Part Thirteen: **NEURAL TISSUES** 531

    31. Central Nervous System 533

Part Fourteen: **SUPPORTING STRUCTURES** 621

    32. Muscular System 623
    33. Skeletal System 629
    34. Adipose Tissue 641

INDEX 647

Part 1

CARDIOVASCULAR SYSTEM

Chapter 1

HEART

EMBRYOLOGY

The primordium of the heart appears in the third week of gestation within the mesoderm in front of, or ventral to, the oral membrane. Here, two short endocardial tubes, a right and a left, develop in the mesenchyme and fuse to form a single median vessel.[1]

In the fourth week the cardiac rudiment is carried ventrally beneath the foregut and behind the oral membrane. At this stage the heart has begun to beat. Its subsequent development consists of folding, differential growth, and the formation of septa in different parts of the original tube.[1]

As the simple tubular heart elongates, it begins to exhibit alternate dilatations and constrictions. At about the twenty-third day a ventricle and an atrium are recognizable, the former lying cranial to the latter.[2]

The arterial (cranial) and venous (caudal) ends of the heart tube are fixed in place by the branchial arches and the septum transversum, respectively. Because the ventricle and its adjacent outflow tract, the bulbus cordis, grow faster than the rest of the heart, the heart bends upon itself to form a V-shaped bulboventricular loop ventrally; later the bend becomes S-shaped.

As the heart bends, the atrium and its inflow tract, the sinus venosus, come to lie dorsally.

All during these stages of the evolution of the organ, the mesenchyme around the heart tubes proliferates and forms a thick *myoepicardial mantle*, which ultimately differentiates to form the myocardium (from myoblasts) and the epicardium. Between the myoepicardial mantle and the endothelial lining is the so-called cardiac jelly, a loose gelatinous connective tissue which forms the subendocardial tissue.[2]

Partitioning of the heart begins about the middle of the fourth week and is virtually complete by the end of the fifth week. Thickenings of the subendocardial tissue, called endocardial cushions, appear in the dorsal and ventral walls of the heart in the region of the atrioventricular canal; they grow toward each other and fuse, dividing the canal into two parts, a right and a left.

The *primitive atrium* is first divided by a thin curtain-like membrane, the septum primum, growing down into it from the dorsocranial wall toward the endocardial cushions; it stops short of that goal, leaving a temporary gap (the foramen primum) between the curtain and the cushion. Just before that opening is obliterated, a second opening (the foramen secundum) appears in the center of the curtain. A little later a second curtain, the septum secundum, grows up from below (from the ventrocranial wall of the atrium), on the right side of the septum primum. As it grows, the septum secundum covers the foramen secundum, leaving only a small oval opening (the foramen ovale). Finally, the upper part of the septum primum disappears and the lower part becomes the valve of the foramen ovale.

Division of the primitive ventricle into two parts occurs concurrently with the division of the atria. It begins with the appearance of a muscular ridge near the apex. This thick crescentic membrane has an upper concave free edge. The two ventricles formed on each side of it dilate as the ridge grows upward to form the muscular portion of the interventricular septum. Until about the end of the seventh week there is a small opening between its free upper edge and the endocardial cushions. This is then closed with the formation of the membranous portion of the interventricular septum.

Meanwhile, the *bulbus cordis* proximally and the *truncus arteriosus* distally, which in continuity with each other constitute the outflow tract of the primitive ventricle, are being divided into two adjacent channels by the junction of a pair of internal opposing spiral ridges. These two channels superiorly (the truncus arteriosus) become the aorta and the pulmonary trunk. The bulbus cordis below is incorporated into the walls of the two ventricles, becoming the infundibulum of the right ventricle and the aortic vestibule of the left.[2]

MORPHOLOGY

The wall of the heart, in both the atria and the ventricles, consists of three main layers: (1) the internal, or endocardium; (2) the intermediate, or myocardium; and (3) the external, or epicardium.

During the greater part of late fetal life and early infancy, the *endocardium* is composed of a single layer of flat endothelial cells beneath which there is, in most sites, a thin connective tissue band containing collagenous and elastic fibers (Fig. 1–16). This so-called subendocardial layer binds the endocardium and the myocardium together and is directly continuous with the interstitial connective tissue of the latter. It contains blood vessels and nerves (Fig. 1–15). In the spaces between the muscle bundles of the atria (Fig. 1–10), the connective tissue of endocardium continues into that of the epicardium. This subendocardial layer is absent from the papillary muscles (Fig. 1–14) and the chordae tendineae.

The *myocardium* is composed of a network of unique striated muscle fibers, the structure of which differs in several respects from that of skeletal striated muscle. The fibers form networks with narrow meshes stretched in one main direction (Fig. 1–7); in cross section they are round or irregular and of various sizes (Fig. 1–4). The *nuclei* are always in the interior of the fiber (Figs. 1–4 and 1–5a), usually in the axial portion. They are scattered in the network of the fibers at various distances from one another. Their shape is short to long oval (Figs. 1–4 to 1–9).

Among the nuclei within the myocardium of the fetus and the newborn, so-called Anitschkow myocyte nuclei are sometimes seen; they appear to be more common in the hearts of immature infants (Figs. 1–8 and

1–9). They are quite different from other myocardial nuclei, and have a characteristic histologic appearance; their chromatin content seems to be clumped together into a single central bar, longitudinally oriented, with a number of small branches projecting out at right angles to the bar on both sides. (These cells have been seen elsewhere in infants; *e.g.*, they are present in the soft tissue of the larynx in the immediate vicinity of a lesion, of unknown etiology, called focal fibrinoid necrosis.)

The myofibrils and sarcoplasm in cardiac muscle are similar to those of ordinary striated fibers. However, in late fetal life and early infancy the heart muscle fibers may appear to be markedly vacuolated (Figs. 1–4 to 1–6, 1–8, and 1–9) because of the fact that they contain abundant glycogen, which washes out during routine preparation of paraffin sections and leaves spaces behind. As early as three weeks after birth, that exceptionally heavy burden of glycogen has virtually disappeared (Fig. 1–7).

The *conduction system* of the heart is composed of specialized tissue, of which the Purkinje fibers are part (Figs. 1–21 to 1–26). During the perinatal period the atrioventricular node and the bundle of His present a very loosely woven microscopic appearance characteristic of this period.[3] They do not, however, show any evidence of *active* degeneration, necrosis, phagocytosis, or replacement fibrosis as has been suggested.

The *epicardium* is covered on its free surface by a single layer of flat mesothelial cells (Fig. 1–17a). Beneath that mesothelium is a layer of connective tissue, which is thin during most of late fetal life (Fig. 1–17b) but which, near term, may be somewhat thickened in places by the appearance within it of islands of adipose tissue (Fig. 1–17a). This layer contains blood vessels and nerves.

The *"skeleton" of the heart* is its central supporting structure, to which most of the muscle fibers are attached and with which the valves are connected (Fig. 1–11). It consists mainly of dense connective tissue. Its main parts are the *membranous septum*, the *fibrous trigone*, and the *annulus fibrosus* of the atrioventricular and arterial foramina. The fibrous trigone and annulus fibrosus in the infant contain islands of chondroid tissue with globular cells resembling chondrocytes, but they lack true capsules (Fig. 1–11); hence, this tissue is not truly cartilage.

The *cardiac valves* (atrioventricular, aortic, and pulmonary) all have the same general histologic structure (Figs. 1–12 and 1–13). Each consists of a plate of connective tissue that begins at the annulus fibrosus and extends out into the lumen. The plate is covered on all free surfaces by a layer of endocardium. The normal valves of fetuses and newborns frequently present a surprisingly myxoid character on microscopic examination (Fig. 1–13).

References

1. Willis, R. A.: The Borderland of Embryology and Pathology. London, Butterworth and Co., Ltd., 1958, pp. 24 and 64–67.
2. Moore, K. L.: The Developing Human, Clinically Oriented Embryology. Philadelphia, W. B. Saunders Co., 1973, pp. 239–264.
3. Valdes-Dapena, M. A., Greene, J., Basavanand, N., *et al.*: The myocardial conduction system in sudden death in infancy. N. E. J. M., 289:1179–1180, 1973.

6 HEART

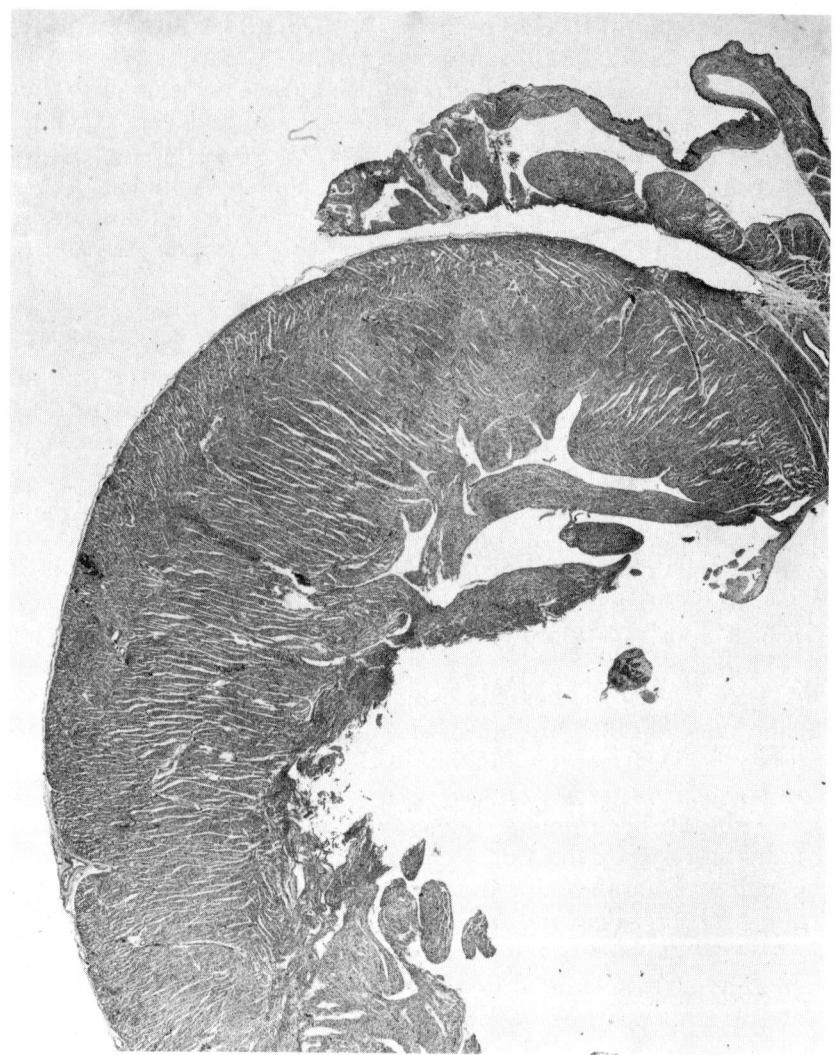

Figure 1-1

Figures 1-1 to 1-3. This set of three illustrations depicts the pattern of the "weave" of myocardium in the wall of the left ventricle. In each, epicardium is to the left and endocardium is to the right. In Fig. 1-1 the atrial appendage is visible at the top and, below that, a cross section of coronary artery and a bit of the mitral valve. In Fig. 1-2 the mitral valve and papillary muscle both appear, and in Fig. 1-3 the addition of adipose tissue to the epicardium (not present in Figs. 1-1 and 1-2) is obvious.

Another feature of the set is the clear increase in the thickness of the wall.

Hematoxylin and eosin stain. Mag. 15×.

Fig.	Wt.	Race	Sex	Gestation	Age
1-1	370 gm.			18 wk.	Stillborn
1-2	1,240 gm.	W	F		15 days of age
1-3	5,000 gm.				

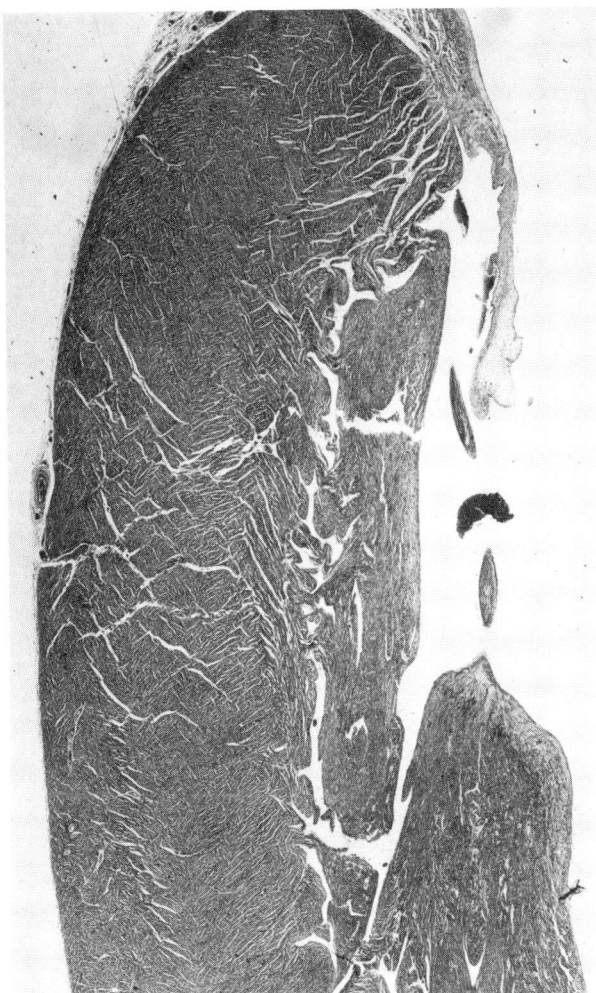

Figure 1-2

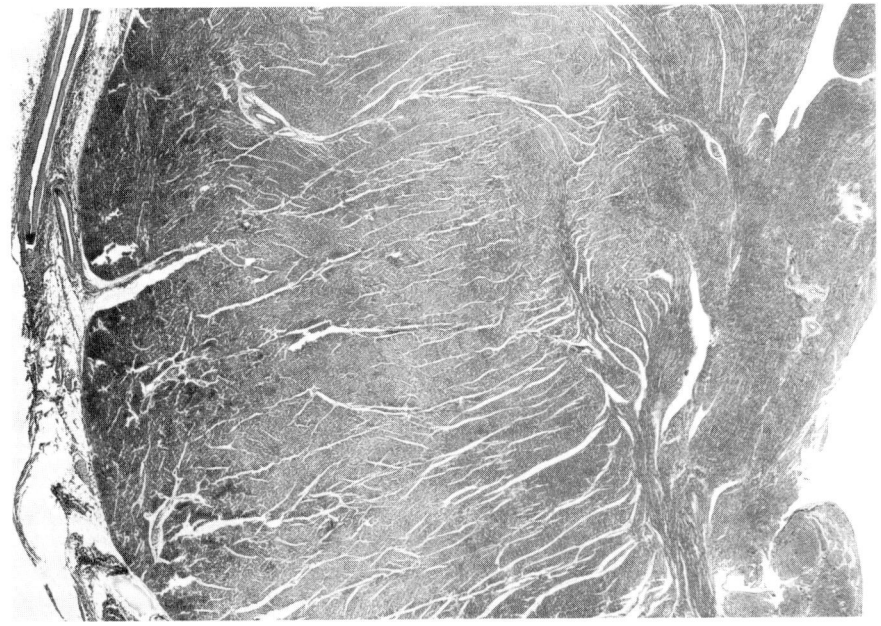

Figure 1-3

Figures 1–4 and 1–5. The myocardial fibers of the fetus, midway through gestation, are heavily laden with glycogen. Inasmuch as routine procedures for the preparation of paraffin sections extract most of the glycogen, the fibers appear in hematoxylin-and-eosin stained sections to be extremely vacuolated; this extensive vacuolization lends the myocardium a lacy appearance at higher magnifications.

See illustrations on the following pages

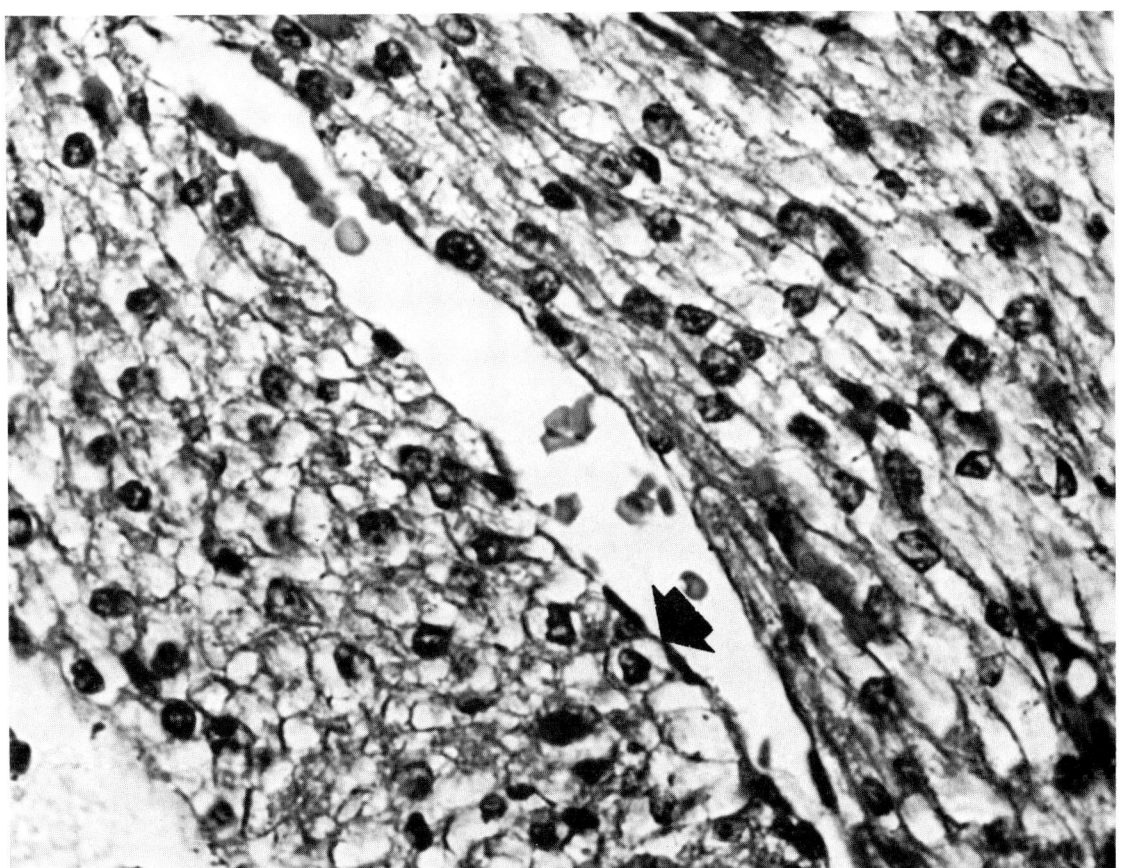

Figure 1-4

Figure 1-4. In the right upper corner of this photograph the myocardial fibers have been sectioned longitudinally; in the opposite corner, they have been sectioned transversely. In both it is apparent that the nuclei lie more or less in the center of the fiber (see black arrow).

Cross striations are faint but apparent in a few scattered portions of the longitudinal section. This is from the ventricular myocardium of a 200 gram female fetus who was born dead. Hematoxylin and eosin stain. Mag. 660×.

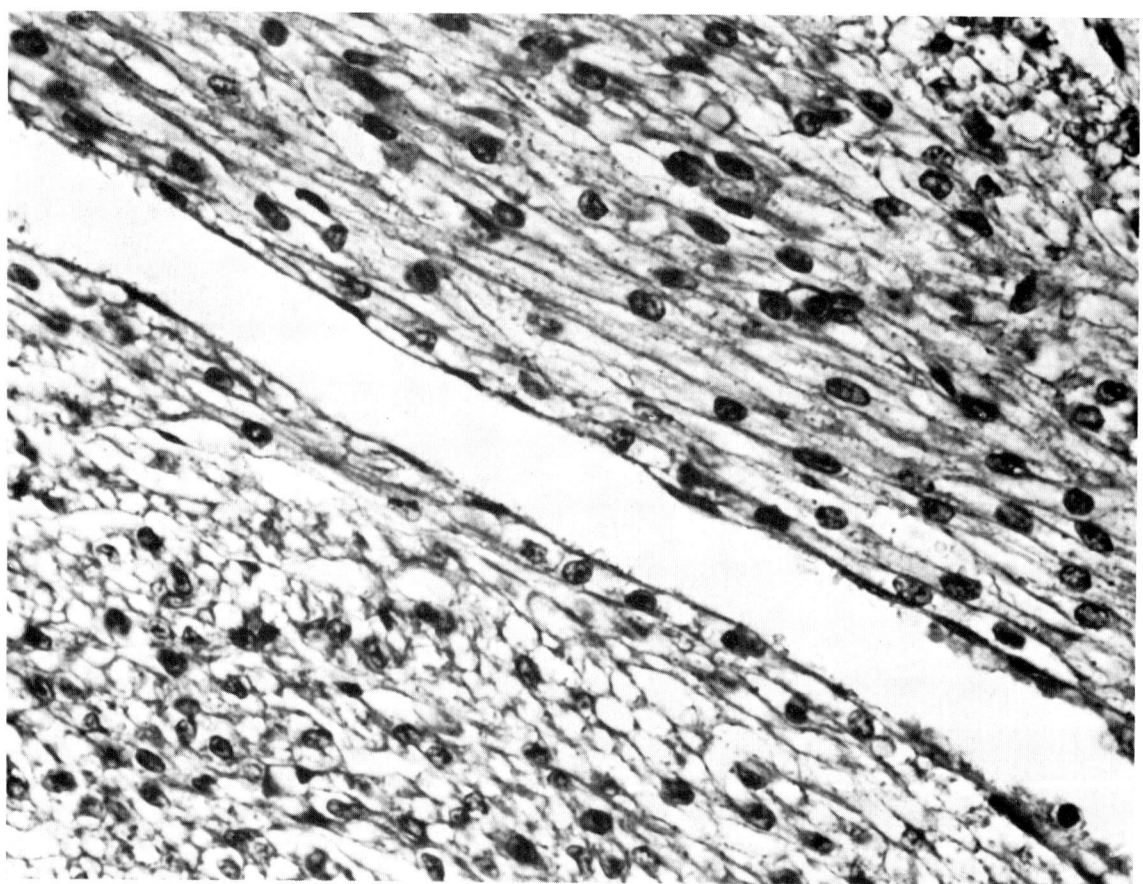

Figure 1–5a

Figure 1–5a. This is a section of the ventricular myocardium from a slightly larger fetus, weighing 320 grams at necropsy. The gestation was said to have been of 16 weeks duration. The infant was stillborn.

Hematoxylin and eosin stain. Mag. 304×.

HEART 11

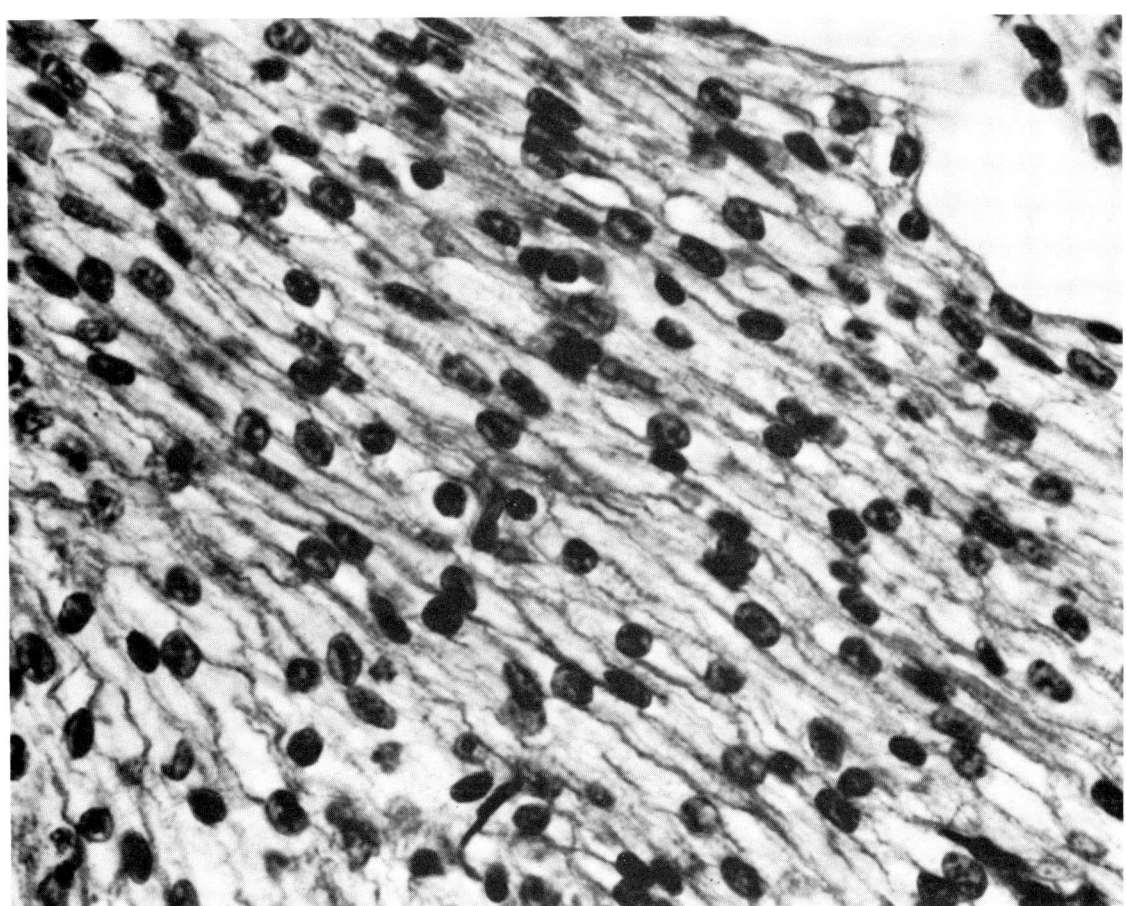

Figure 1–5b

Figure 1–5b. This is a section of the heart depicted in Fig. 1–5a, but seen here at higher magnification. Delicate cross striations are apparent in at least two fibers above and to the left of center and another two below and to the right of center.
Hematoxylin and eosin stain. Mag. 660×.

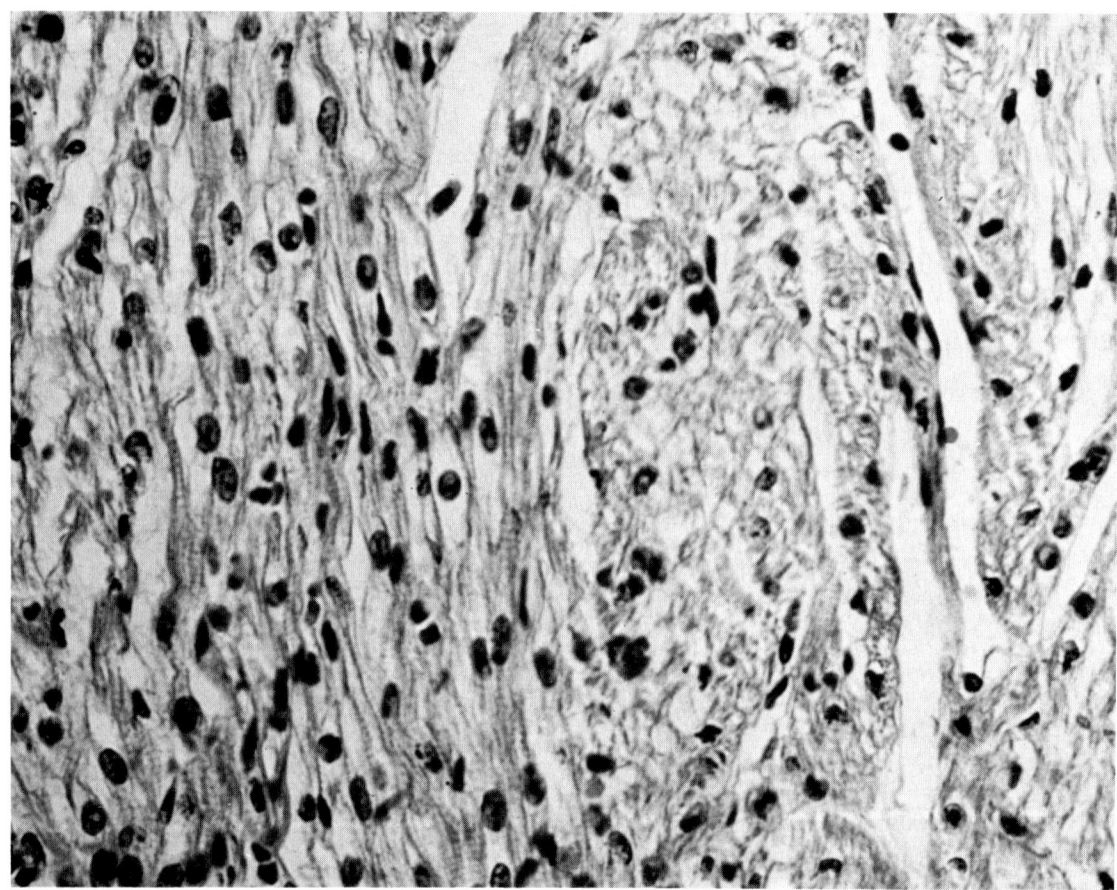

Figure 1–6

Figure 1–6. The myocardial fibers of the newborn may retain their prominent burden of glycogen for a surprisingly long period of time.

This is a histologic section from the ventricular myocardium of a liveborn female, the product of a 29 week gestation, whose body weight at autopsy was 3,100 grams. She lived for 1 day and 20 hours.

Most of the fibers on the left have been sectioned longitudinally, while those on the right are a mixture of longitudinal, transverse, and oblique orientations.

Hematoxylin and eosin stain. Mag. 471×.

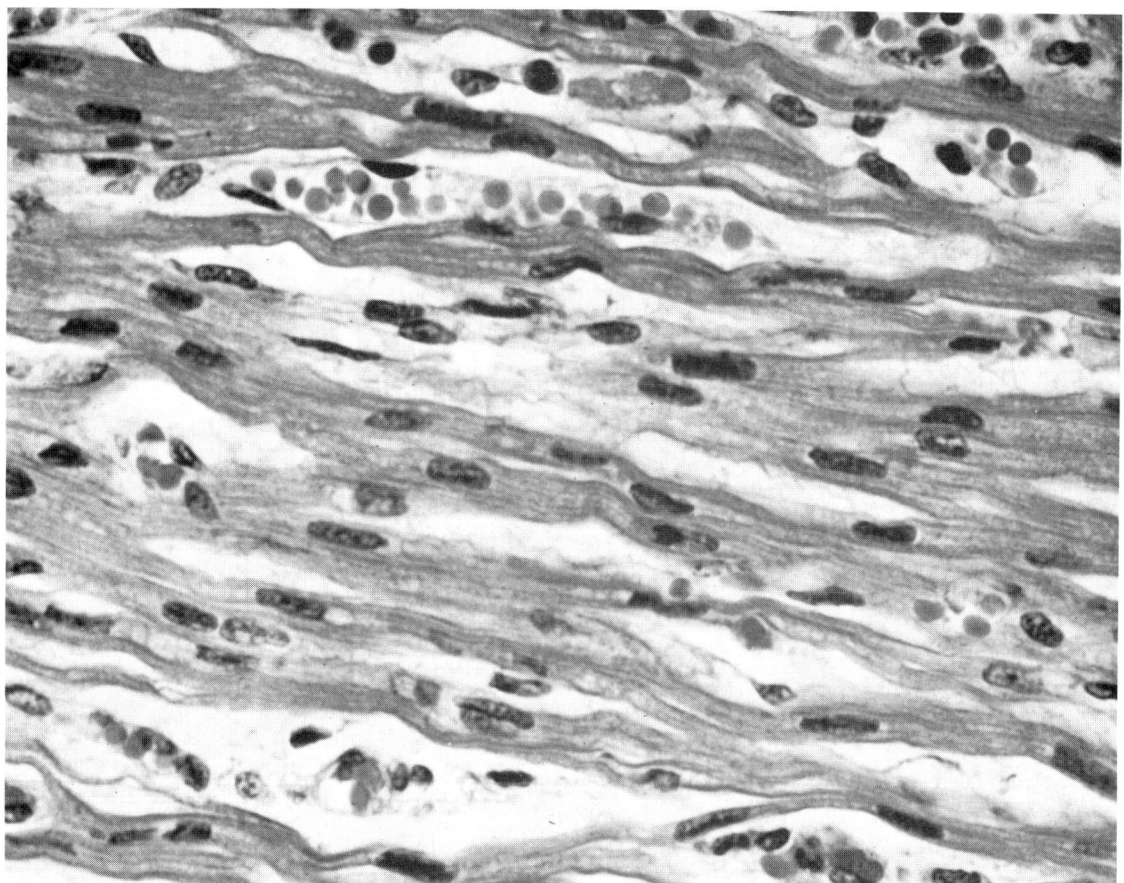

Figure 1-7

Figure 1-7. By the time a term infant has attained an age of even three weeks of extra-uterine life, the myocardial fibers have lost most of their visible glycogen vacuolization, a state apparent in this photograph.

This illustration shows clearly the branching and joining together typical of the histologic pattern of the myocardium.

This female infant was born after 36 weeks gestation. She survived for six weeks after birth and her body weight at postmortem examination was 4,080 grams.

Hematoxylin and eosin stain. Mag. 555×.

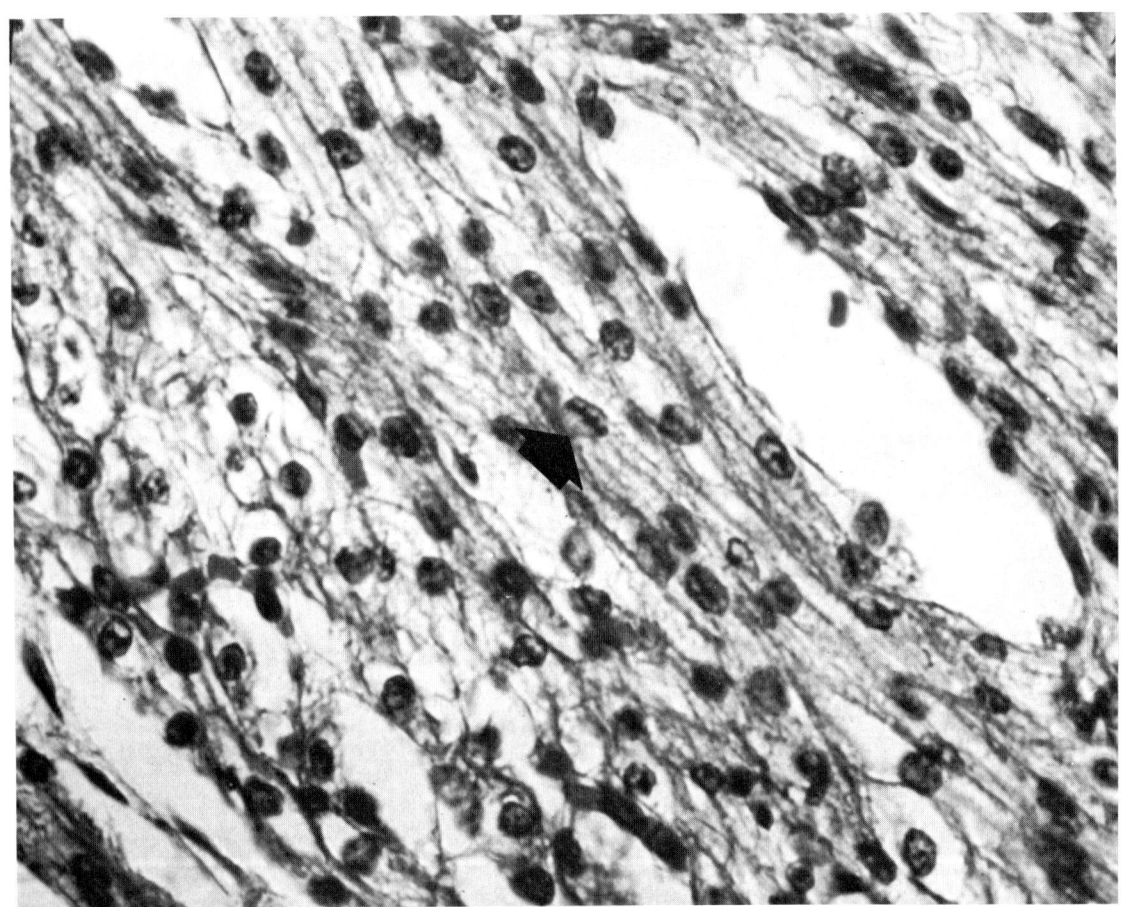

Figure 1–8

Figures 1–8 and 1–9. Among the myocardial fibers, especially of the premature infant, many so-called Anitschkow myocytes can be found. They are characterized by a unique arrangement of chromatin, seen here at medium and high magnification; the chromatin appears in the form of a longitudinally oriented central bar, with delicate branches projecting out perpendicularly to both sides.

Figure 1–8. This is the ventricular myocardium of a 200 gram stillborn female infant of 18 weeks gestation. Arrow indicates one of the Anitschkow myocytes.
Hematoxylin and eosin stain. Mag. 555×.

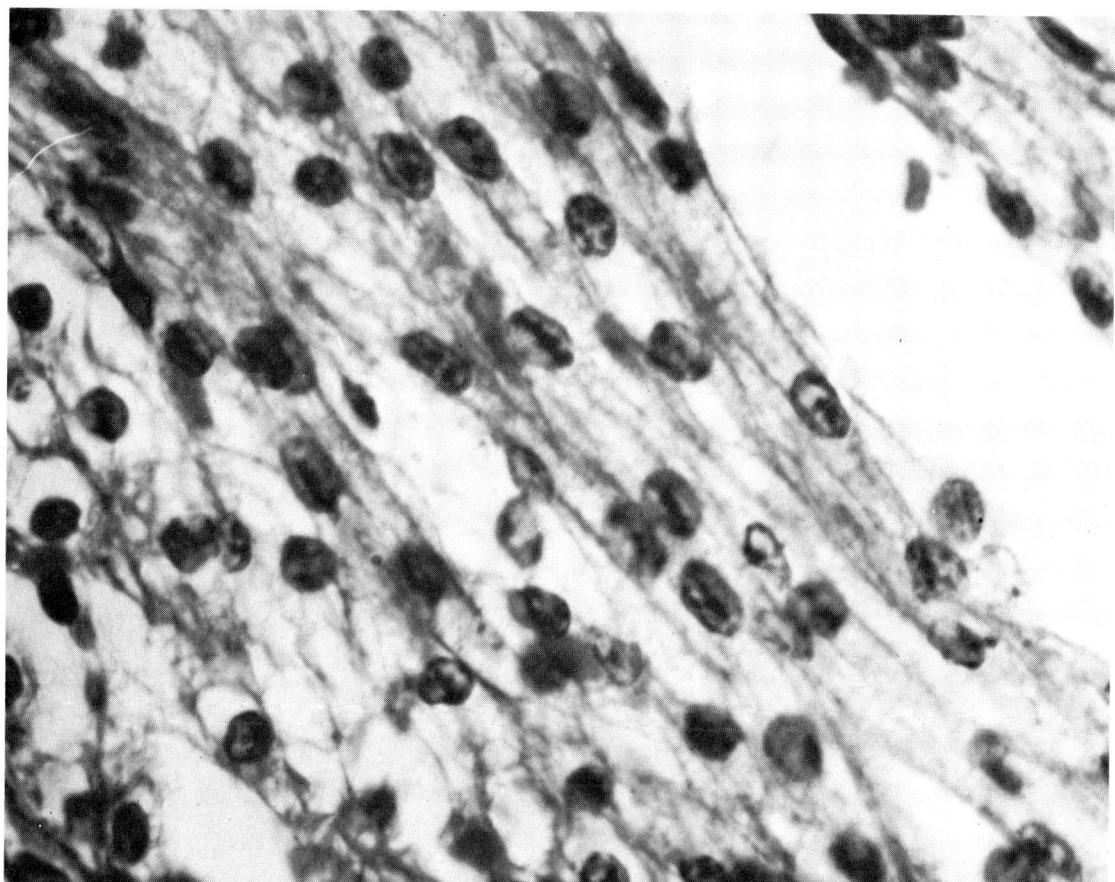

Figure 1-9

Figure 1-9. Detail of Fig. 1-8 (center of photo). Hematoxylin and eosin stain. Mag. 660×.

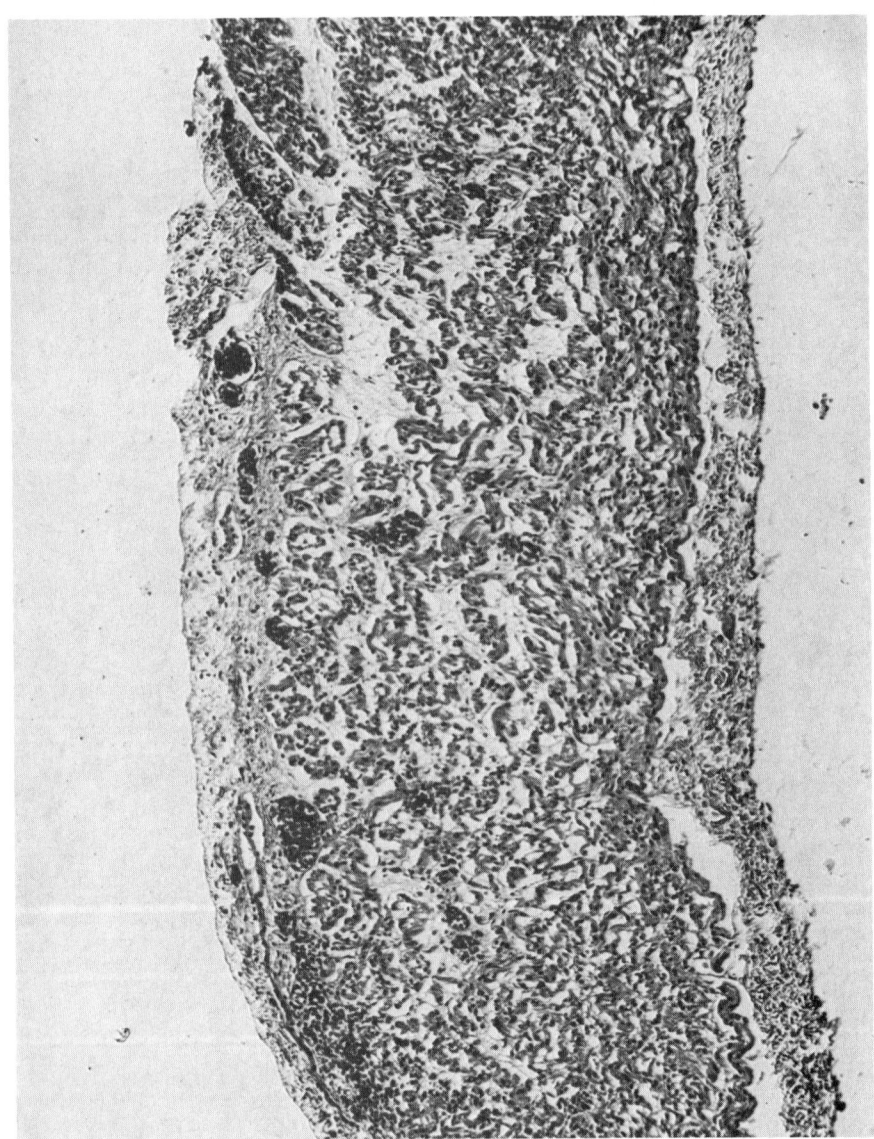

Figure 1–10

Figure 1–10. Seen here, at rather low magnification, is the interatrial septum. The endocardium is relatively thick on both sides, and the myocardial fibers are variously oriented.

The subject was a 230 gram female fetus, born after 20 weeks of gestation; she lived for 5 minutes after birth.

Hematoxylin and eosin stain. Mag. 124×.

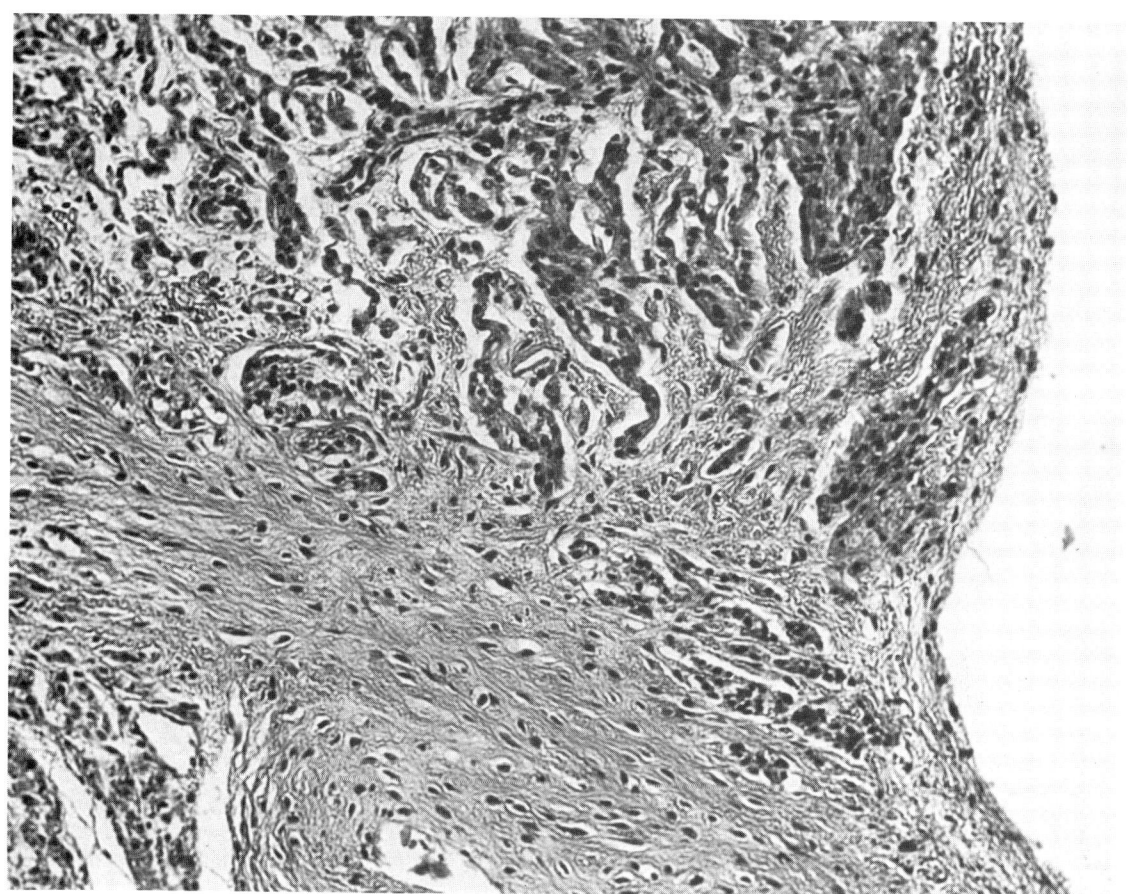

Figure 1-11

Figure 1-11. This photograph depicts atrial myocardial fibers above, blending into the ring of the mitral valve below (going off toward the lower right corner of the illustration). The fibrous tissue here at the base of the valve and in the vicinity of the bundle of His frequently bears a close resemblance to cartilage, although it is not cartilage.

This section was removed from the heart of a prematurely born female infant who died 10 minutes after birth (estimated gestational age, 29 weeks). Her body weighed 1,610 grams at autopsy.

Hematoxylin and eosin stain. Mag. 208×.

18   HEART

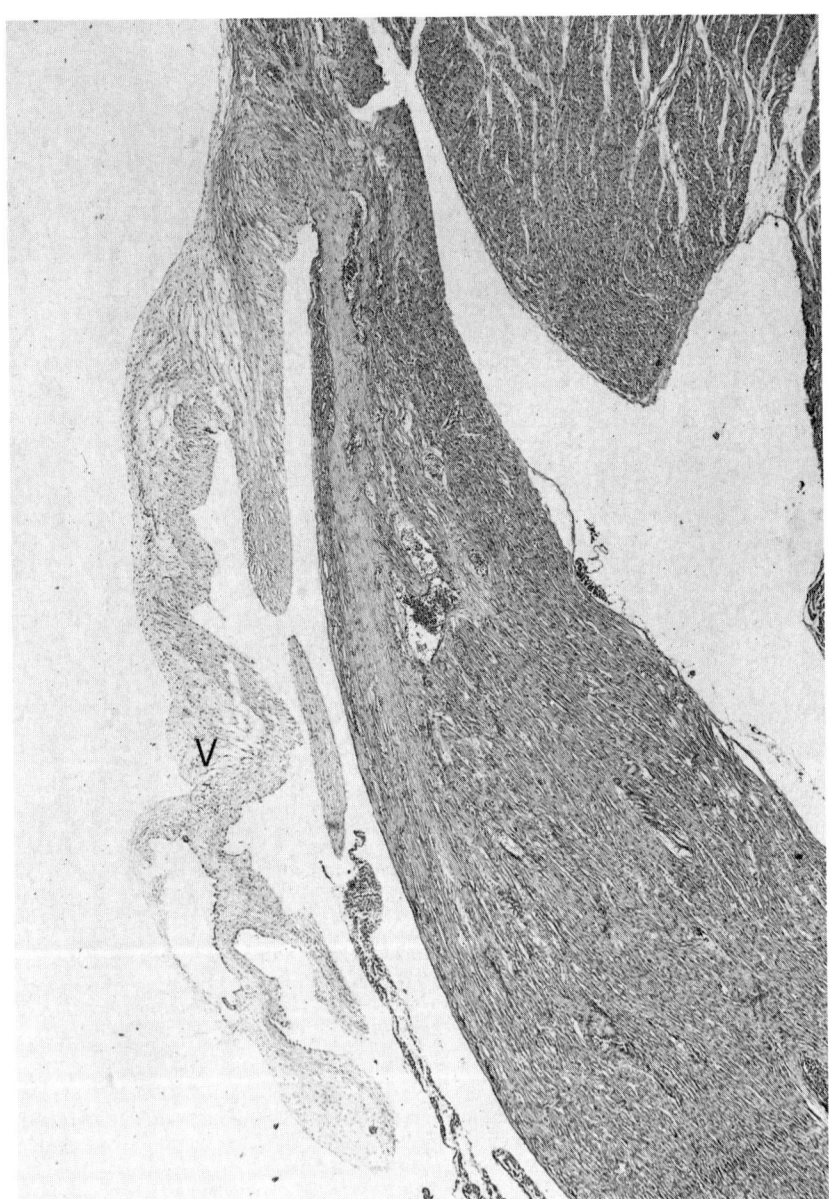

Figure 1–12

Figure 1–12. Seen here, at very low magnification, is a section of the mitral valve, as well as a papillary muscle and a portion of the wall of the left ventricle.

The patient was a 27 hour old black male infant, born at term, who weighed 4,225 grams at autopsy.

Hematoxylin and eosin stain. Mag. 38×.

HEART 19

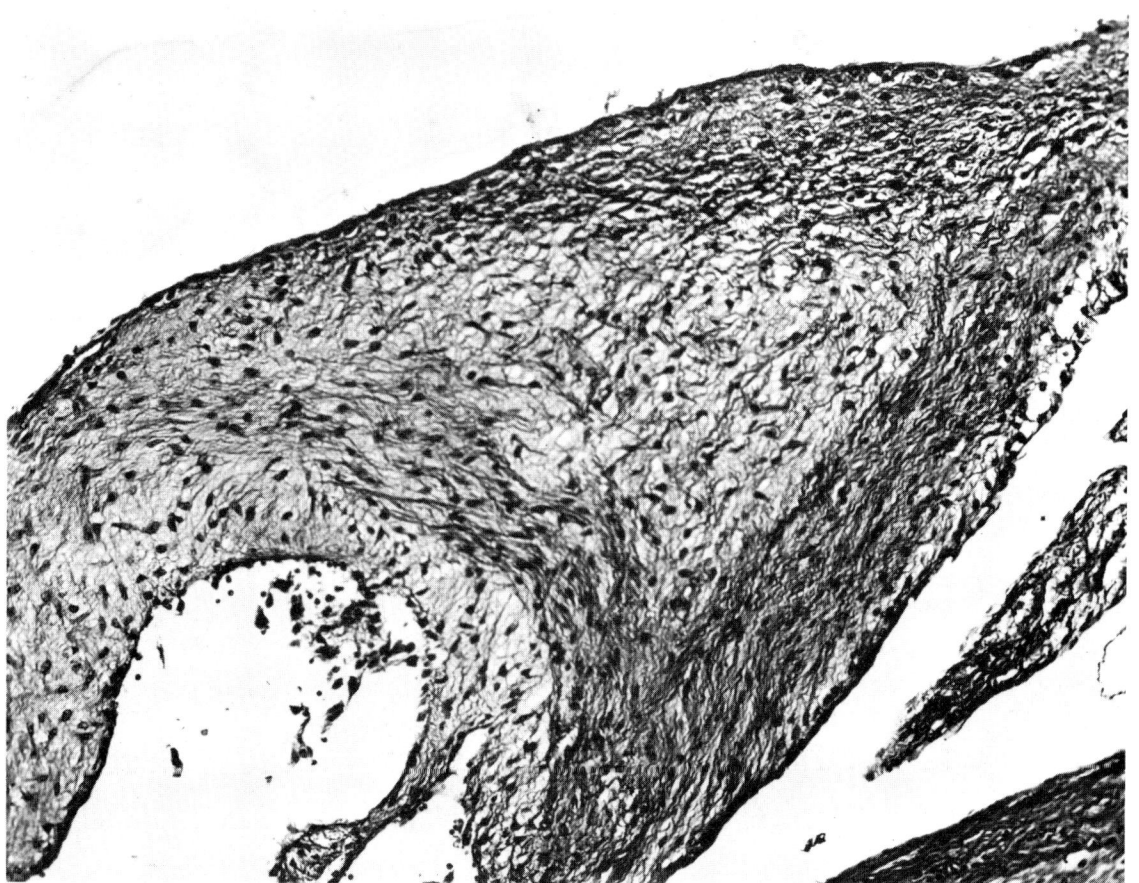

Figure 1–13

Figure 1–13. The substance of the valve leaflet in the fetus and the infant is surprisingly loosely woven fibrous connective tissue. In certain instances it even has a myxoid appearance, as illustrated here.

This is a section of the mitral valve of an 18 day old white female infant, born at 40 weeks gestation, whose body weighed 3,010 grams at autopsy.

Hematoxylin and eosin stain. Mag. 164×.

20 HEART

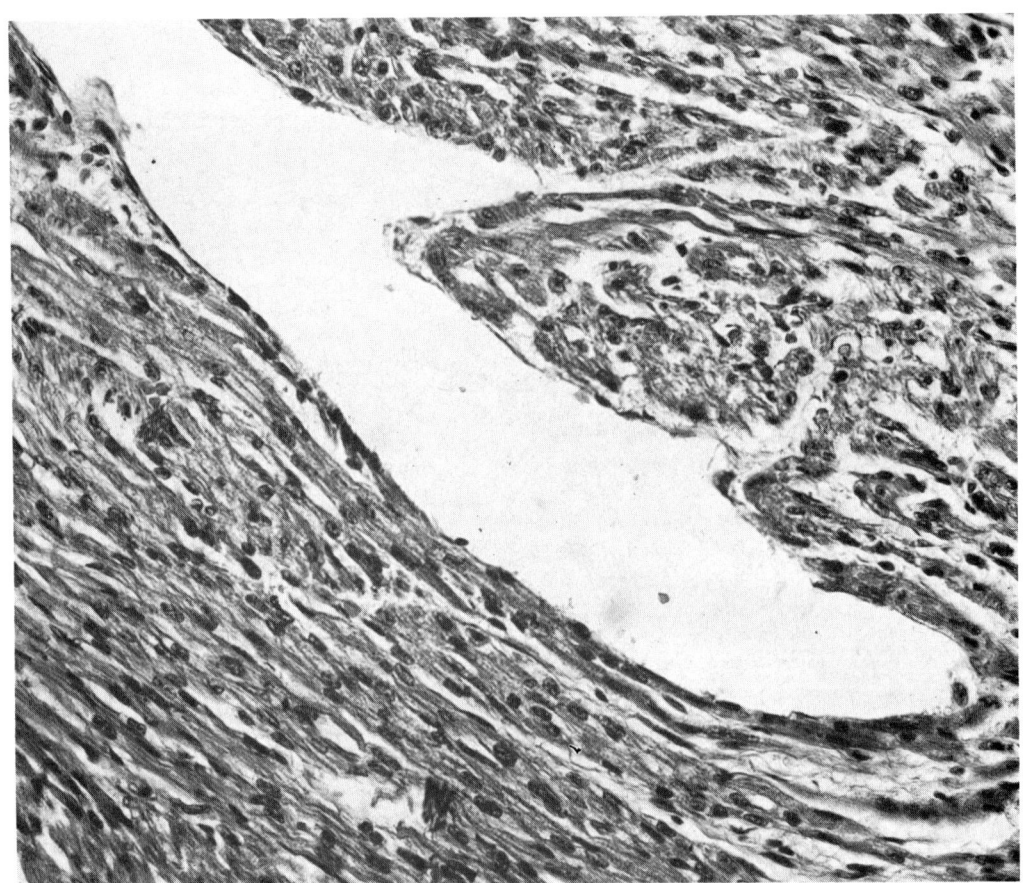

Figure 1–14

Figures 1–14 to 1–16. The normal endocardium of the fetus and the infant varies considerably from site to site. It is very thin, little more than a single layer of endothelium over papillary muscles and in the crevices between muscle bundles in the wall of the ventricle; it is apt to be stouter elsewhere, with a relatively thick subendothelial layer of connective tissue, as depicted in Figs. 1–15 and 1–16. (These three photographs all represent sections taken through the wall of the ventricle.)

Figure 1–14. The endocardium here appears to consist of only a single layer of flat endothelial cells.

This is a section of the wall of the ventricle of a liveborn black male infant who lived for 9 hours and 47 minutes. His body weight at necropsy was 1,010 grams. (Estimated gestational age, 26 weeks.)

Hematoxylin and eosin stain. Mag. 270×.

HEART   21

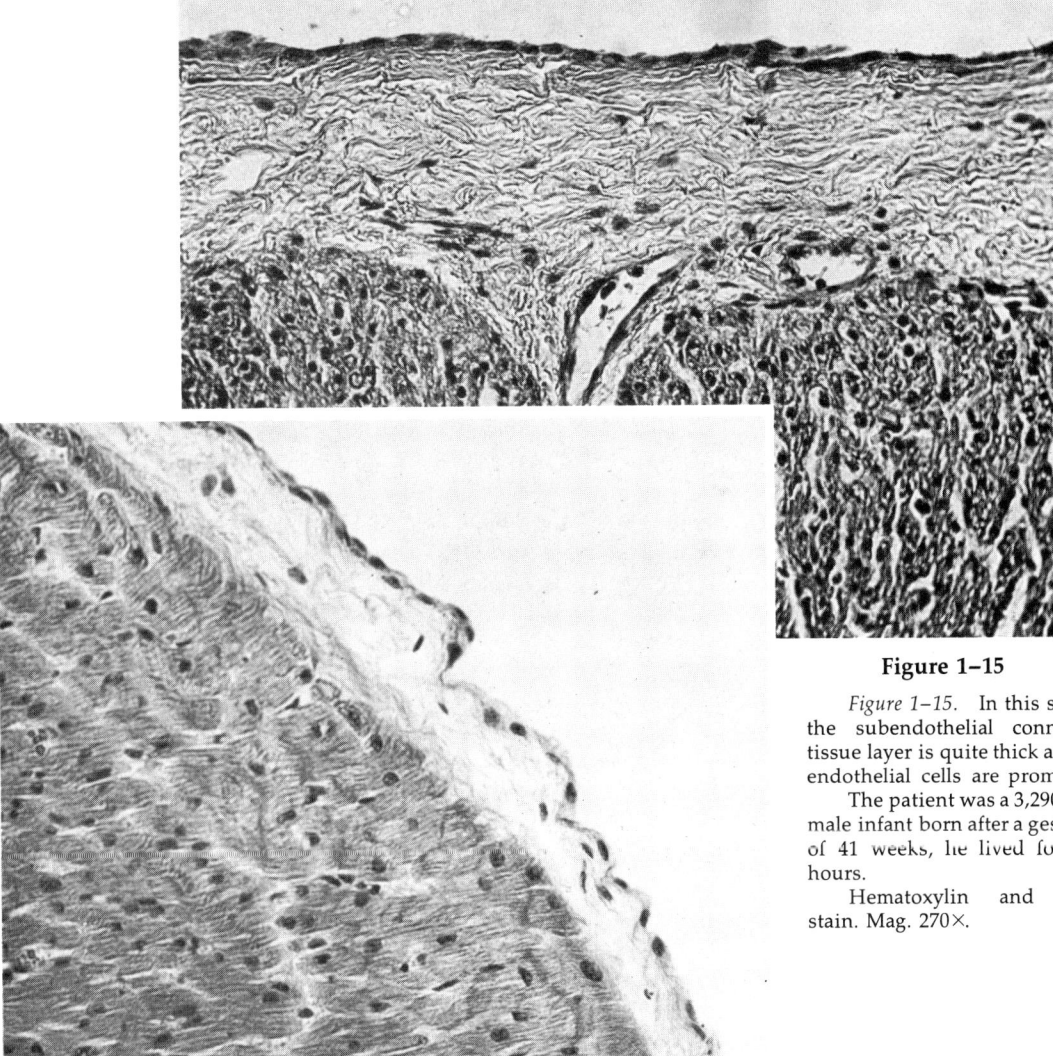

Figure 1–15

Figure 1–15. In this section the subendothelial connective tissue layer is quite thick and the endothelial cells are prominent.

The patient was a 3,290 gram male infant born after a gestation of 41 weeks, he lived for 12¼ hours.

Hematoxylin and eosin stain. Mag. 270×.

Figure 1–16

Figure 1–16. Although this patient is much older than that from which Fig. 1–15 was taken, the endocardium here is somewhat more delicate. This subject was a 3 year old child.
Hematoxylin and eosin stain. Mag. 250×.

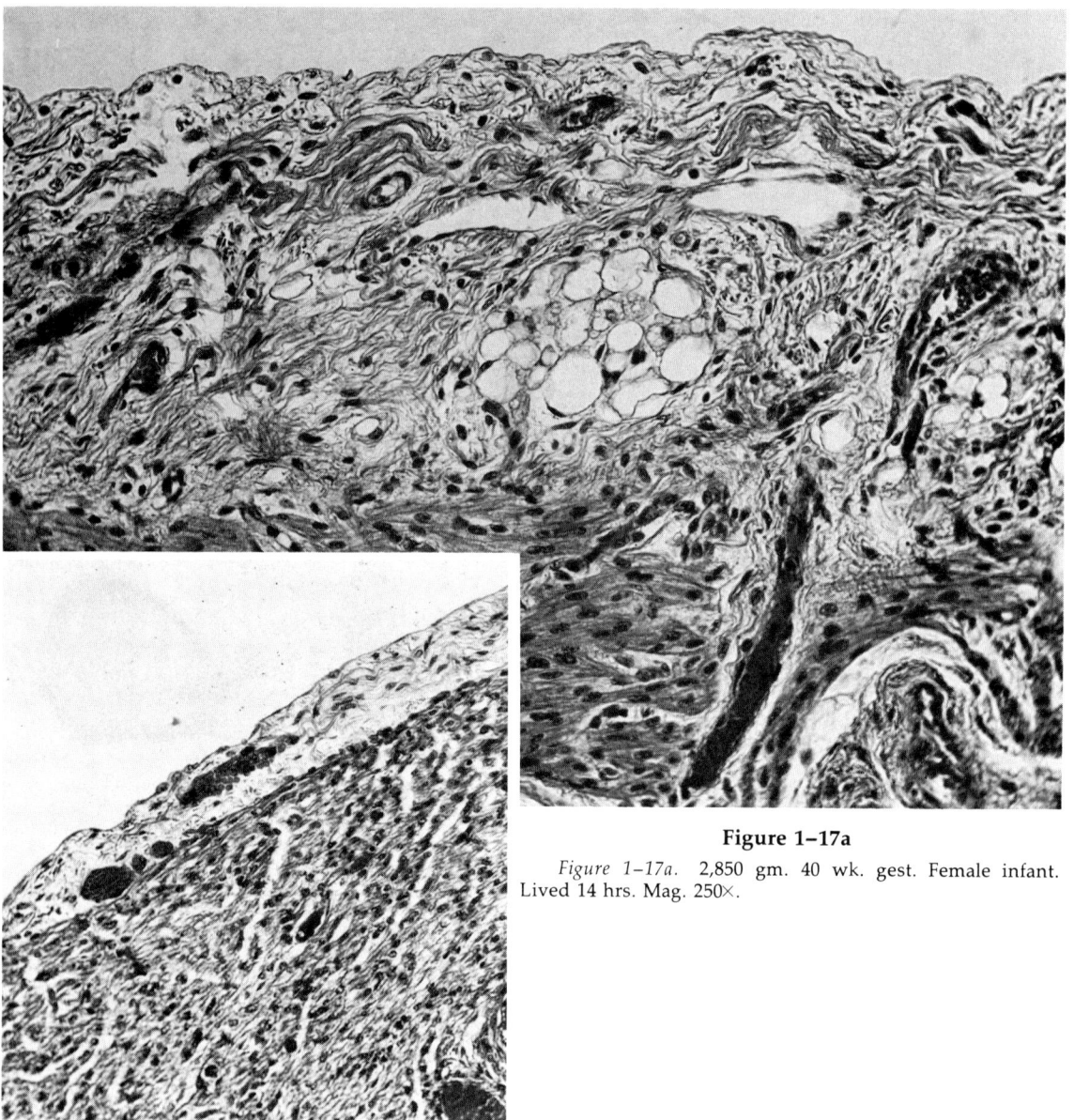

Figure 1–17a

Figure 1–17a. 2,850 gm. 40 wk. gest. Female infant. Lived 14 hrs. Mag. 250×.

Figure 1–17b

Figure 1–17b. 370 gm. 16 wk. gest. Stillborn. Mag. 175×.

Figures 1–17a and 1–17b. In the fetus, one does not expect to observe any adipose tissue within the epicardium. It usually consists of nothing more than a single layer of flat mesothelial cells on the surface and, beneath that, a stout band of connective tissue containing networks of elastic fibers, blood vessels, and nerves (Fig. 1–17b). Near term, however, scattered islands of adipose tissue may begin to appear within it, as illustrated in Fig. 1–17a. They tend to persist at that site thereafter.

Hematoxylin and eosin stain.

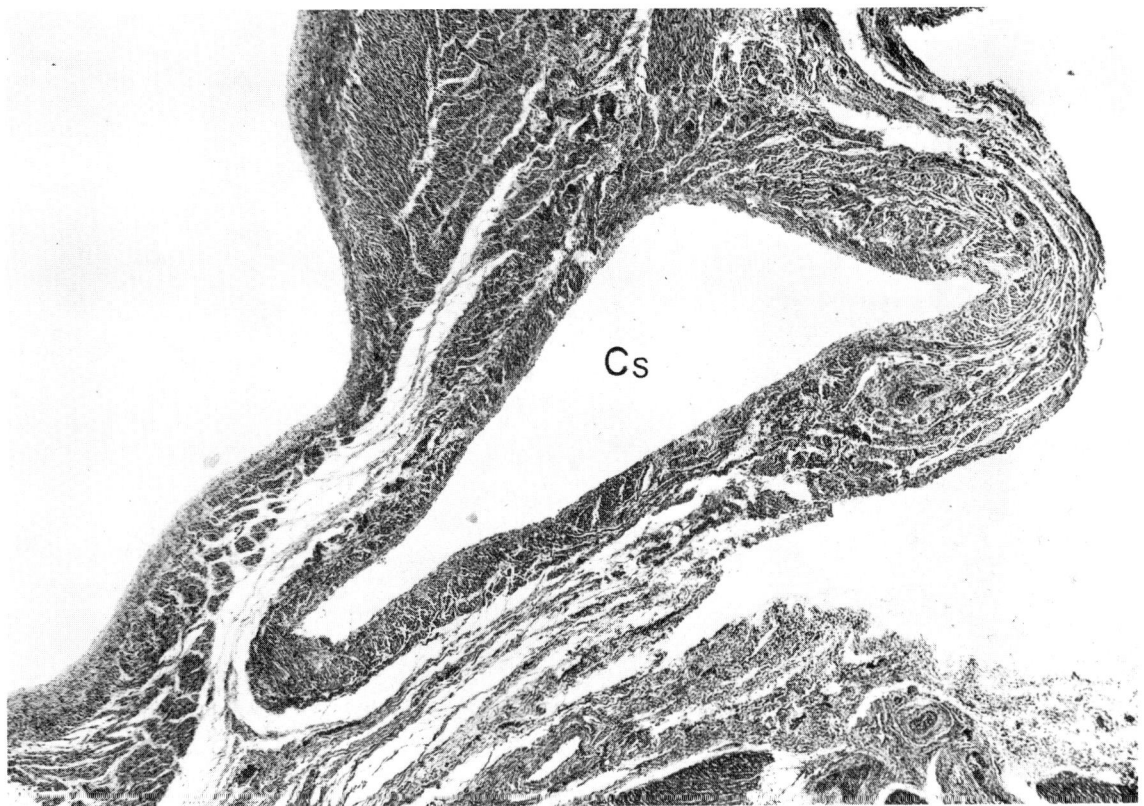

Figure 1–18

Figure 1–18. As it winds around the perimeter of the base of the left atrium, the coronary sinus often appears to be very prominent in the newborn infant.

On the left side of this photograph is the endocardium of the left atrium; on the right is the corresponding epicardium. The large triangular space between them is the coronary sinus cut transversely.

The subject was a 1,030 gram white male infant whose stated gestational age was 26 weeks. He survived for 7 hours.

Hematoxylin and eosin stain. Mag. 45×.

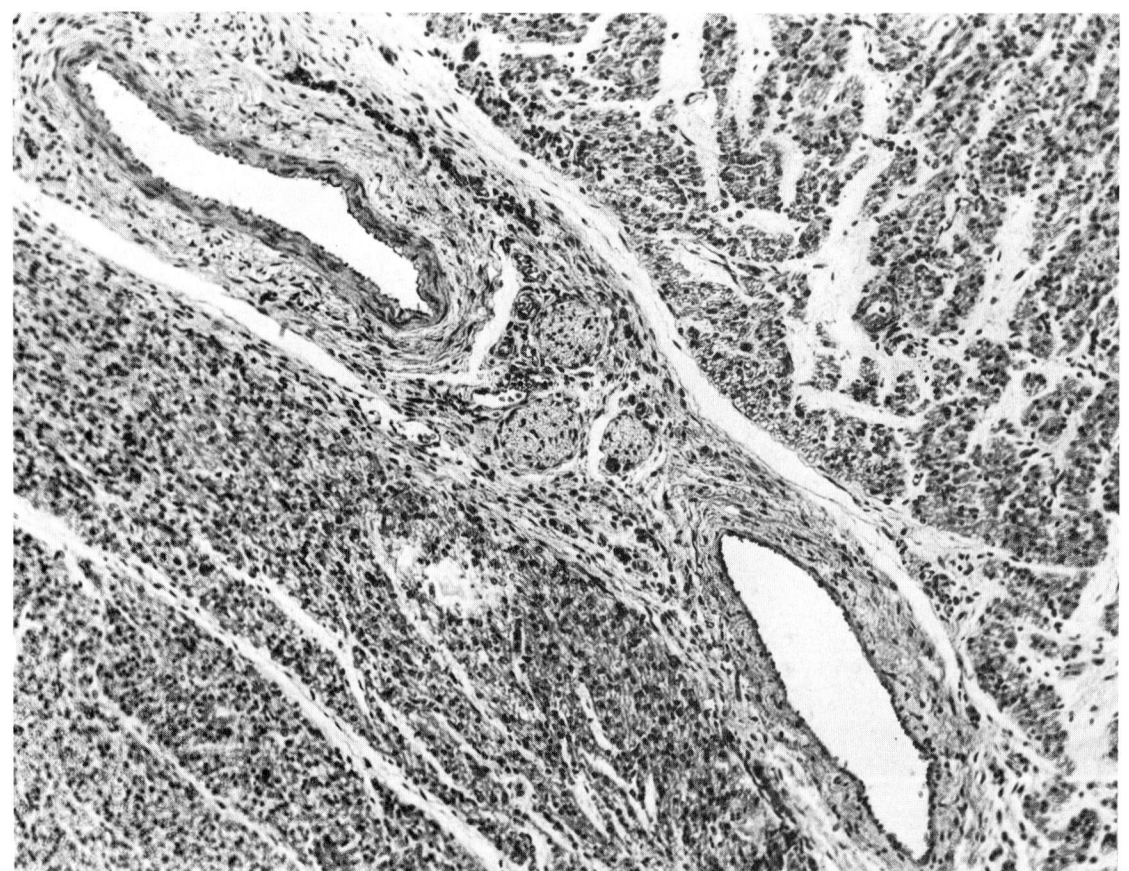

Figure 1–19

Figure 1–19. Depicted here are sections of the coronary artery and vein of a 370 gram stillborn fetus delivered at 16 weeks of gestation. In each instance the vessel has been cut tangentially but all layers are clearly visible.

Hematoxylin and eosin stain. Mag. 142×.

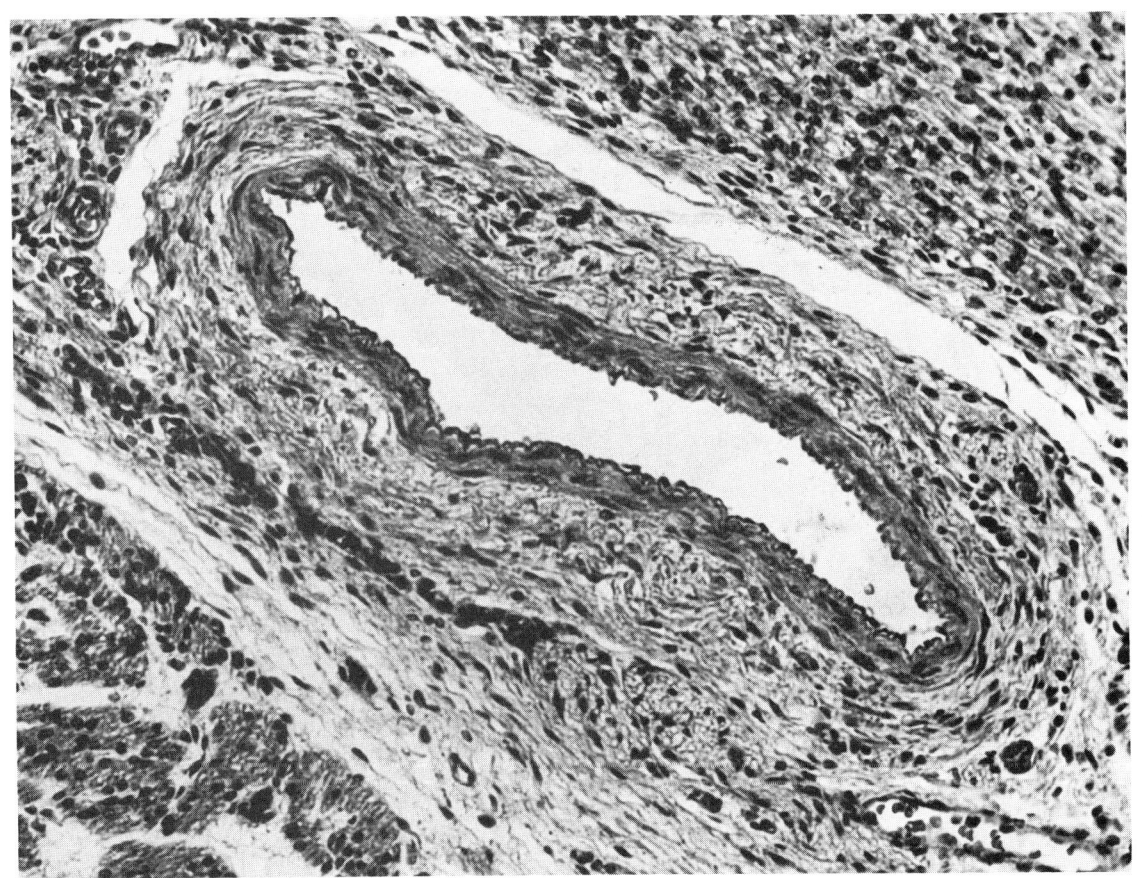

Figure 1–20

Figure 1–20. This is a photomicrograph of the same histologic section as was employed in the preparation of Fig. 1–19. The internal elastic lamina appears here as a fine but rather prominent undulating black line. Only the nuclei of a few endothelial cells are visible as small black knob-like projections (lower right). The media stains much more darkly than the adventitia.

Hematoxylin and eosin stain. Mag. 243×.

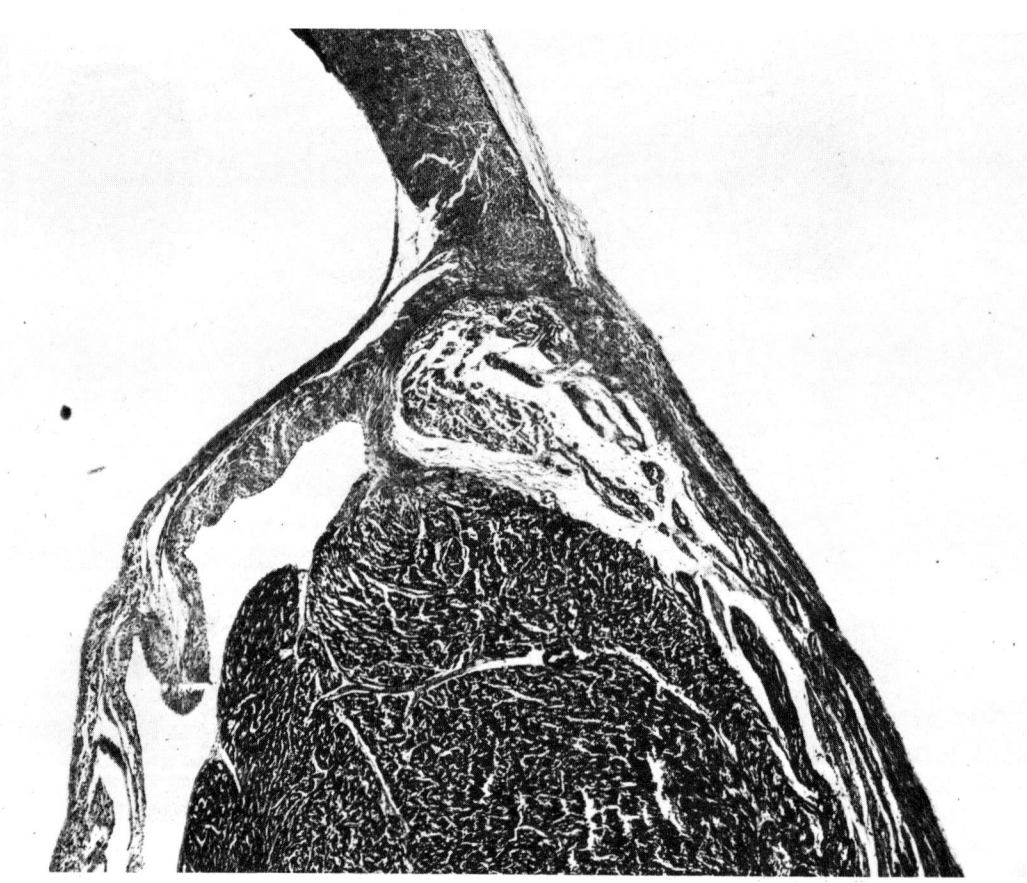

Figure 1–21

See legend on the opposite page

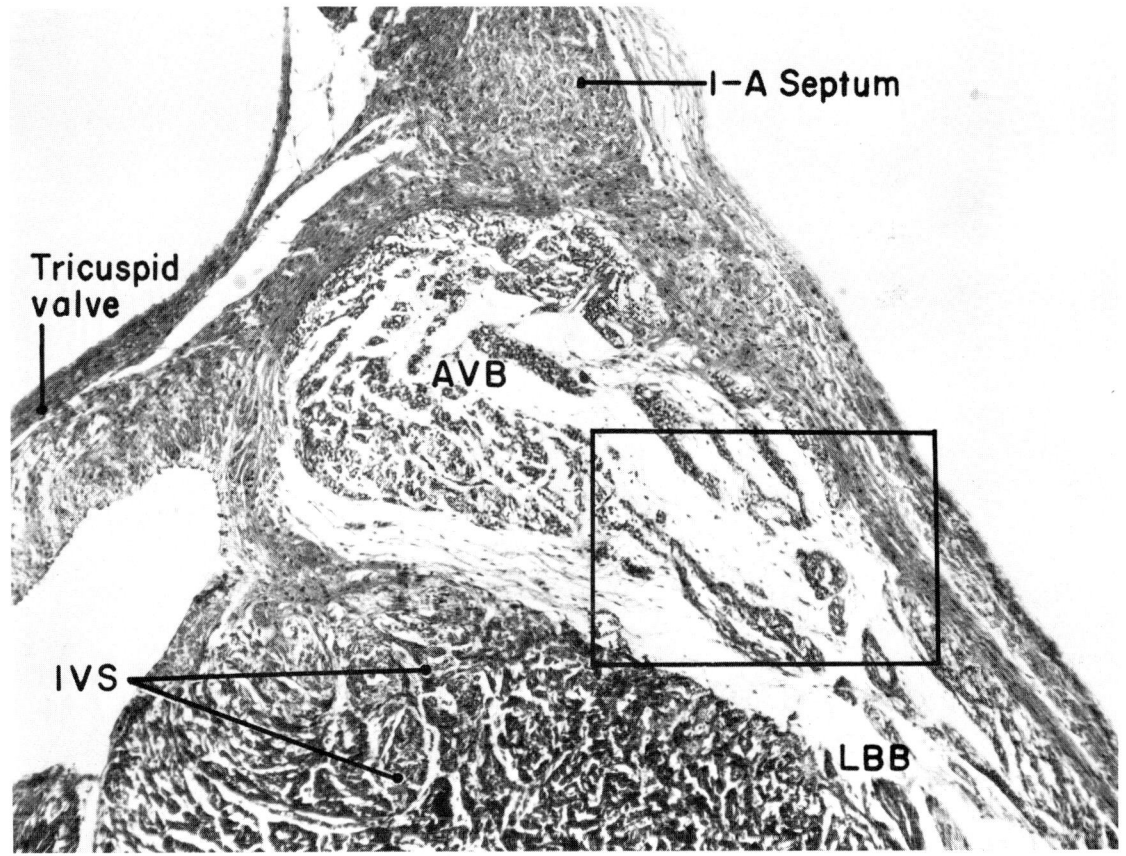

Figure 1-22

Figures 1-21 to 1-23. These sections were taken through the interventricular septum in the coronal plane to illustrate certain portions of the infant myocardial conduction system. Fig. 1-22 represents the central portion of Fig. 1-21, at higher magnification. In each, the interatrial septum is seen at the top and the interventricular septum is at the bottom. AVB: atrioventricular bundle. LBB: left bundle branch. Details of the boxed portion of Fig. 1-22 appear in Fig. 1-23, where collagen supporting fibers are marked with arrows.

The patient, a 2 month old black male, died of bronchopneumonia. His body weighed 3,690 grams at autopsy.

Masson's trichrome stain with aniline blue counter-stain.

Fig. 1-21 Mag. 45×.
Fig. 1-22 Mag. 104×.
Fig. 1-23 Mag. 330×.

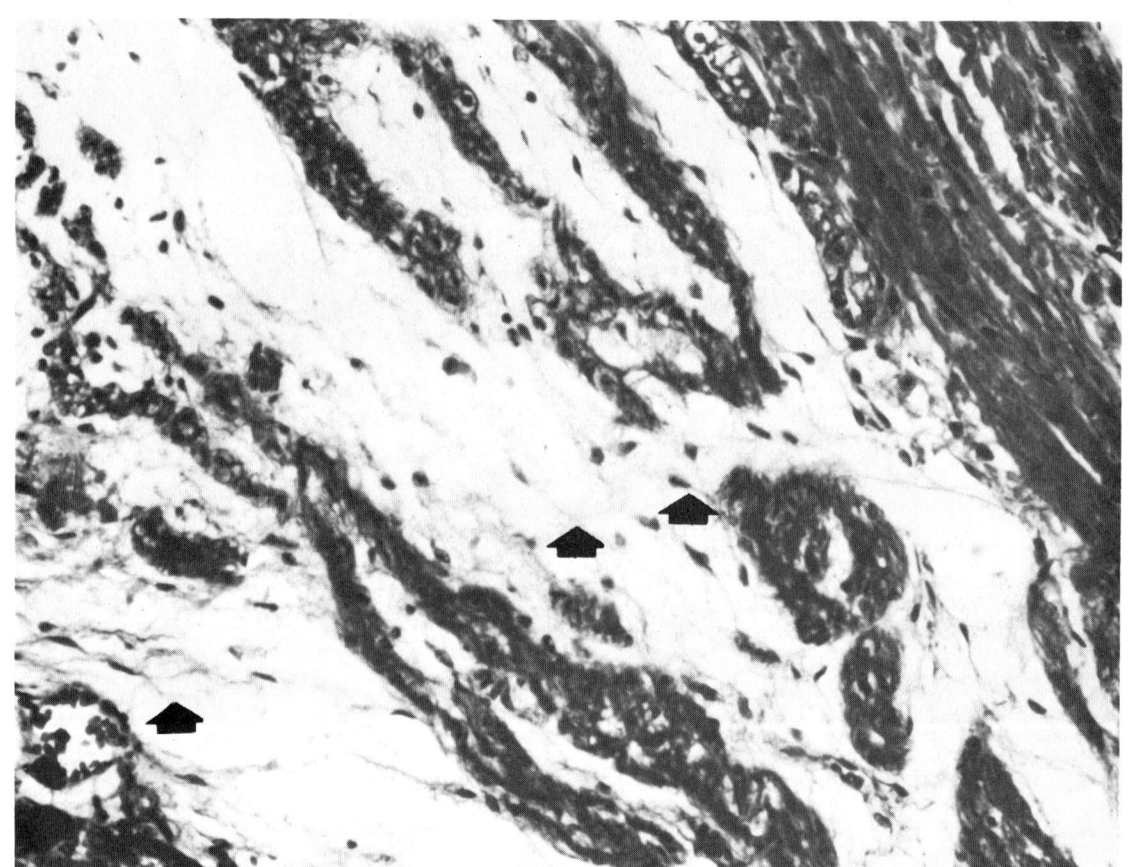

Figure 1–23

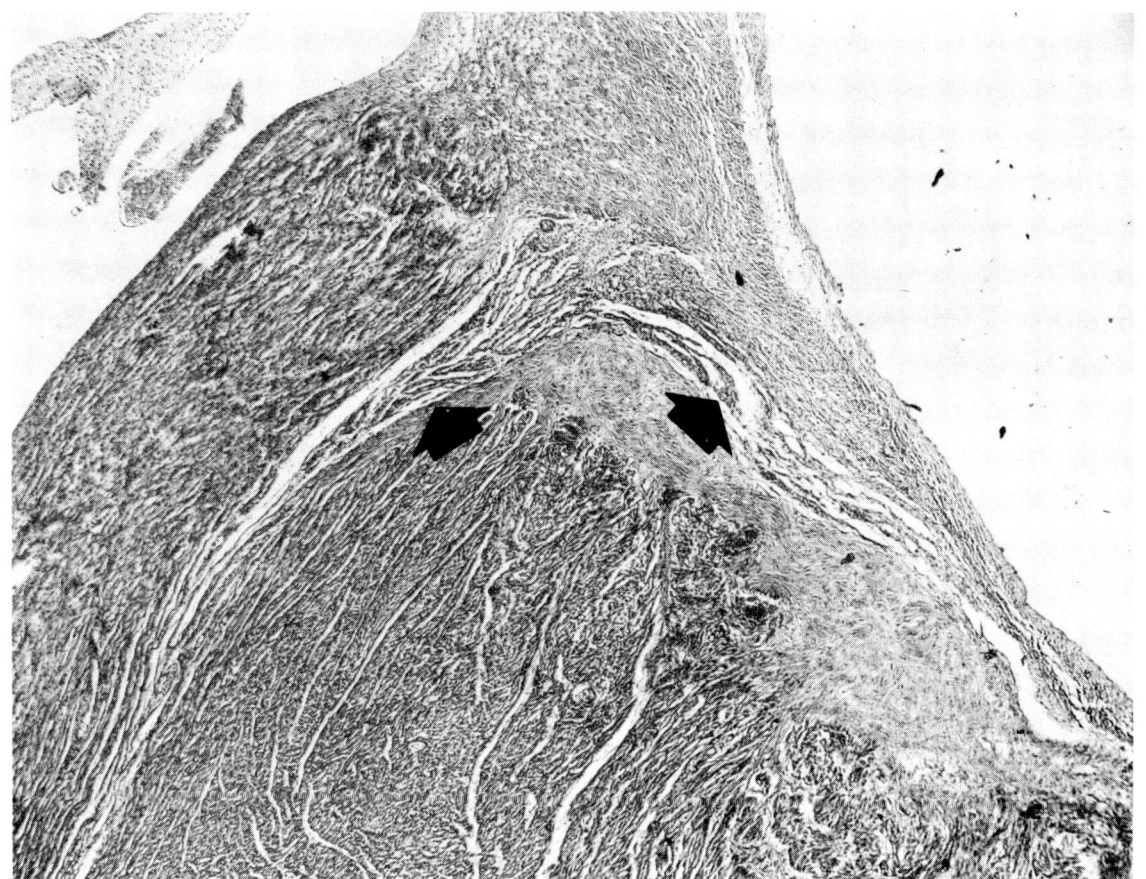

Figure 1–24

Figure 1–24. This represents another coronal section in the same orientation as, but somewhat anterior to, that illustrated in Figs. 1–21 to 1–23. (The patient is the same.)

The atrioventricular bundle is no longer present at this level; instead, only the right and left bundle branches appear, as indicated by the arrows.

As is often the case, the right bundle branch is embedded deep in the myocardium, whereas the left branch is rather superficial.

Hematoxylin, phloxine, and saffranin stain. Mag. 45×.

30 HEART

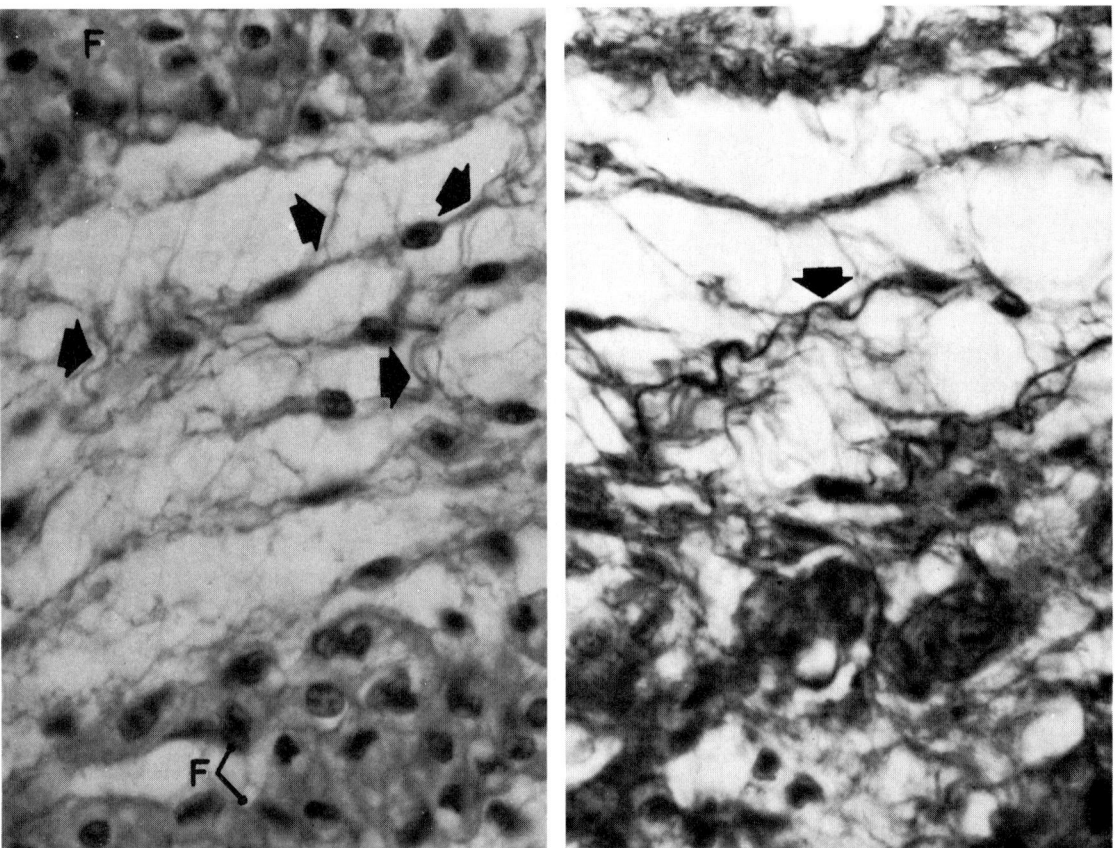

Figure 1-25 **Figure 1-26**

Figures 1-25 and 1-26. These two sections illustrate the supporting "skeleton" of the myocardial conduction system, collagen, and elastic fibrils. Both photographs were taken from sections in the immediate vicinity of that seen in Fig. 1-23. (The patient is the same.)

Figure 1-25. This photomicrograph depicts the collagen fibers as stained with van Gieson stain. The fibers of the myocardial conduction system itself are labeled F.

Figure 1-26. Here the elastic fibers are accentuated by a Weigert's methenamine silver stain. The arrow indicates one fiber.
Mag. 555×.

Chapter 2

BLOOD VESSELS

EMBRYOLOGY

In the fourth week of gestation (when the embryo is 5 mm. long, with 42 somites), as the central nervous system, the skeleton, and the mouth begin to appear, tiny spaces become evident within the mesenchyme. Ultimately they join one another, linking to form a vascular network that spreads out into the chorion, the yolk sac, and the embryo itself. This network is destined to give rise to the heart, the blood vessels, and the lymphatics.[1] (Each of the initial vessels consists only of a single layer of lining endothelial cells.) A little later, as the heart takes shape, the paired system of blood vessels is established and a functional circulation begins. The first indications of the paired vessels are solid cell clusters and mesenchymal clefts, which are aligned longitudinally in four incompletely joined courses. The medial pair are for the dorsal aortae; they continue cranially through what will become the first pair of aortic arches to join the primordia of the heart. From the heart a second pair of alignments extend caudally and ventrally, organizing the vitelline and umbilical veins. Later there is a complete circuit of arteries and veins for the yolk sac (the vitelline circuit) and a placental circuit of the umbilical arteries and vein that uses the body stalk to reach the chorion. The vitelline circulation lasts but a short time, while the umbilical remains functional until birth.

These sets of paired symmetrical vessels represent the primitive vascular plan. This is later profoundly altered and made rather asymmetrical by fusions, certain localized enlargements, atrophy, and emergence of new vessels and routings as organ systems develop.

As the primitive blood vessels grow, the neighboring mesenchyme adds accessory coats about the endothelium: the tunica intima (endothelial and fibrous), the tunica media (fibrous and muscular), and the tunica externa or adventitia (fibrous). Through folding, the tunica intima of the veins gives rise to pocket-like valves.[1]

The aorta eventually develops six pairs of arches which, on each side, join the ventral aortic sac (formed by the fusion of the ventral aortae) with the dorsal aortae. The most caudal of these, the sixth, is called the pulmonary arch. On the right side it loses its connection with the right dorsal aorta; but on the left side its distal segment remains as the ductus arteriosus.

The aortic sac and the primitive truncus split into the aortic and pulmonary stems in such manner that the aortic trunk remains continuous with the third and fourth arches, and the pulmonary with the left sixth.[1]

ANATOMY

The anatomy of the aorta and the great vessels arising from it, in the fetus and the newborn, is quite like that of the adult with the possible exception of a slight relative narrowing of the isthmus in the arch, between the origin of the left subclavian artery and that of ductus arteriosus. The umbilical arteries are patent throughout their entire course (as in the umbilical vein).

The ductus arteriosus, late in the third trimester, is visibly different from the aorta and from the pulmonary artery. The intima, when seen laid out flat, is of a somewhat darker tan hue and is definitely wrinkled rather than smooth, as though it were beginning to contract. (This does not seem to be true in those instances of congenital heart disease in which the ductus arteriosus is destined to remain open.)

The umbilical vein is relatively large; its lining intima is shiny and white. The two umbilical arteries, flanking the urachus and urinary bladder, are smaller and firmer. Each is cylindrical, with a tiny round lumen and glistening intima.

HISTOLOGY

The wall of the aorta (Figs. 2-1, 2-2, 2-3, and 2-5) in the fetus and newborn has three recognizable tunicae or coats: the intima, media, and adventitia. The tunica intima is extremely thin at this age and generally consists of little more than a single layer of endothelial cells.

The tunica media consists largely of elastic tissue in the form of many concentric fenestrated elastic laminae. Adjacent laminae connect by slanting bands to form complex elastic networks. In the spaces between the laminae are thin layers of connective tissue bearing delicate collagenous and elastic fibers, fibroblasts, and smooth muscle cells, mostly arranged circumferentially. Between these elements is a certain amount of amorphous ground substance.

The tunica adventitia of the aorta in infants is relatively thicker than it is in adults. It is made up of collagenous connective tissue and bears the vasa vasorum (Fig. 2-3).

The ductus arteriosus is as different from the aorta histologically as it is macroscopically (Figs. 2-3 to 2-6). Both the intima and the media are thicker. The intima is far more cellular. In addition, the arrangement of fibers in the media is distinctive. In the ductus one is not impressed by striking, concentrically arranged lamina, tightly packed, one against another. Instead, fibers are arranged in various directions and there are many irregularly shaped gaps between fibers, even at the time of a premature delivery (Fig. 2-6).

The histology of medium-sized muscular arteries is like that of the adult (Fig. 2-7).

With birth and the interruption of placental circulation, the umbilical vein and the umbilical arteries undergo gradual involution. The flow of blood ceases immediately with ligation of the cord, but obliteration of the lumen is likely to take from three to five weeks, and isolated segments may retain a vestigial lumen for much longer. Ultimately, they become fibrous cords; the umbilical vein is represented by the ligamentum teres extending from the umbilicus to the liver and by the ligamentum venosum within the liver. In the interim, between birth and its obliteration, it remains a relatively stout vessel with rather a large lumen and thick media, in which numerous discrete bundles of smooth muscle are easily discernible (Fig. 2–8).

The proximal portions of the umbilical arteries become the hypogastrics; their fibrous continuations in the direction of the umbilicus are known as the lateral umbilical ligaments.[2]

References

1. Arey, L. B.: Developmental Anatomy. Philadelphia, W. B. Saunders Co., 1974, pp. 94, 97, 348–350.
2. Patten, B. M.: Human Embryology, 2nd ed. New York, McGraw-Hill Book Co., Inc., 1953, pp. 696–697 and 704.

34 BLOOD VESSELS

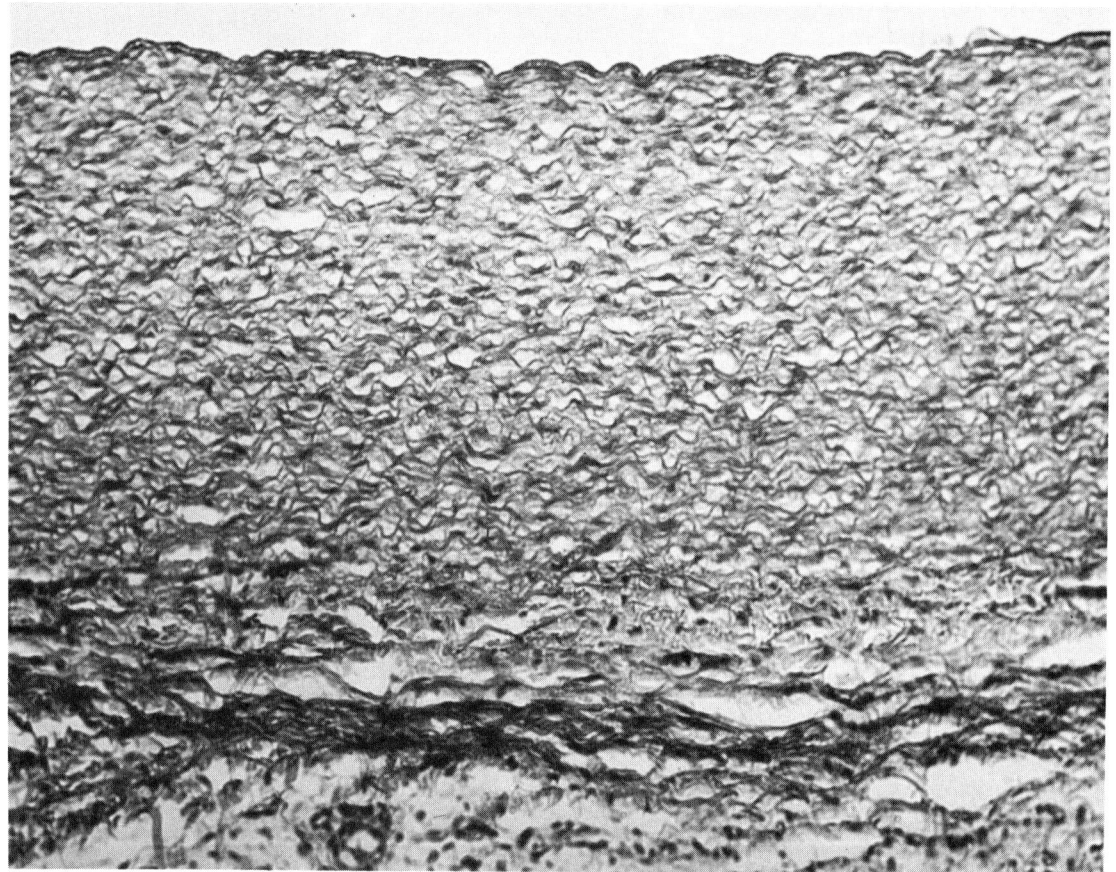

Figure 2–1

Figures 2–1 and 2–2. These two illustrations are for purposes of comparison of the aorta in immature and term infants. Both have been taken at the same magnification, and both are stained with hematoxylin and eosin stain.

Figure 2–1. This is a section through the wall of the aorta of a very immature infant. The baby, a black female, was born in the 24th week of gestation. Her body weight was 865 grams; she survived for $8^{1}/_{2}$ hours.

The delicate, wavy, more or less horizontally oriented black lines represent the elastic laminae. They appear to be relatively loosely woven.

Hematoxylin and eosin stain. Mag. 186×.

BLOOD VESSELS 35

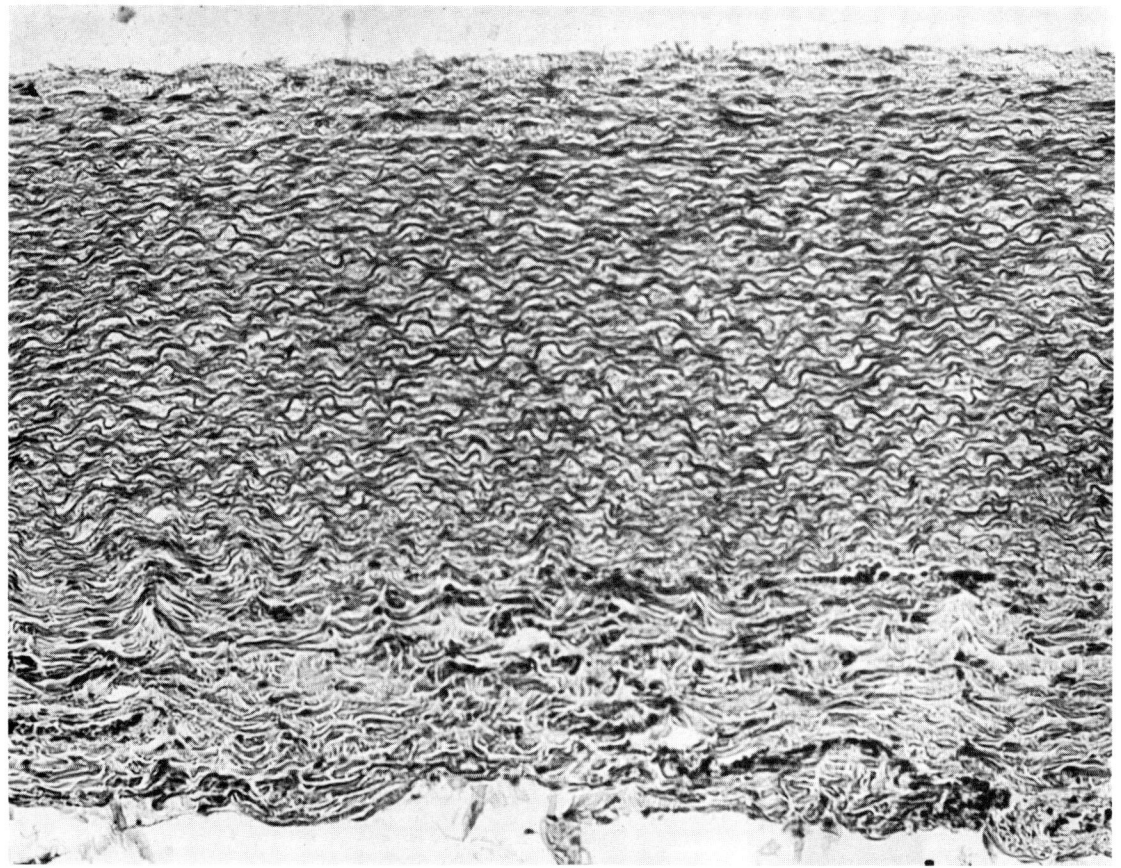

Figure 2–2

Figure 2–2. Taken at the same magnification as Fig. 2–1, this photomicrograph illustrates the wall of the aorta of an infant delivered near term. This baby, a black male weighing 2,850 grams, lived for 25½ hours.

The elastic fibrils in the media appear to be a little coarser than those in the less well developed infant, and their horizontal orientation is more marked. Further, the density of the weave seems to be a little greater; the spaces between elements are not so clear.

Hematoxylin and eosin stain. Mag. 186×.

36 BLOOD VESSELS

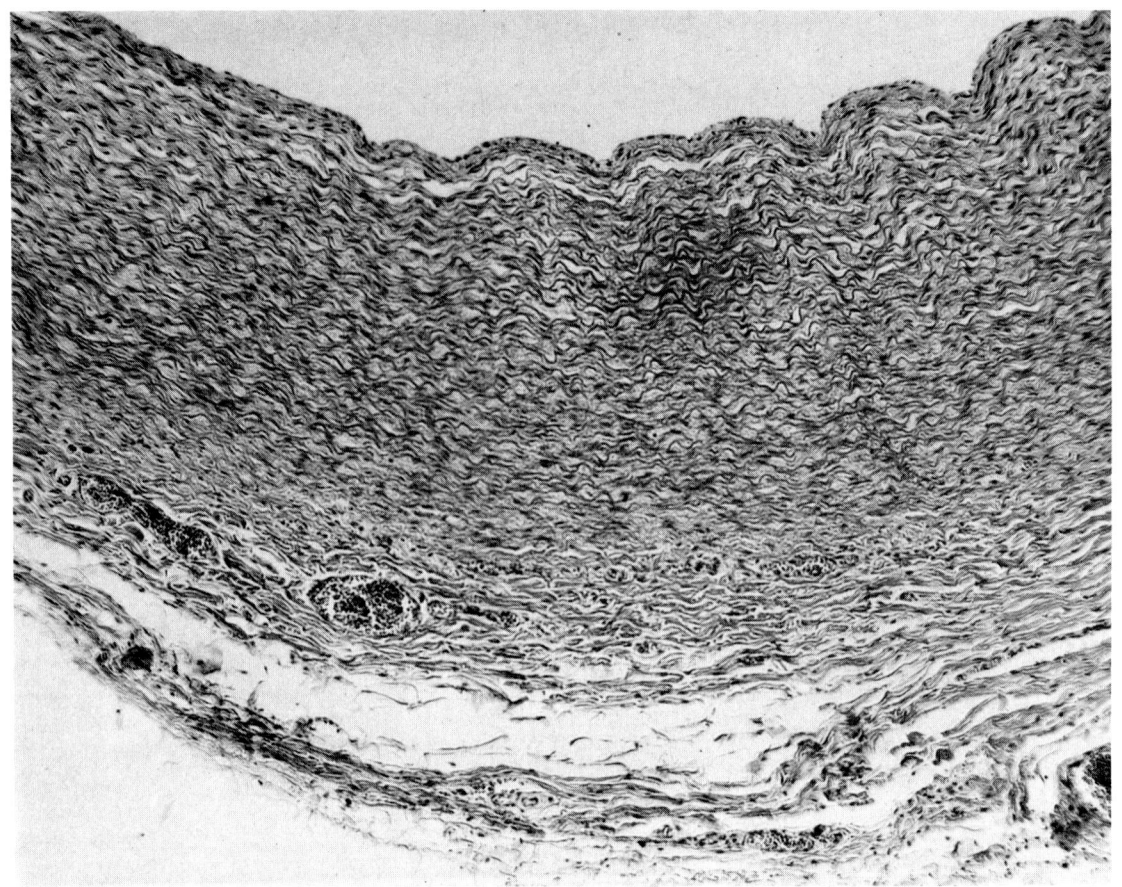

Figure 2–3

Figures 2–3 and 2–4. Taken at the same magnification, these two illustrations constitute a matched pair. Figure 2–3 is of the aorta of this infant and Figure 2–4 shows the ductus arteriosus. They were prepared in this manner to show the clear morphological differences between the two. The elastic laminae of the aorta are far more orderly and compactly laminated than those of the ductus, where the weave is open.

The infant was a twin, twin "A," a black female weighing 1,200 grams, of unknown gestation, whose mother was only 14 years old. The baby survived for 35 hours and 55 minutes.

Hematoxylin and eosin stain. Mag. 108×.

Figure 2–3. This is a section through the wall of the aorta. The tunica intima, at the top, is extremely thin. The tunica media consists largely of elastic tissue in the form of concentric laminae, which here appear as wavy parallel black lines. The tunica adventitia, at the bottom, is moderately vascular.

BLOOD VESSELS 37

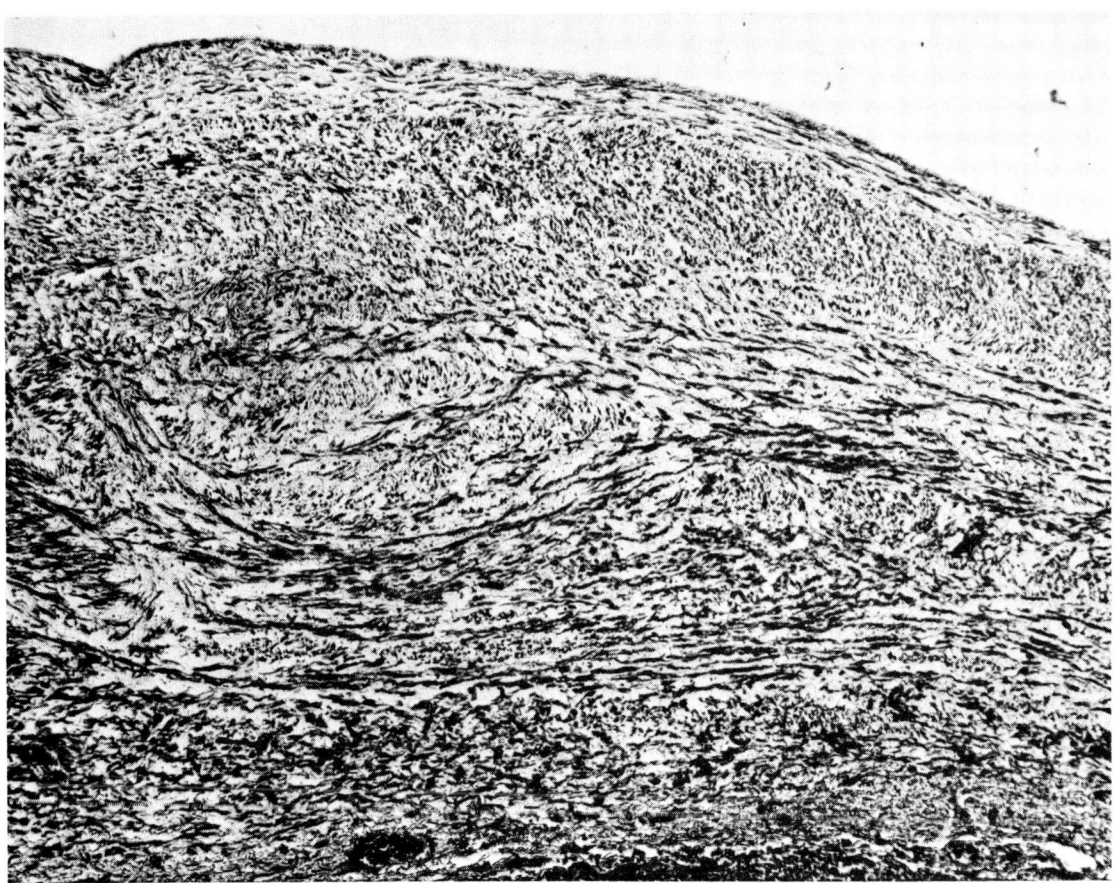

Figure 2-4

Figure 2-4. This photograph shows clearly the different arrangement of the elements of the media, apparently appropriate for contraction and closure after birth. In addition, it shows the very much thicker tunica intima, an additional asset, presumably, for potential closure of the vessel.

38 BLOOD VESSELS

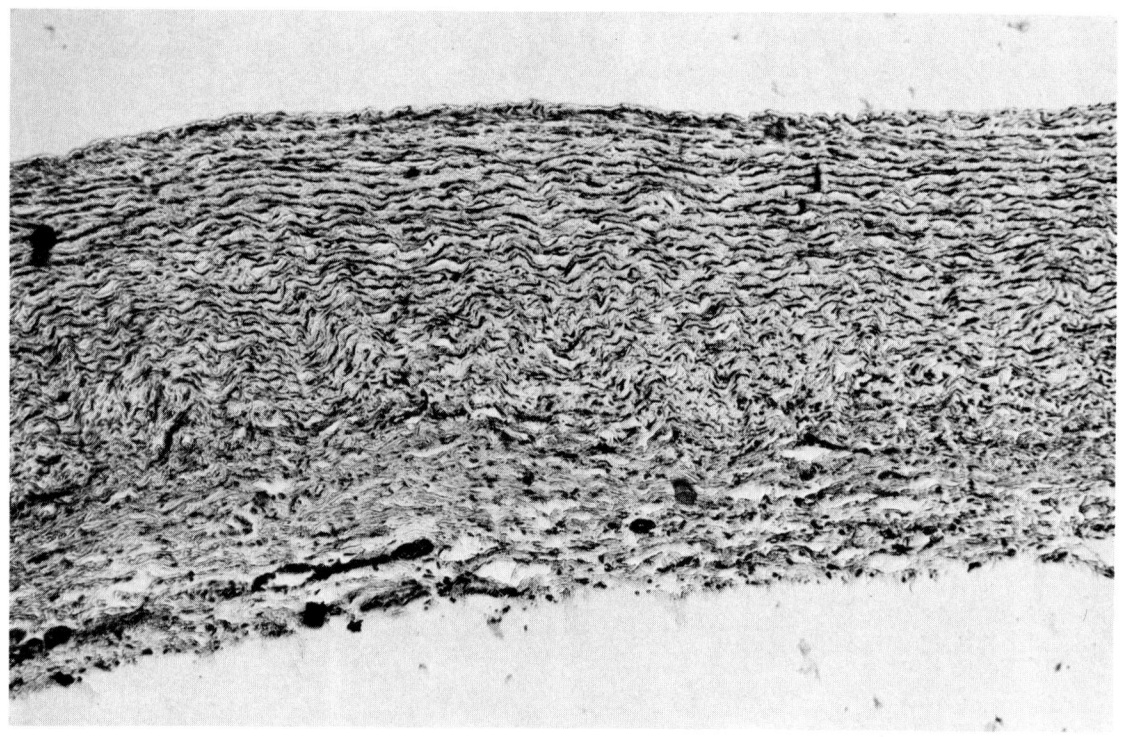

Figure 2-5

Figures 2-5 and 2-6. These two photomicrographs were taken from different infants, but the two are of comparable gestational age. The magnification in each is the same.
Hematoxylin and eosin stain. Mag. 116×.

Figure 2-5. This is a section of the aorta from a 1,200 gram black female infant, a twin, who lived for 35 hours and 55 minutes. Note the very delicate intima and the compact, clearly laminated tunica media. Vessels of the loosely woven adventitia are engorged.

BLOOD VESSELS 39

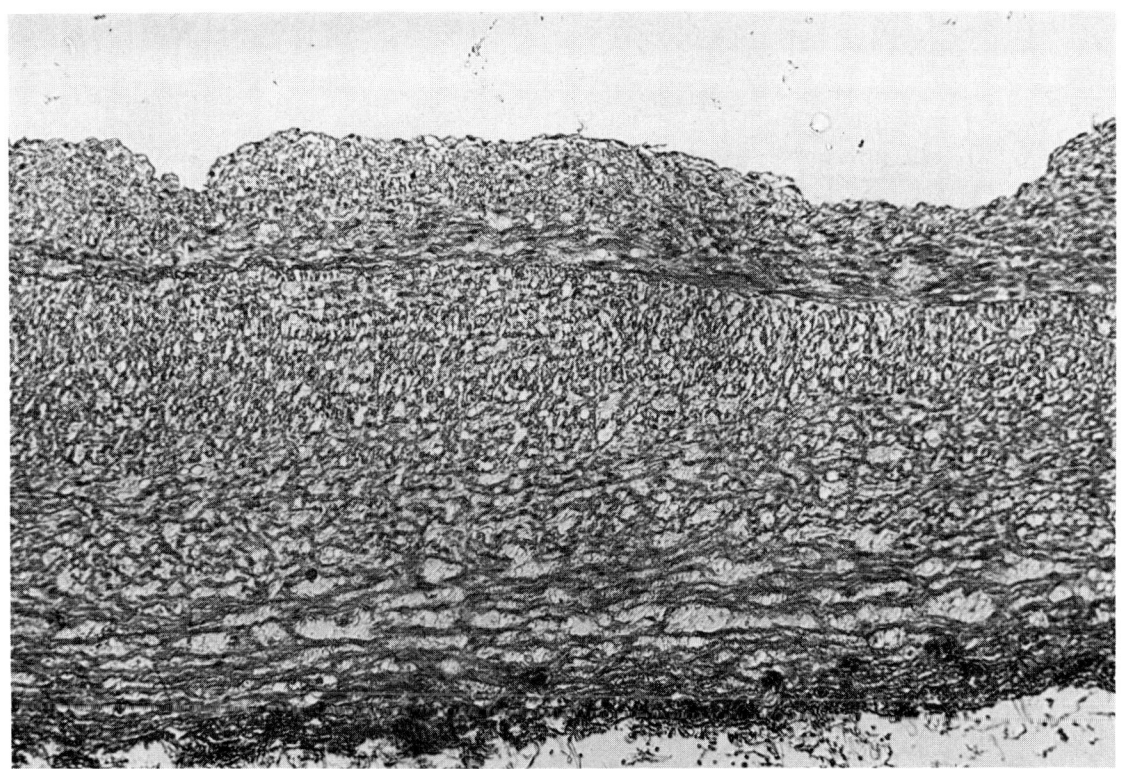

Figure 2–6

Figure 2–6. This is a section of the ductus arteriosus from a 1,550 gram black male infant of unknown gestational age, who lived for only 15 minutes.

The tunica intima is relatively thick, in comparison with that of the aorta at the same developmental stage (Fig. 2–5), and the tunica media has many open spaces in it, apparently as a result of initial tentative contraction.

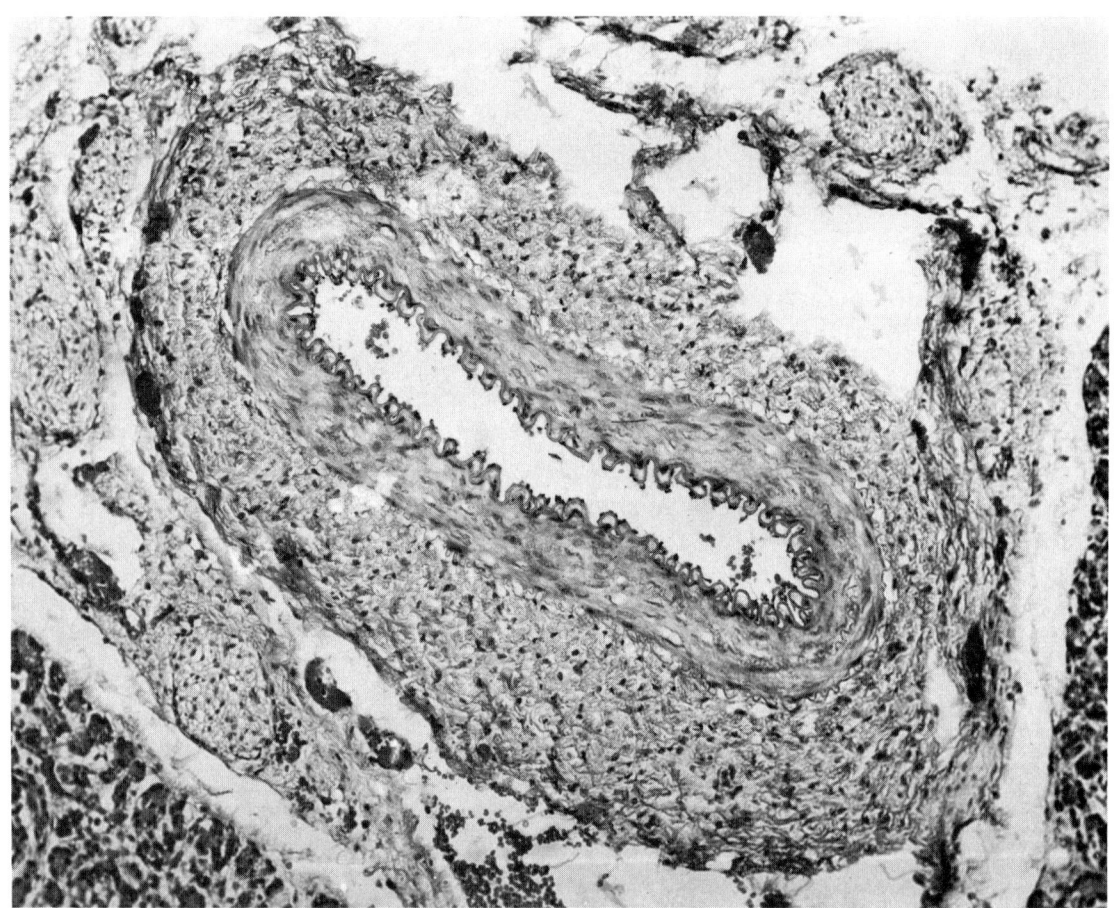

Figure 2–7

Figure 2–7. This photograph illustrates the character of the wall of a medium-sized or muscular artery in an infant.

This is a section of the wall of the splenic artery as it lies immediately adjacent to the pancreas. It is a clear cross section and shows well the delicate, almost invisible, tunica intima; the prominent, broad, wavy internal elastic lamina; the muscular media, and the fibrous tunica adventitia. There are four nerve bundles and numerous vessels surrounding the artery, and two portions of the pancreas in the right and left lower corners.

Hematoxylin and eosin stain. Mag. 142×.

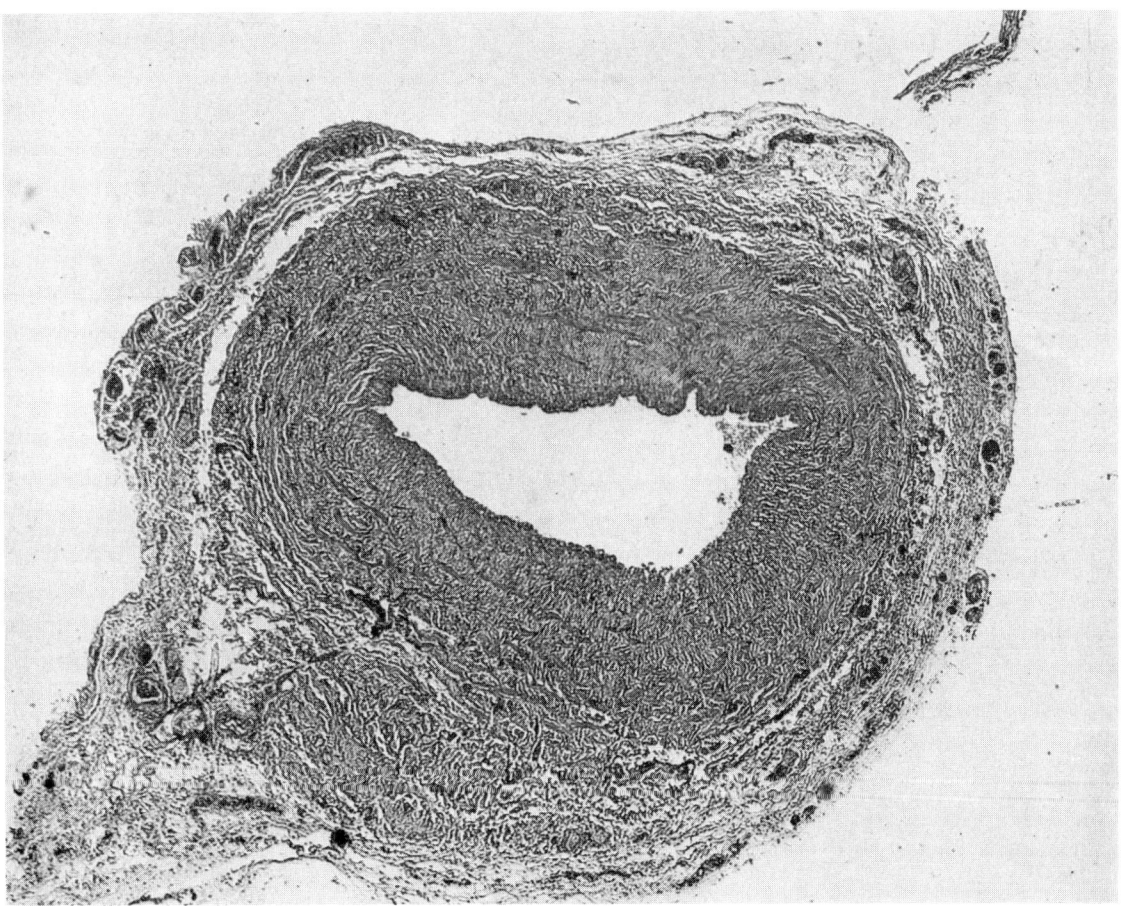

Figure 2–8

Figure 2–8. This is a cross section of the umbilical vein from an infant born prematurely. This baby was delivered in the 28th week of gestation and lived for 6½ hours. The infant was a female whose body weighed only 1,180 grams at postmortem examination.

The umbilical vein is a large vessel with a large lumen and relatively thick wall. Bundles of smooth muscle are arranged in almost haphazard fashion in the media. The tunica intima is very thin, and the adventitia is rather thick.

Hematoxylin and eosin stain. Mag. 45×.

Part 2

LYMPHOID TISSUE

Chapter 3

THYMUS

EMBRYOLOGY

Most embryologists believe the thymus to be derived solely from the endodermal thymic outgrowths of the third and fourth pharyngeal pouches at about the sixth week of gestation; some maintain that it is mainly from the third.[1] At least one investigator believes that it receives an ectodermal contribution from the cervical sinus,[2] but this cannot be regarded as proved.[3]

The third pouch develops into a diverticulum directed laterally on each side from the pharynx with a narrow duct-like neck and a flask-shaped fundus oriented caudally. Most of the endoderm of that fundus forms the rudiment of half of the thymus, a small dorsal part forming the inferior parathyroid.

The duct of the thymic diverticulum then becomes solid and disappears, leaving the thymic rudiments separate from the pharyngeal wall. At this stage it is a purely epithelial structure made up of anastomosing cords of columnar epithelial cells. Remnants may persist, however, giving rise to the very common accessory nodules of thymic tissue seen so often, particularly in the vicinity of the lower poles of the lateral lobes of the thyroid.

After the thymic rudiment becomes separated from the pharyngeal wall, it loses its lumen, becomes solid, and proliferates rapidly. During the seventh week it moves caudally into surrounding mesenchyme with the heart, as the head extends and the neck is formed.[1] About this time the epithelial cells change their character, becoming more and more like reticular cells, and lymphocytes invade this network in great numbers from surrounding mesenchyme. The parts that remain in the neck may appear as separate accessory glands or may remain in continuity with the mediastinal portion. In the middle of the eighth week the lower portion of the organ slides under the sternum to become intimately united with the anterior surface of the parietal pericardium.

Ventral to the aortic sac, the two thymic rudiments meet and are subsequently united by connective tissue only; the rudiments themselves never fuse.[4]

Early in the third month, then, the primordium is a bilobed mass of closely packed epithelial cells.[4] The margins soon show lobulation as a result of the ingrowth of surrounding mesenchyme. At the same time, the epithelial cells differentiate to form a loosely arranged cytoreticulum, into the interstices of which lymphocytes migrate from the mesenchyme.

The peripheral part of each lobule is densely populated by the immigrant lymphocytes, while the central medulla remains a loose epithelial reticulum with few lymphocytes.[4]

Hassall's corpuscles, which are squamoid foci in the epithelial reticulum often partially keratinized and frequently containing eleidin granules, are seen by the end of the third month.

MORPHOLOGY

As previously mentioned, thymic tissue may appear not only in the bilobed major structure within the anterior mediastinum, but also in anterior cervical extensions or lobes; in entirely independent round or oval nodules near the lower poles of the lateral lobes of the thyroid; and tucked into the cleft between the lateral aspects of the esophagus and mid-portions of the lateral lobes of the thyroid. In both of the last mentioned positions, the thymic nodule frequently embraces a single parathyroid, usually as a rather coral-colored discoid subcapsular nodule.

In all of these various positions, thymic tissue has the same histological appearance. It is basically a branching structure, best appreciated in sections of the thymus of premature infants and fetuses (Figs. 3–1 and 3–2). Each branch or lobule, attached to its neighbors by a stout cord of medullary tissue, is composed of a peripheral portion (the cortex) and a central core (the medulla).

The *cortex* consists of lymphocytes which are densely and uniformly packed, obscuring the sparse reticular framework (Figs. 3–3 to 3–7). The cortex has no lymph nodules. These lymphocytes are said to arise by division of stem cells that have originally migrated to the thymus from the bone marrow.[4]

The majority of thymic lymphocytes have a short life span of three to five days and degenerate while still in the thymus,[4] while the remainder leave to form part of the circulating pool of lymphocytes that are as yet immunologically uncommitted. In the perivascular regions and near the capsule and trabeculae, it is said that, at least in adults, a number of true phagocytic macrophages may be found. This may not be true in the perinatal period.

The medulla stains less intensely because of the few lymphocytes that it contains (Figs. 3–3 to 3–7). Here reticular cells predominate, and the characteristic Hassall's thymic corpuscles are found (Figs. 3–8 to 3–16). The thymic reticular cells are not members of the reticuloendothelial system in that they do not phagocytose diffusible dyes or particulates.[1]

There is an epithelial framework throughout the thymus, which is almost certainly derived from the original endodermal thymic diverticulum from the embryonic pharynx. These cells have oval, pale-staining nuclei and vary in size and shape in different parts of the thymus. They form flattened, incomplete sheets that extend under the connective tissue capsule and ensheath trabeculae and vessels. The framework of the medulla is made up of a system of incomplete anastomosing sheets of similar but larger eosinophilic epithelial cells.

The concentric corpuscles of Hassall are first formed in early fetal life and are thereafter continuously formed throughout the life of the thymus (Figs. 3–8 to 3–16). A medullary epithelial cell enlarges and develops an intense eosinophilia (Figs. 3–8 and 3–9). It then follows a train of further degenerative changes as it becomes larger. Progressive vacuolization of its cytoplasm and fragmentation of its nucleus are followed by engulfment of the nuclear debris by the vacuoles, which then become confluent.[4] Adjacent epithelial cells increase in size and become arranged as a series of eosinophilic concentric cellular lamellae around a central mass (Fig. 3–12). As the corpuscle grows, further degenerate epithelial cells are added to the central mass, together with the products of cortical lympholysis carried there by macrophages[4] (Fig. 3–13). They pass between the epithelial covering cells to reach the center. The core may become hyalinized or may break apart, as though solubilized or quite necrotic (Fig. 3–14). Corpuscles seem to increase in size and number during periods of intense lympholysis and during thymic involution.

Even during early infancy, episodes of stress may result in considerable reduction in the number of lymphocytes in the thymus or involution. In the process the thymus becomes histologically quite atypical and loses much of its dark staining propensity; at the same time, Hassall's corpuscles appear to be far more numerous and larger. Possibly some of this latter alteration is an artifact, the result of their becoming crowded together as the organ diminishes in size.

One of the histologic features of the thymus in the infant, and particularly in the fetus as early as 18 weeks — but not apt to be observed in later life — is the presence of islands of hematopoietic elements within connective tissue septa between lobules (Fig. 3–17). The developing cells include both erythrocytic and granulocytic elements. As in other hematopoietic sites in the fetus, members of the eosinophilic series are often quite prominent among these cells.[5] In the normal full term infant little of this remains.

References

1. Willis, R. A.: The Borderland of Embryology and Pathology. London, Butterworth and Co., Ltd., 1958, pp. 112–114 and 272.
2. Norris, E. H.: The morphogenesis and histogenesis of the thymus gland in man: in which the organ of the Hassall's corpuscles in the human thymis is discovered. Contribs. Embryol., No. 166, 27: 191–208, 1938.
3. Garrett, F. D.: Development of cervical vesicles in man. Anat. Rec., 100:101–113, 1948.
4. Warwick, R., and Williams, P. L.: Gray's Anatomy, 35th British ed. Philadelphia, W. B. Saunders Co., 1973, pp. 170 and 723–727.
5. Valdes-Dapena, M. A.: An Atlas of Fetal and Neonatal Histology. Philadelphia. J. B. Lippincott Co., 1957, pp. 163–171.

Note: For good accounts of thymic histological differentiation, see references mentioned in Willis (as above), pp. 112–113.

48 THYMUS

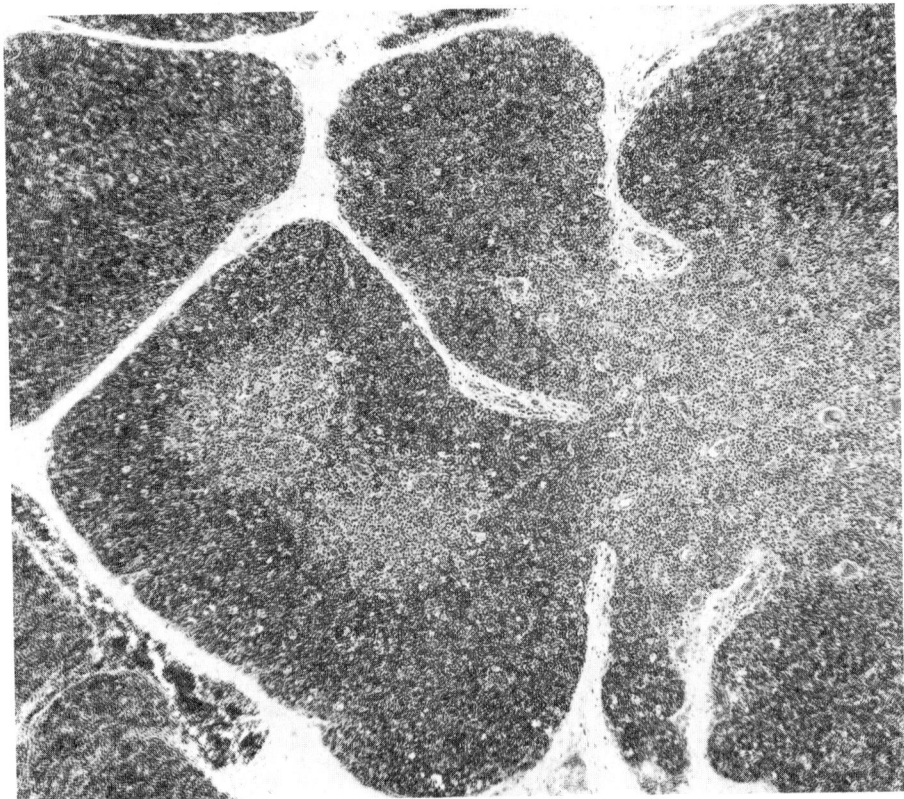

Figure 3–1

Figures 3–1 and 3–2. These two photomicrographs, both taken at the same magnification, illustrate the basic branching architecture of the thymus. The core of each "branch" or lobule is the pale-staining medulla in which Hassall's corpuscles are located. The peripheral portion, or cortex, is composed of myriads of uniform, densely packed, small lymphocytes with darkly stained nuclei and almost no visible cytoplasm.

Figure 3–1. This section was taken from the thymus of a 1,505 gram male infant, born after seven months of gestation, who lived for 26 hours. (Estimated gestational age: 29 weeks.)
Hematoxylin and eosin stain. Mag. 81×.

THYMUS 49

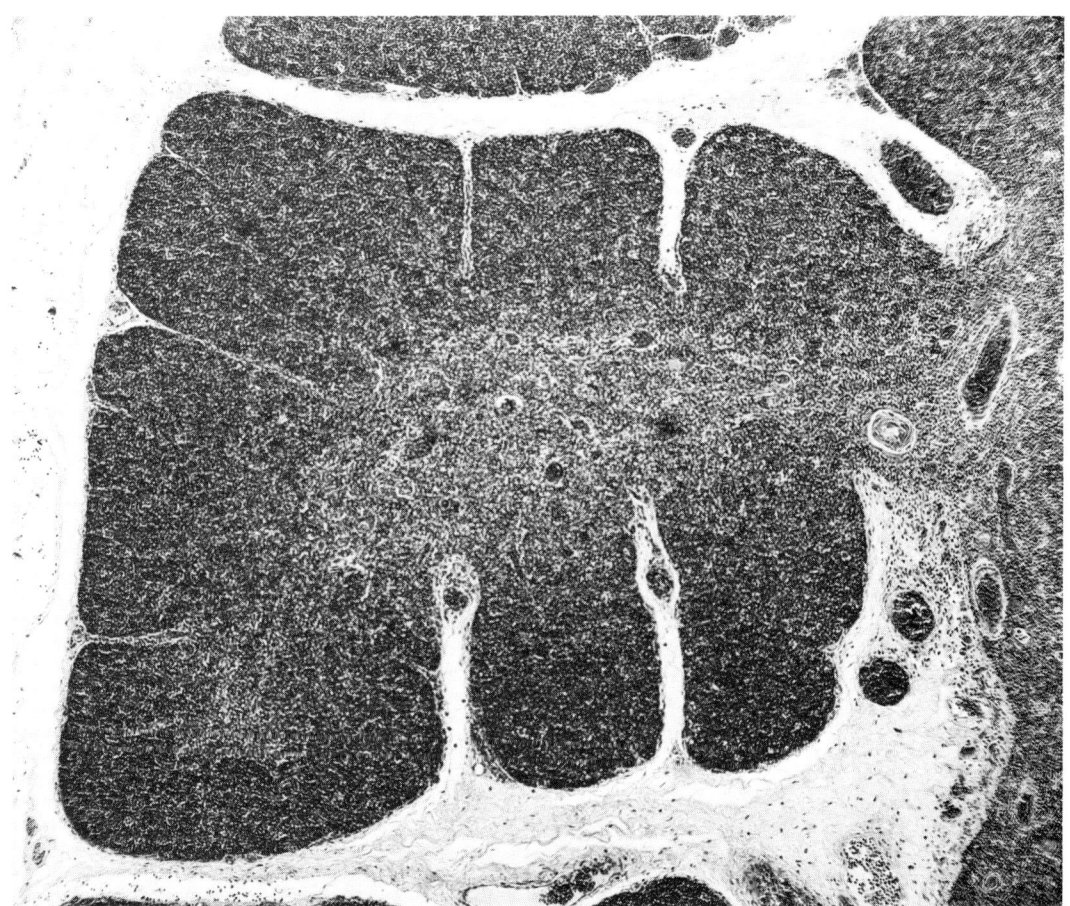

Figure 3–2

Figure 3–2. This represents a section from the thymus of an infant who weighed 1,587 grams at necropsy. The infant was the product of a 28 week gestation and survived for 12 days, 9½ hours. Hematoxylin and eosin stain. Mag. 81×.

50 THYMUS

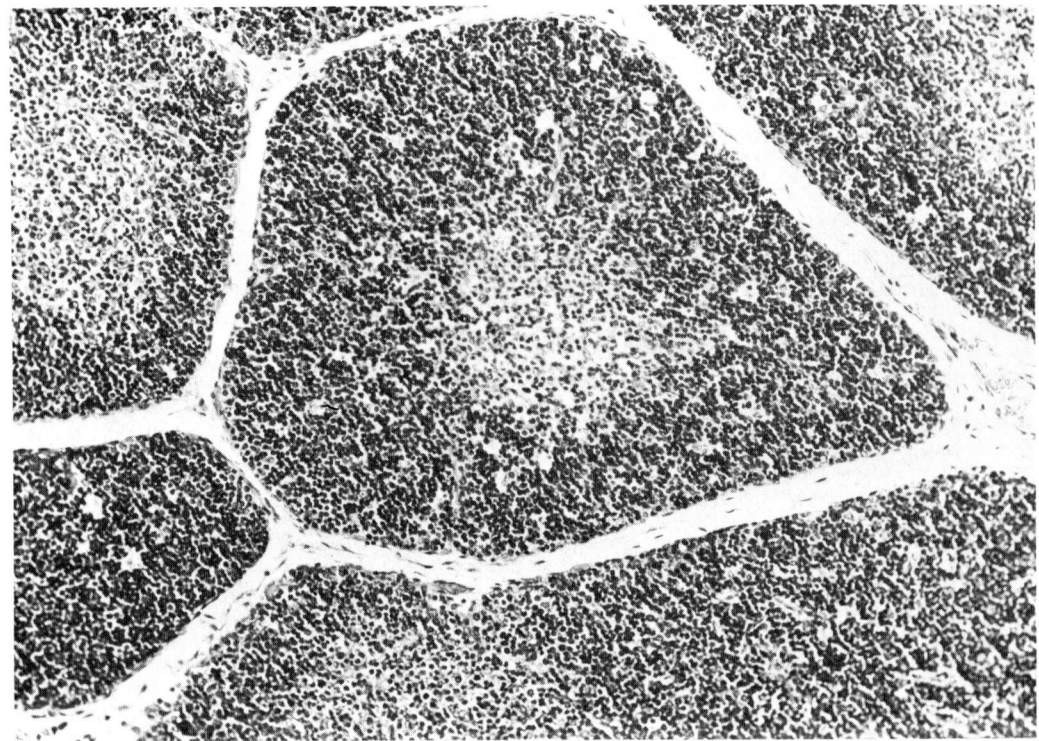

Figure 3–3

Figures 3–3 to 3–5. This set of three photographs illustrates the variability in the size of lobules apt to be seen in the infant thymus, and the fact that the lobules individually tend to be larger as the development of the infant progresses.

In this group of pictures the magnification diminishes progressively from 153× (Fig. 3–3) through 76× (Fig. 3–4) to 72× (Fig. 3–5). (This diminution, to a certain extent, lessens the visual impression of the marked difference which, in fact, exists between them.)

Figure 3–3. Section from a 200 gram female stillborn infant (gestational age uncertain, stated to be 26 weeks). Hematoxylin and eosin stain. Mag. 153×.

Figure 3–4. Section from a 2,000 gram white female infant of 32 weeks gestation who lived for 13 hours and 18 minutes. Hematoxylin and eosin stain. Mag. 76×.

Figure 3–5. Section from a 3,373 gram male infant of 40 weeks gestation who survived for 1½ hours. Hematoxylin and eosin stain. Mag. 72×.

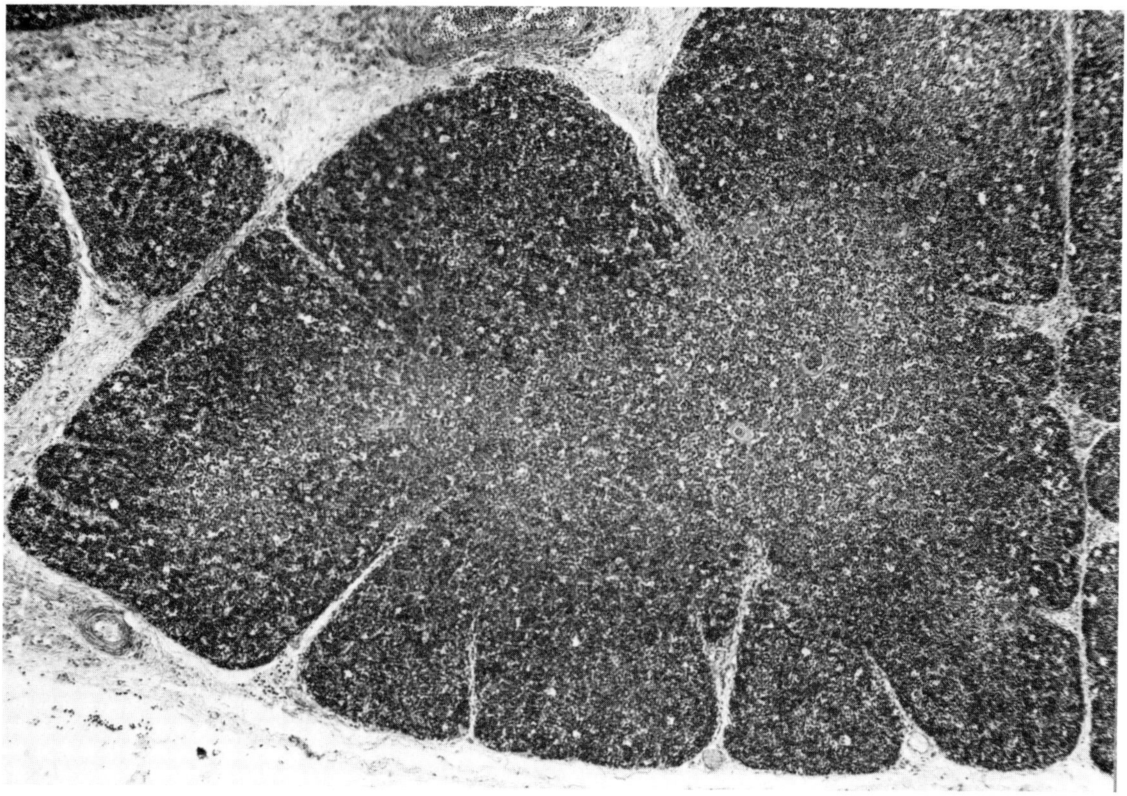

Figure 3-4

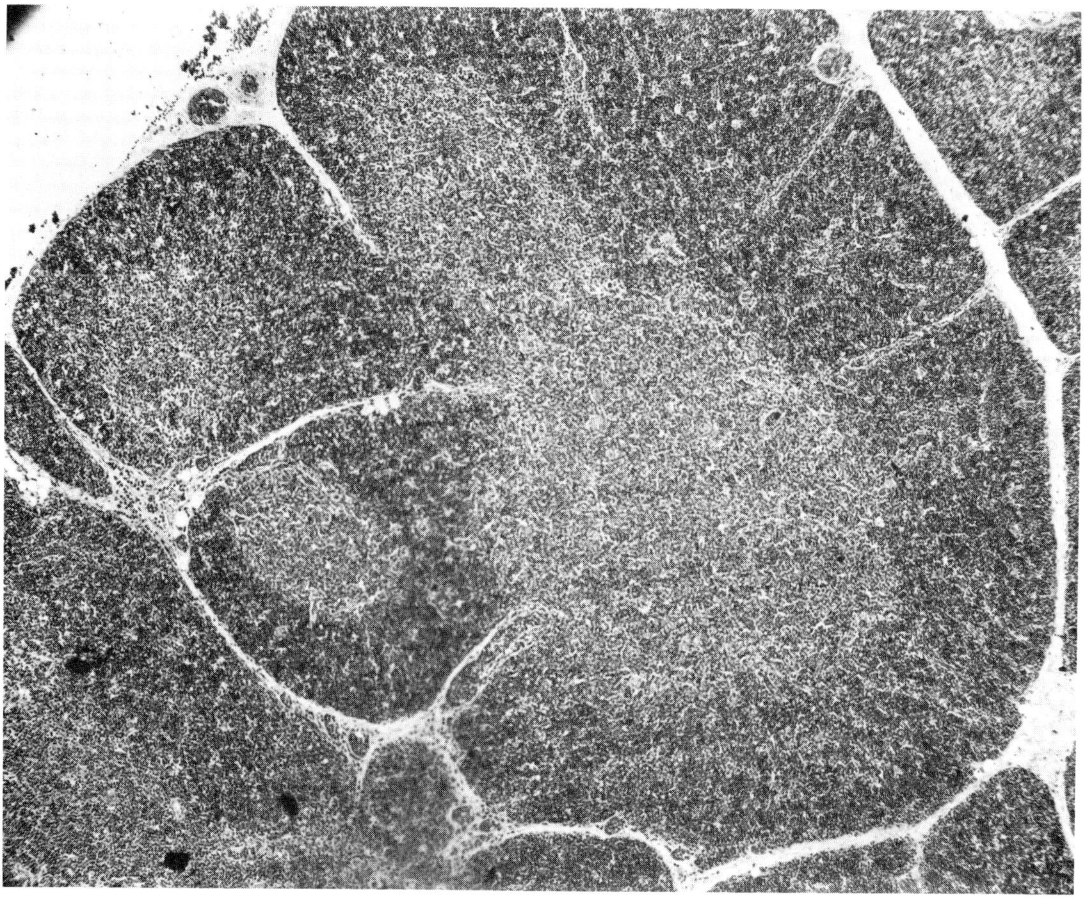

Figure 3-5

52 THYMUS

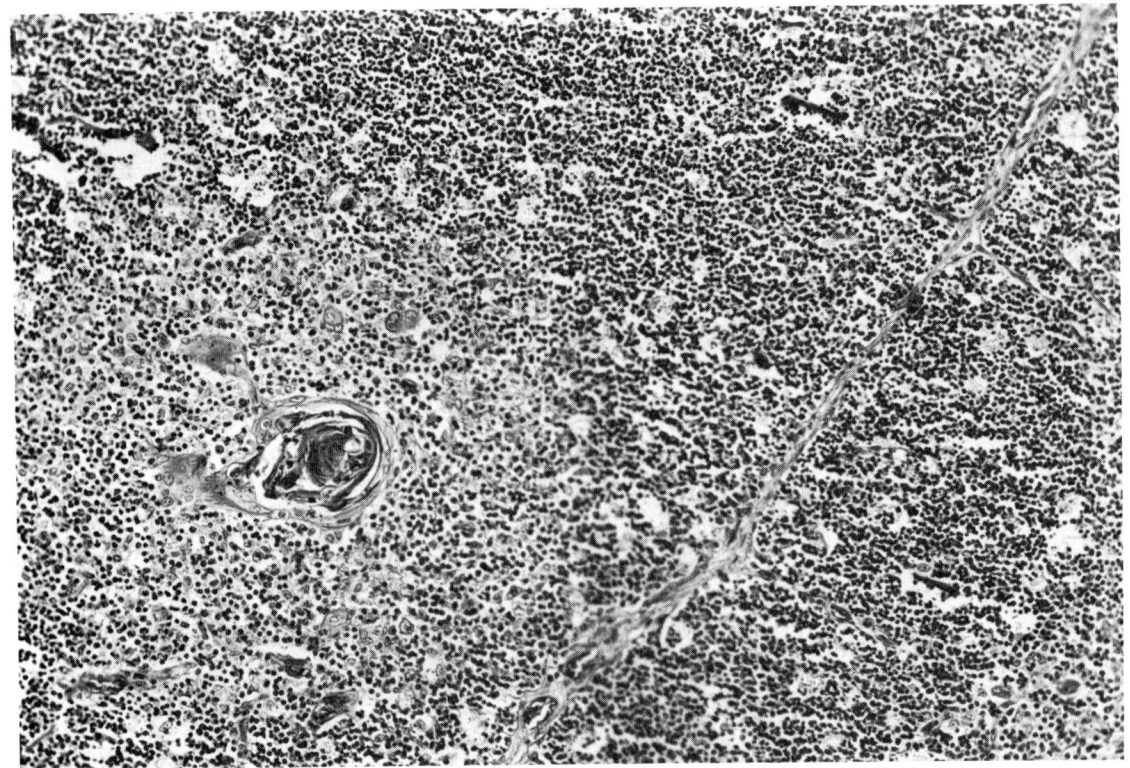

Figure 3–6

Figures 3-6 and 3-7. These two photomicrographs illustrate the differences that exist between the densely packed, small lymphocytes which populate the cortex of the infant thymus and the larger, pale-staining cells of the medulla.

Figure 3-6. Here the cortex occupies an arc at the upper margin of the photograph, most of the right side, and a slender band at the inferior margin. The medulla, confined to the central lower section of the left side, bears a large Hassall's corpuscle.

Section is from a 21 hour old black male infant weighing 1,270 grams. (Estimated gestational age: 28 weeks.)

Hematoxylin and eosin stain. Mag. 153×.

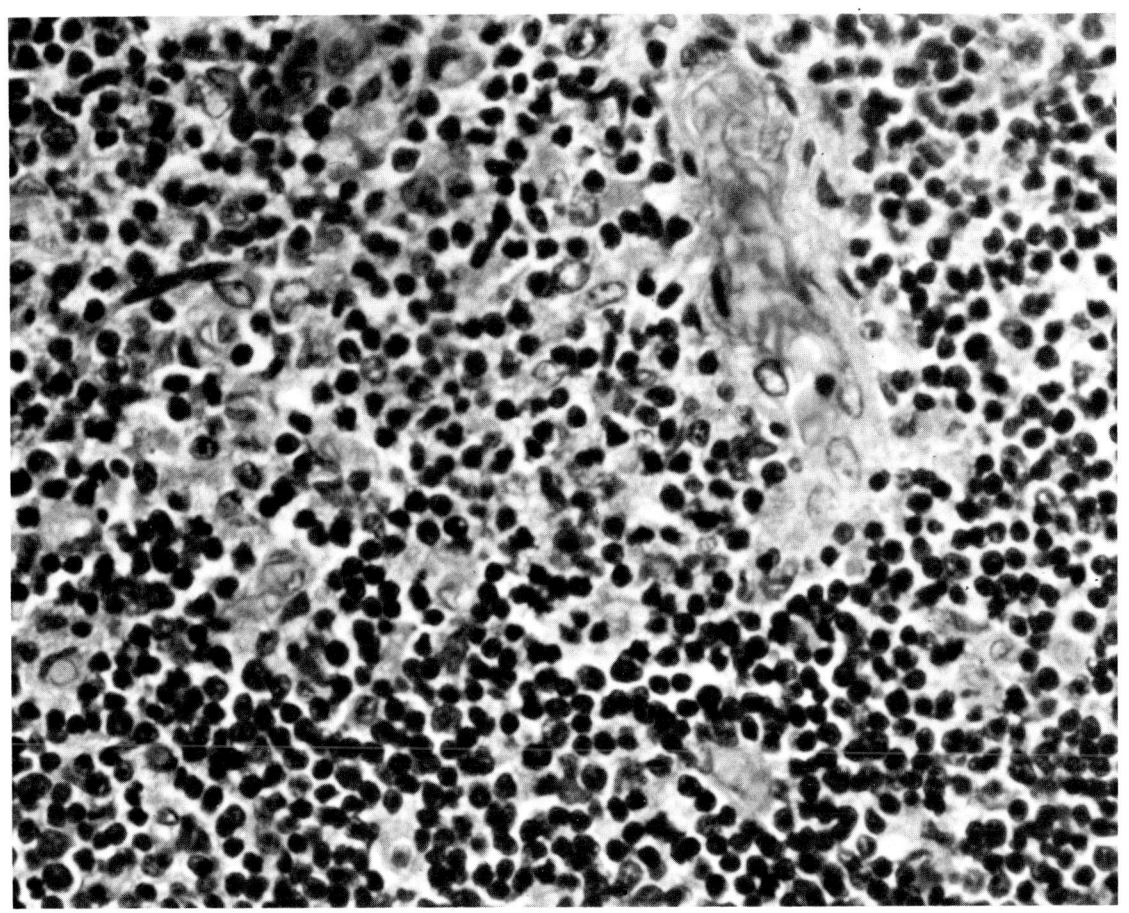

Figure 3–7

Figure 3–7. Here the crowded, tiny lymphocytes of the cortex occupy the lower third of the illustration, and the cells of the medulla form the upper two-thirds.

Section is taken from a 1,000 gram female infant of 29 weeks gestation who lived for 8 hours. Hematoxylin and eosin stain. Mag. 597×.

54 THYMUS

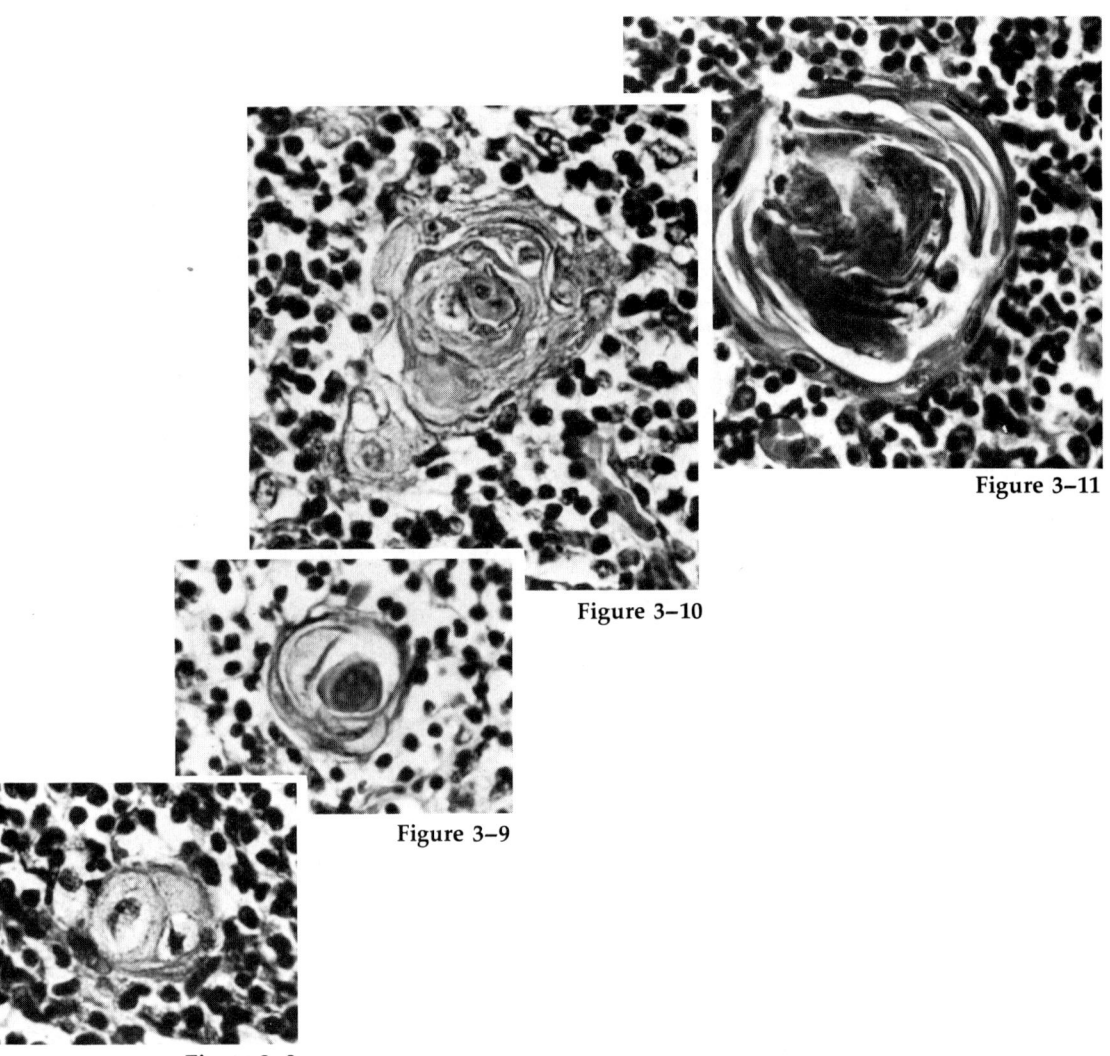

Figure 3–11

Figure 3–10

Figure 3–9

Figure 3–8

Figures 3–8 to 3–14. This continuous arc of photomicrographs illustrates the stages in the evolution of a Hassall's corpuscle from a tiny structure of one or two cells in Figures 3–8 and 3–9, to a huge body, the center of which is filled with debris, in Figure 3–14.
Hematoxylin and eosin stain. Mag. 440×.

Fig.	Wt.	Race	Sex	Gestation	Age
3–8	312 gm.	B	F	30 wk.	37 min.
3–9	2700 gm.	W	M	34 wk.	2 wk.
3–10	620 gm.	B	F	20 wk.	2 hr. 2 min.
3–11	2270 gm.	W	F	33 wk.	Stillborn
3–12	1900 gm.	?	F	28 wk.	5 hr.
3–13	2850 gm.	W	M	36 wk.	4 hr.
3–14	4120 gm.	?	?	39 wk.	16 mo.

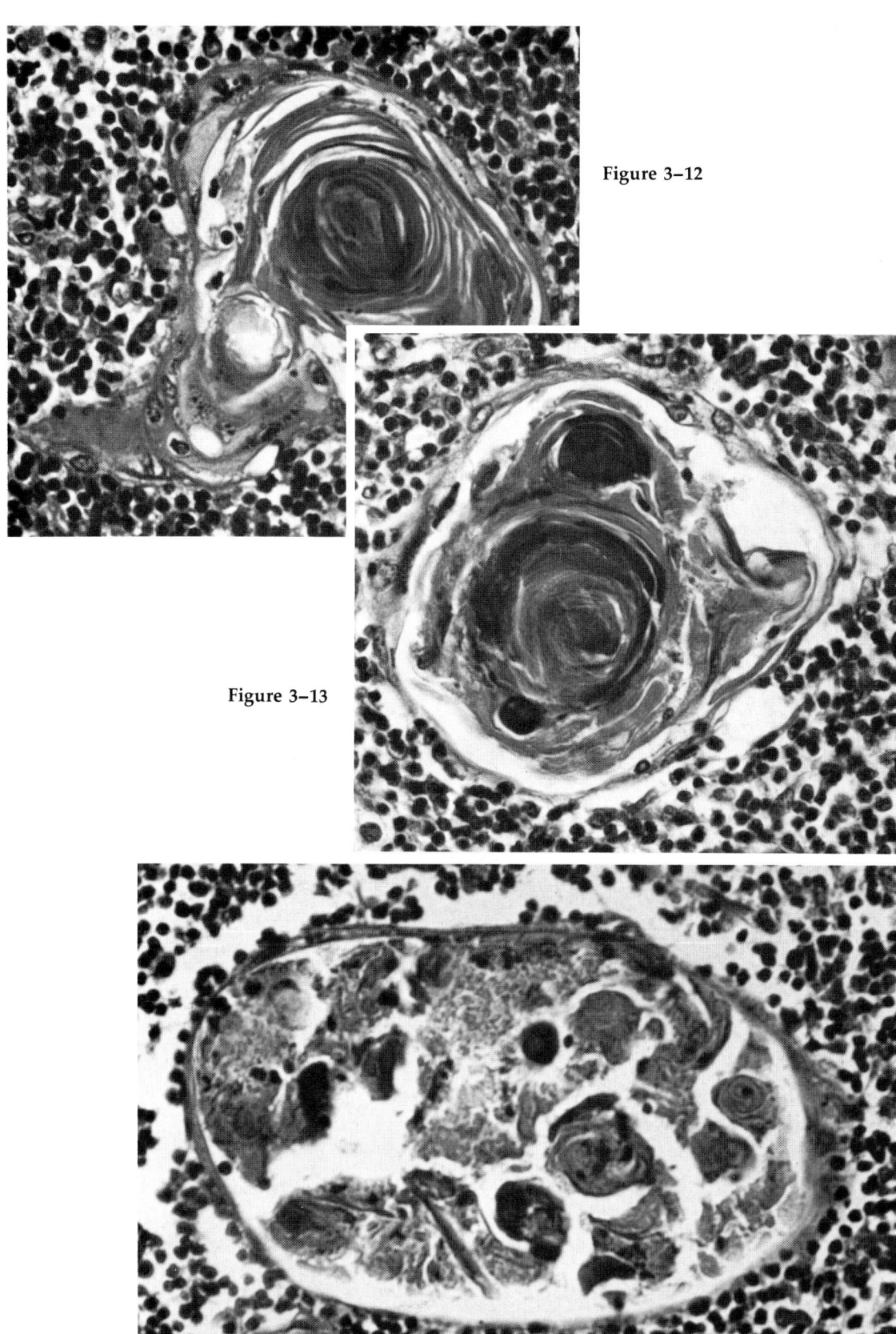

Figure 3–12

Figure 3–13

Figure 3–14

56 THYMUS

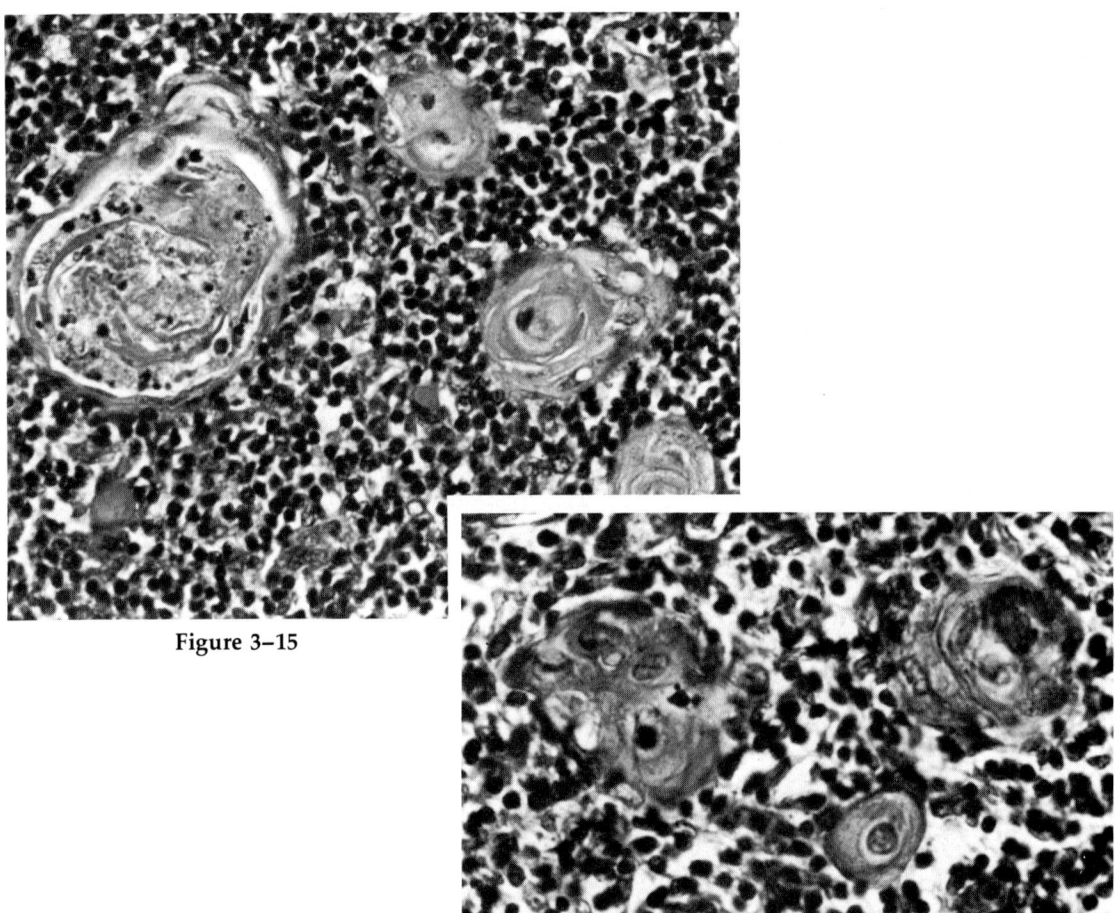

Figure 3–15

Figure 3–16

Figures 3–15 and 3–16. These two micrographs depict typical clusters of Hassall's corpuscles of various sizes and stages of development within the medulla of the infant thymus.

Figure 3–15. Section from a 1,670 gram female infant, the product of 30 weeks gestation, who survived for 1 month and 1 day.
Hematoxylin and eosin stain. Mag. 370×.

Figure 3–16. Section from the thymus of a 6 day old white female infant who, at autopsy, weighed 2,800 grams. (Estimated gestational age: 36 weeks.)
Hematoxylin and eosin stain. Mag. 440×.

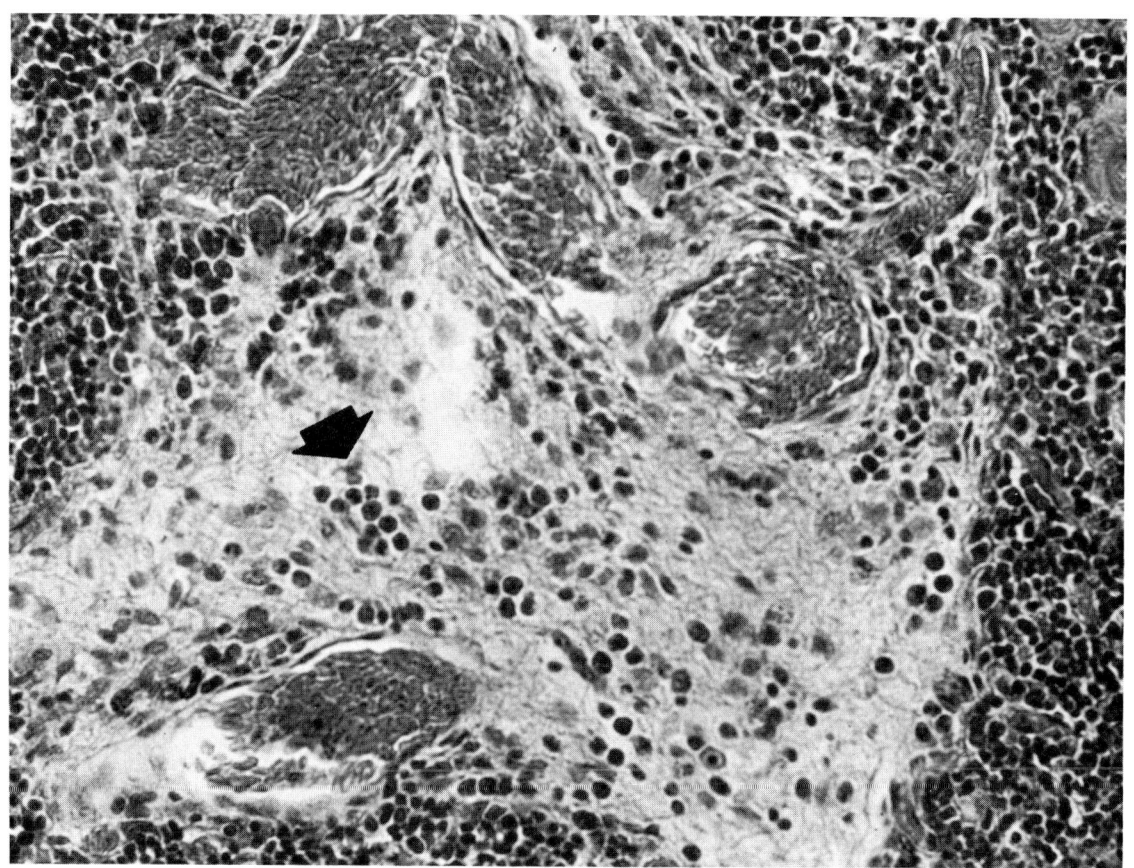

Figure 3–17

Figure 3–17. Extramedullary hematopoiesis is commonly encountered within the connective tissue septa of the thymus during the perinatal period. Here, several clusters of hematopoietic elements are apparent within the vascular loose connective tissue between lobules. One of the clumps is marked by an arrow.

This is a section of the thymus of a male infant who weighed 1,520 grams at necropsy. Gestational age: 32 weeks. Age: 34 hours.

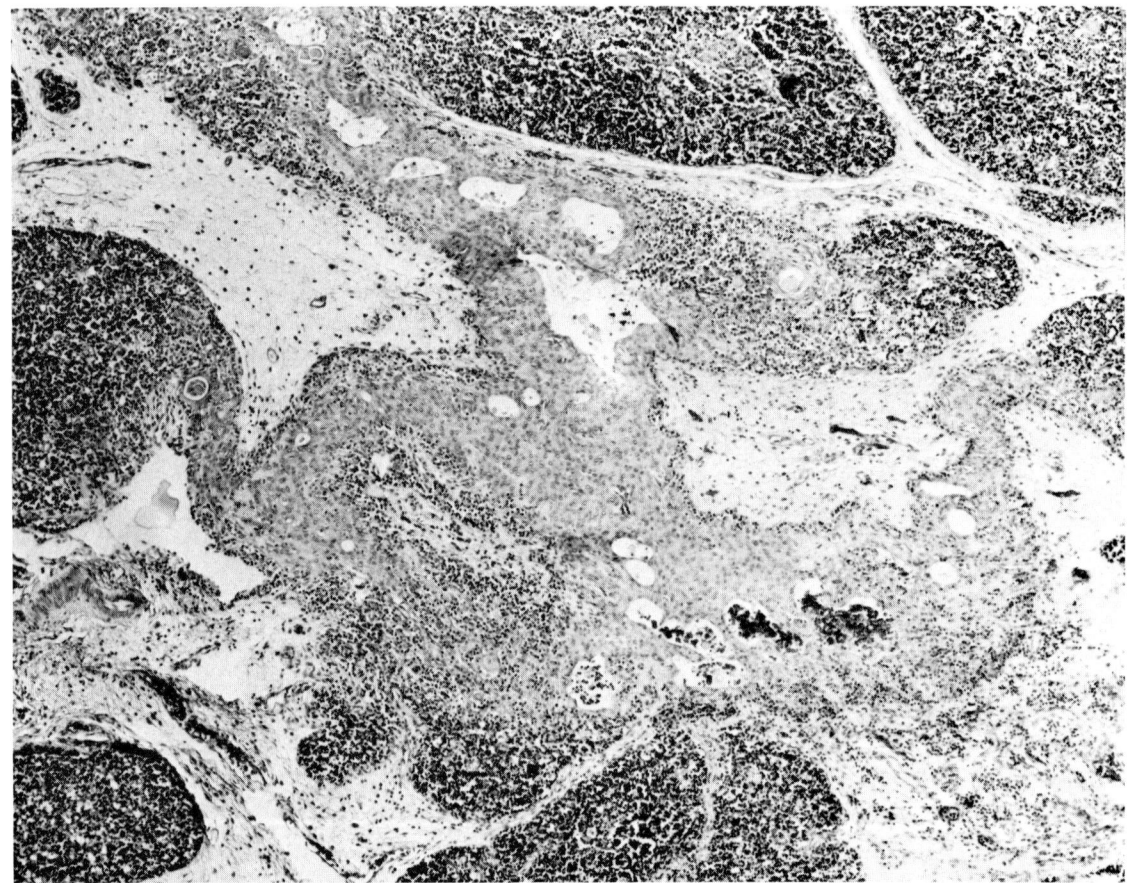

Figure 3–18

Figure 3–18. Uncommonly, in the thymus of a prematurely born infant, one may find small and very irregular islands of pure epithelial tissue, such as is seen in the center of this photograph. In hematoxylin and eosin stains its color is pale pink, and the cells appear to be rather squamoid. In this illustration, slender elongate projections are noted, which attach the island to individual surrounding lobules.

We are no longer able to identify the infant from whom this section was taken.

Hematoxylin and eosin stain. Mag. 83.6×.

Chapter 4

PALATINE TONSILS

EMBRYOLOGY

The second pharyngeal pouch, embryologically, gives rise to the fossa and covering epithelium of the palatine tonsil[1]; the pouch persists as the fossa, while its entoderm furnishes the epithelium covering the tonsil and lining its crypts.

The crypts arise progressively in fetuses of three to six months as solid ingrowths from the surface epithelium. They branch and hollow secondarily. Lymphocytes appear deep to the epithelium in the third month and organize as nodules[1] after the sixth month (Figs. 4–2 and 4–3).

ANATOMY

The palatine tonsils are two oval masses of lymphoid tissue, situated in the lateral walls of the oropharynx. Each is located in a triangular recess, known as the tonsillar fossa, between the palatoglossal and palatopharyngeal arches. The medial surface of each is free and projects somewhat into the pharynx. In the perinatal period, however, that projection is minimal. The magnitude of the projecting portion in no way reflects the size of the organ as a whole, because much of its mass is embedded deeply in the wall of the pharynx where its margins blend rather indistinctly with surrounding connective tissue. Its deep aspects extend upward, downward, and forward beyond the limits of the medial surface. Inferiorly it reaches out into the dorsum of the tongue; superiorly it invades the soft palate; anteriorly, it may extend for some distance beneath the palatoglossal arch.

The medial surface of the tonsil presents twelve to fifteen orifices leading into deep, narrow recesses, termed the tonsillar crypts (Figs. 4–2 and 4–3). These crypts penetrate nearly the whole thickness of the tonsil.

The lateral or deep aspect is covered by a layer of fibrous tissue termed the capsule.[2]

HISTOLOGY

The stratified squamous epithelium of the free surface overlies an indistinct thin layer of connective tissue (Figs. 4–1 and 4–3). The crypts, when they appear, are of simple branching form[3] (Figs. 4–2 and 4–3).

Almost all of the small round cells that populate the tonsil in this period of life are small lymphocytes. Lymphoid nodules, although present near the time of term birth, are not nearly so conspicuous at this time as they are in childhood. The lumens of the crypts, as they develop, may contain sizeable accumulations of desquamated squamous epithelial cells, but not much in the way of other debris such as cells or microorganisms (Figs. 4–2 and 4–3) which, of course, they do contain in later life.

Many small glands are connected with the palatine tonsils (Fig. 4–3). Their bodies are outside the capsule and their ducts open, for the most part, on the free surface.[3]

References

1. Arey, L. B.: Developmental Anatomy, 7th ed. Philadelphia, W. B. Saunders Co., pp. 237 and 238.
2. Warwick, R., and Williams, P. L.: Gray's Anatomy, 35th British ed. Philadelphia, W. B. Saunders Co., 1973, pp. 1244 and 1245.
3. Bloom, W., and Fawcett, D. W.: A Textbook of Histology. Philadelphia, W. B. Saunders Co., 1975, pp. 615–617.

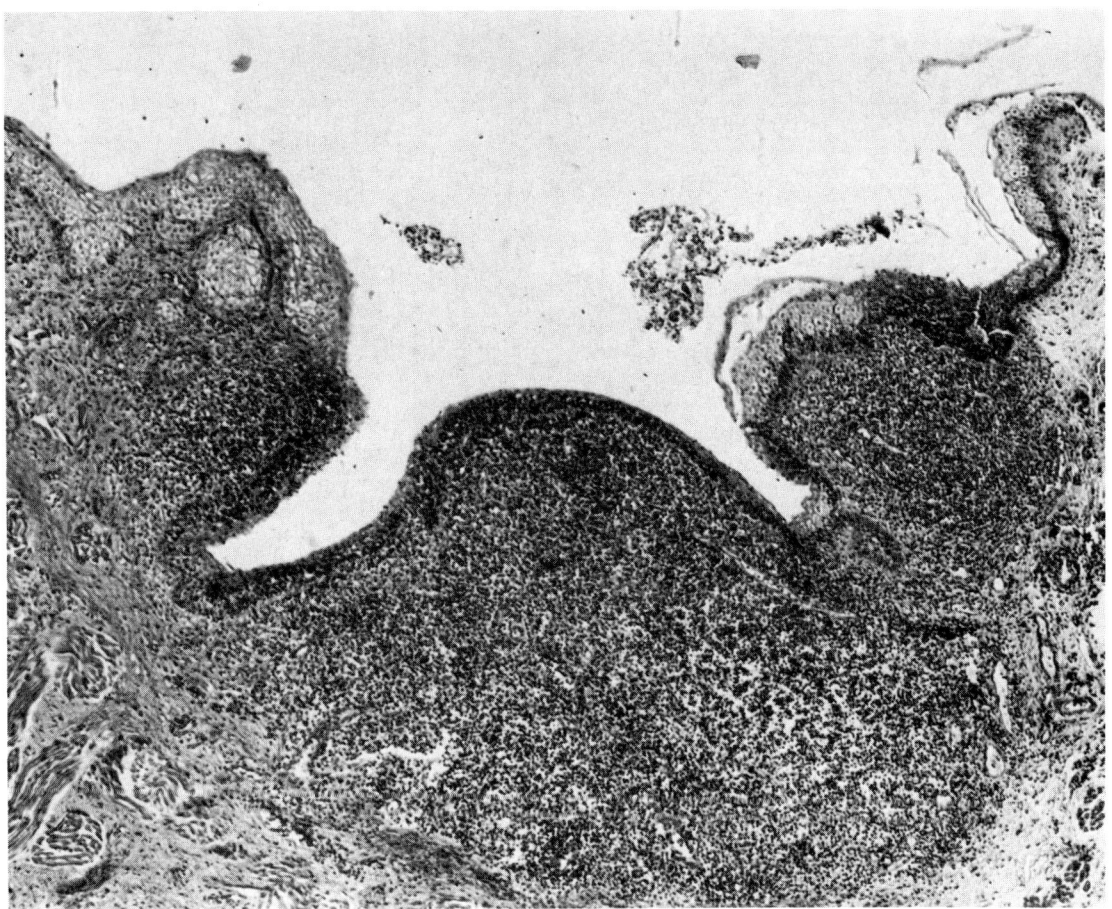

Figure 4–1

Figure 4–1. Pictured here is the tonsil of an infant born prematurely. The infant is not now otherwise identifiable.

Note that there is a complete covering of stratified squamous epithelium, continuous on both sides with that of the oropharynx. However, as it clothes the central mound of the palatine tonsil itself, the epithelium is distinctly thinner than it is in the pharynx.

At this stage of development there are no crypts, but there is a substantial body of lymphoid tissue comprising the tonsil. A tonsil of this size is visible to the naked eye.

Hematoxylin and eosin stain. Mag. about 90×.

62 PALATINE TONSILS

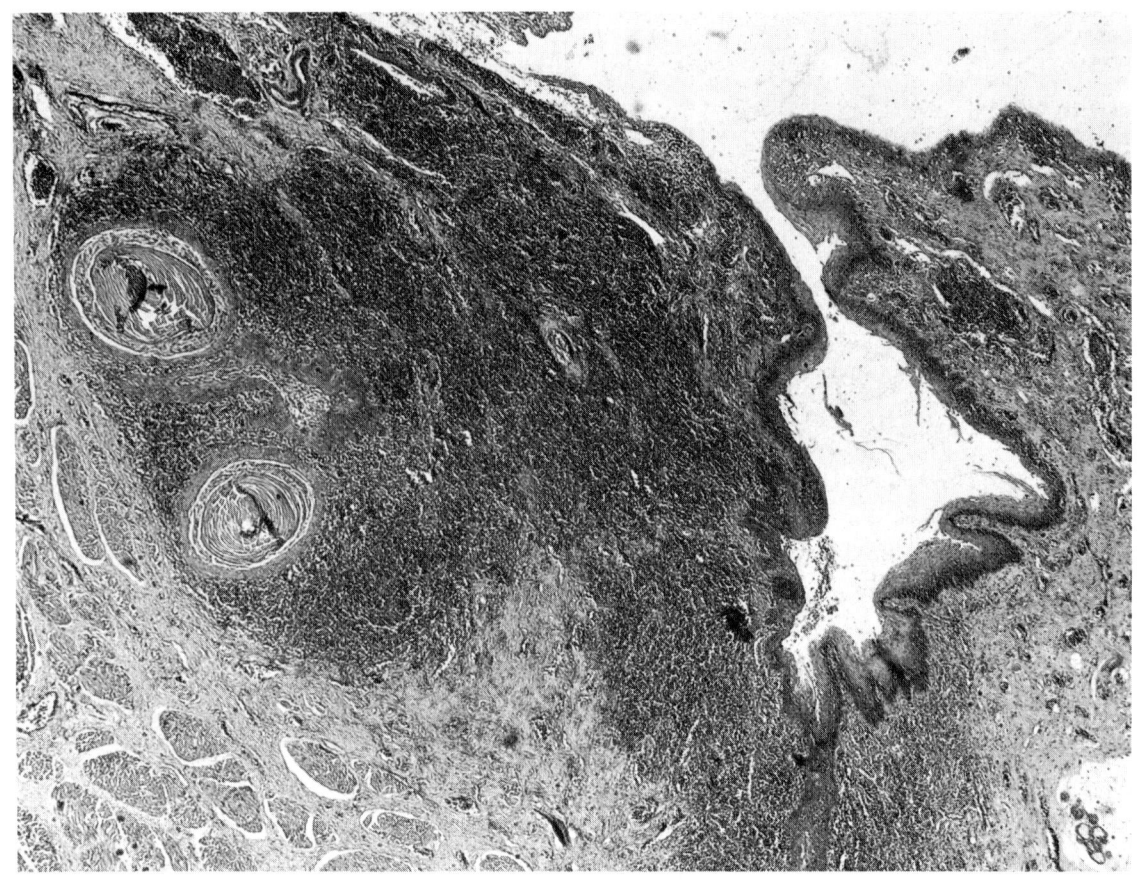

Figure 4–2

Figure 4–2. By contrast with Fig. 4–1, this is a section of the tonsil from an infant born at term. (The magnification is approximately half of that in Fig. 4–1.)

This infant, a black male, was born at term and weighed 4,225 grams at autopsy. He lived for 27 hours.

Note that at this stage there are crypts not only easily visible but filled with packed, laminated layers of sloughed-off squamous cells. Numerous bundles of skeletal muscle appear in the left lower corner, embracing the depths of the tonsil.

Hematoxylin and eosin stain. Mag. 45×.

PALATINE TONSILS 63

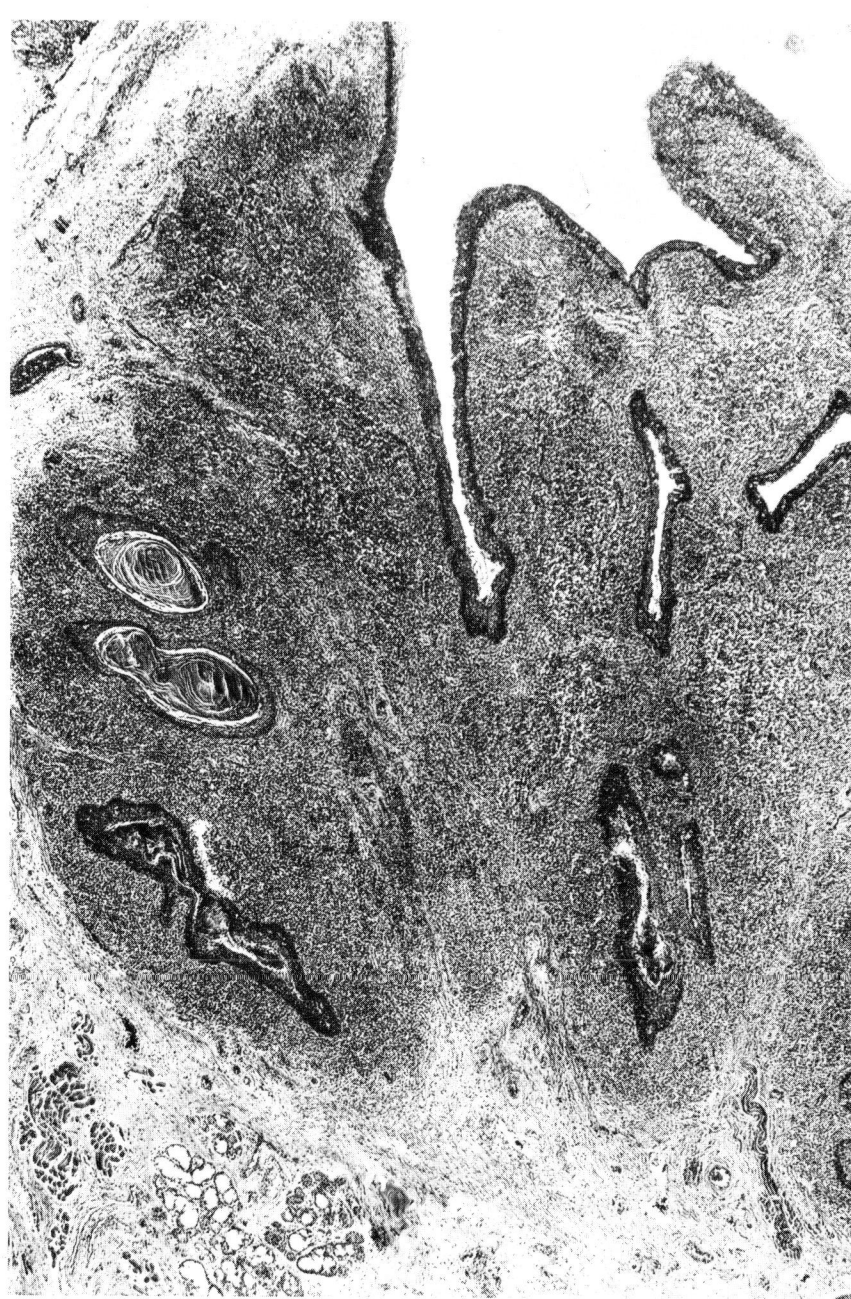

Figure 4–3

Figure 4–3. This section also is from an unidentified infant, but probably one born near term. Seven of the tonsillar crypts are apparent in this photograph. Two contain laminated debris. In the left lower corner there are bundles of striated muscle and also accessory salivary glands. Hematoxylin and eosin stain. Mag. 45×.

Chapter 5

LYMPH NODES

EMBRYOLOGY

The lymphatics develop quite independently of the blood vessels. They originate as discrete spaces in the mesenchyme. The mesenchymal cells bordering each space flatten into an endothelial lining. By progressive fusion, these locally formed clefts link into continuous channels which also grow and branch, extending the system further.[1]

The first plexus of lymphatics is distributed along the primitive main venous trunks. The dilatation and coalescence of these lymphatic networks at definite regions give rise to six lymph sacs. In embryos of about 10 mm., in approximately the fifth week of gestation, the right and left jugular lymph sacs can be recognized. A little later others appear: the subclavian duct in the axillary region, the thoracic duct along the dorsal body wall, the cisterna chyli retroperitoneally in the lumbar region, and, ventral to it, the retroperitoneal lymph sac.[2]

The extension of small channels from the primary sacs and trunks takes place by the growth of endothelial sprouts, which are at first solid and then, as they extend, become hollow to form lymphatic vessels.[2]

When the lymphatic vascular channels have been fairly well sketched out, the lymph nodes begin to make their appearance in the system. The earliest, or primary, lymph nodes appear during the third month. Secondary lymph nodes develop later along the course of the peripheral lymphatics. The first stage of development is marked by a lymphatic plexus that lies in association with strands of mesenchymal tissue. These areas are colonized by lymphoblasts, and then lymphocytes are formed in large numbers in the loose meshes of the young connective tissue. Such aggregates of lymphocytes inserted on the course of a lymphatic channel break it up into a meshwork of tortuous, smaller channels (Fig. 5–12). Beyond the developing node, these small channels reconverge as the efferent vessels. At the same time, small blood vessels follow along in the connective tissue framework in which the lymphocytes are proliferated.

Gradually, as the node takes shape, cords of dense lymphoid tissue develop along the vascular strands of connective tissue, producing the characteristic picture ordinarily seen in the medulla of a lymph node.[2]

The true cortex appears much later, and definitive cortical nodules with germinal centers become visible, for practical purposes, only after birth.[1]

ANATOMY

The lymph nodes are small, oval or bean-shaped bodies (in the perinatal period they range from less than 0.1 to about 3 mm. in greatest diameter) situated in the course of lymph vessels so that the lymph passes through them on its way to the blood. Generally, each presents with a slight depression on one side known as the hilus; through the hilus the blood vessels enter and leave. The efferent lymph vessel emerges from the node at this spot, while the afferent vessels enter it at different parts of the periphery.

A lymph node has a cortex and a medulla, with no clear demarcation between the two. The cortex is deficient at the hilus so that there the medulla reaches the surface of the node. Thus, the efferent vessel is derived from the medulla while the afferent vessels empty into the cortex. In the perinatal period, lymph nodes are most prominent and numerous in the mesentery and to a lesser extent in the thoracic mediastinum.

Each lymph node is supported by a framework consisting of the capsule, the fibrous trabeculae which enter into the node from the capsule, and the reticular tissue; the lymphoid cells are enmeshed in that system and supported by it.

The capsule is composed mainly of collagen fibers with a few fibroblasts (Figs. 5–6, 5–8, 5–9, and 5–11). The capsule covers the outside of the node. Trabeculae extending into the node are not seen in the fetus or neonate. Beneath the capsule is the peripheral sinus (Figs. 5–1, 5–4, 5–9, and 5–11).

After birth, lymphoid follicles or cortical nodules may appear as more or less isolated masses of lymphocytes, especially deep to the peripheral sinus. As the follicles develop, the central portions become less deeply staining than the peripheral portions. These central areas are called germinal centers (Fig. 5–9).

HISTOLOGY

The lymph node is basically a mass of lymphoid tissue traversed by specialized lymph vessels or sinuses. Its collagenous framework begins with the capsule, which invests the entire organ (Figs. 5–1, 5–2, 5–6, 5–8, 5–9, and 5–11). In older children and adults, a number of trabeculae extend into the substance of the node from the capsule; but these are not ordinarily seen in the nodes of infants in the perinatal period.

The lymphoid parenchyma of the node is supported by a three-dimensional network of reticular fibers with associated reticular cells. The meshes of that network are filled with lymphocytes; cells are few to rare in the newborn plasma, but macrophages may be seen. The lymph sinuses are irregular channels forming a labyrinth of intercommunicating chambers (Figs. 5–12 and 5–13).

In the newborn it is difficult if not impossible to ascertain any boundary between cortex and medulla (Figs. 5–2, 5–3, 5–6, 5–7, and 5–8).

The afferent lymphatic vessels enter into the peripheral or subcapsular sinus (Fig. 5–12). The peripheral sinus separates the cortical parenchyma from the capsule. It communicates at the hilus with the lumens of efferent lymph vessels. Arising from the marginal sinus are radially directed lymph channels, called intermediate or cortical sinuses, which penetrate the cortical parenchyma (Figs. 5–12 and 5–13). These continue into the medulla as medullary sinuses — large, tortuous, irregular channels that branch and anastomose repeatedly, fragmenting the lymphoid parenchyma into a number of medullary cords. The sinuses of the medulla are confluent with the marginal sinus at the hilus and form there a plexus of tortuous vessels, which penetrate the thickened capsule and continue into the efferent lymphatics.

The framework of the sinuses is a layer of reticular fibers continuous with the parenchymal reticulum. There are also fibers, traversing the sinuses, which are completely clothed in luminal stellate cells.[4] Some of these are probably macrophages while others are endothelial cells.

The cortex is ordinarily said to contain primary nodules or follicles, secondary nodules, and diffuse lymphoid tissue. The primary nodules are located at the periphery (Fig. 5–9). "Secondary nodule" refers to either the germinal center itself or the germinal center with its cap of small lymphocytes (Fig. 5–9). Primary and secondary nodules compose the outer cortex. The deep cortex (or paracortical area) consists of diffuse lymphoid tissue (Fig. 5–9). There is no clear-cut boundary between the two, and the latter continues without demarcation into the medullary cords. The relative proportions of the two are variable in different nodes.

The medullary cords consist of aggregates of lymphoid tissue organized around small blood vessels. The cords branch and anastomose freely with one another, and near the hilus they terminate blindly or form loops continuing into other cords. These medullary cords are not prominent in resting nodes.

The capsule consists of collagenous fibers with a moderate number of fibroblasts (Fig. 5–11). Its outer aspect blends into the fat or loose connective tissue surrounding the node. Its inner aspect is lined by the endothelium of the marginal sinus.[4]

References

1. Arey, L. B.: Developmental Anatomy, rev. 7th ed. Philadelphia, W. B. Saunders Co., 1974, pp. 370–372.
2. Patten B. M.: Human Embryology, 2nd ed. New York, McGraw-Hill Book Co., Inc., 1953, pp. 649-655.
3. Warwick, R., and Williams, P. L.: Gray's Anatomy, 35th British ed. Philadelphia, W. B. Saunders Co., 1973, pp. 716-717.
4. Bloom, W., and Fawcett, D. W.: A Textbook of Histology. Philadelphia, W. B. Saunders Co., 1975, pp. 471-480.

68   LYMPH NODES

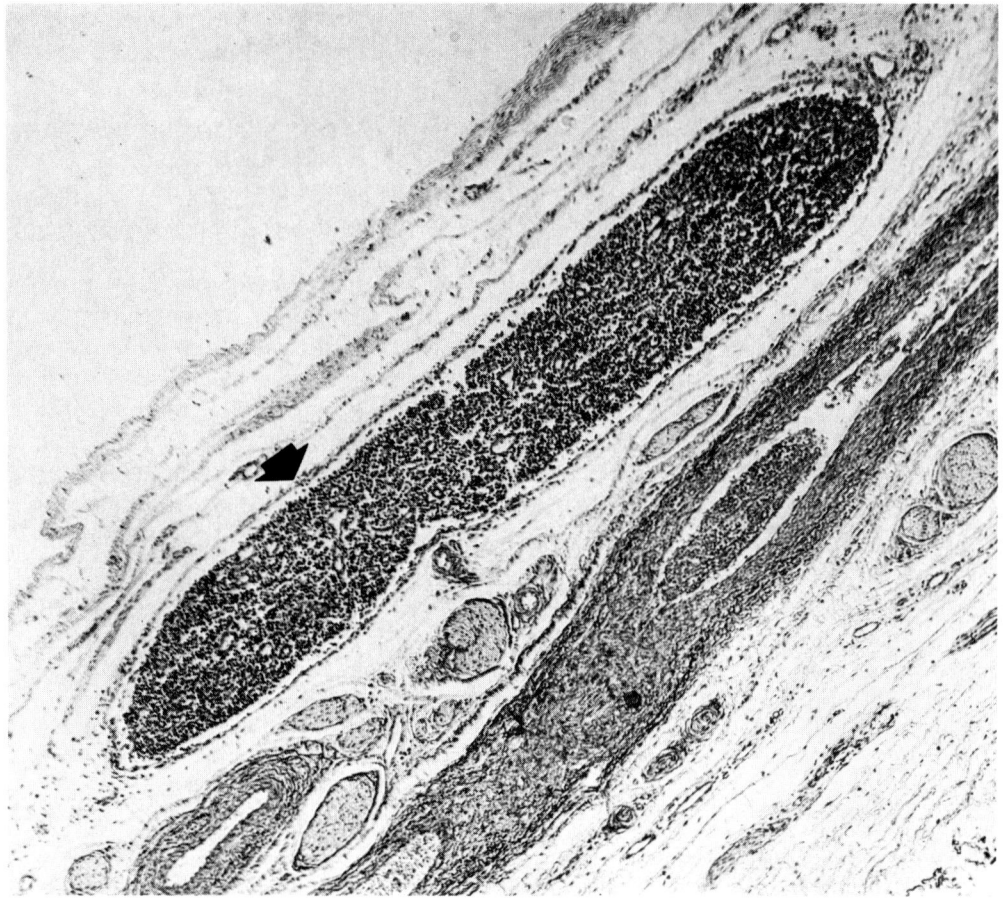

Figure 5–1

Figures 5–1 to 5–5. This set of five photomicrographs depicts—at moderately low magnification—the early phases of the development of lymph nodes both in infants born prematurely and in those born at term.

Figure 5–1. This structure is typical of a very young lymph node. About the perimeter (marked by an arrow) is a delicate collagenous connective tissue capsule. Immediately internal to that is an open peripheral lymph sinus, completely encircling the node. At this stage there are no cortical nodules. The infant was a one day old black female weighing 755 grams (29 weeks gestation).
Hematoxylin and eosin stain. Mag. 55×.

Figures 5–2 and 5–3. These two nodes are slightly more advanced in their development than that depicted in Fig. 5–1. They are larger and more cellular. The capsule is thicker but the peripheral sinus is less clear. No follicles are apparent.
Hematoxylin and eosin stain. Mags. 6× and 12×.

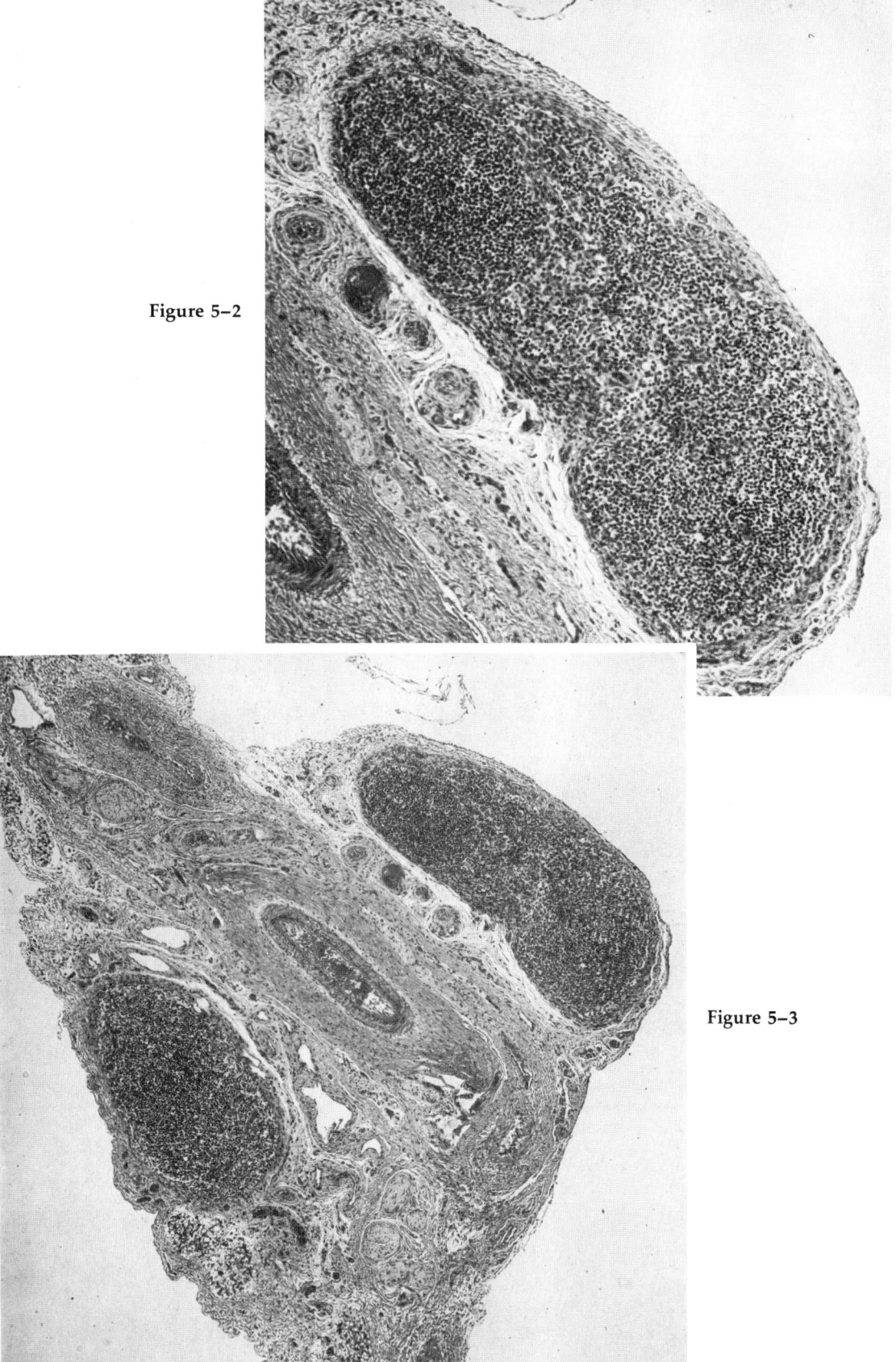

Figure 5–2

Figure 5–3

70 LYMPH NODES

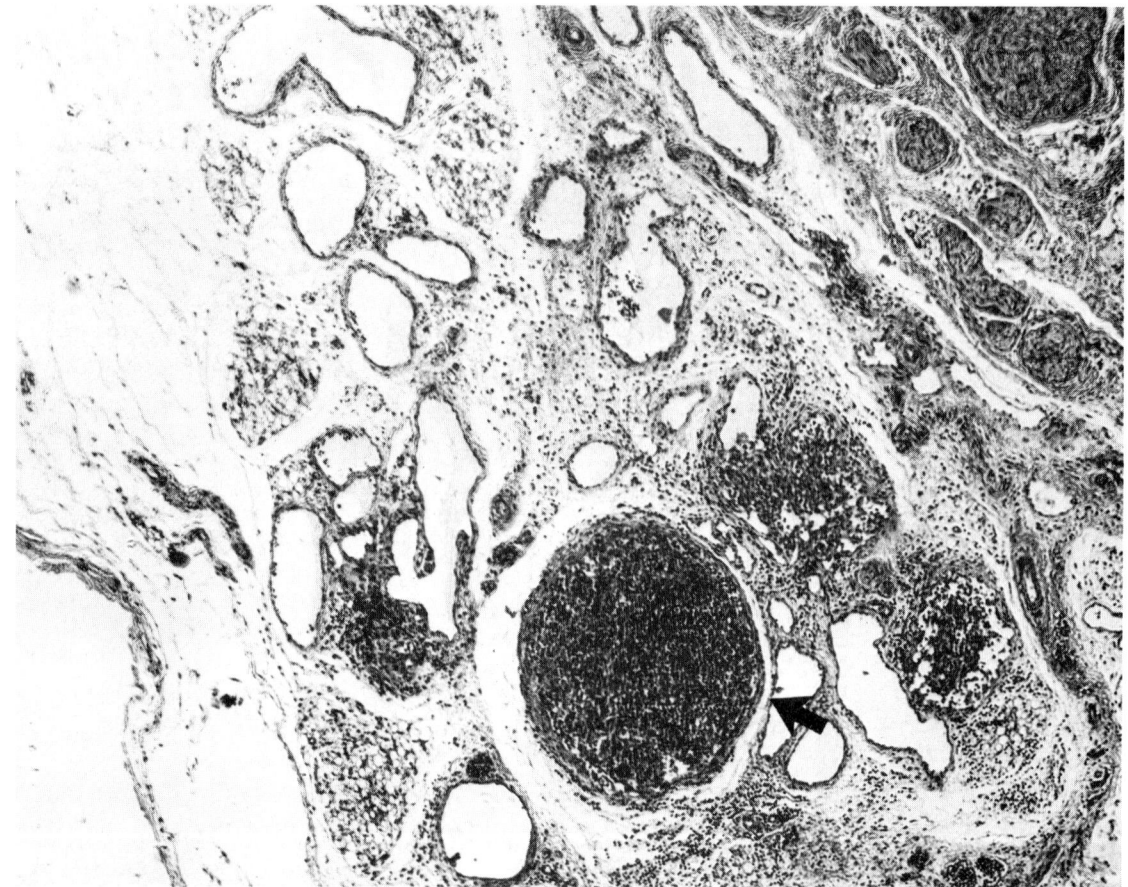

Figure 5–4

Figure 5–4. At moderately low magnification, this photomicrograph depicts the earliest phases in the development of a lymph node. A number of thin-walled dilated vascular channels are distributed in a broad band across the central portion of the picture. Clusters of lymphoid tissue are forming at four sites in their midst. One of them, the largest, has already developed a clear-cut peripheral sinus (marked by arrow).

This infant was born at term. He was a white male who lived for three weeks. His body weight at autopsy was 3,850 grams.

Hematoxylin and eosin stain. Mag. 50×.

LYMPH NODES 71

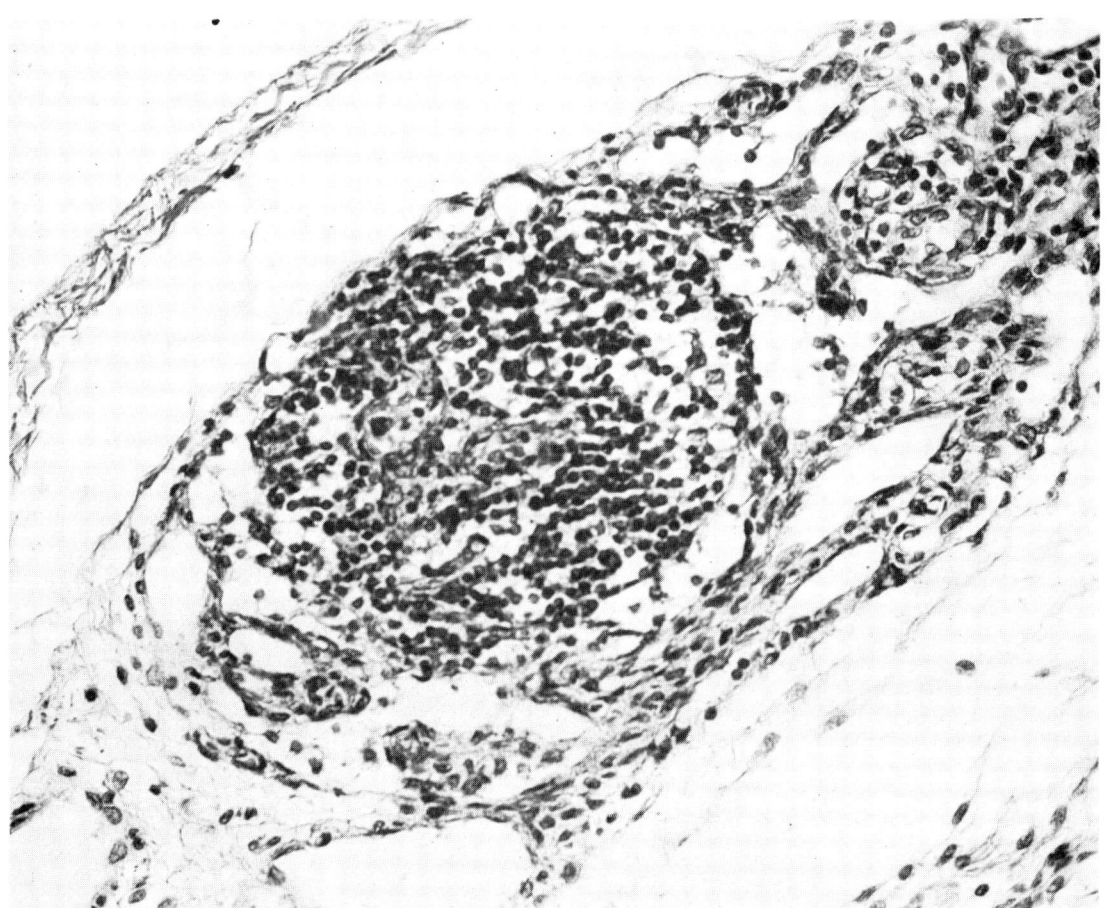

Figure 5-5

Figure 5-5. At much higher magnification than any of the preceding four photographs in this set, this picture illustrates in some detail small lymphocytes which populate the earliest nodes. A delicate capsule is visible at some points about the perimeter of the node, as are some tiny lymph channels just deep to it. Three small blood vessels, probably capillaries, appear in the center of the node.

The patient was a six hour old black female, born at 32 weeks of gestation. Body weight at postmortem examination was 1,680 grams.

Hematoxylin and eosin stain. Mag. 290×.

72 LYMPH NODES

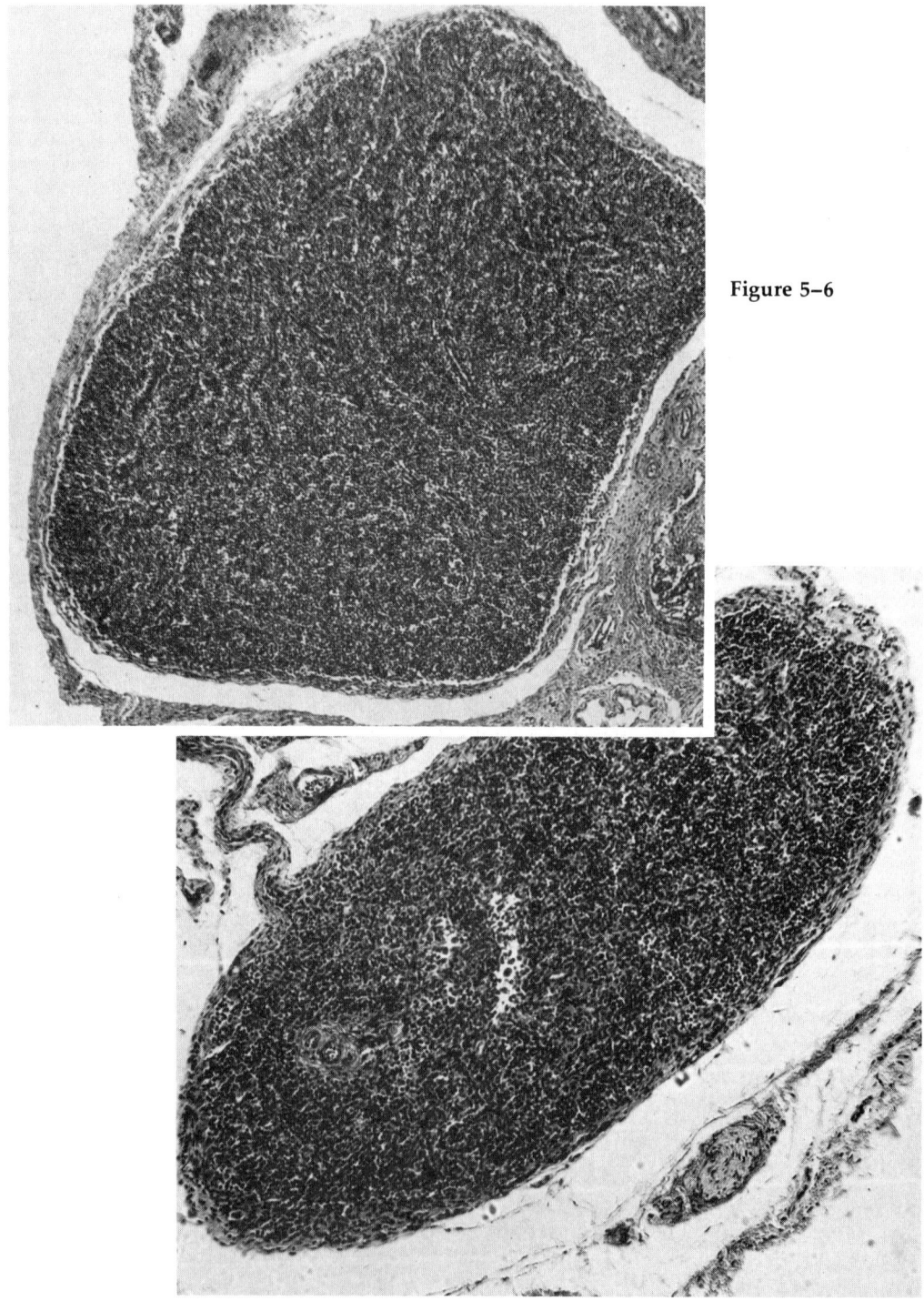

Figure 5-6

Figure 5-7

Figures 5–6 to 5–8. This set of three pictures illustrates somewhat larger, better developed lymph nodes in infants of different gestational ages. In Figs. 5–6 and 5–7 there are no visible follicles, whereas in Fig. 5–8 there is the slightest suggestion of the formation of two follicles on the extreme right end.

LYMPH NODES 73

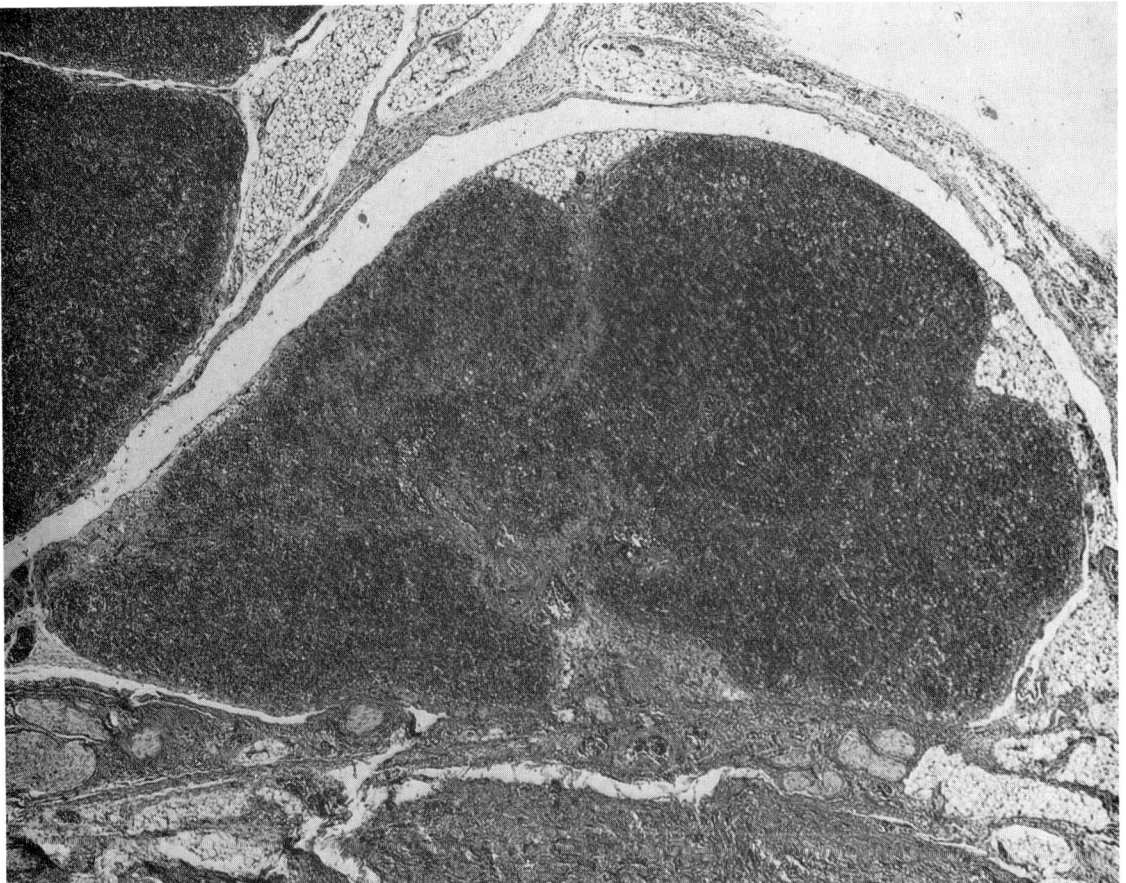

Figure 5–8

Figure 5–6. This is a photograph of a mesenteric lymph node from an 800 gram infant born at the 23rd week of gestation, a black female who lived for 19 minutes.
Hematoxylin and eosin stain. Mag. 55×.

Figure 5–7. This is an entire node from an infant of unknown gestational age who survived for seven days. It was a black male who, at autopsy, weighed 1,100 grams.
Hematoxylin and eosin stain. Mag. 116×.

Figure 5–8. This also is a mesenteric lymph node. The infant was born at term. He was a black male who lived for 27 hours and whose weight at autopsy was 4,225 grams.
Hematoxylin and eosin stain. Mag. 45×.

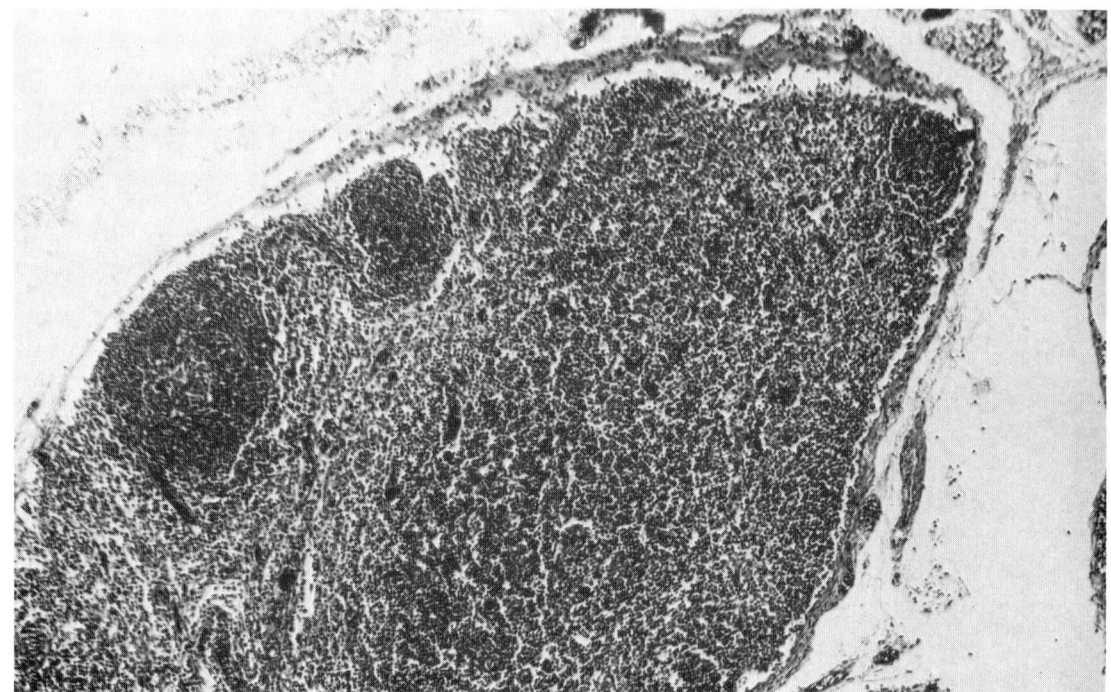

Figure 5–9

Figures 5–9 to 5–11. This group of three illustrations depicts the development of cortical nodules, virtually all of which appear after birth.

Figure 5–9. This is a section of a mesenteric lymph node from a white female infant born at 39 weeks of gestation. She lived for three weeks. Her body weight at autopsy was 2,700 grams.

Several cortical nodules of various sizes can be seen. They are just deep to the peripheral sinus. The largest has a pale staining center, the first evidence of a germinal center.

Hematoxylin and eosin stain. Mag. 60×.

Figure 5–10. At a slightly lower magnification, this is a mesenteric node from a six day old white female. Weight at postmortem examination was 3,090 grams. Many follicles are present, and some of them have germinal centers.

Hematoxylin and eosin stain. Mag. 55×.

Figure 5–11. At very high magnification, a single cortical nodule is shown here. The capsule of the node is apparent at the top and, just below that, the peripheral sinus. The nodule itself is not clearly defined but appears as an oval cluster of uniformly small, darkly stained cells, its long axis oriented in the long axis of the photograph.

Hematoxylin and eosin stain. Mag. 279×.

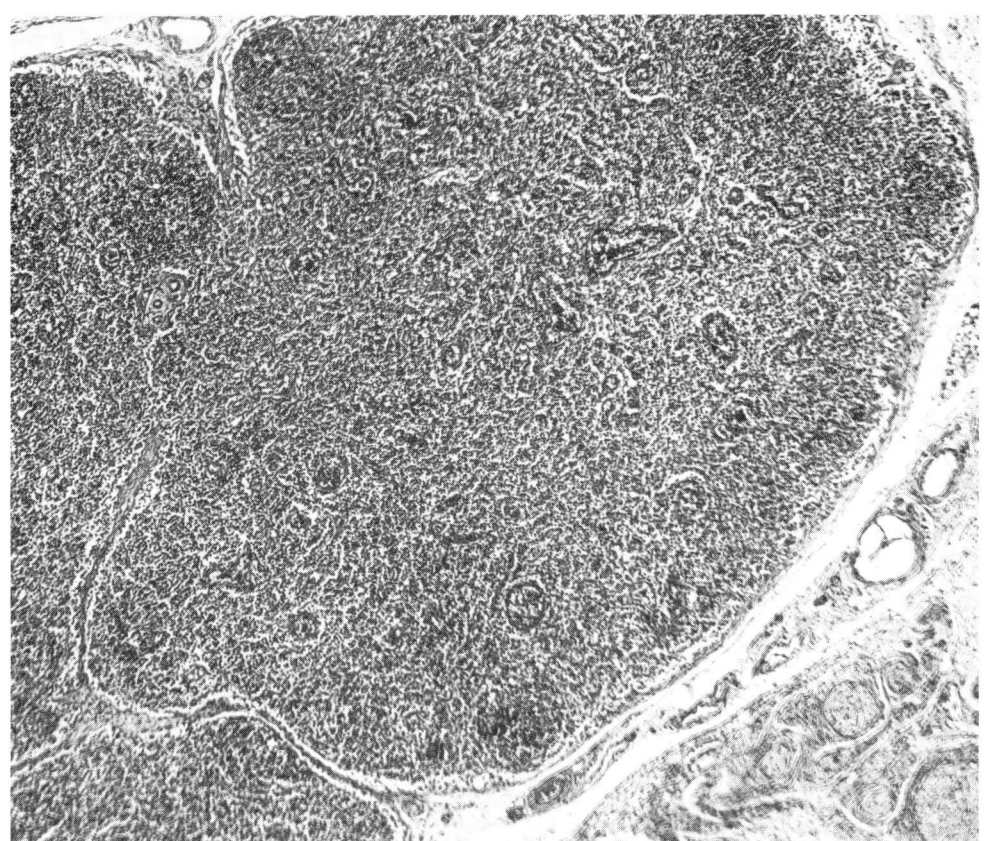

Figure 5–10

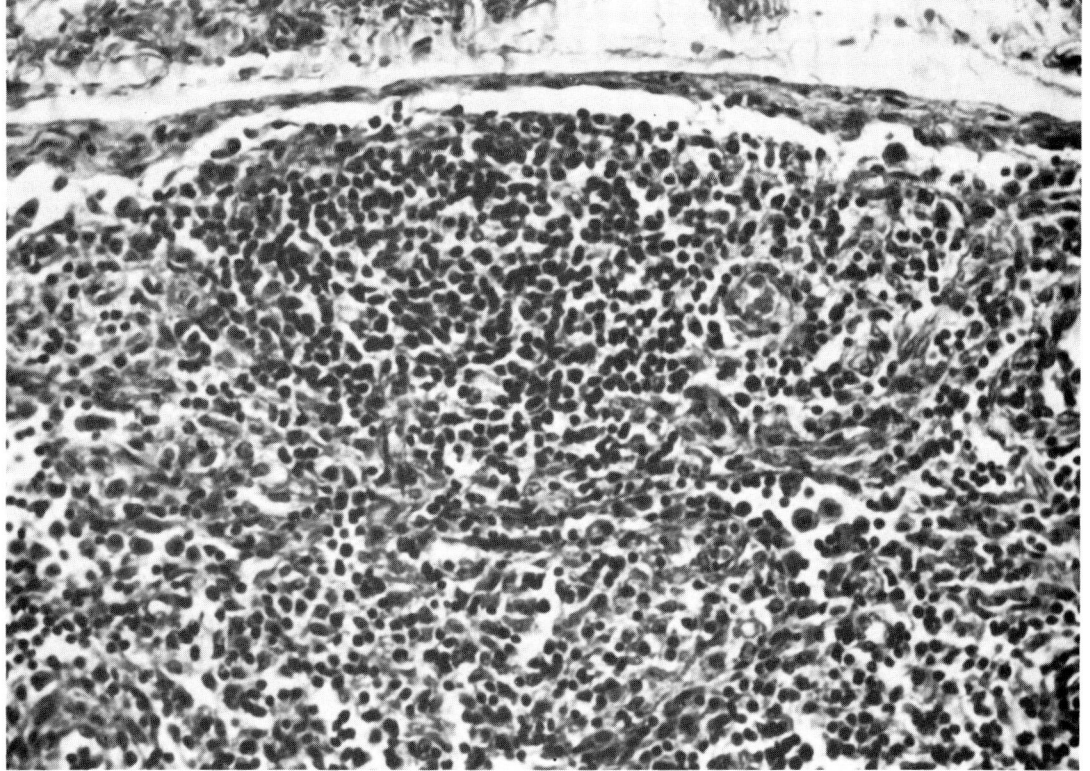

Figure 5–11

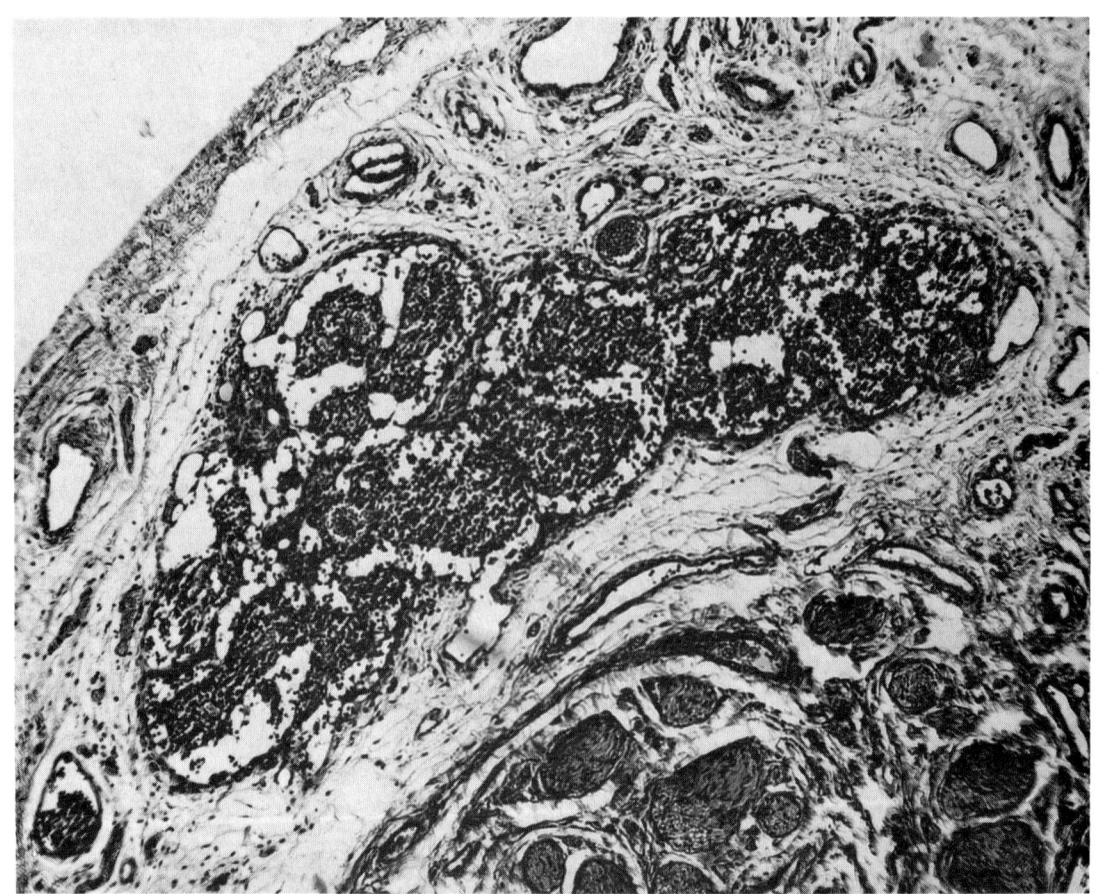

Figure 5–12

Figure 5–12. This developing lymph node, taken from the mesentery, illustrates rather dramatically the configuration of small lymphatic channels coursing throughout the body of the node. A number of them clearly communicate with the peripheral sinus. One thin-walled channel, possibly at the hilus, is either entering or leaving the node.

This patient was a 13 hour old black male of unknown gestational age who, at postmortem examination, weighed 1,310 grams.

Hematoxylin and eosin stain. Mag. 124×.

LYMPH NODES 77

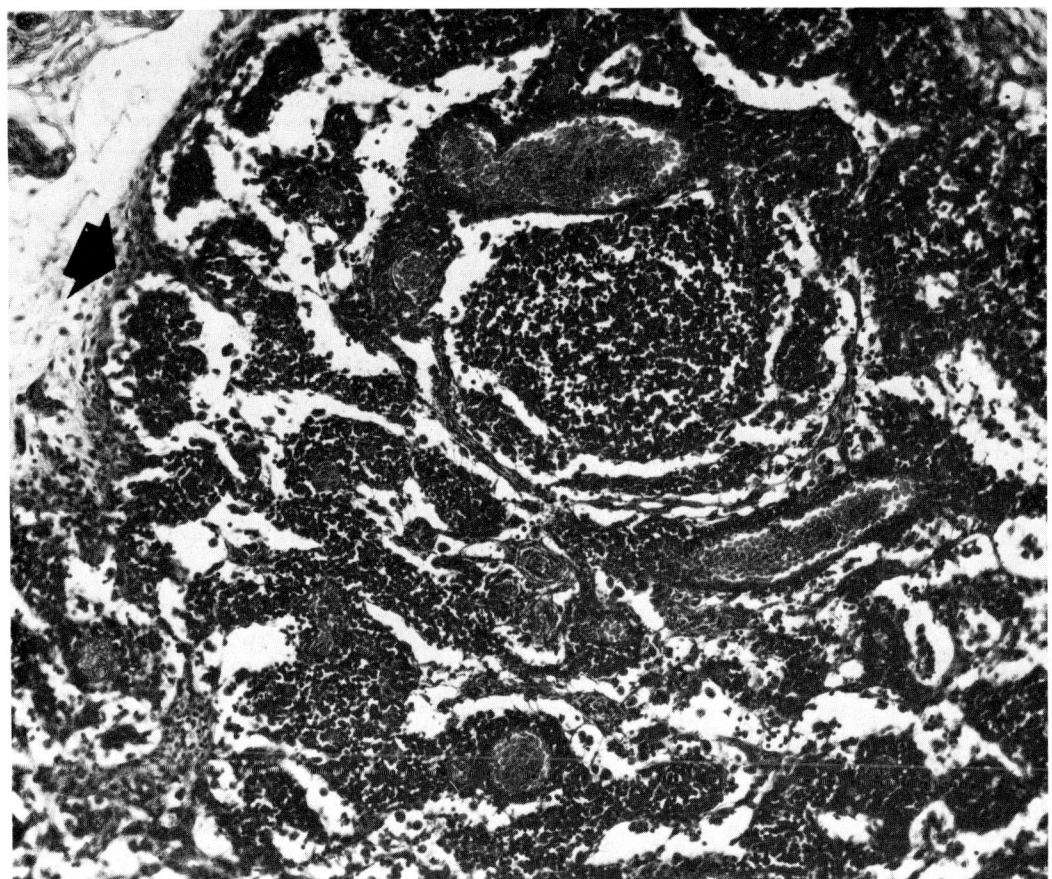

Figure 5–13

Figure 5–13. Within a mass of lymphoid tissue arranged about open channels, a single cortical nodule with germinal center is apparent, with a blood vessel on either side. Particularly in the vicinity of the arrow one can see the flat endothelial cells lining the slender lymphatic channels.

This patient was a four day old white male. We do not know the length of his gestation. At autopsy he weighed 1,175 grams.

Hematoxylin and eosin stain. Mag. 142×.

Part 3

SPLEEN

Chapter 6

SPLEEN

EMBRYOLOGY

The spleen makes its first appearance as a mass of undifferentiated mesenchymal cells within the dorsal mesogastrium during the sixth week of gestation. These cells multiply by mitosis; as the mass enlarges, it bulges out to the left side and dorsally toward the body wall, to the left side of the stomach and a little dorsal to it.

The mesothelium covering the cell mass continues to proliferate and add to the splenic blastema until the seventh week,[1] when the mesothelial cells become cuboidal and separated from the splenic tissue by a membrane that later becomes the splenic capsule.

The elements of the primary mesenchymal primordium differentiate in two directions. Some remain connected with one another by means of processes, and form the reticular framework of both the red and white pulp. Others become isolated as free cells within the meshes of that framework.[2] At first they all have the character of basophilic wandering elements.[3] Later they give rise to red cells, leukocytes, and megakaryocytes. However, very little myeloid and lymphoid hematopoiesis occurs in the spleen during fetal life. Lymphoid nodules begin to appear at about 24 weeks of gestation.

ANATOMY

The spleen in the perinatal period is fundamentally of the same shape as it is in the adult. Its position is the same and so is its size relative to the liver. Ordinarily its caudal tip is located at the costal margin; in immature infants it is sometimes cranial to that point.

The color is deep purple and the consistency quite firm, at least equivalent to that of the liver. What is at times surprising is the intimate adherence of the spleen at its hilus to the tip of the tail of the pancreas; occasionally sharp dissection is required to separate the two. Not uncommonly, a little spherical nodule of accessory splenic tissue may be embedded in the tail of the pancreas. Such nodules range from 1 to 2 mm. in diameter. Very often, independent accessory nodules of the splenic tissue can be found in the vicinity of the hilus, of about that same size. Although I have never conducted a systematic search for them, I estimate that they can be found, if one really looks, in 90 per cent of autopsies on infants in the perinatal period. They are characteristically maroon to purple and invariably spherical.

The fresh cut surface of the spleen in the infant is maroon; in most instances follicles are difficult or impossible to identify with the naked eye, especially in the prematurely born. When they do appear in infants at term, they are uniformly distributed, light grey, ill-delineated and slightly protuberant. Each is a little less than one millimeter in diameter.

HISTOLOGY

At the histologic level the spleen is composed, basically, of two kinds of tissue, the red pulp and the white pulp. The former derives its name from its appearance on naked eye examination of a fresh cut surface; the red pulp predominates and seems to form the background upon which the white pulp is set.

The red pulp consists of innumerable irregularly shaped sinusoids and the slender bands of tissue supporting them, the splenic cords of Billroth. The red color observed in a gross fresh cut surface is due to the presence of red cells within these myriads of sinusoids.

The white pulp is composed of lymphoid tissue arranged in many small compact masses and branching cords scattered evenly throughout the organ.

The spleen has a collagenous capsule, with inward extensions known as trabeculae that penetrate the parenchyma.

The Red Pulp

The red pulp comprises a vast network of branching and anastomosing, tortuous sinuses, separated from one another by delicate cellular partitions, the splenic cords (Figs. 6–11, 6–12, and 6–13). The splenic cords are supported by a framework of reticular fibers.[3] The collagenous fibers of the trabeculae continue directly into the reticular fibers of the red pulp, which, in turn, merge with material supporting the sinus endothelium.[3] The meshes of the reticulum in the pulp cords contain many free cells, including macrophages and circulating elements of the blood.

The White Pulp

The white pulp, which first appears in the form of nodules or sheaths at about the twenty-fourth week of gestation (Figs. 6–14 to 6–21), is arranged about the arteries where they leave the trabeculae to penetrate the parenchyma. The periarterial lymphoid sheaths follow peripherally along the vessels almost to the point where they break up into capillaries.[3] In infants, after birth, germinal centers begin to appear at intervals along the course of the lymphoid sheath (Figs. 6–14 to 6–19). The lymphoid sheath and the germinal center are morphologically different; the former consists predominantly of small and medium sized lymphocytes (Figs. 6–20 and 6–22), while the latter comprises larger cells with more abundant pale-staining cytoplasm (Figs. 6–17 to 6–19).

The white pulp is supported by a loose network of reticular fibers with associated reticular cells, which, at the periphery of the sheath, become circumferentially arranged to form concentric layers.[3]

The Capsule and Trabeculae

The capsule and trabeculae of the spleen consist of dense connective tissue with some smooth muscle elements and elastic networks.[4] The external layer is covered by a single layer of mesothelial cells (Fig. 6–10b).

The trabeculae (Fig. 6–10c) are projections of this same connective tissue from the capsule into the parenchyma. They tend to be cylindrical and they carry the arteries, veins, and lymphatics. They contain many elastic fibers and little smooth muscle.[3]

Arteries

Branches of the splenic artery enter at the hilus (Fig. 6–7) and pass along the trabeculae, in which they branch repeatedly, becoming ever smaller in diameter. These muscular arteries leave the trabeculae when their dichotomous branching has reduced their diameter to a very small size. At that point the adventitia is replaced by a sheath of lymphoid tissue[3] (Fig. 6–21) and the vessel is referred to as a central artery or arteriole. When germinal centers appear, the central arteriole is definitely displaced to the opposite side of the lymphoid aggregate (Figs. 6–17 and 6–18); they are almost never truly centrally located (Fig. 6–22). The central artery is of the muscular type, with prominent endothelial cells and one or two layers of smooth muscle in the media in older infants and children (Fig. 6–23).

These central arterioles give rise to capillaries that supply the lymphoid tissue of the sheath. They, in turn, pass into the marginal zone around the lymphoid aggregate, and the manner in which they end is uncertain.[3]

Venous Sinuses and Veins

As previously mentioned, the venous sinuses permeate the entire red pulp. They are particularly numerous around lymphoid aggregates.[3] They have wide, irregular lumens, depending upon the amount of blood in the organ[3] (Figs. 6–11 to 6–13). They are lined by endothelial cells, sometimes called *stave cells*,[5] oriented parallel to the longitudinal axis of the sinus.

Outside the endothelium, the wall of the sinus is supported by a system of circumferential ribs like hoops around the staves of a barrel[3]; these are continuous with the reticular fibers of the splenic cords.

The venous sinuses empty into the veins of the pulp; these coalesce to form the veins of the trabeculae, which, in turn, are drained by the veins at the hilus (Fig. 6–7), tributaries of the splenic vein.

References

1. Willis, R. A.: The Borderland of Embryology and Pathology. London, Butterworth and Co., Ltd., 1958, pp. 73–74.
2. Maximow, A. A., and Bloom, W.: A Textbook of Histology, 7th ed. Philadelphia, W. B. Saunders Co., 1957, pp. 263–275.
3. Bloom, W., and Fawcett, D. W.: A Textbook of Histology. Philadelphia, W. B. Saunders Co., 1975, pp. 487–502.
4. Bergman, R. A., and Afifi, A. K.: Atlas of Microscopic Anatomy. A Companion to Histology and Neuroanatomy. Philadelphia, W. B. Saunders Co., 1974, pp. 202–205.
5. Warwick, R., and Williams, P. L.: Gray's Anatomy, 35th British ed. Philadelphia, W. B. Saunders Co., 1973, pp. 718–723.

84 SPLEEN

Figures 6–1 to 6–6. This series of six photographs illustrates quite clearly the evolution of the adult pattern of splenic histology. In Fig. 6–1 there are no malpighian corpuscles. They are seen faintly in Fig. 6–2 but become gradually more sharply defined in Figs. 6–3 and 6–4, and are of nearly adult proportions in Fig. 6–6.

Hematoxylin and eosin stain. Mag. 55×.

Fig.	Wt.	Race	Sex	Gestation	Age
6–1	320 gm.	?	?	16 wk.	Stillborn
6–2	900 gm.	B	M	24 wk.	54 hr.
6–3	1,300 gm.	?	M	31 wk.	19 hr.
6–4	2,000 gm.	?	F	31 wk. (est.)	13 days
6–5	3,090 gm.	W	F	37 wk.(est.)	6 days
6–6	4,225 gm.	B	M	40 wk. (est.)	27 hr.

See illustrations on the following pages

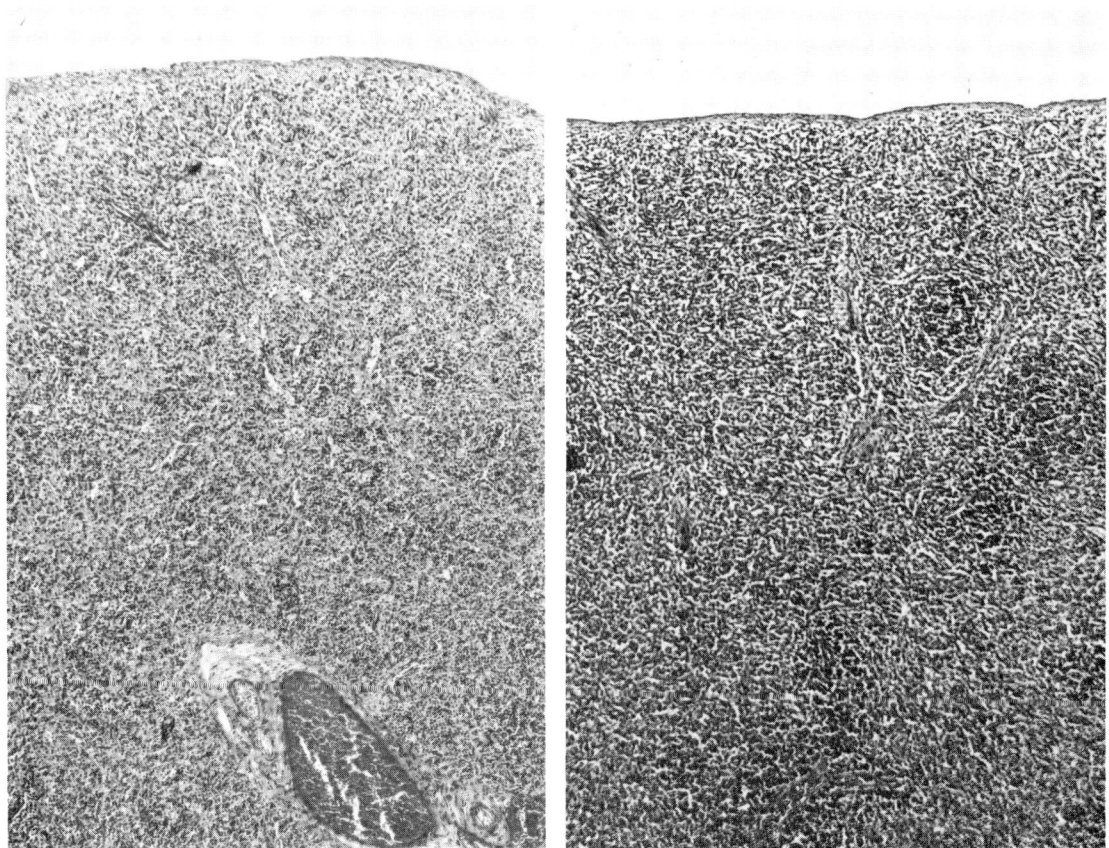

Figure 6–1

Figure 6–2

See legend on the opposite page

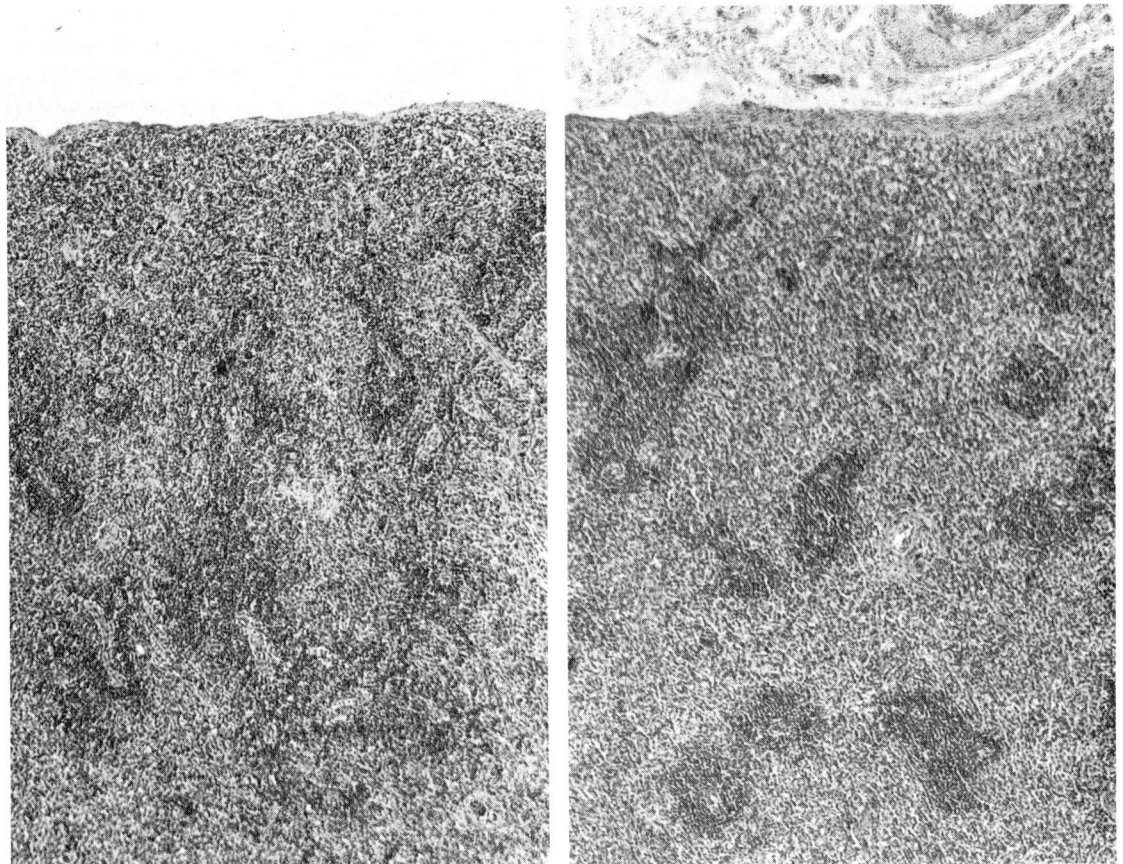

Figure 6–3

Figure 6–4

SPLEEN 87

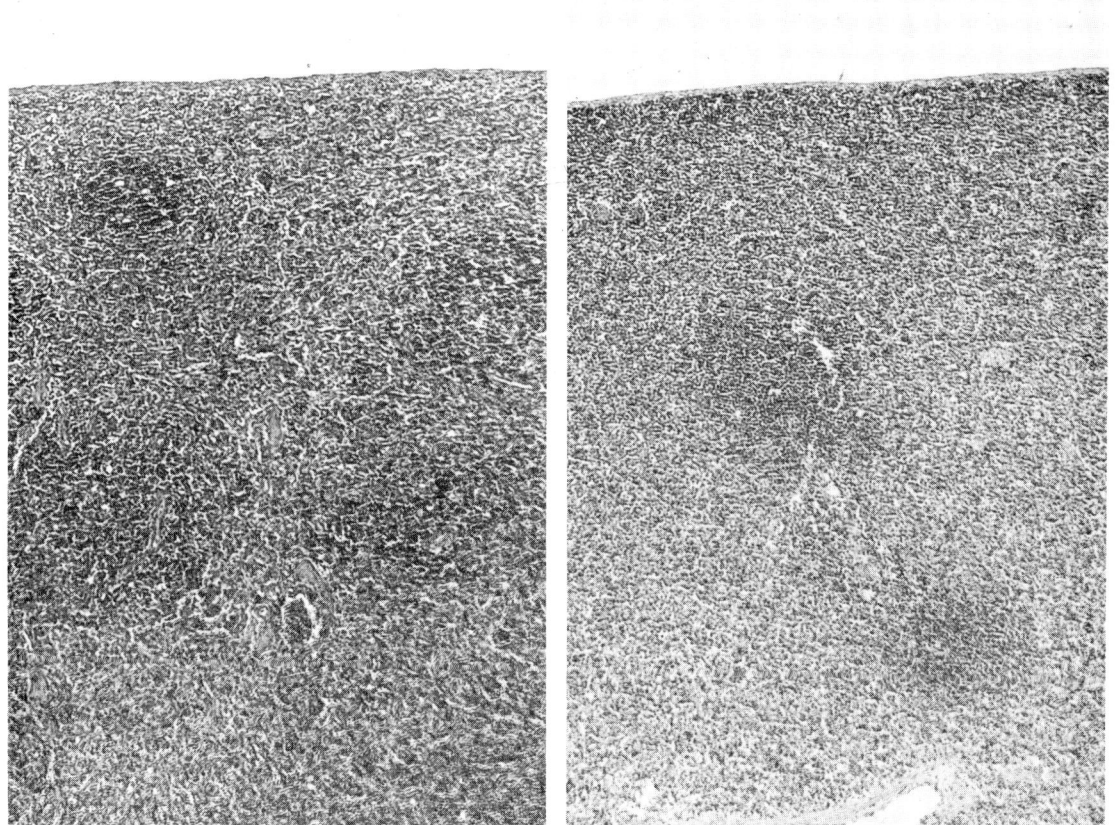

Figure 6–5

Figure 6–6

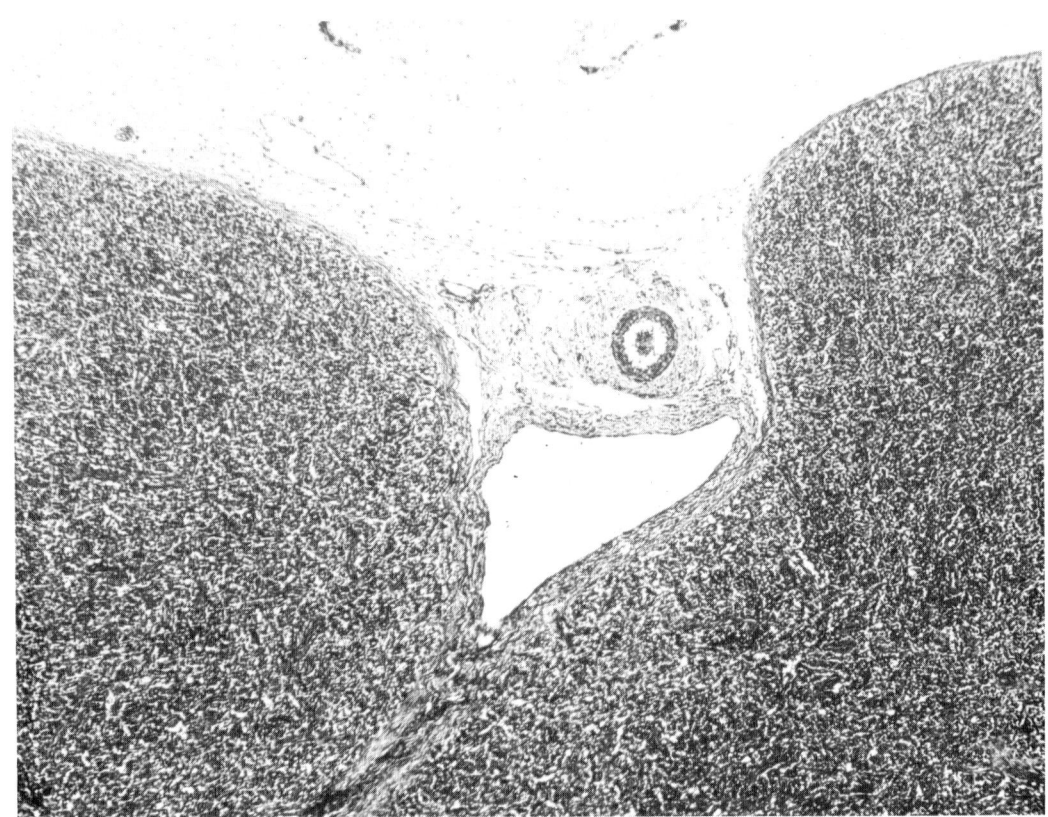

Figure 6–7

Figure 6–7. This section passes through the hilus of the spleen, in which an artery and a large vein are seen.

This was from a black male baby who weighed 760 grams at necropsy. He had been born after a 26 week gestation and survived 12 hours and 7 minutes.

Hematoxylin and eosin stain. Mag. 55×.

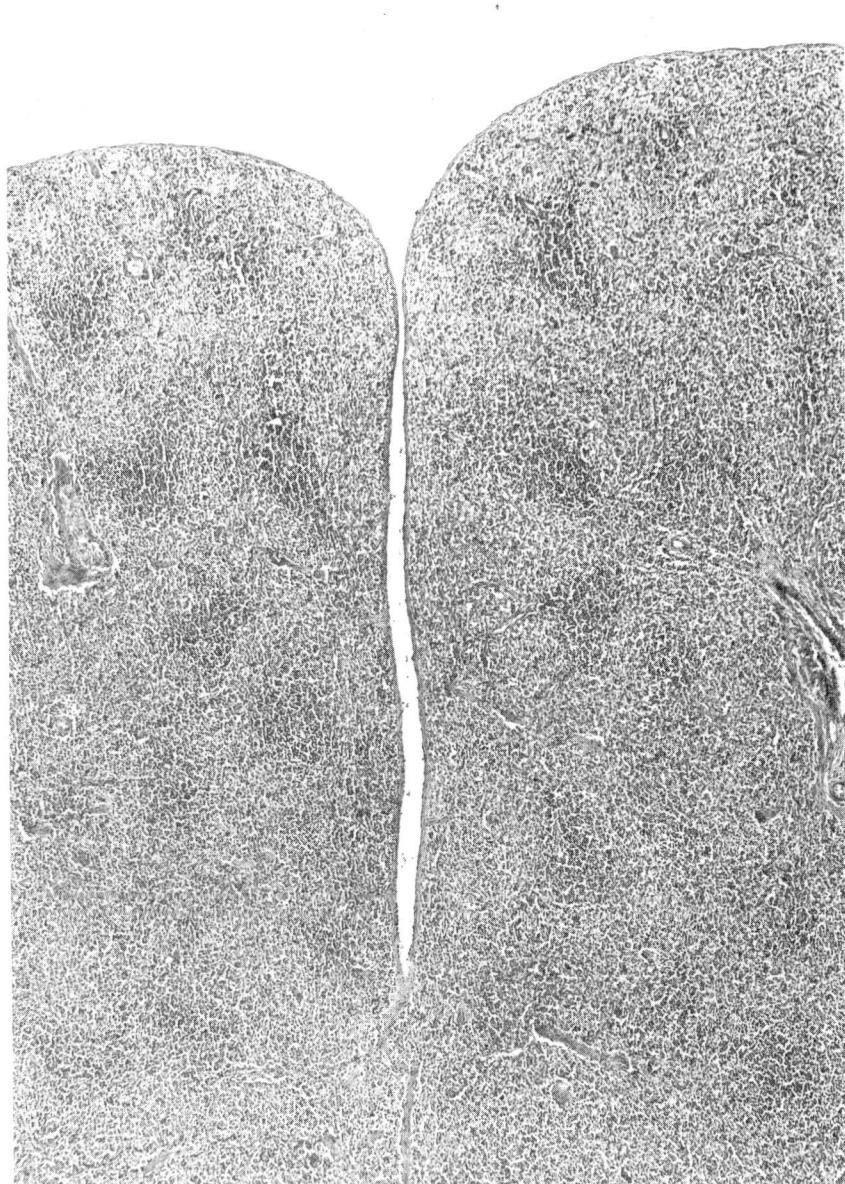

Figure 6–8

Figure 6–8. In contrast to the hilus, through which the nutrient vessels pass, this is one of the natural clefts or notches which so commonly appear on the superior border of the spleen, even in infants.

The patient was a 29 hour old black female carried to term, whose body weight at postmortem examination was 2,930 grams.

Hematoxylin and eosin stain. Mag. 45×.

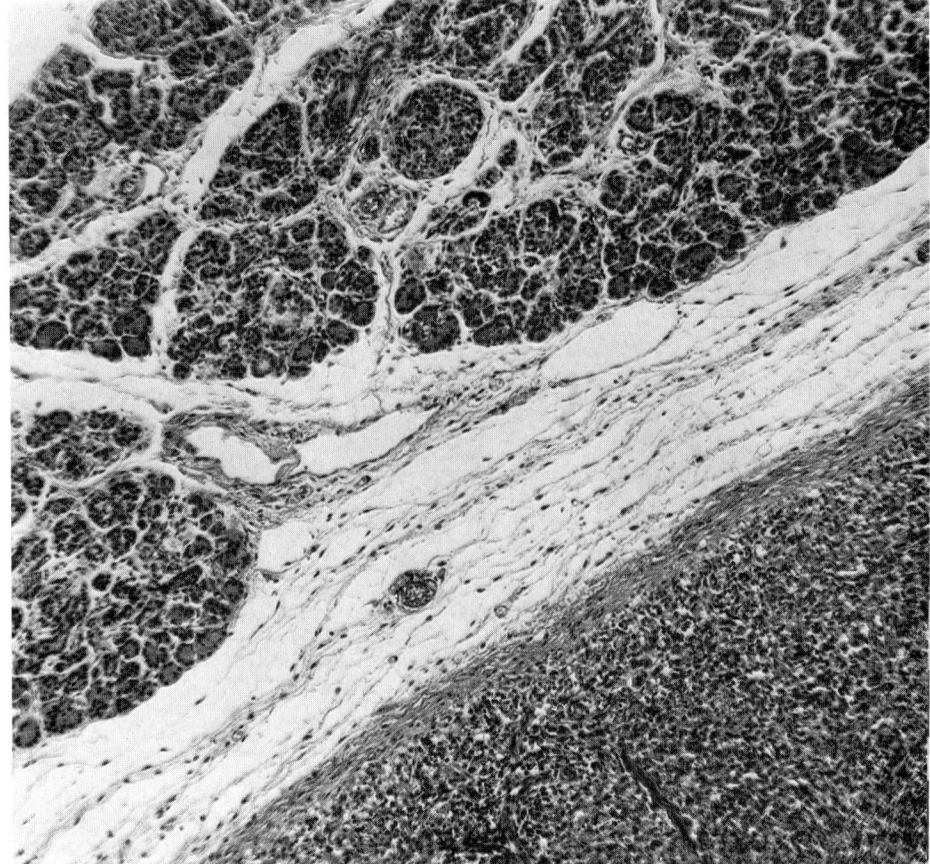

Figure 6–9

Figure 6–9. The so-called pancreatic impression of the spleen is often intimately united to the tail of the pancreas in infants. At times, splenic tissue is actually embedded in the tail of the pancreas, either as an extension of the organ or as a spherical encapsulated accessory nodule. Not uncommonly, one encounters considerable difficulty in dissecting the two organs away from each other at this site.

This photograph illustrates the close approximation of the two; in this instance they are separated by a band of connective tissue.

The subject was a 6 hour old black female, the product of a 32 week gestation, who weighed 1,680 grams at autopsy.

Hematoxylin and eosin stain. Mag. 124×.

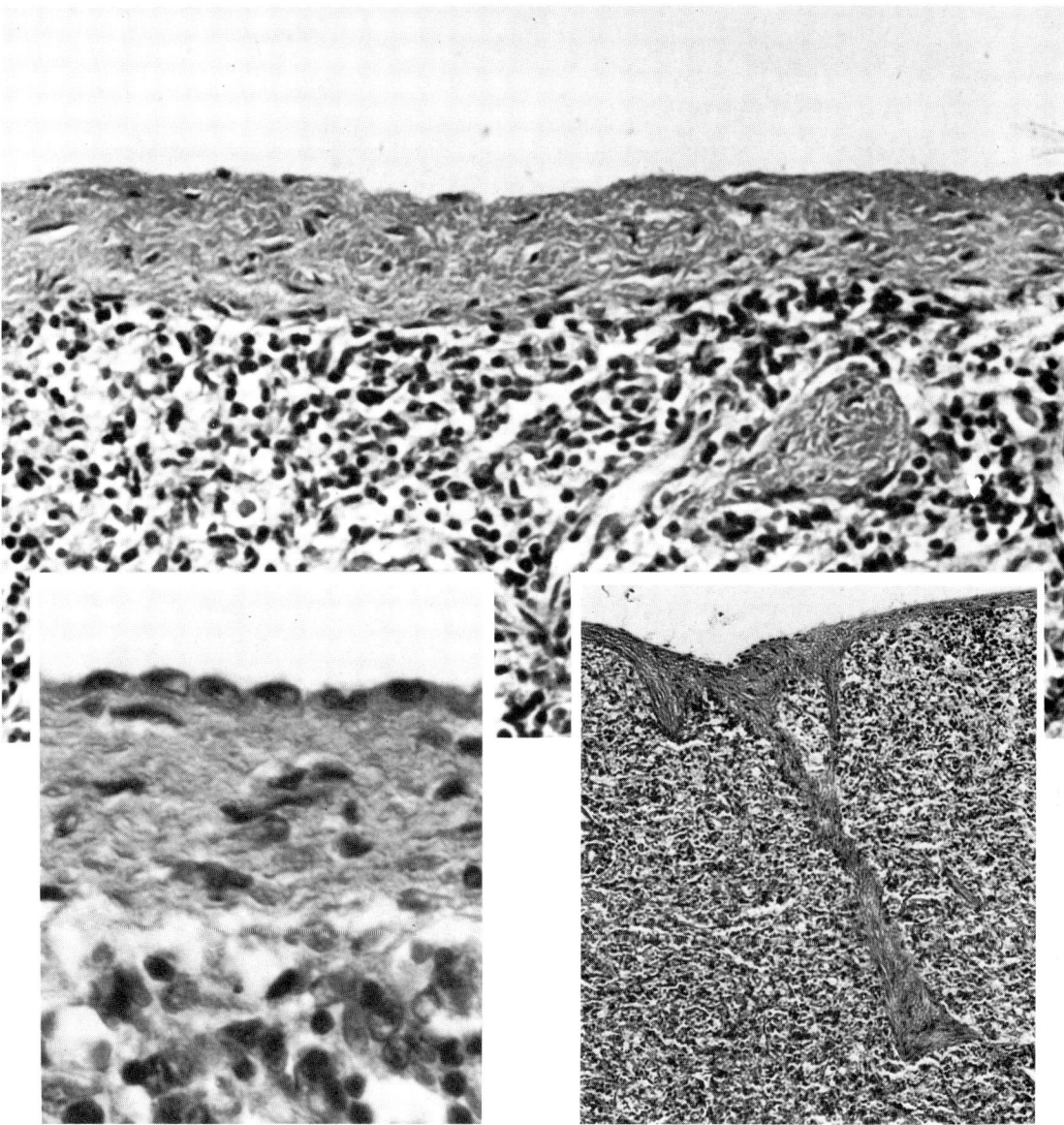

Figure 6–10a

Figure 6–10b

Figure 6–10c

Figure 6–10. The capsule, or fibroelastic coat, investing the spleen is depicted here. It consists of collagenous white fibrous tissue and yellow elastic fibers. It appears here as a band stretched over the spleen. The capsule is, in turn, covered by a delicate serous coat. The mesothelial cells of the serous coat are not well preserved in Fig. 6–10a but are prominent in the inset, Fig. 6–10b.

A single trabecula penetrates the organ from the capsule in Fig. 6–10c.

Hematoxylin and eosin stain.

Fig.	Wt.	Race	Sex	Gestation	Age	Mag.
6–10a	2,960 gm.	B	M	40 wk.	1 hr. 25 min.	382×
6–10b	2,410 gm.	?	?	40 wk.	5 wk.	660×
6–10c	2,180 gm.	B	M	42 wk.	10½ hr.	108×

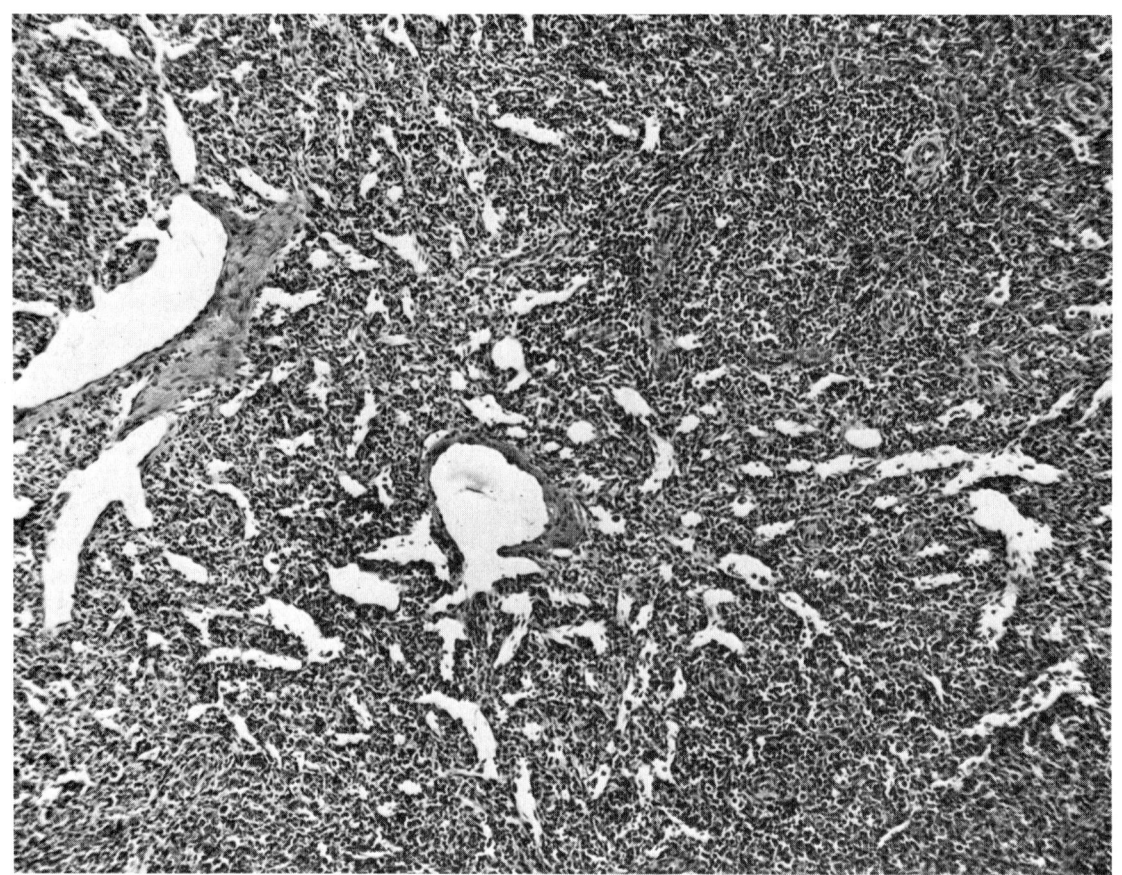

Figure 6–11

Figures 6–11 to 6–13. This set of three photomicrographs, taken at progressively increasing magnification, depicts the red pulp of the spleen. As is apparent here, the contained sinusoids are large and numerous. They are lined by flattened endothelial cells and are supported on their outer surfaces by strands of circularly arranged reticulum.

Hematoxylin and eosin stain.

Fig.	Wt.	Race	Sex	Gestation	Age	Mag.
6–11	2,560 gm.	B	M	40 wk.	11 hr.	124×
6–12	2,560 gm.	B	M	40 wk.	11 hr.	267×
6–13	3,240 gm.	?	F	40 wk.	46 hr.	660×

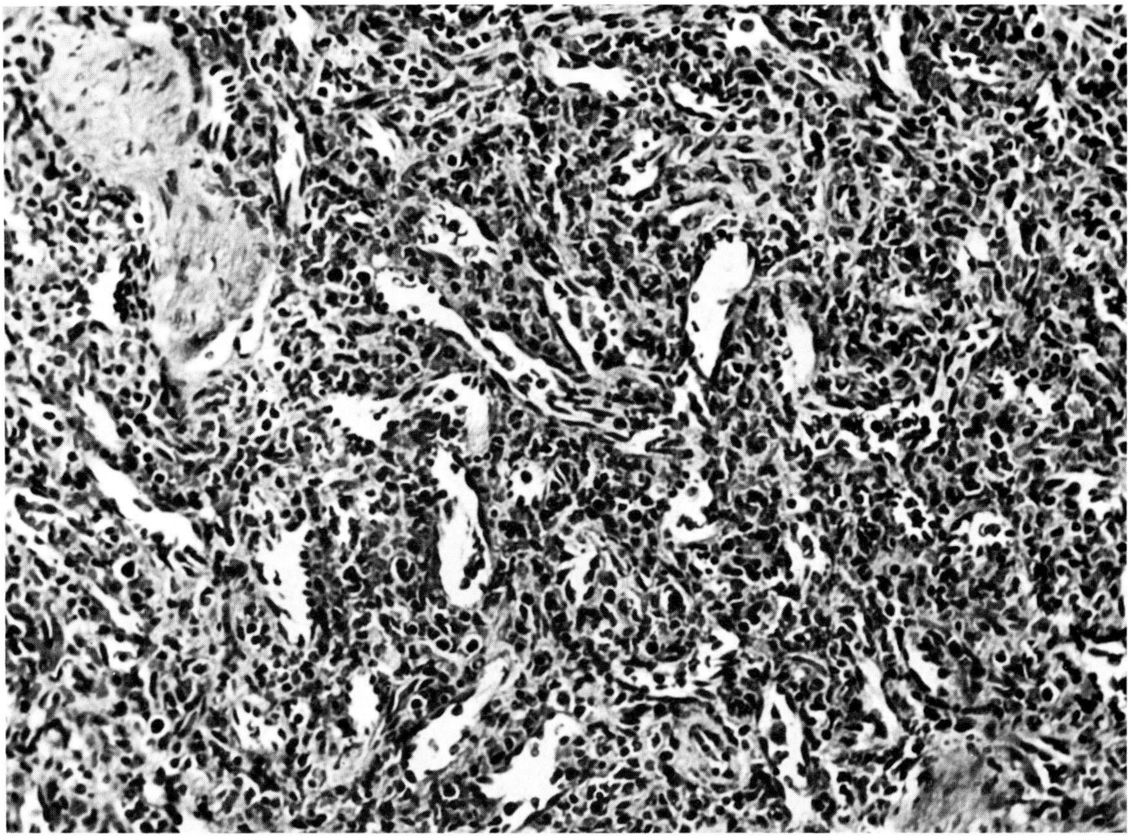

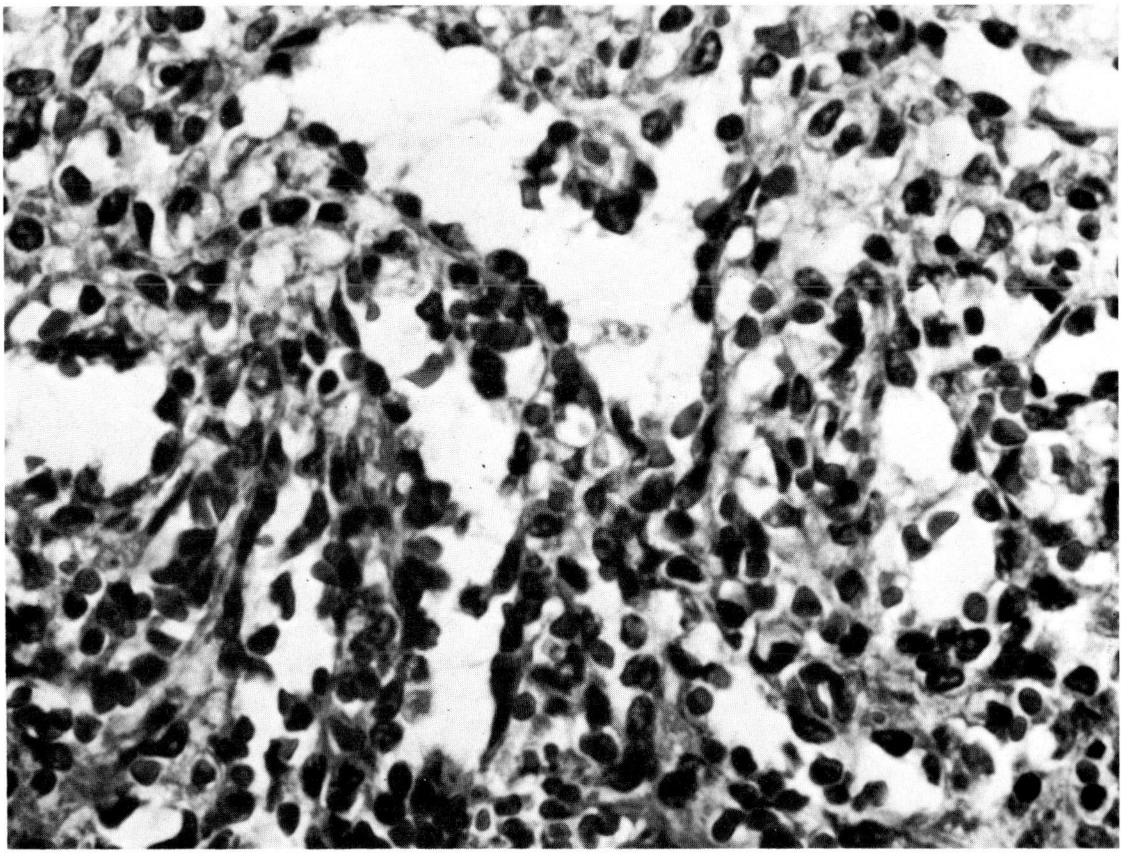

Figures 6–12 and 6–13

94 SPLEEN

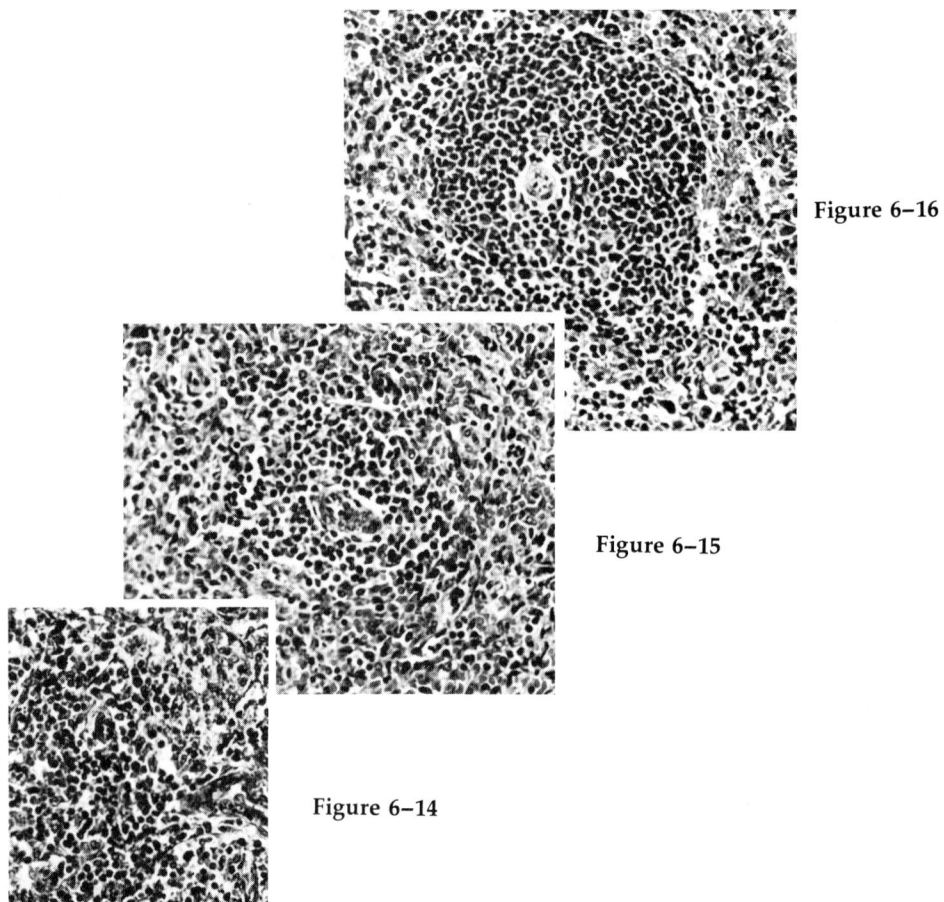

Figure 6–16

Figure 6–15

Figure 6–14

Figures 6–14 to 6–19. This arc of photographs illustrates the evolution of the perivascular lymphatic aggregates from their first appearance to their full-blown state. In the infant of less than 20 weeks gestation, as seen in Fig. 6–1, the aggregates are really not discernible. By 20 weeks (Fig. 6–14) they are just barely distinguishable; germinal centers make their appearance at about 32 weeks.

There is a trend toward progressive increase in size (overall diameter) throughout the latter half of gestation and infancy.

Hematoxylin and eosin stain.

Fig.	Wt.	Race	Sex	Gestation	Age	Mag.
6–14	460 gm.	B	F	?	1 hr. 15 min.	175×
6–15	865 gm.	?	F	20 wk.	10 min.	197×
6–16	1,685 gm.	?	F	30 wk.	34 hr.	197×
6–17	2,836 gm.	?	?	32 wk.	4 mo.	175×
6–18	?	?	?	38 wk.	2 yr. 9 mo.	197×
6–19	?	?	?	40 wk.	3 yr.	175×

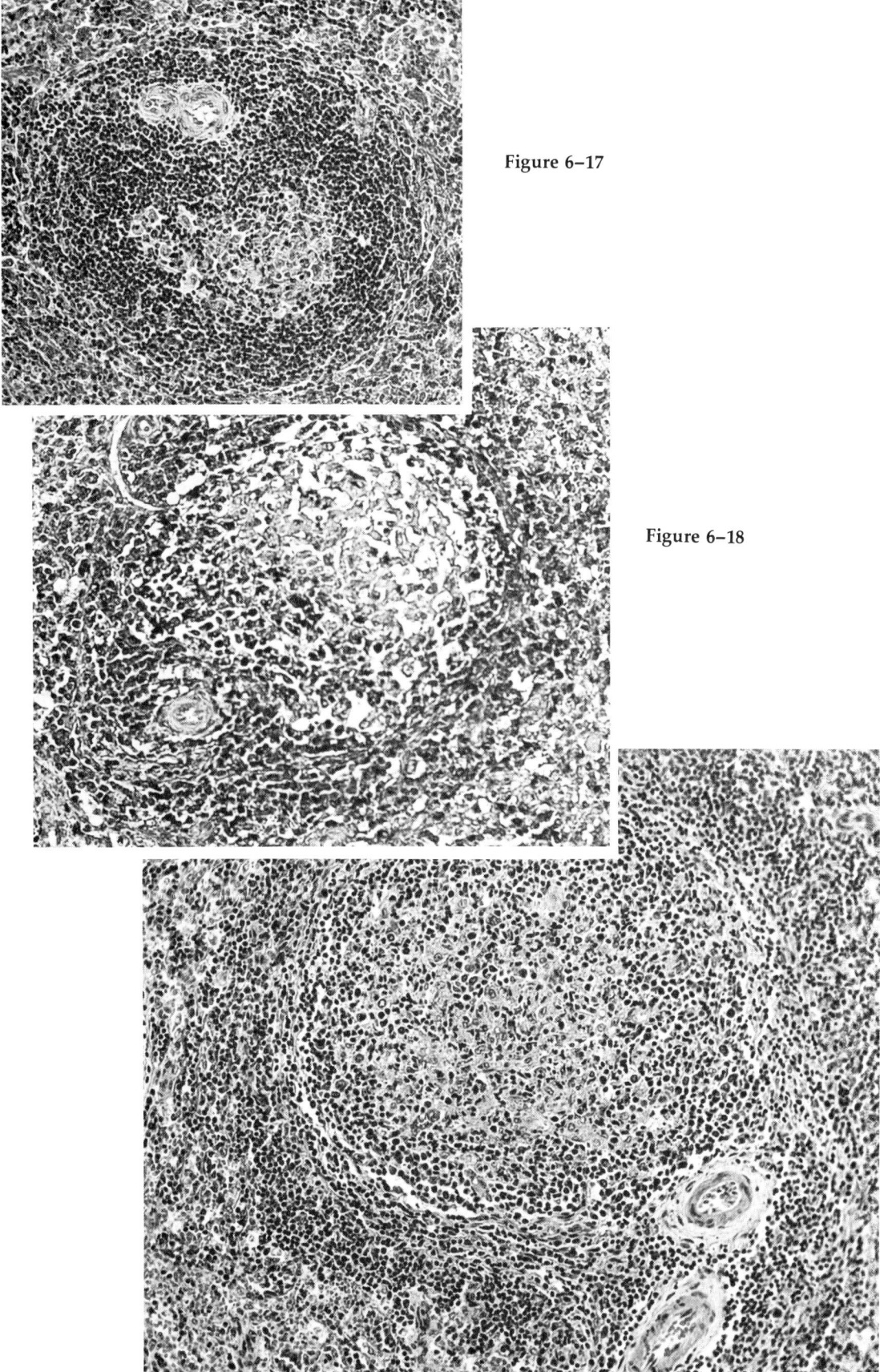

Figure 6–17

Figure 6–18

Figure 6–19

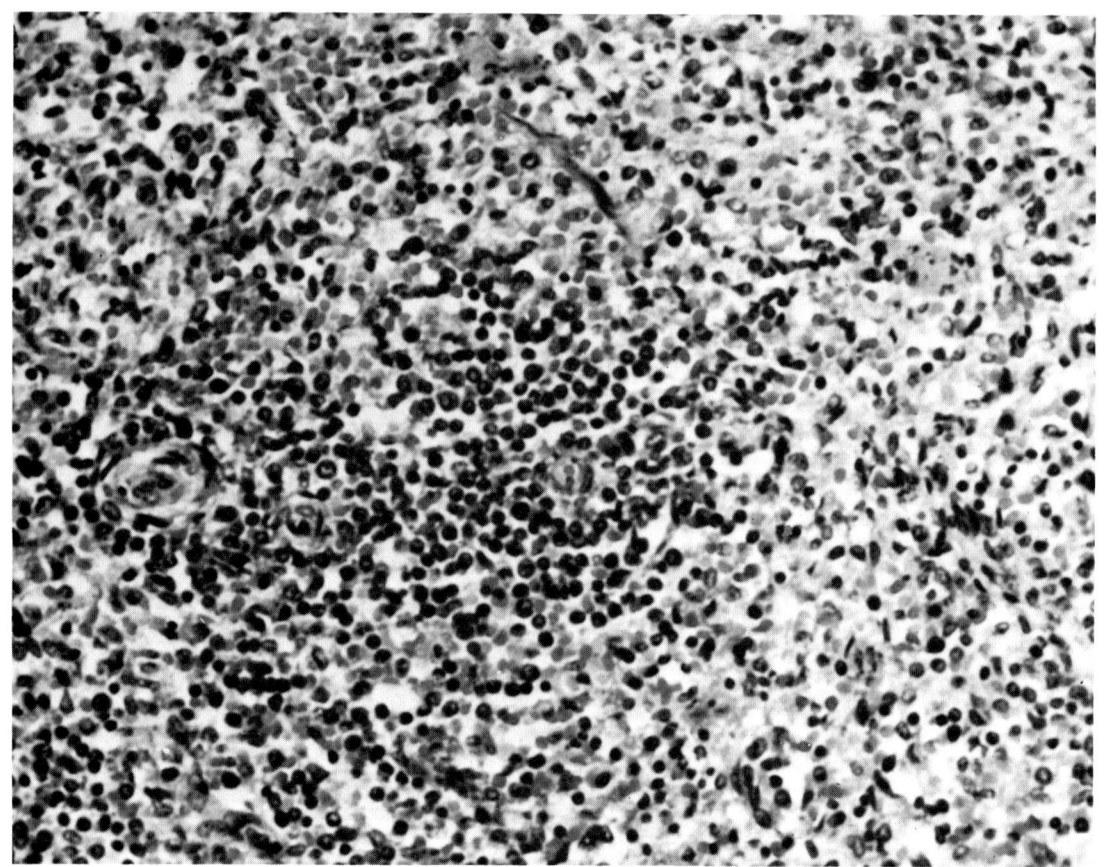

Figure 6–20

Figure 6–20. This illustration depicts the appearance of a single "young" perivascular lymphocytic aggregate in some detail because of the relatively high magnification.

The patient was a ½ hour old black male whose body weight at necropsy was only 680 grams. (Estimated gestational age: 23 weeks.)

Hematoxylin and eosin stain. Mag. 382×.

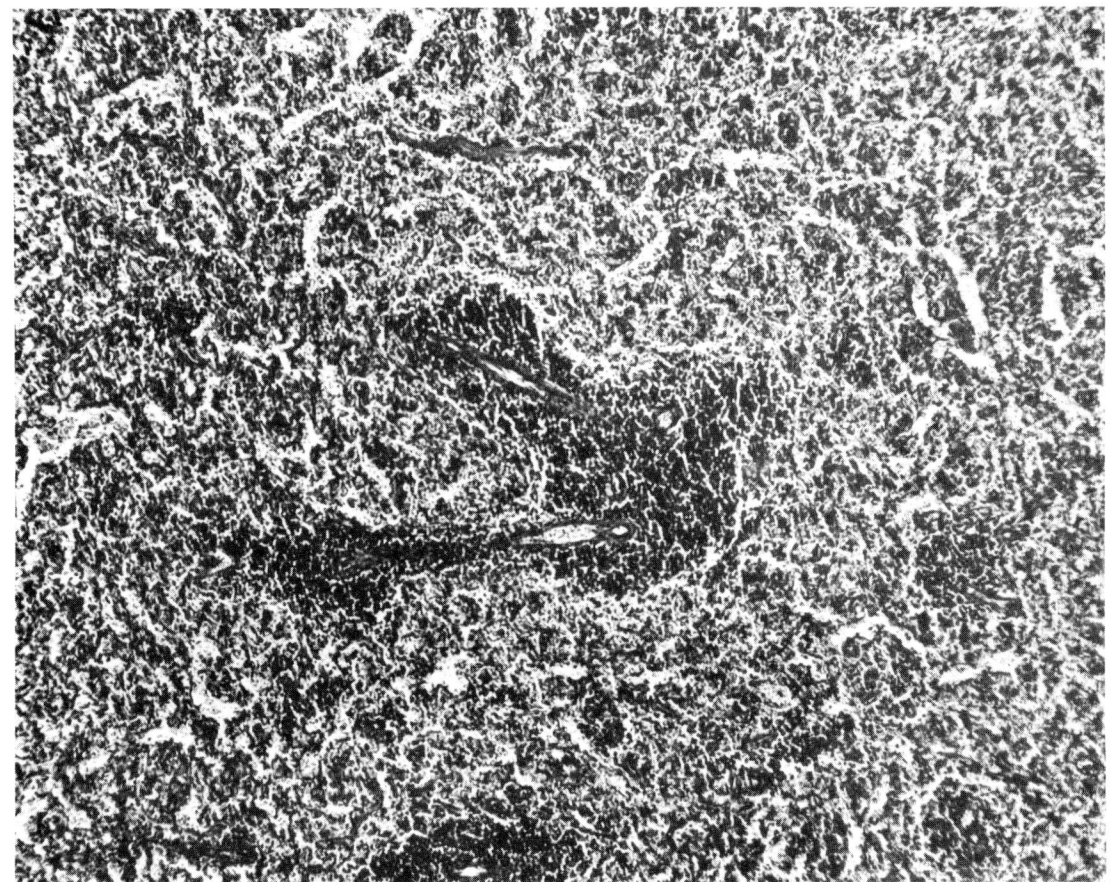

Figure 6–21

Figure 6–21. This photomicrograph illustrates the fact that the white pulp of the spleen is indeed composed of *sheaths* of lymphatic tissue which accompany splenic arterioles and their branches. Here a single sheath is seen at the site of its branching.

This section is from the autopsy of a 2 day old white female infant whose body weighed 1,890 grams at postmortem examination. (Estimated gestational age: 31 weeks.)

Hematoxylin and eosin stain. Mag. 132×.

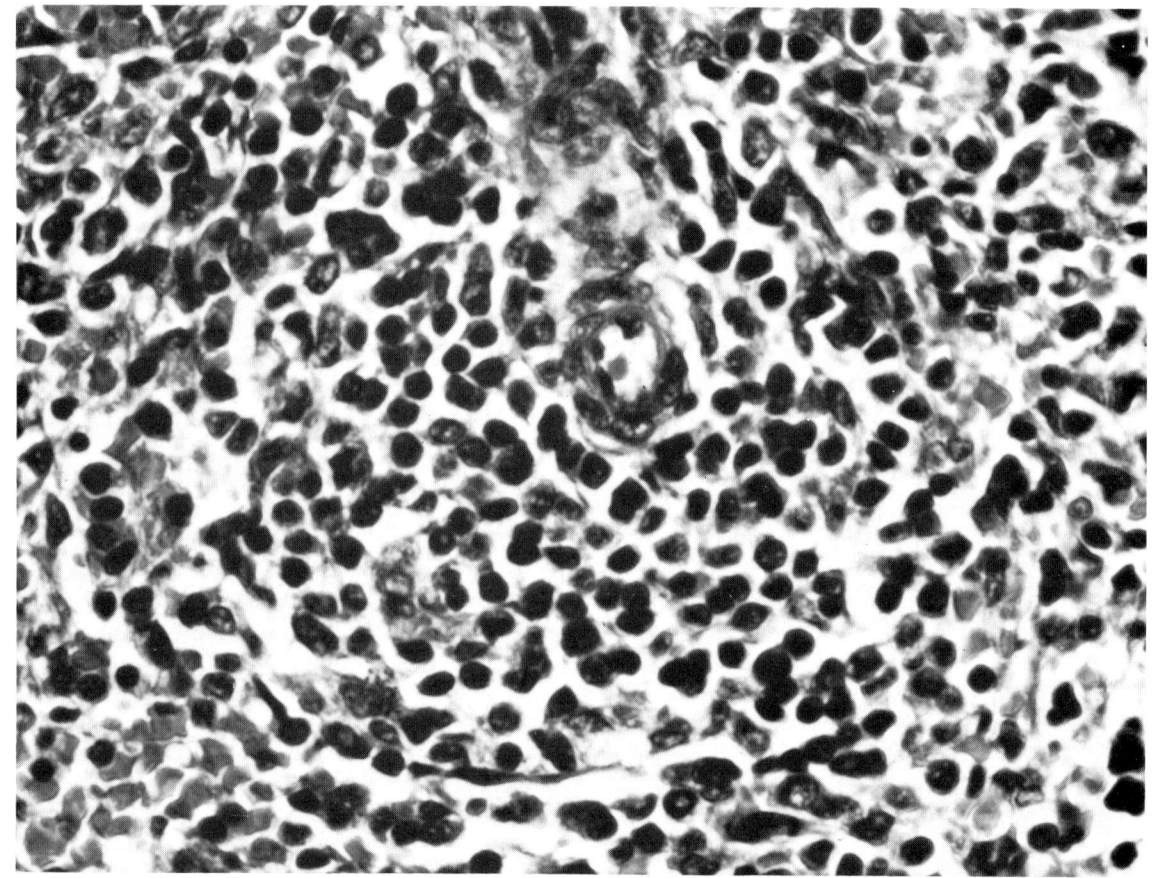

Figure 6–22

Figures 6–22 and 6–23. These two photomicrographs were taken at the same magnification and illustrate the marked change that takes place in the so-called central arteriole between mid-gestation and the end of infancy.

Figure 6–22. This central arteriole is typical of those in the section as a whole. The section is from the spleen of an 865 gram female infant, the product of a 20 week gestation, who survived for 10 minutes.

Hematoxylin and eosin stain. Mag. 660×.

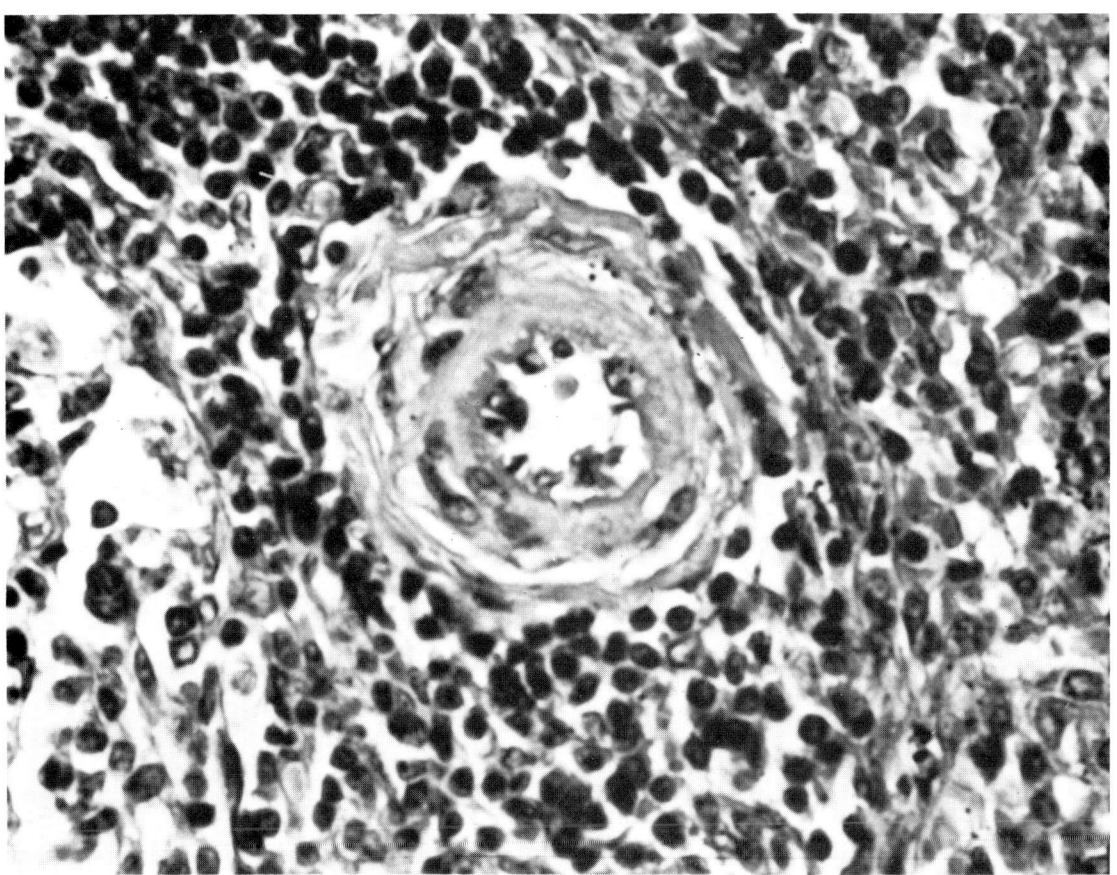

Figure 6–23

Figure 6–23. Note the much larger size of this arteriole, also typical of those in the section. The patient was 2 years and 9 months old (38 week gestation). Hematoxylin and eosin stain. Mag. 660×.

Part 4

ENDOCRINE GLANDS

Chapter 7

PITUITARY GLAND

EMBRYOLOGY

The pituitary gland (hypophysis) develops from two different sources, the ectoderm of the primitive mouth cavity and the neuroectoderm of the diencephalon. This double origin explains the presence of two completely disparate types of tissue in the adult gland. The glandular portion arises from oral ectoderm and the neural portion from the neuroectoderm.

At about the middle of the third week of embryonic life, a diverticulum, Rathke's pouch, arises from the roof of the primitive mouth cavity and grows upward toward the brain.[1] By the fifth week it has become elongated and constricted at its attachment to oral epithelium. At this stage its upper end has come into contact with the infundibulum that has developed from the neurohypophyseal bud. The bud originates as a ventral diverticulum from the floor of the diencephalon.

During the sixth week, the narrowing connection of Rathke's pouch with the oral cavity disappears. Subsequently, cells of its anterior wall proliferate and give rise to the pars distalis or anterior lobe.[1]

Later, a small cranial extension of the anterior lobe, the pars tuberalis, projects upward around the infundibular stem. The proliferation of cells within the anterior wall of Rathke's pouch reduces the lumen behind to a mere slit or cleft, which is often still visible microscopically in the pituitary of the fetus and the newborn (Fig. 7–5), but is usually obliterated in the adult. The cells of the posterior wall do not proliferate but remain as the thin, poorly defined pars intermedia (Fig. 7–5).

The infundibulum, coming down from above, gives rise to the pars nervosa or posterior lobe, the infundibular stem, and the median eminence. Although the infundibulum is originally a thin plate, its distal end soon becomes a solid mass as the neuroepithelial cells there proliferate. These cells later differentiate into *pituicytes* resembling neuroglial cells (Fig. 7–8). Nerve fibers grow into the pars nervosa from the hypothalamic area to which the infundibular stem is attached.[1]

ANATOMY

The completely developed gland consists of two major portions, a larger anterior segment (the adenohypophysis) and a smaller posterior segment (the neurohypophysis) (Figs. 7–1 and 7–2). The pituitary is suspended from above by a slender stalk, the infundibulum, to which both lobes contribute. This stalk consists primarily of a neural core, the infundibular stem, which contains the neural connections of the pituitary and which is in turn continuous with the median eminence of the tuber cinereum above. Within the infundibulum there is also an extension of the adenohypophysis, largely surrounding the neural core; this is the pars tuberalis.[2]

The adenohypophysis consists of the large pars distalis or anterior lobe, and, posterior to that, the pars intermedia (Fig. 7–5). In fetal and early postnatal life, these two are separated by the hypophyseal cleft, a vestige of Rathke's pouch; as previously mentioned, this usually becomes obliterated during childhood, leaving behind only clusters of cystic cavities at that site in some instances.

HISTOLOGY

The adenohypophysis is a highly vascular structure (Figs. 7–3 and 7–4) consisting of epithelial cells of varying size, shape, and staining capacity, arranged in cords and irregular masses that are separated from one another by delicate vascular sinusoids and supported by a complex network of reticular tissue.

In general, these epithelial cells are considered to be of three types: (1) the chromophil cells, which include (a) the acidophilic cells and (b) the basophilic cells; and (2) the chromophobe cells.

Originally these three cell types were distinguished from one another by their staining reactions, using the simple criterion of their differential binding affinities for mixtures of acidic and basic dyes such as Orange-G and aldehyde fuchsin. Modifications of these techniques using multistage staining methods further distinguished subcategories. These more sophisticated techniques, applied to pituitary glands from patients with known hormonal defects, were used to correlate specific cell types with specific hormones.[2]

More recently, the methods of immunochemistry have been brought to bear on differentiation, and it has been possible to identify sites of hormone synthesis by means of immunofluorescence. Furthermore, electron microscopy has delineated the unique ultrastructural characteristics of each cell type.[2]

The *acidophilic* cells (alpha cells) (Figs. 7–3 and 7–4) are large, with prominent cytoplasmic granules that stain bright red with eosin and in general bind other acidic dyes such as acid fuchsin, Congo red, and azocarmine.[3] Their nuclei are spherical or round and are eccentrically placed. Each nucleus has one or two nucleoli. The cells vary not only in size but also in form, chromatin content, and number of cytoplasmic granules.

The cytoplasmic granules of the *basophilic* cells (beta cells) stain strongly with basic dyes such as hematoxylin, aniline blue, resorcin fuchsin, and mucicarmine. These cells are larger than the alpha cells and are round, oval, or angular. Their cytoplasmic granules are less numerous than those of the alpha cells[2] (Fig. 7–4).

The *chromophobe* cells (reserve cells, chief cells, or simply C cells) are present as inconspicuous clusters of small elements with scanty, poorly stained cytoplasm (Figs. 7–3 and 7–4) devoid of alpha or beta granules. It is thought that they may represent only a non-secretory phase in the activity cycle of the two other cell types.[2]

There is no particular discernible pattern in the distribution of these three cell types within the lobe.

The *pars intermedia* is poorly delimited (Fig. 7–5). In many fetuses and newborns it presents as a cleft enclosed by an anterior and a posterior wall.

The *anterior wall* comprises an irregular layer, one or two cells thick, of undifferentiated alpha, beta, and C cells that blend into the anterior lobe[3] (Fig. 7–5).

The *posterior wall* is thicker, with several layers of small undifferentiated cells. Numerous beta cells, somewhat smaller than those of the anterior lobe, may extend for a variable distance from the pars intermedia into the neural lobe (Fig. 7–6).

Cysts full of "colloid" may appear chiefly in that portion of the pars intermedia farthest removed from the stalk (Fig. 7–7). The cells that line the cysts are undifferentiated small cells without granules and C cells. In addition, branched tubules of pale-staining columnar cells may extend upward into the infundibular process.[3]

Nerve fibers and capillaries are numerous in the pars intermedia.

The *neurohypophysis* is composed of thin nonmyelinated nerve fibers and associated cells that are the terminal ramifications of the hypothalamo-hypophyseal tract (Fig. 7–8). Within the infundibulum the fibers are ensheathed by typical astrocytes; but in the posterior lobe another cell type, the pituicyte, appears (Fig. 7–8). This is a dendritic cell with variable morphology, often possessing long processes that lie parallel to adjacent axons and form the bulk of the tissue there[2] (Fig. 7–8). These are probably modified glial cells, and they appear singly or in small or large groups.

Some fine collagen fibers are often interspersed between the pituicytes and the endothelial cells of nearby sinusoids.

References

1. Moore, K. L.: The Developing Human. Clinically Oriented Embryology. Philadelphia, W. B. Saunders Co., 1973, pp. 320–322.
2. Warwick, R., and Williams, P. L.: Gray's Anatomy, 35th British ed. Philadelphia, W. B. Saunders Co., 1973, pp. 1368–1371.
3. Maximow, A. A., and Bloom, W.: A Textbook of Histology, 7th ed. Philadelphia, W. B. Saunders Co., 1957, pp. 293–303.

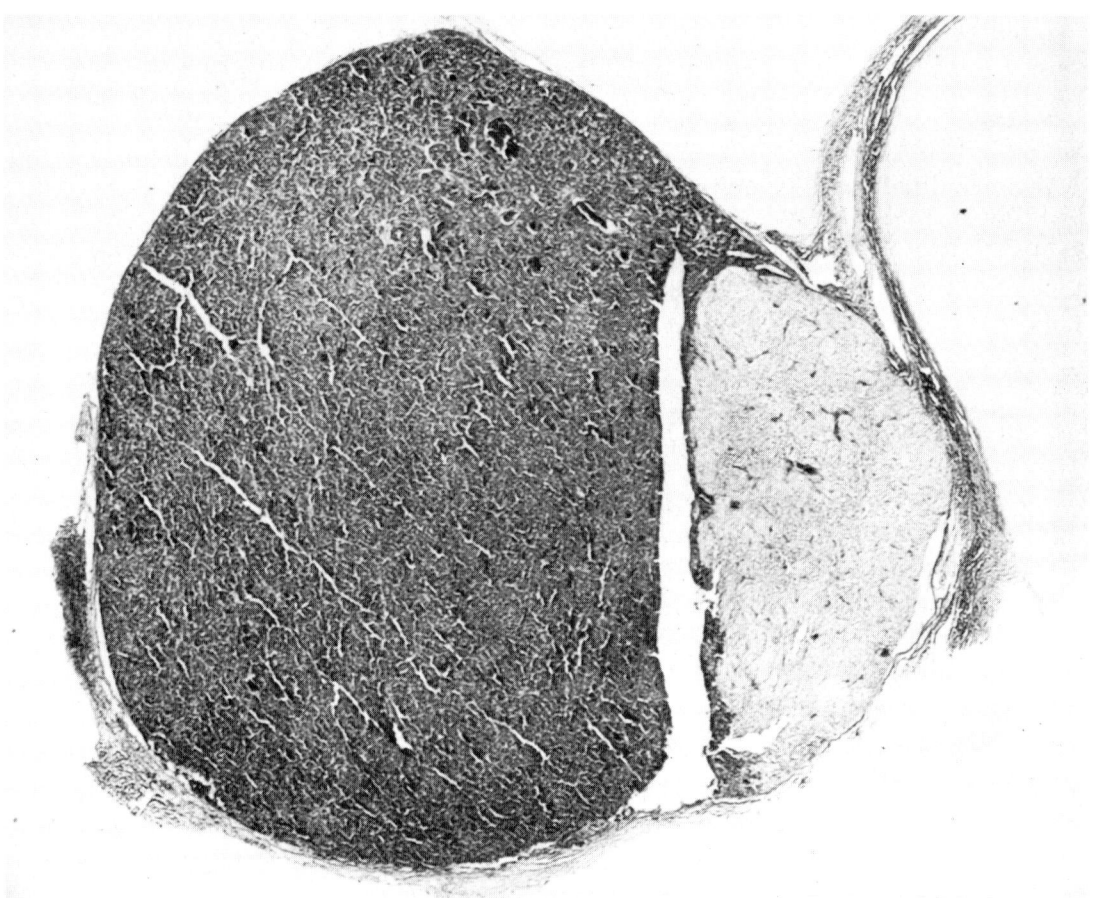

Figure 7–1

Figure 7–1. This is a survey view of the pituitary sectioned in the mid-line sagittal plane. To the left is seen the adenohypophysis, centrally the cleft so frequently encountered in the infant in relation to the pars intermedia, and, to the right, the neurohypophysis. A bit of the sella turcica appears posterior to the posterior lobe.

This is a section of the pituitary from a male infant, born at 41 weeks of gestation. He lived 12¼ hours and his body, at autopsy, weighed 3,290 grams.

Hematoxylin and eosin stain. Mag. 27.5×.

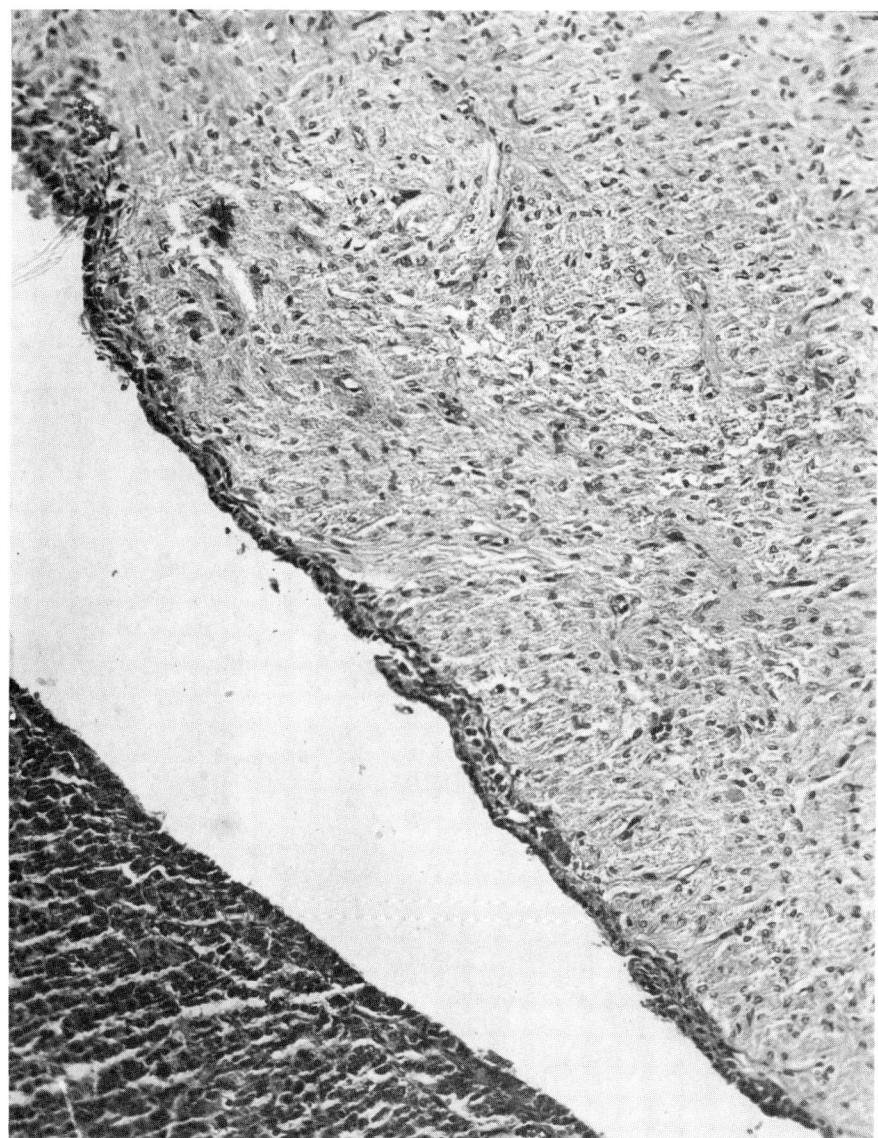

Figure 7–2

Figure 7–2. Seen here is the prominent cleft commonly encountered within the pars intermedia of the hypophysis in infants and children. In the left lower corner, constituting its anterior wall, is the pars distalis or anterior lobe. Above and to the right is the neurohypophysis or posterior lobe with its typical, rather whorled pattern of intertwined pituicytes.

The patient was a 1 month old black male who weighed 4,005 grams at autopsy.

Hematoxylin and eosin stain. Mag. 153×.

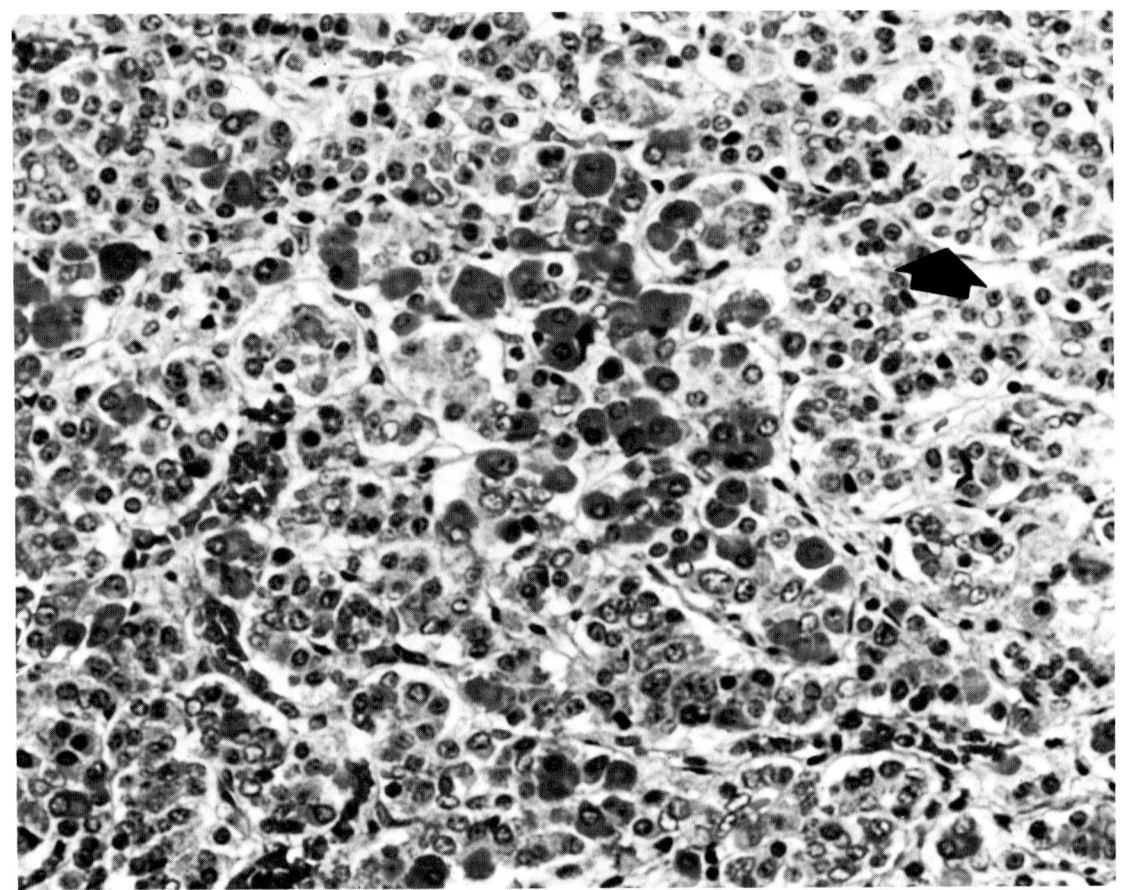

Figure 7-3

Figures 7-3 and 7-4. These photomicrographs both depict the cells of the anterior pituitary or pars distalis. They were taken from the same section from a 4½ month old male infant, the product of a 9 month gestation, whose body weight at autopsy was 6,510 grams.

Figure 7-3. The very intensely stained cells (which are bright red in hematoxylin and eosin preparations), with eccentrically placed nuclei, represent the alpha cells. The large cells with somewhat lighter cytoplasm are the beta cells. In the upper right corner, the arrow indicates C cells or chromophobes. They are angular and their cytoplasm is devoid of alpha or beta granules.
Hematoxylin and eosin stain. Mag. 382×.

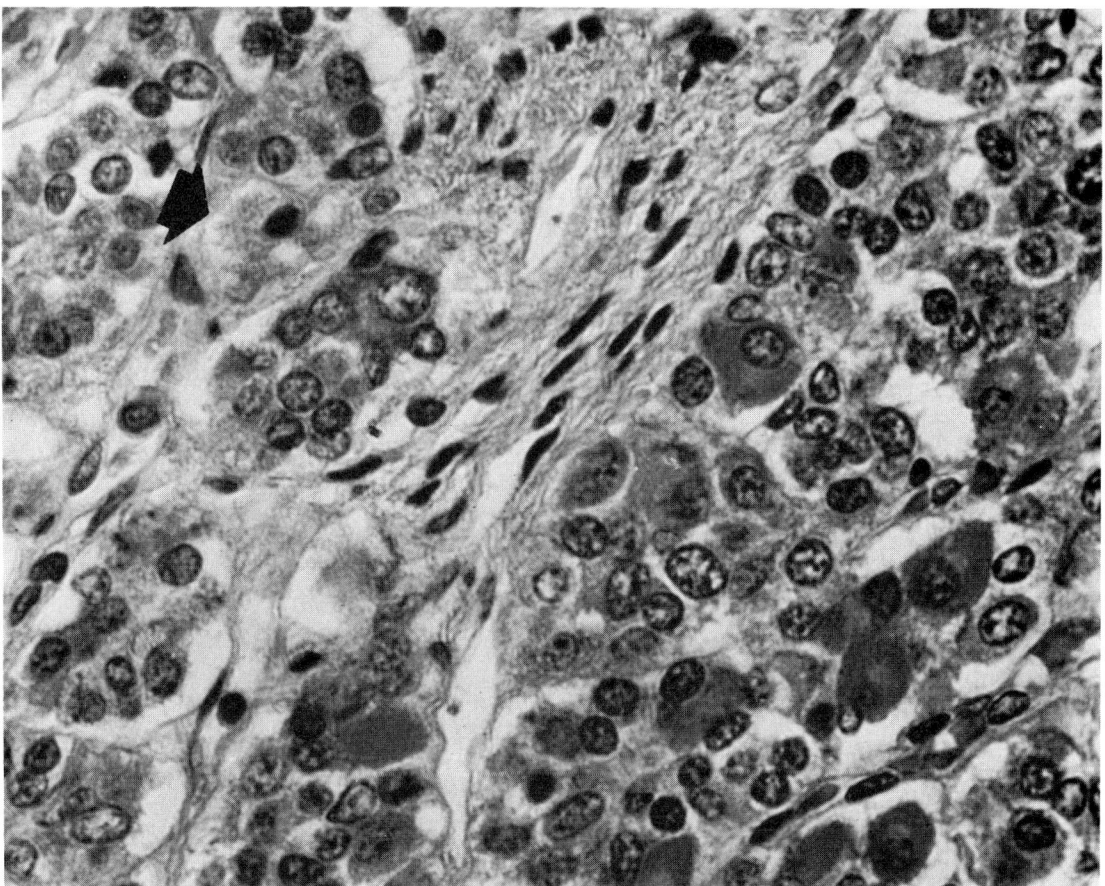

Figure 7–4

Figure 7–4. Different types of cells within the adenohypophysis are depicted here. The arrow indicates what is probably a large beta cell. On the right side are a number of intensely stained acidophilic cells and an occasional small, poorly stained chromophobe.
Hematoxylin and eosin stain. Mag. 828×.

Figure 7–5. In this photomicrograph is seen again the cleft which so frequently appears within the pars intermedia of the fetus and the newborn. The cells of its posterior wall, in juxtaposition to the neurohypophysis, are characteristic; they are predominantly of the basophilic type, polygonal and morphologically like the basophils of the adenohypophysis. They tend to form follicles and clefts, one of which is seen at the top of the band to the right of center, vertically oriented.

This section is from a female infant weighing 3,080 grams, of 40 weeks gestation and 21 hours of age.

Hematoxylin and eosin stain. Mag. 231×.

See illustration on the opposite page

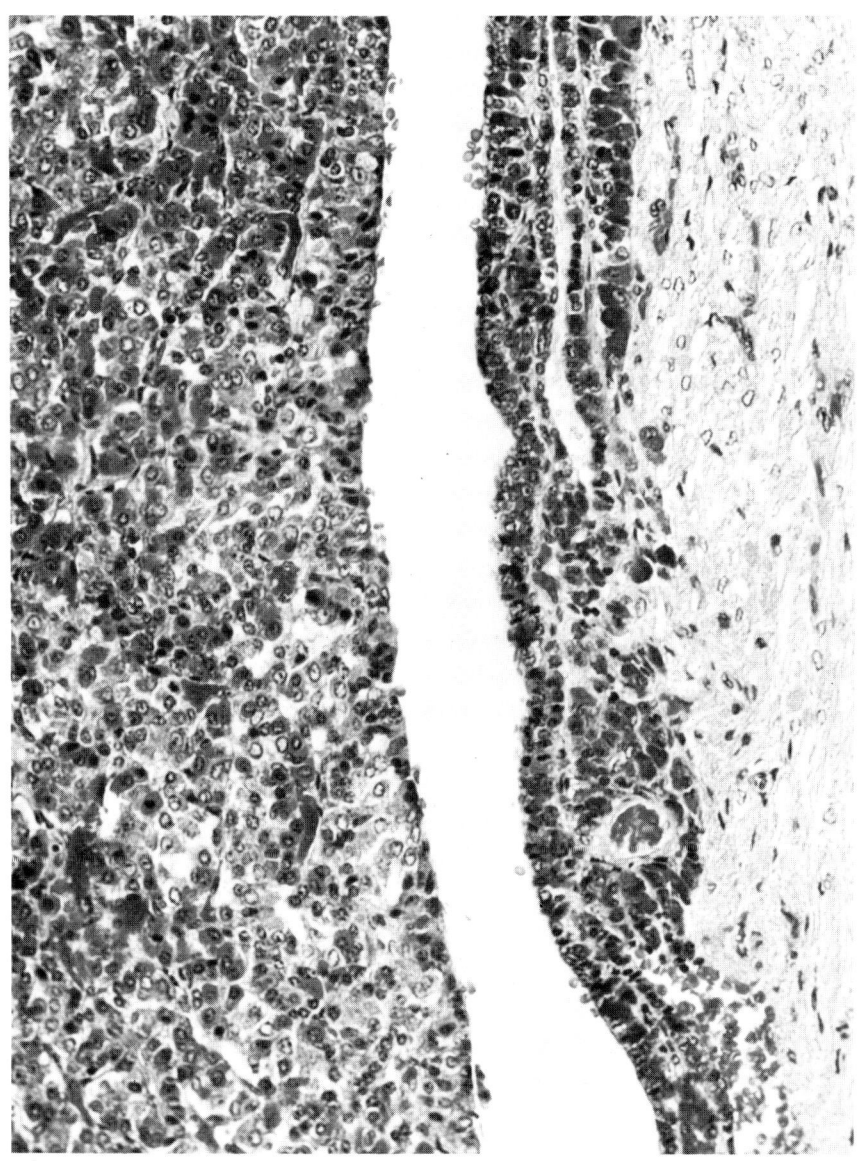

Figure 7-5

See legend on the opposite page

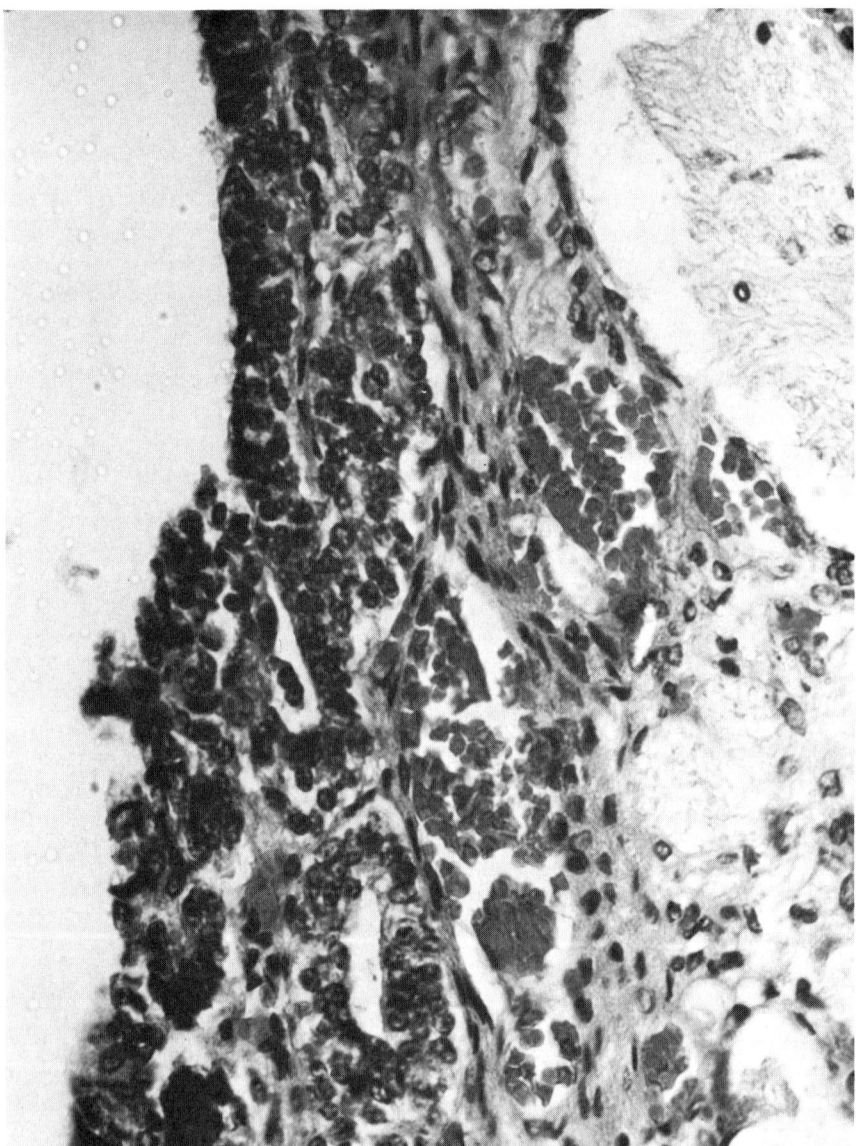

Figure 7–6a

Figure 7–6a. The basophilic cells of the pars intermedia are depicted here at higher magnification. Two of the epithelial-lined follicles they so frequently exhibit are illustrated here, to the left of center in the lower half of the photograph.

The patient was a 2 week old black male. His weight and gestational age were not recorded. Hematoxylin and eosin stain. Mag. 410×.

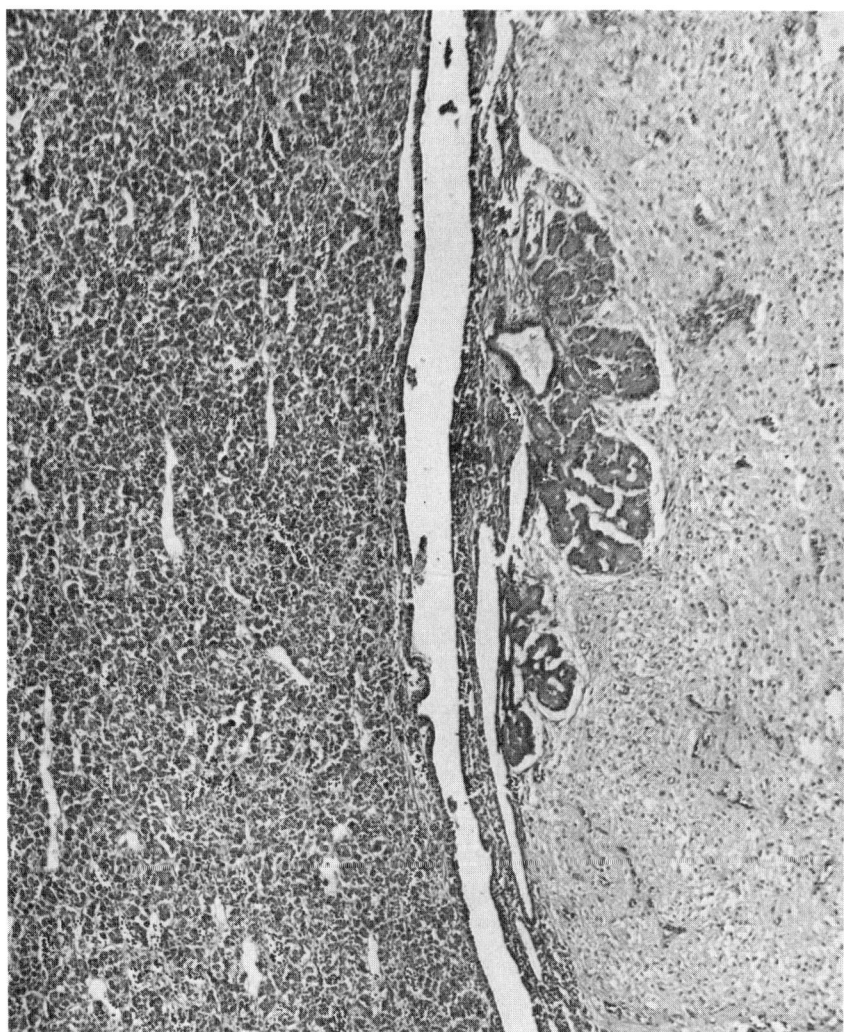

Figure 7–6b

Figure 7–6b. This figure also illustrates the pars intermedia and the clusters of small gland-like structures commonly included in that area in the perinatal period.

This infant was a female of unknown race, whose body weight at autopsy was 3,100 grams and who lived for 1 hour and 32 minutes.

Hematoxylin and eosin stain. Mag. 50×.

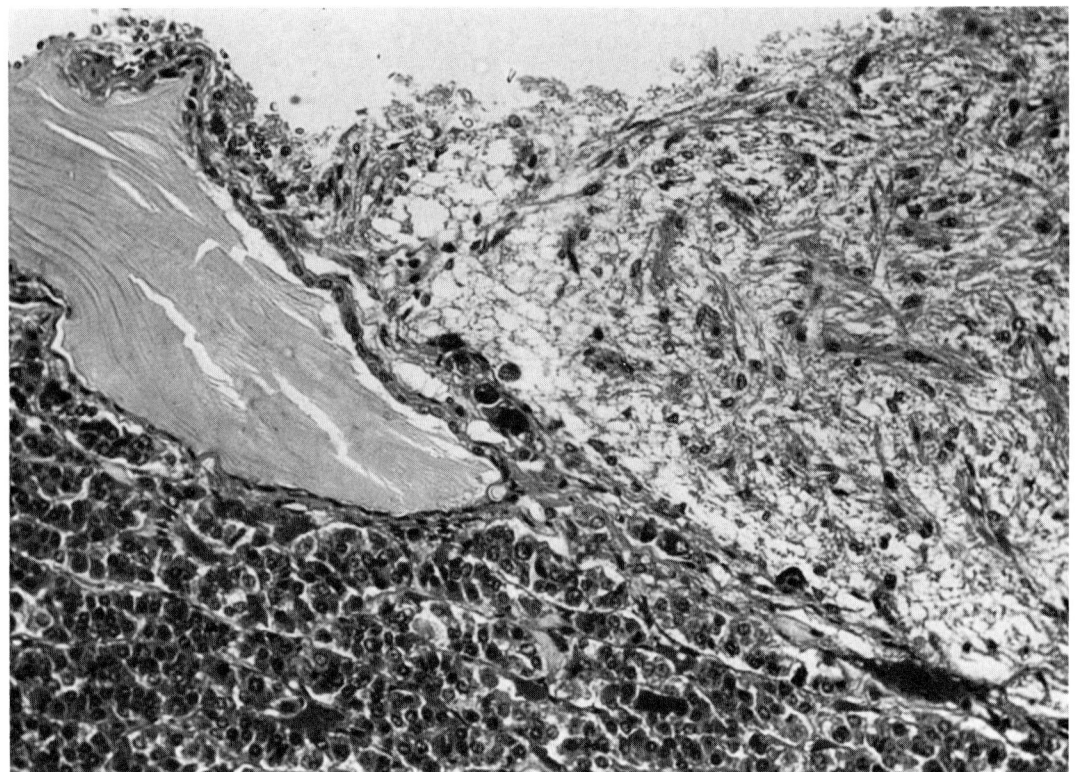

Figure 7–7

Figure 7–7. Between the anterior lobe, lower left, and the posterior lobe, upper right, there is a cyst, probably a remnant of Rathke's pouch (Rathke's cyst). These are common in the pars intermedia of both infants and adults. They may be lined by tall columnar and even ciliated epithelium. They contain colorless to yellow colloid material, which varies in consistency from a thin to a highly viscous fluid.

The subject was a female infant, born at 23 to 25 weeks of gestation. The infant survived for 48 hours despite the fact that the body weight, at autopsy, was only 450 grams.

Hematoxylin and eosin stain. Mag. 219×.

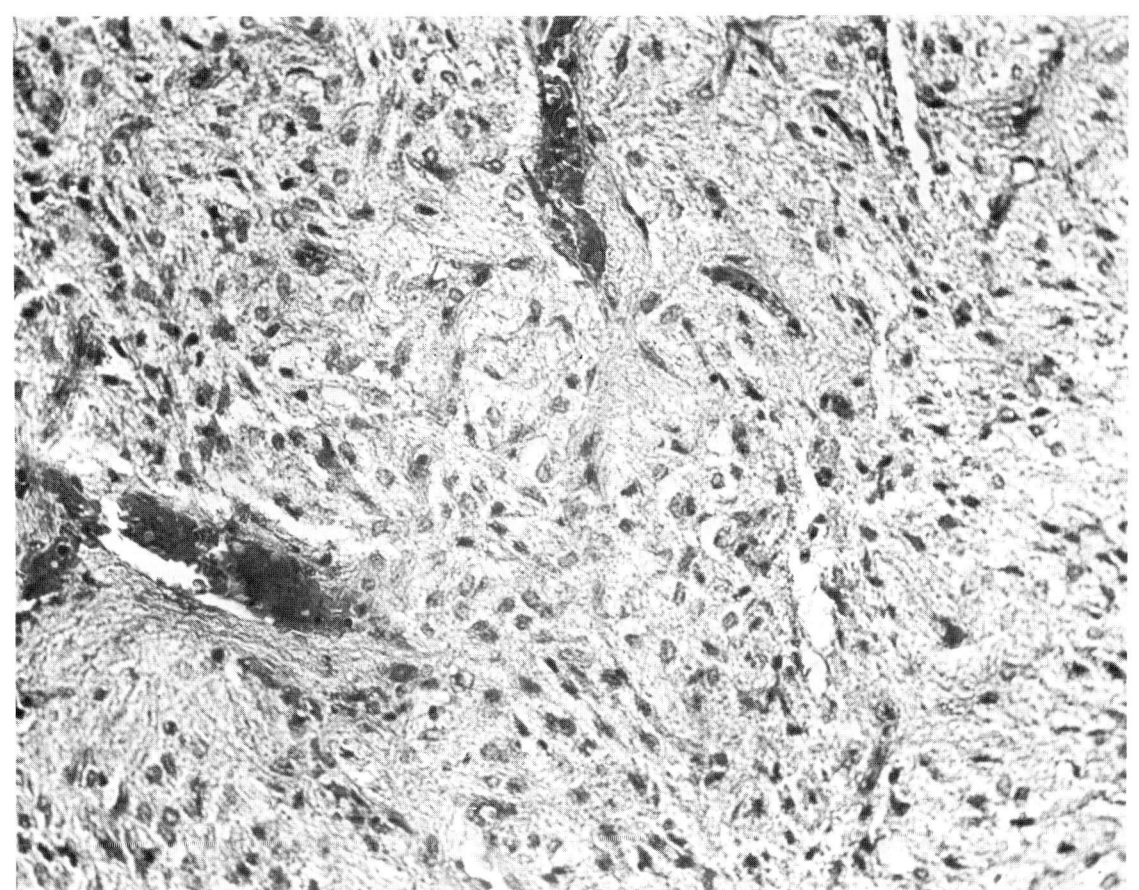

Figure 7–8

Figure 7–8. Illustrated here, in some detail, is the histologic architecture of the posterior lobe of the pituitary. It is composed of thin, nonmyelinated nerve fibers and associated cells which are the terminal ramifications of the hypothalamo-hypophysial tract. The pituicyte is a dendritic cell with variable morphology, but often possessing long processes that lie parallel to the adjacent axons and form the bulk of this lobe.

The patient was a 3,290 gram infant, born at 41 weeks of gestation, who survived for $12\frac{1}{4}$ hours.

Hematoxylin and eosin stain. Mag. 250×.

Chapter 8

THYROID GLAND

EMBRYOLOGY

The thyroid is the earliest glandular structure to appear in the embryo.[1] Even an embryo 2 mm. long shows an external bulge on the ventral floor of the foregut indicating the site of its origin. A distinct endodermal outpocketing there, the thyroid diverticulum, soon protrudes downward to lie between the first pair of pharyngeal pouches. The narrow neck of this diverticulum is known as the thyroglossal duct, so named because it is hollow at first and connects the primitive thyroid with the base of the tongue, which is taking shape from the pharyngeal floor at the same time. The duct soon becomes a solid stalk and then fragments in the sixth week, but its point of origin on the dorsal surface of the tongue is permanently indicated by a large pit named the foramen cecum.[1]

The thyroid sac or diverticulum quickly becomes converted into a solid mass that lies against the primitive aortic stem. Early it is bilobed; when released by atrophy of its stalk, it begins to change into an irregular mass of epithelial plates.

By the seventh week the gland has attained its final position anterior to the trachea, has become crescent-shaped, and has settled into a transverse position with one lobe on each side of the airway. (Actually it only appears to have shifted caudally because the pharynx has grown forward, leaving the thyroid behind.) The ventral elongate part of each fourth pharyngeal pouch (or, as classified by some, the rudimentary fifth pouch) develops into an ultimobranchial body, which fuses with the thyroid. Some believe that these bodies subsequently disseminate within the gland to give rise to the parafollicular or C cells.[2] Others feel that they simply degenerate, while still others describe their ultimate conversion into thyroid tissue.[1]

The pyramidal lobe, present in about fifty per cent of thyroids, is a derivative or remnant of the lowermost segment of the thyroglossal duct.

In the eighth week, isolated cavities begin to appear in swollen or beaded portions of the solid thyroid plates; these represent the earliest formation of follicles or acini, which begin to acquire colloid in the third month.[1]

By the end of the fourth month, that conversion into follicles ceases; thereafter new follicles arise only by the budding and subdivision of those already present.[1]

THYROID GLAND

The capsule and vascular stroma of the thyroid are derived from local mesenchyme.

By the twenty-fourth week of gestation, the acini generally are larger (Figs. 8–3 and 8–6), and by 29 weeks the histologic appearance of the gland resembles very closely that of the adult (Figs. 8–4 and 8–8).

Throughout this entire stage of development, from the very first appearance of follicles with lumina to 40 weeks of gestation, there is a tendency toward a discrepancy between the sizes of centrally and peripherally located follicles. Those in the heart of each lobe are generally much smaller than those nearer the capsule, and there is a gradual progression from one size to the other. Although it is not quite so striking later, this unique disproportion is maintained until the age of 2 to 3 years.[3]

The epithelial cells lining the follicles of the premature infant's thyroid tend to be rather tall (Fig. 8–9), but by 32 weeks of gestation they become low cuboidal (Figs. 8–10 and 8–11).

ANATOMY

The thyroid of the newborn is tightly adherent to the trachea on both sides and anteriorly. The shape is quite like that of the adult, and the size is similarly appropriate to that of the trachea.

The color is reddish tan and the consistency firm. Cut surfaces are also firm, tan, and slightly translucent. The entire organ is enveloped by a thin, translucent, fibrous capsule. The external surface is ordinarily quite smooth.

HISTOLOGY

In the fetus of 12 weeks much of the thyroid, at first glance, might appear microscopically to be an almost solid structure composed of closely packed tiny rounded clusters of epithelial cells.

By the sixteenth week of gestation, however, a moderate number of follicles, especially those about the perimeter, have opened up and have developed colloid-containing lumina (Figs. 8–1, 8–2, and 8–5).

References

1. Arey, L. B.: Developmental Anatomy. A Textbook and Laboratory Manual of Embryology, 7th ed., revised. Philadelphia, W. B. Saunders Co., 1974, pp. 241–242.
2. Moore, K. L.: The Developing Human. Clinically Oriented Embryology. Philadelphia, W. B. Saunders Co., 1973, pp. 145–146.
3. Valdes-Dapena, M. A.: An Atlas of Fetal and Neonatal Histology. Philadelphia, J. B. Lippincott Co., 1957, pp. 153–162.

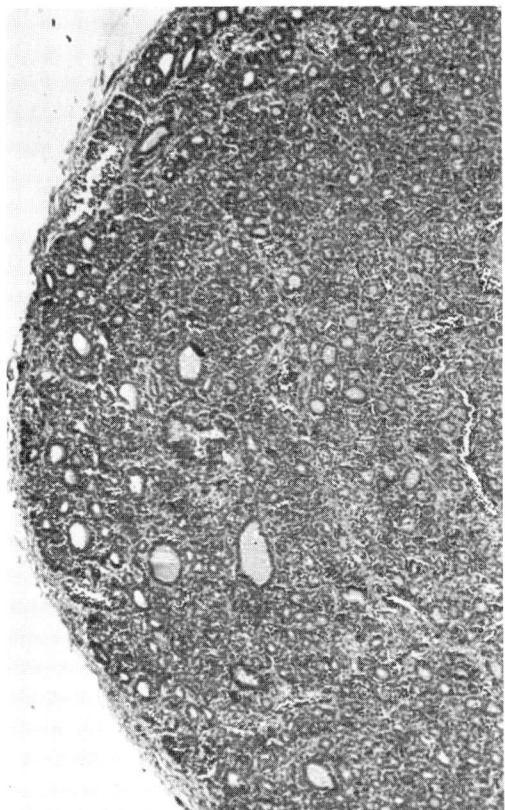 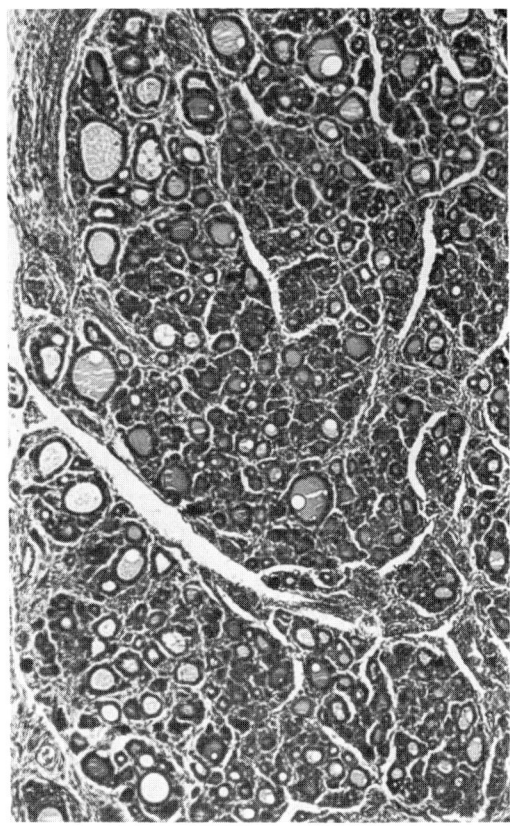

Figure 8–1   Figure 8–2

Figures 8–1 to 8–4. This set of four photographs depicts, at very low magnification, the changing histologic pattern of the fetal and neonatal thyroid.

With increasing gestational age there is, as might be expected, a progressive increase in the average diameter of acini, expansion of the lumina of acini, and filling of those lumina with colloid. (Some acini contain colloid even in the thyroids of fetuses of only 16 weeks gestation.)

At 19 weeks of gestation, Fig. 8–1, some centrally placed acini appear to be almost solid epithelial structures without lumina. (See right-hand margin of this photograph.) There is a general tendency, most marked at this stage in the development of the gland but also apparent later (see Figs. 8–2 and 8–3), toward relative enlargement of acini peripherally, so that in any given section there is apt to be an obvious difference between the average diameter of the acini located in the center of the lobe and the diameter of those beneath the capsule. (In Figs. 8–2, 8–3, and 8–4, compare acini in the right lower corner of the photograph with those in the upper left.)

This difference may still be apparent in the thyroids of children 2 and even 3 years of age.
Hematoxylin and eosin stain. Mag. 81×.

Figure 8–1. Section from the thyroid of a 430 gram twin, a black male infant, born at 19 weeks of gestation, who lived for 13 minutes.

Figure 8–2. Section of the thyroid of a 250 gram female infant born at 16 weeks of gestation, who lived for 1 hour.

120 THYROID GLAND

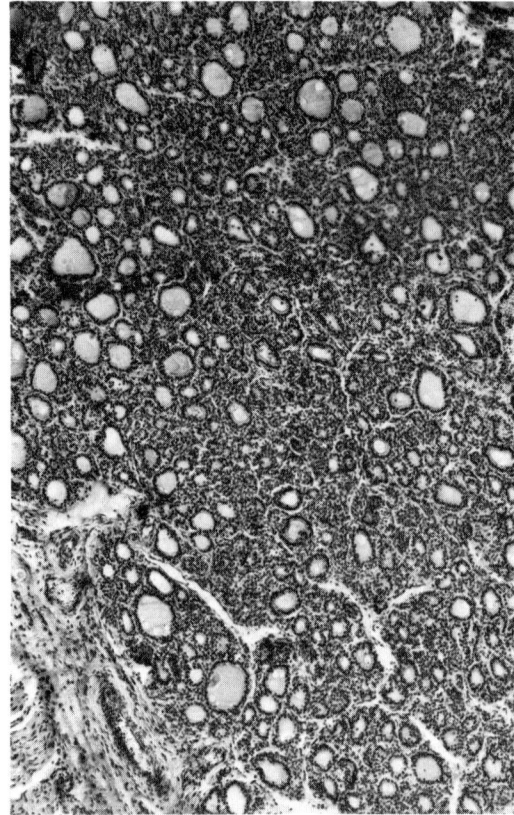

Figure 8-3

Figure 8-3. Section of the thyroid of a 930 gram female infant of 24 weeks gestation, who survived for 3 days.

THYROID GLAND 121

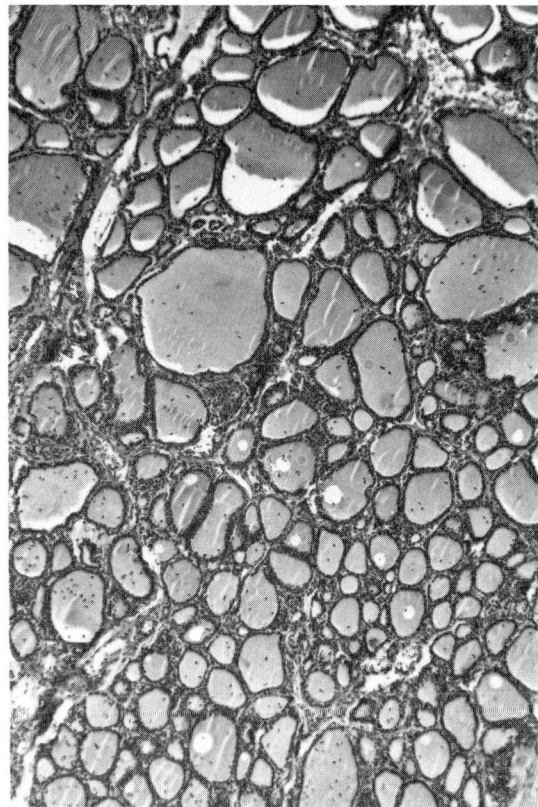

Figure 8–4

Figure 8–4. Section of the thyroid of an infant born after 29 weeks of gestation. The infant weighed 1,895 grams and died at 18 hours of age.

122 THYROID GLAND

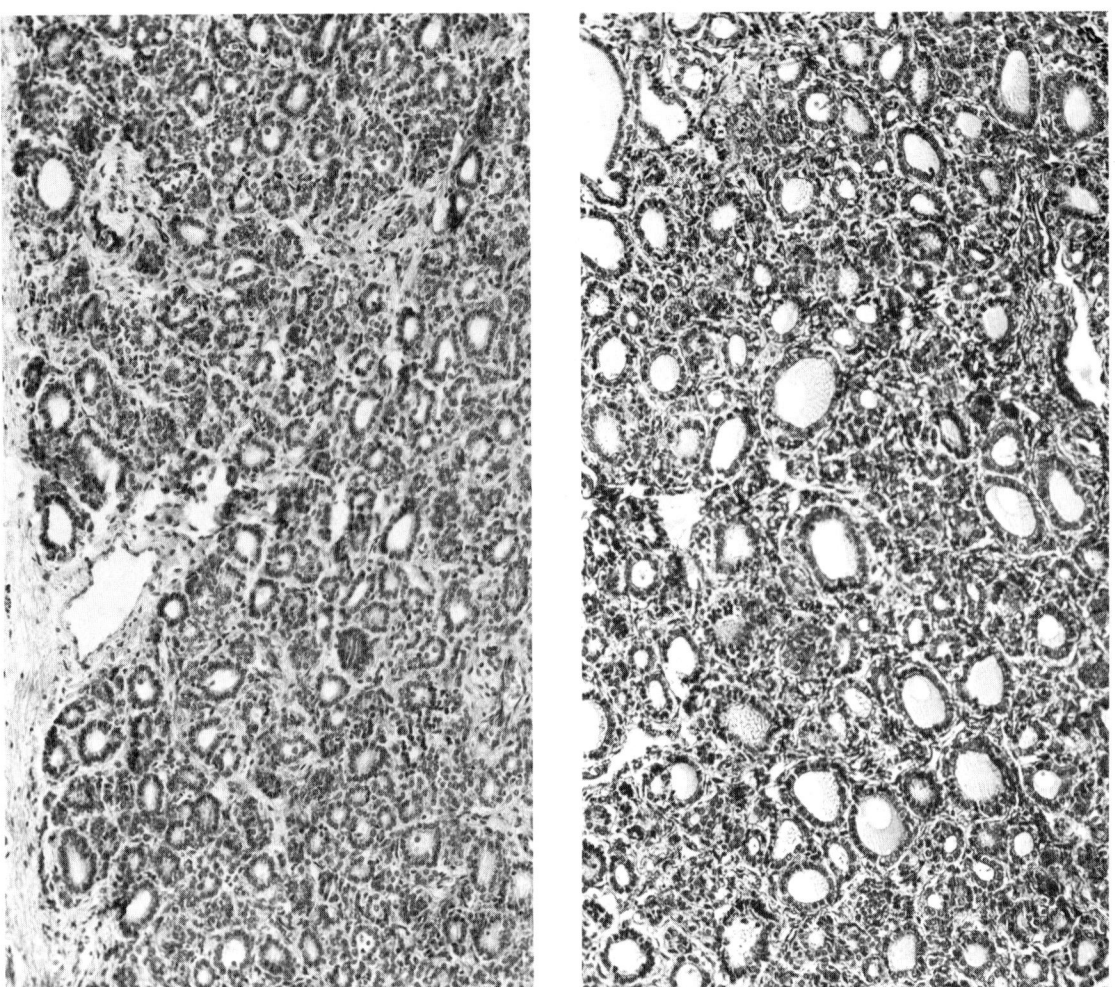

Figure 8-5   Figure 8-6

Figures 8–5 to 8–8. In this set of four photomicrographs, the changing histologic appearance of the thyroid, through late fetal life and early infancy, is again displayed—but in this instance at somewhat higher magnification. (All four pictures were taken at the same magnification.)

In Fig. 8–5, the acini are relatively and generally small; through Figs. 8–6, 8–7, and 8–8, the average diameter of the acini increases, the lumina enlarge and filling of the acini with colloid becomes more uniform.

Hematoxylin and eosin stain. Mag. 142×.

Figure 8–5. Section of the thyroid of a black male prematurely born infant, born at 19 weeks of gestation, a twin, weighing 430 grams. The infant survived for 13 minutes.

Figure 8–6. Section of the thyroid of a 615 gram white male infant born at 22 to 24 weeks of gestation, who lived for 5 hours and 42 minutes.

THYROID GLAND 123

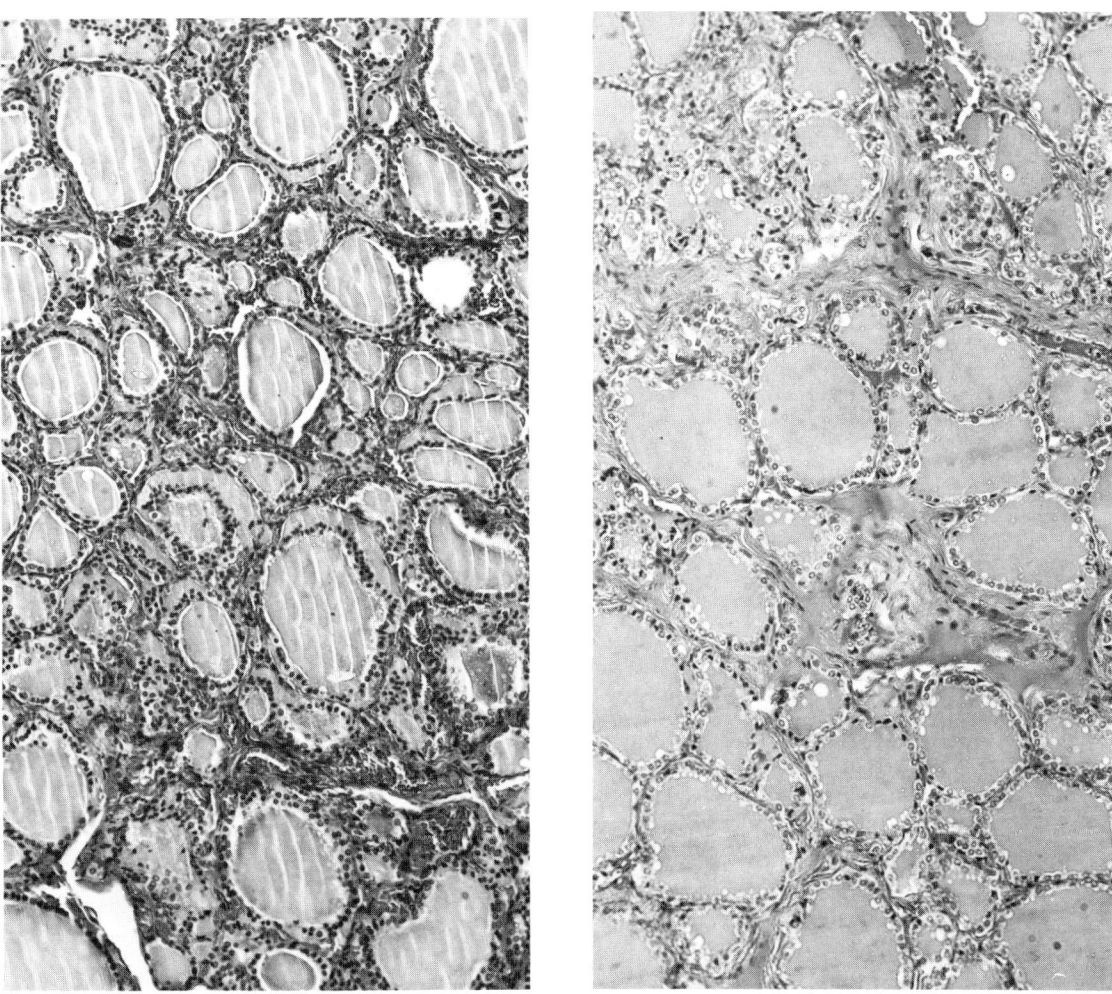

Figure 8–7   Figure 8–8

Figure 8–7. Section of the thyroid of a 2 day old white female infant, who weighed 2,275 grams at autopsy. (Estimated gestational age: 32 weeks.)

Figure 8–8. Section of the thyroid of an infant, the product of a 36 week gestation, who died at the age of 4½ months.

124 THYROID GLAND

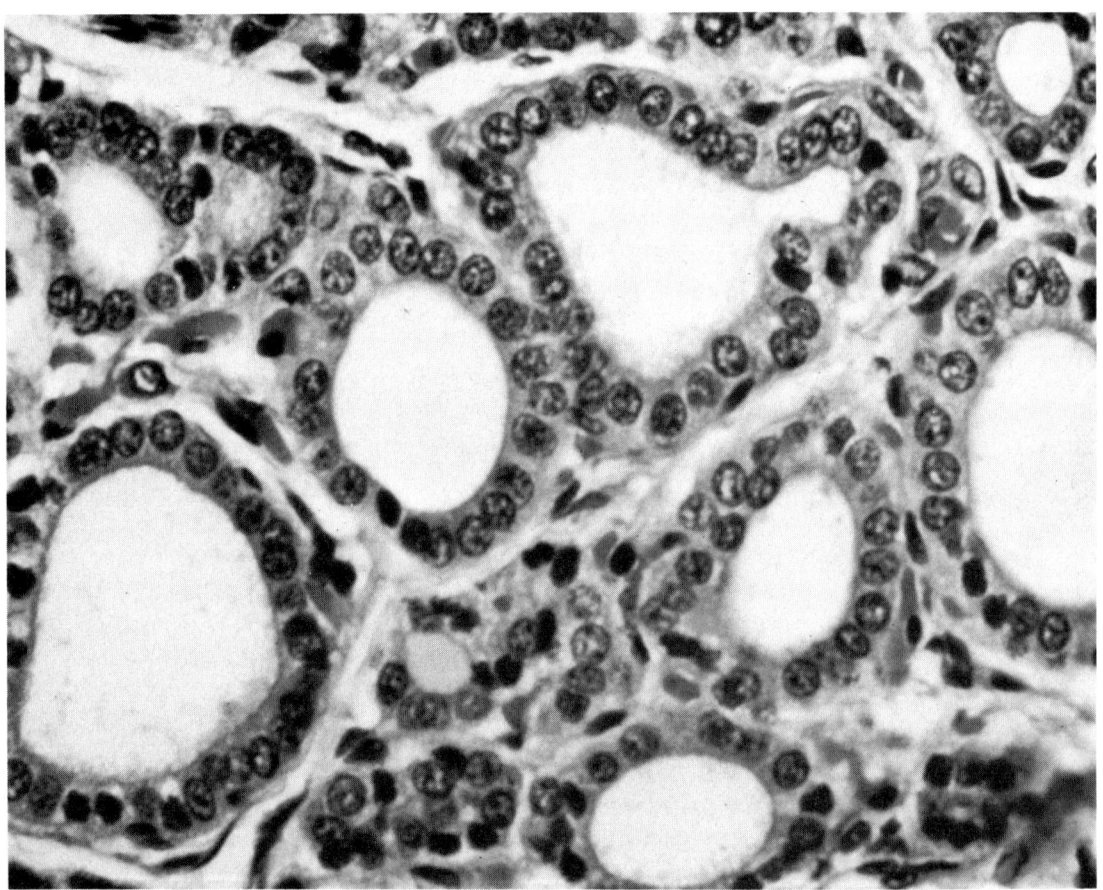

Figure 8–9

Figures 8–9 to 8–11. In this set of three photomicrographs, all taken at the same relatively high magnification, finer details of acinar structure are more apparent.

In Fig. 8–9, a section from the thyroid of a prematurely born baby, the acini represented are rather small; their lining epithelial cells are relatively tall.

In contrast, in Figs. 8–10 and 8–11 (sections of thyroid from infants 4 months and 23 days of age, respectively), many acini are very large and their lining epithelial cells are considerably flattened. Variability in size of acini is greater.

Hematoxylin and eosin stain. Mag. 660×.

Figure 8–9. This is a section of the thyroid of a 660 gram male infant, the product of a 24 week gestation, who weighed 570 grams at autopsy and who lived for 1 hour.

Figure 8–10

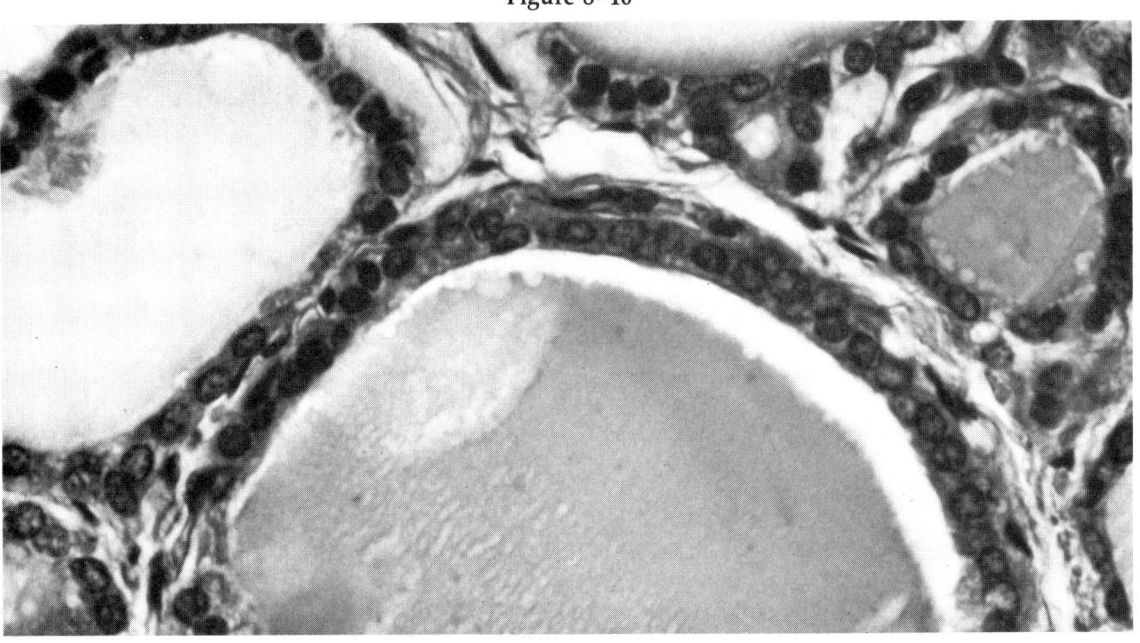

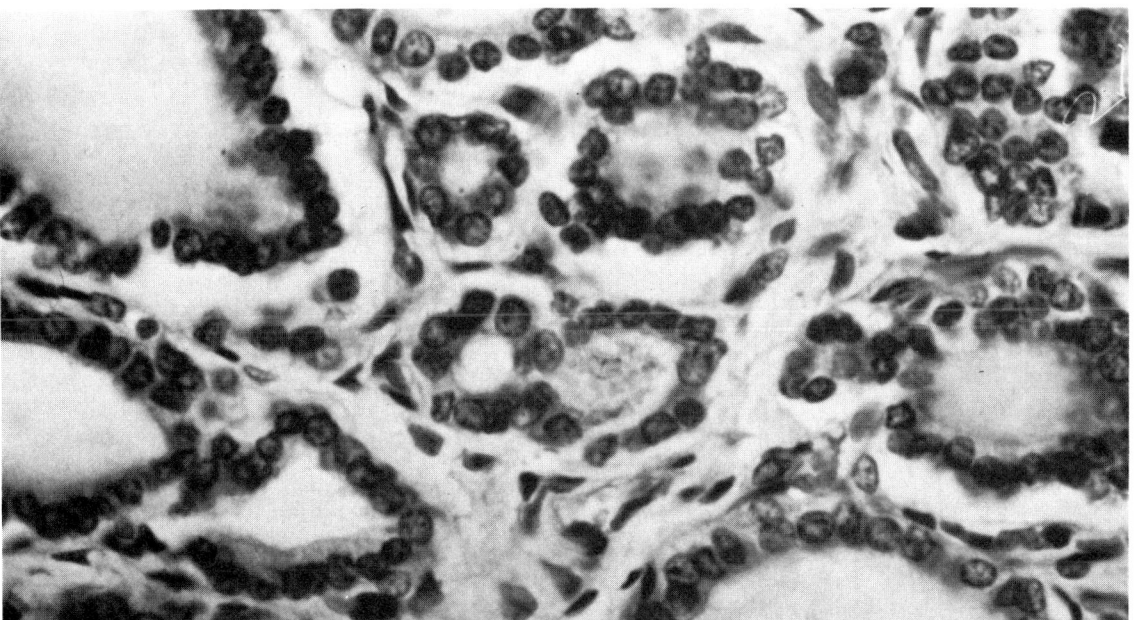

Figure 8–11

Figure 8–10. This is a section of the thyroid of a 2,834 gram infant, born after 32 weeks of gestation. The infant died at the age of 4 months.

Figure 8–11. This is a section of the thyroid of a 2,507 gram infant, born at term, who survived for 23 days.

Chapter 9

PARATHYROID GLANDS

EMBRYOLOGY

The two parathyroid glands on each side are derived embryologically from two pharyngeal pouches. The tissue that ultimately becomes the upper gland is derived from pharyngeal pouch IV, and the lower, from III; the latter passes the former during its caudal migration.

The lower pair are always intimately associated with the uppermost portion of the thymus during fetal life and early infancy because of their common origin from pharyngeal pouch III.

The epithelium of the dorsal portion of the third and fourth pouches proliferates during the fifth week of embryonic life.[1] It expands into a solid dorsal bulbar portion and a hollow ventral elongate part. Its connection with the pharynx is reduced to a narrow duct, which soon disappears. By the sixth week each dorsal bulbar portion begins to differentiate into the parathyroid gland. A vascular network grows into the nodule, forming its capillary network.

ANATOMY

Grossly, the parathyroids during late fetal life and early infancy have a distinctive light coral color. Under the dissecting microscope one can often see their prominent subcapsular net of tiny engorged vessels. Petechiae are common within them. Their shape tends to be discoid and they are plump centrally. The upper pair are usually tucked neatly into the vertical cleft between the lateral lobe of the thyroid (two-thirds of the distance up from lower pole to upper) and the immediately adjacent esophagus. Commonly, they are partially or completely embedded in adipose tissue. They tend to be about 4 mm. in greatest diameter. Their position, size, and appearance are relatively uniform.

The lower parathyroids have the same general morphologic characteristics of size, shape, and color. Like the upper glands, they are almost always independent of the thyroid and embedded to some degree in adipose tissue; at times one (or both) will appear as a coral-colored *subcapsular* disc at the top of a discrete oval nodule of pale pink aberrant thymic tissue near the lower pole of the infant thyroid. Their location is much more variable than that of the upper parathyroids; they may be attached to the capsule of the lower pole of the thyroid inferiorly, or removed from that gland by several centimeters.

HISTOLOGY

Almost from their very first appearance in the fifth week of gestation[2] these glands show distinctively differentiated "water clear" (chief or principal) cells (Fig. 9–2). Their cytoplasm is rich in glycogen and contains numerous fat droplets.[3] (The oxyphil cells do not differentiate until the child has attained an age of 4.5 to 7 years.) The constituent chief cells usually form a continuous mass as in Figs. 9–1 and 9–2; less commonly, they are arranged as anastomosing cords.

When the parathyroid is intimately applied to thymic tissue, histologic section of the line of approximation may reveal that the two tissue types are completely separated from each other by a connective tissue capsule. However, there may be no capsule whatsoever between them, their two cell types intermingling freely at the site.[4]

References

1. Moore, K. L.: The Developing Human. Clinically Oriented Embryology. Philadelphia, W. B. Saunders Co., 1973, pp. 144–145.
2. Willis, R. A.: The Borderland of Embryology and Pathology. London, Butterworth and Co., Ltd., 1958, p. 108.
3. Maximow, A. A., and Bloom, W.: A Textbook of Histology, 7th ed. Philadelphia, W. B. Saunders Co., 1957, pp. 310–313.
4. Valdes-Dapena, M., and Weinstein, D.: The parathyroid glands in sudden, unexpected death in infants. Acta Path. et Micro. Scand., 79:228–32, 1971.

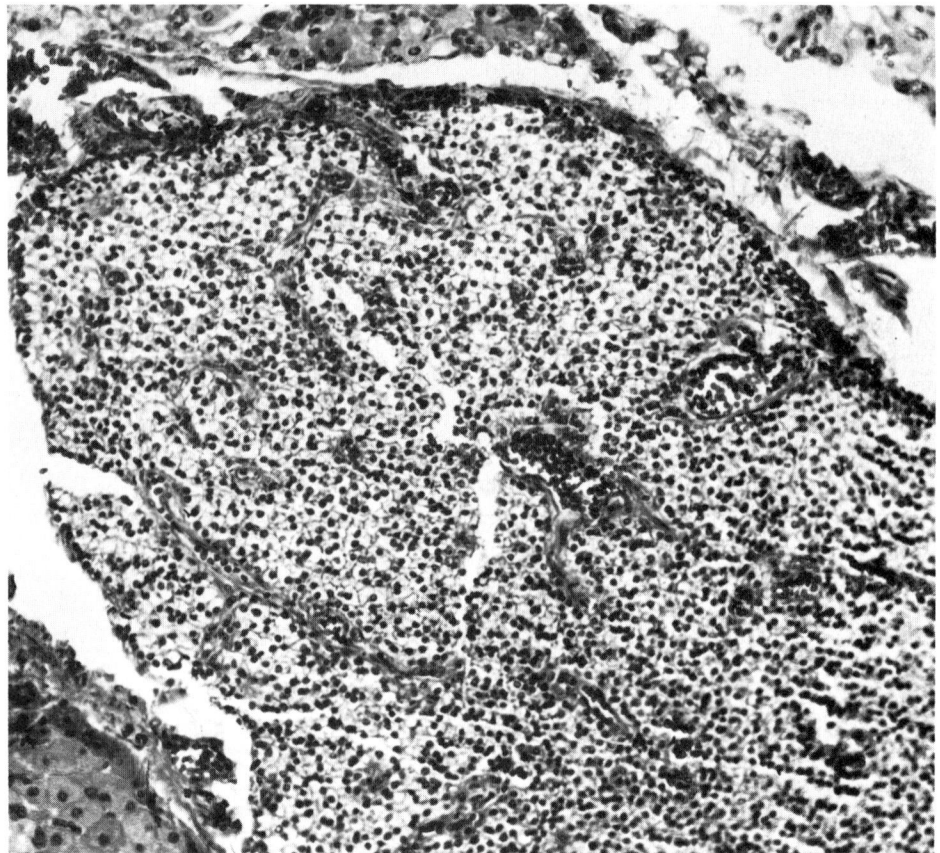

Figure 9–1

Figure 9–1. This photomicrograph illustrates the typical histologic appearance of the parathyroid gland during late fetal life and early infancy. There is no adipose tissue within the gland, and its capsule is extremely delicate. (Note the brown fat cells in clusters about the periphery, at the top and lower left.)

All of the constituent cells of the parathyroid look the same, with centrally placed nucleus, clear cytoplasm and a sharply delineated cell border.

The patient was a two week old black female, said to have been born prematurely. Her body weight at autopsy was 1,600 grams.

Hematoxylin and eosin stain. Mag. 186×.

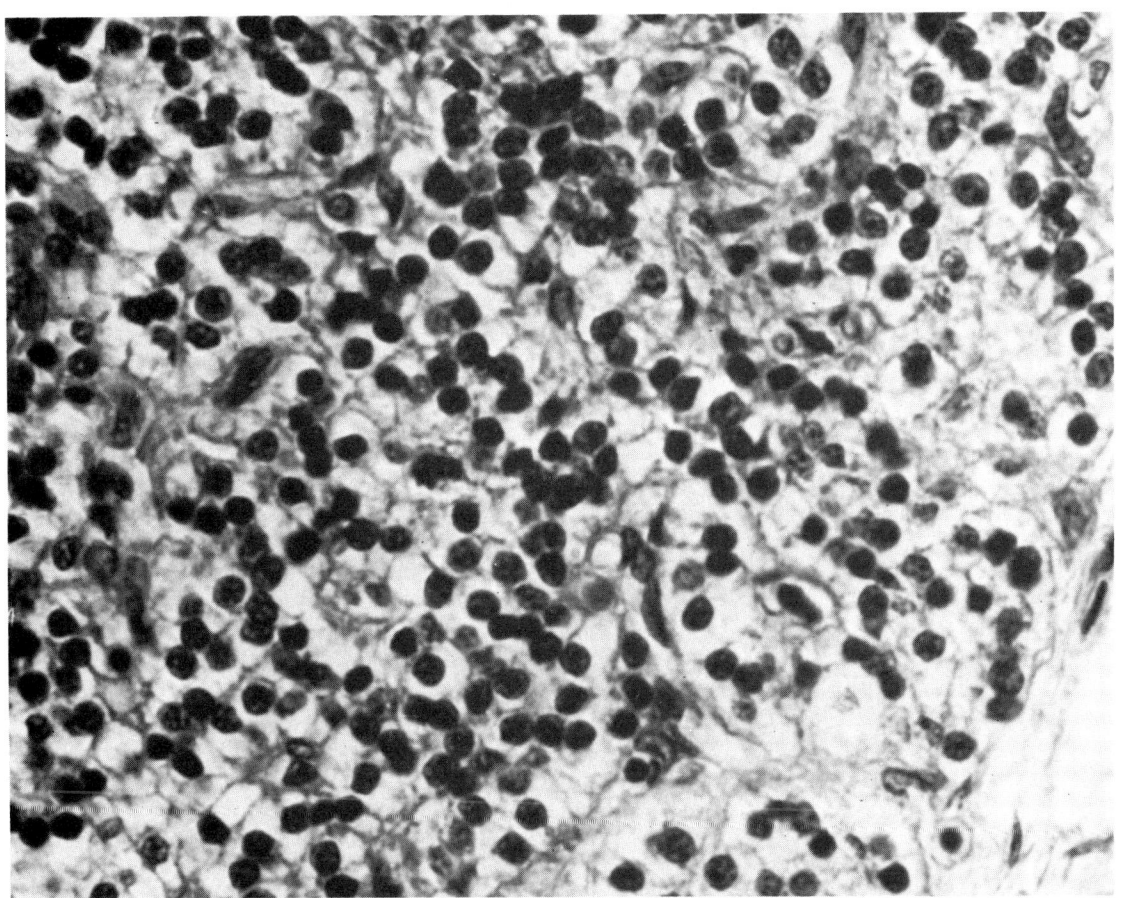

Figure 9-2

Figure 9-2. The individual cells of the parathyroid during the perinatal period are seen here at much higher magnification. Note the round, darkly stained nucleus in each, and the clear, almost unstained cytoplasm. Cell margins are delicately and sharply demarcated.

The cord- or plate-like arrangement of these cells that is apparent in the adult is not present during the perinatal period.

The subject was a female infant, 21 hours of age at death. Her body weight at postmortem examination was 1,270 grams.

Hematoxylin and eosin stain. Mag. 660×.

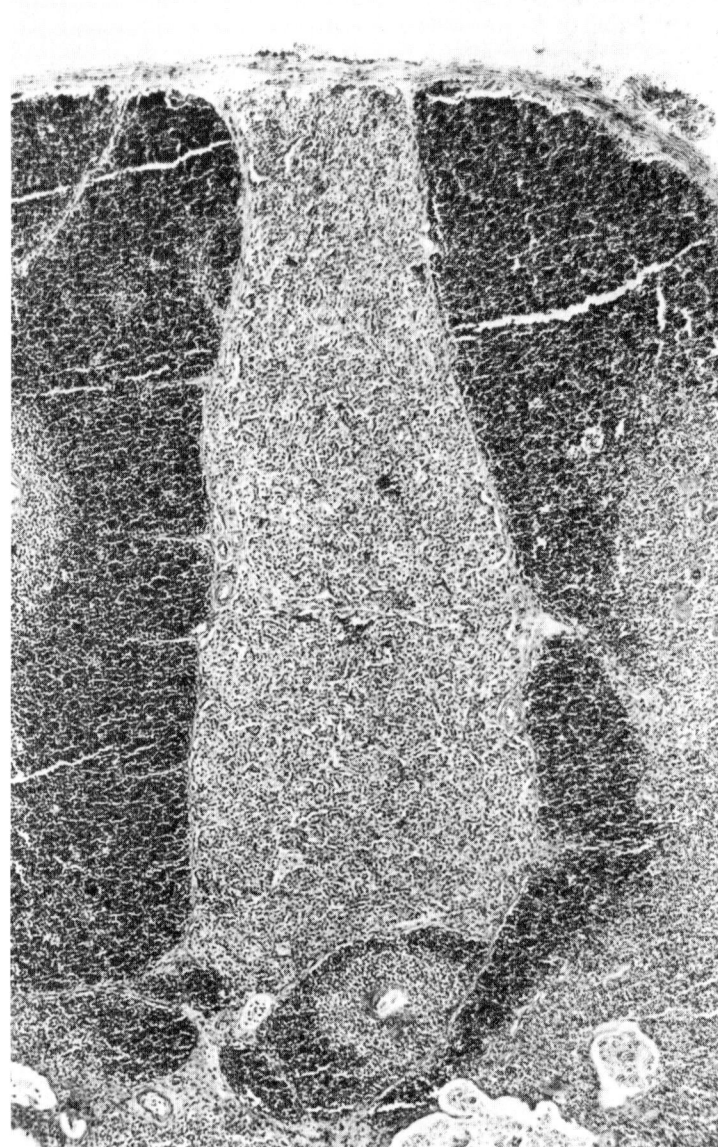

Figure 9-3

Figure 9-3. Rather frequently, one or several parathyroids will be embedded within "aberrant" nodules of thymic tissue in the neck of the infant, in the vicinity of the thyroid. Often they can be seen with the naked eye as coral-colored plaques of rounded shape just beneath the thymic capsule (of a slightly darker as well as different color from the pallid thymic tissue).

Sometimes the clue is the presence of petechiae in the parathyroid—a very common marker for that organ in the newborn.

In this instance, the parathyroid is embedded so very deeply that it is doubtful that it would have been detected from without, even with the use of a dissecting microscope.

This is from a 2 month old white female who succumbed to crib death. The body weight at autopsy was 3,046 grams. (Estimated gestational age: 30 weeks.)

Hematoxylin and eosin stain. Mag. 51×.

In fetuses and newborns the glomerular zone fairly commonly exhibits a series of spaces, round to oval or quite irregular in shape, which lend it a glandular appearance (Figs. 10–13 and 10–14). This alteration has been referred to as an "adenoid" change. The spaces contain a slightly proteinaceous fluid and seem to be lined by a single layer of cortical cells of cuboidal to low columnar character.

Just central to the glomerular zone, a fasciculate zone may be recognizable at times (Fig. 10–5).

The fetal cortex itself is composed of anastomosing columns of polyhedral cells; the cells appear either singly on the columns or, at times, in pairs. The columns radiate away from the central vessels toward the periphery and are separated from one another by sinusoids lined by flattened littoral cells (Figs. 10–9 and 10–10).

Giant cortical cells are occasionally observed within the fetal cortex (Figs. 10–11 and 10–12). They and their nuclei may be as much as three times the size of their neighbors. These cytomegalic cells appear more frequently toward the center of the gland; they are encountered more often in smaller fetuses than in infants at term. Such giant cells are apparently a normal part of the evolution of the early fetal cortex but fail to disappear, for reasons unknown, in certain instances. Although their numbers are great in a few recognized pathologic states such as congenital adrenal hypoplasia, one cannot explain their presence in most cases. (They are not related to cytomegalic inclusion disease.)

Islands of hematopoietic cells may be found between the columns of the fetal cortex, especially in premature infants (Fig. 10–15).

Spherical to oval extracapsular nodules of cortical tissue (Fig. 10–16) are observed fairly frequently, both grossly and microscopically, in fetuses and infants.

Accessory nodules of adrenal cortical tissue, adjacent to the main gland, as above, or near the genital organs are among the most familiar of heterotopic tissues (Fig. 26–17, p. 460).

The aberrant tissue usually occurs as a discrete, encapsulated, round yellow nodule about 2 to 3 millimeters in diameter. Many are identified around the upper pole of the kidney, near the hilus of the ovary in the female, and along the course of the spermatic cord in the male down to the hilus of the testis (where they are apt to be discovered by surgeons in the course of hernia repair and/or orchidopexy).

The explanation for the genital relationships is the fact that the embryonic adrenal cortical rudiment is close to the genital ridge, and thus accessory cortical nodules can easily be carried caudally with the descent of the gonad and its ducts.[4]

In virtually all instances the nodule consists of cortical tissue only, which is without distinct zones and is composed of cells resembling those of the zona glomerulosa or zona fascicularis.

The medulla of the adrenal in the perinatal period is exceedingly scanty; there may be none apparent in numbers of sections taken from a normal gland.

The irregular small cells of the medulla are arranged in rounded, rather ill-defined groups; they tend to be more darkly stained and smaller than adjacent cells of the cortex (Fig. 10–5).

Within the fetal adrenal medulla and scattered through the cortex may occur clusters of small round cells with dense, darkly stained nuclei, the sympathochromaffin cells (Fig. 10–18). These cells migrate, during this period of life, from the perimeter to the center of the organ; they are the forerunners of the sympathetic and medullary cells.

References

1. Warwick, R., and Williams, P. L.: Gray's Anatomy, 35th British ed. Philadelphia, W. B. Saunders Co., 1973, p. 144.
2. Arey, L. B.: Developmental Anatomy. A Textbook and Laboratory Manual of Embryology, 7th ed., revised. Philadelphia, W. B. Saunders Co., 1974, pp. 518–519.
3. Benner, M. C.: Studies on involution of the fetal cortex of the adrenal glands. Am. J. Path., *16*:787–798, 1940.
4. Willis, R. A.: The Borderland of Embryology and Pathology. London, Butterworth and Co., Ltd., 1958, p. 111.

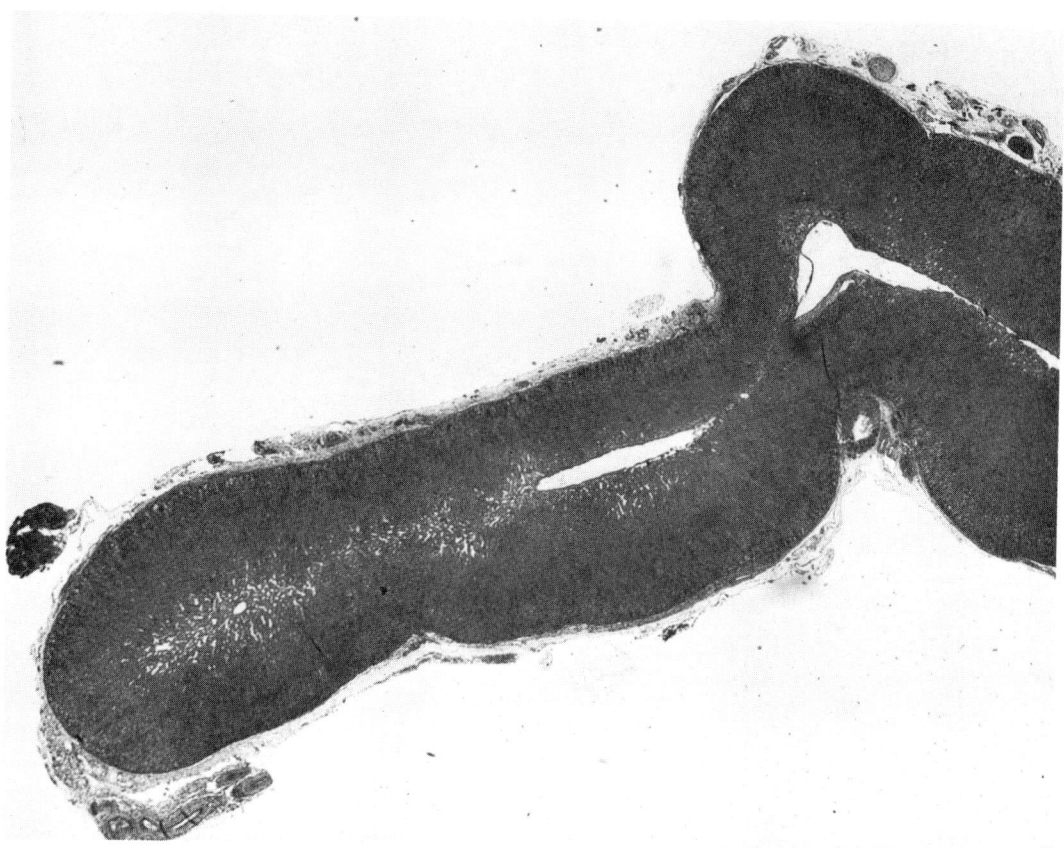

Figure 10–1

Figures 10–1 and 10–2. These two photographs illustrate, at very low magnification, the histologic appearance of the adrenal in the perinatal period. Even at this magnification, particularly in Fig. 10–2, one can appreciate the breadth of the so-called fetal cortex (extending from the apex of one white arrow above to that of the other below — center of photo) as well as the "adenoid" alteration in the subcapsular portion of the definitive or adult cortex (black arrow).

Figure 10–1. This is a section of the adrenal from a prematurely born male infant who survived for 14½ hours and whose body weight at autopsy was 1,570 grams. (Estimated gestational age: 29 weeks.) The bulk of the visible cortex here is fetal cortex; the distinction between that which is fetal and that which is adult is apparent over the vertex of the bulge in the upper right corner of the photograph.

Hematoxylin and eosin stain. Mag. 18.8×.

Figure 10-2. This is a section of the adrenal gland from a male liveborn infant who died with pulmonary hyaline membrane disease at the age of 13 hours. His body weight at necropsy was 1,360 grams. (Estimated gestational age: 28 weeks.)
Hematoxylin and eosin stain. Mag. 18.8×.

See illustration on the opposite page

ADRENAL GLAND 137

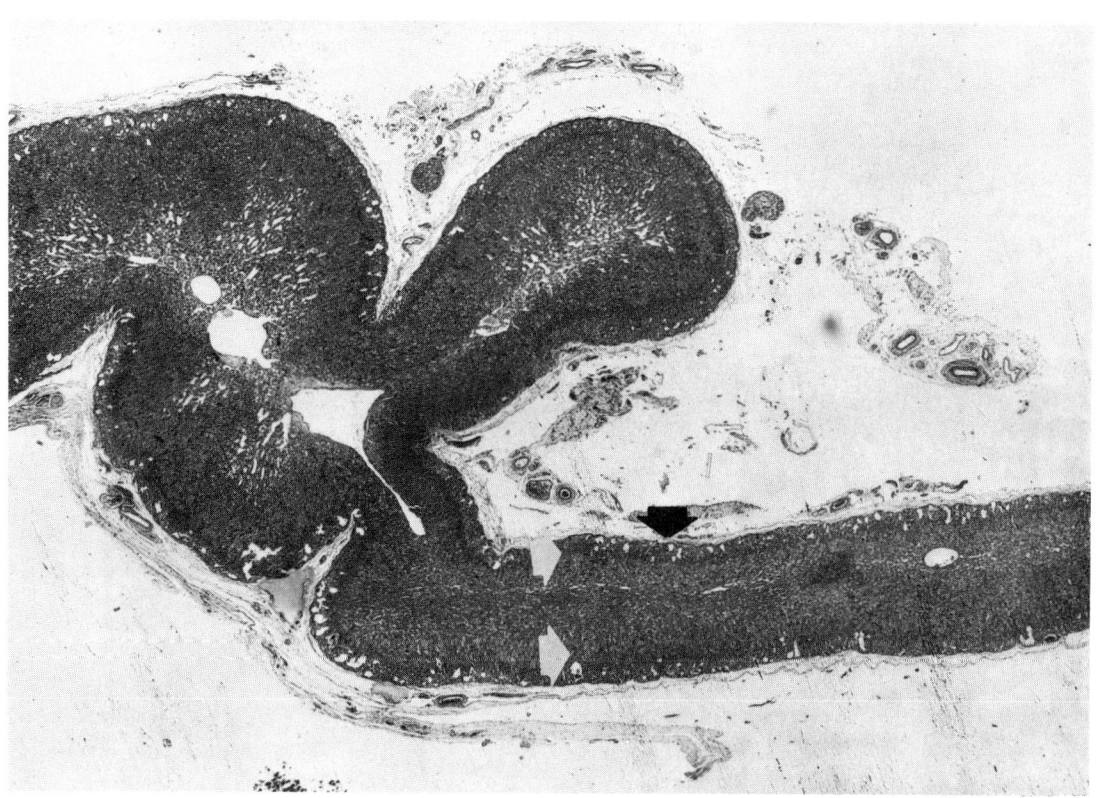

Figure 10-2

See legend on the opposite page

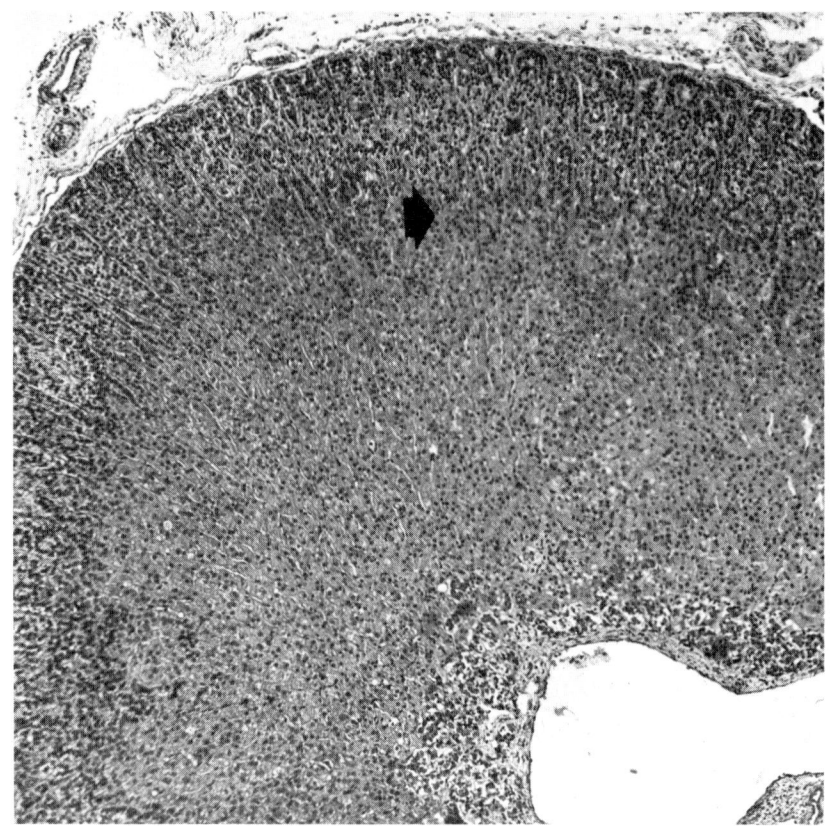

Figure 10-3

Figures 10-3 to 10-5. These three photomicrographs illustrate, at somewhat higher magnification, the histologic architecture of the adrenal during the perinatal period. The line of demarcation between fetal and adult cortex is indicated in each by a black arrow.

The clusters of small dark cells around the central vein in Figs. 10-3 and 10-5 represent medulla, of which there is relatively little at this age.

Figure 10-3. This is a detailed view of the breadth of the gland at medium magnification, from the central vein (lower right) to the capsule (top). The cells extending from the black arrow upward to the capsule constitute the definitive cortex, and those from the arrow downward to the clusters of small, darkly stained cells around the central vein are fetal cortex.

Hematoxylin and eosin stain. Mag. 100×.

Figures 10-4 and 10-5. These two illustrations, both taken at slightly higher magnification than Fig. 10-3, show the difference between the histologic appearance of the cortex of the adrenal of a small infant (1,360 grams) and that of a term infant (2,875 grams).

Fig.	Wt.	Sex	Est. Gestation	Age
10-3	1,570 gm.	M	30 wk.	14.5 hr.
10-4	1,360 gm.	M	28 wk.	13 hr.
10-5	2,875 gm.	F	40 wk.	17 hr.

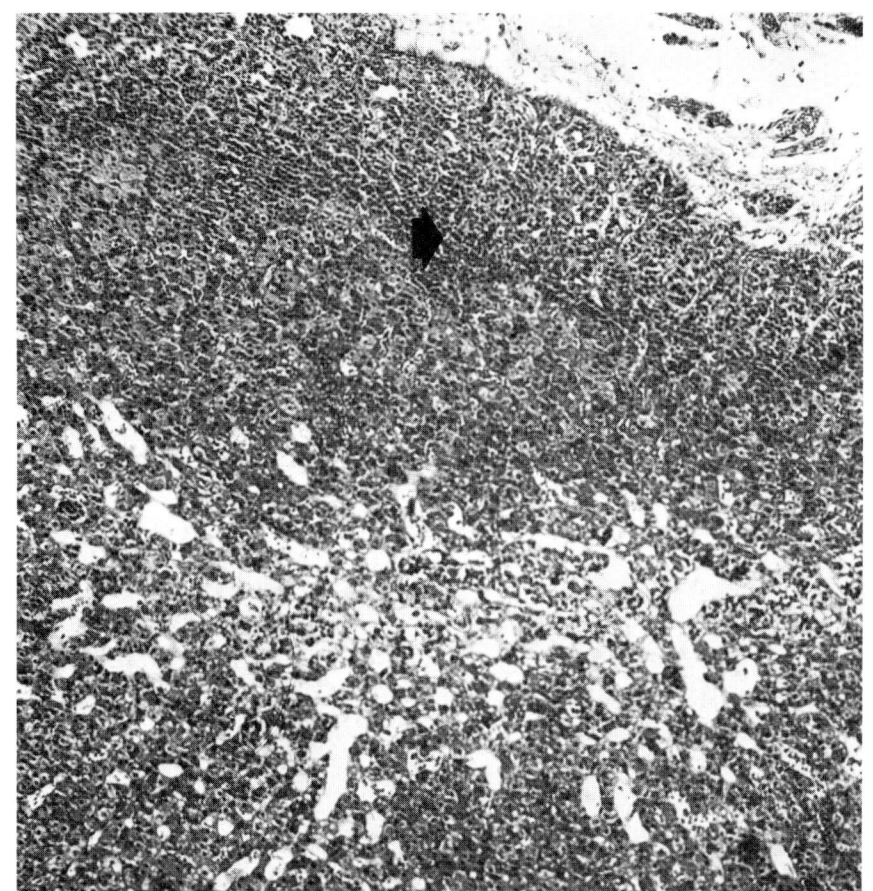

Figure 10-4

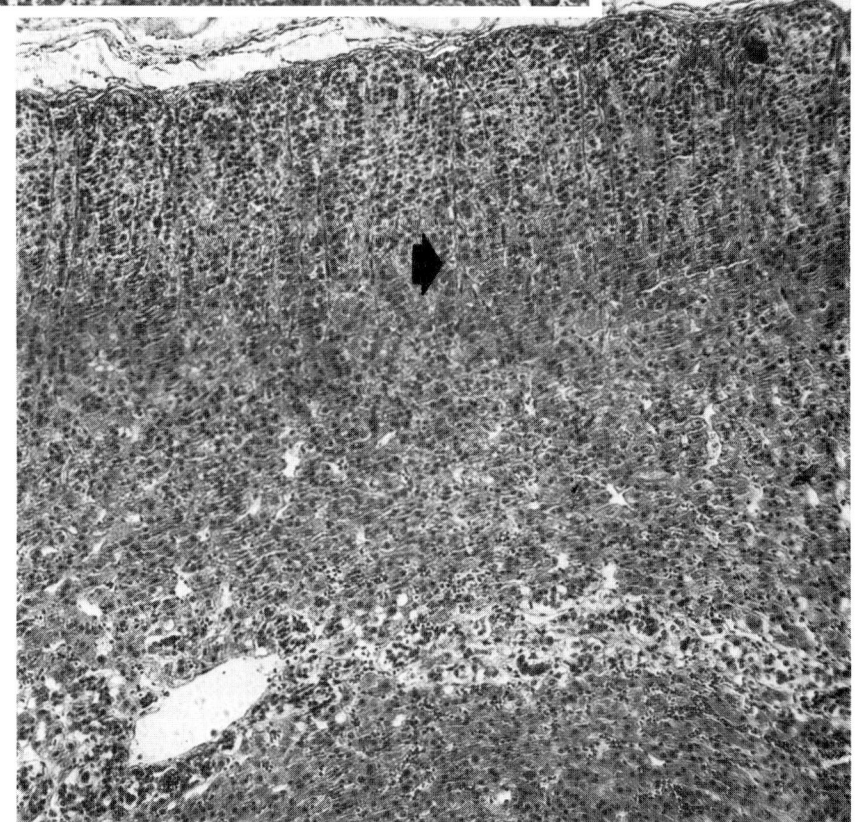

Figure 10-5

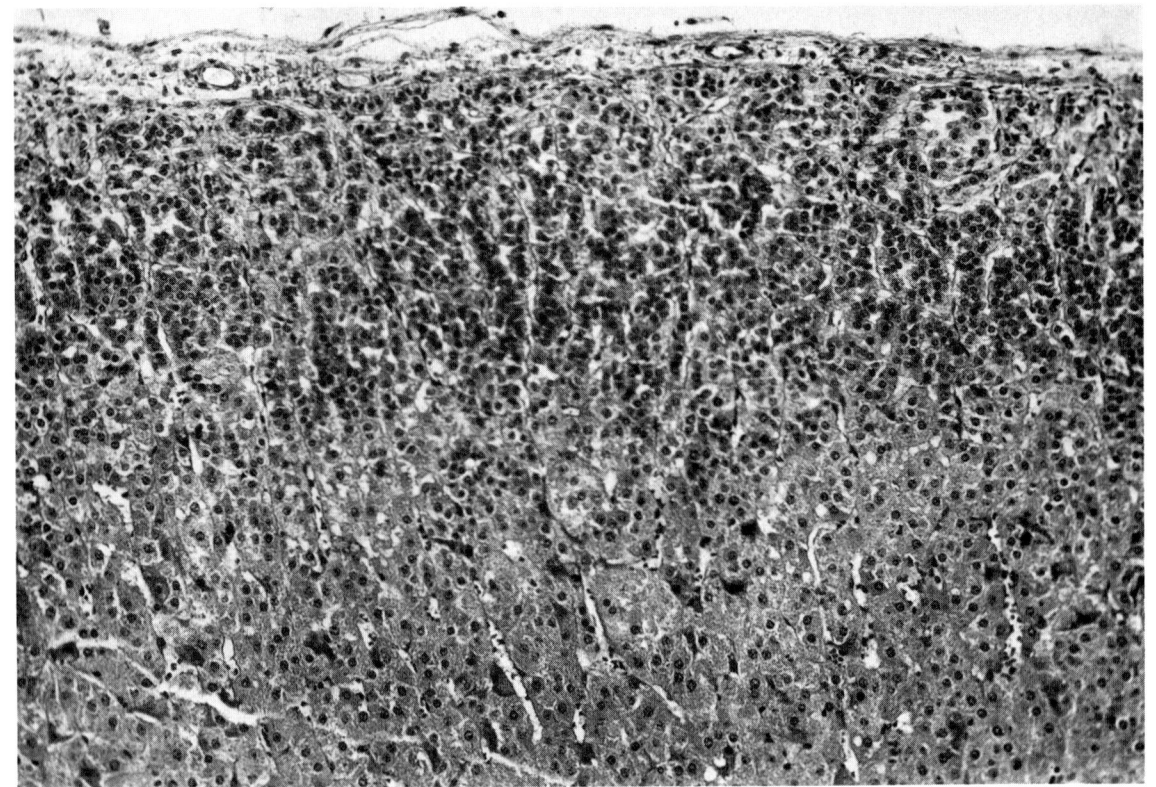

Figure 10–6

Figures 10–6 to 10–8. This set of three illustrations, taken at progressively increasing magnification, depicts the more intimate details of the adult or definitive cortex. (In Figs. 10–6 and 10–7, it occupies approximately the upper half of the picture; in Fig. 10–8 it is slightly more than that.)

Figure 10–6. This represents much of the breadth of the adrenal cortex of a 930 gram female liveborn infant who died at 8¼ hours of age. (Gestation: 28 weeks.)
Hematoxylin and eosin stain. Mag. 142×.

Figure 10–7. The lighter staining cells beneath the capsule are the adult cortex; most superficially they do have a rather "glomerular" aspect. This is a section from the adrenal of a black female infant who lived for 2 days, 1 hour and 4 minutes. Her birth weight was 6 pounds and 1 ounce and her weight at autopsy was 2,610 grams. (Estimated gestational age: 34 weeks.)
Hematoxylin and eosin stain. Mag. 219×.

Figure 10–8. The adult cortex of a 7 day old male infant whose body weight at postmortem examination was 1,965 grams. (Estimated gestational age: 31 weeks.)
Hematoxylin and eosin stain. Mag. 330×.

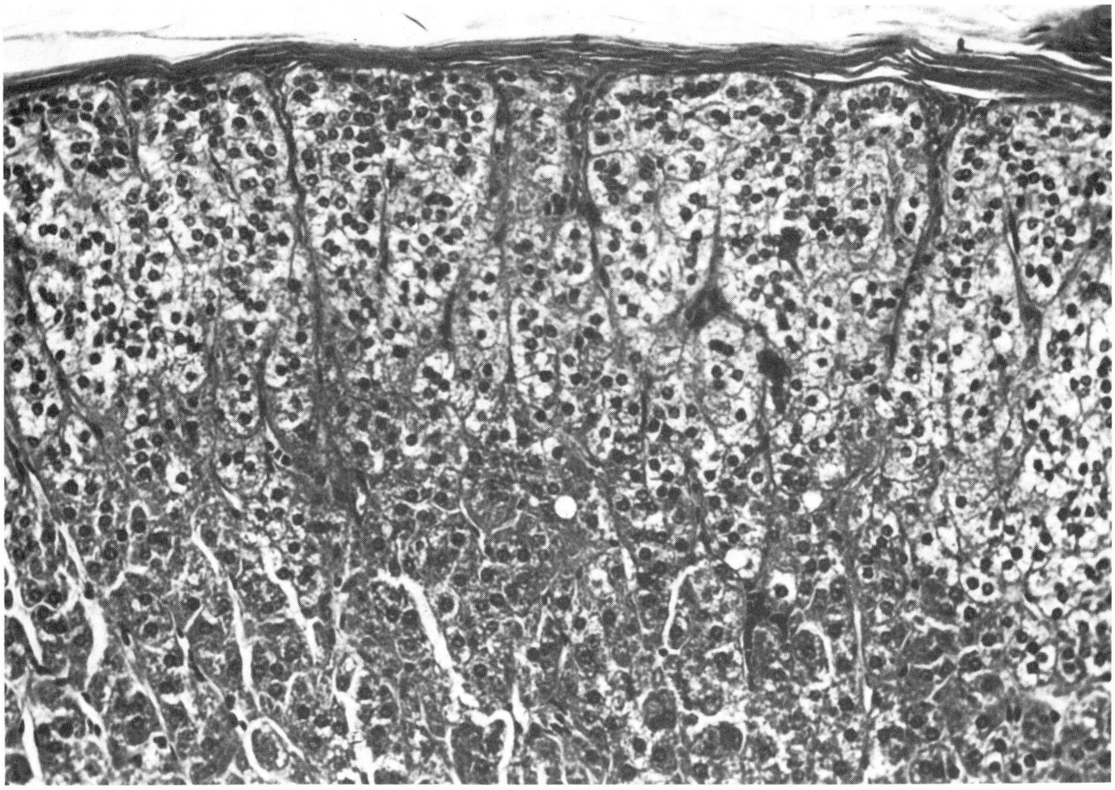

Figure 10-7

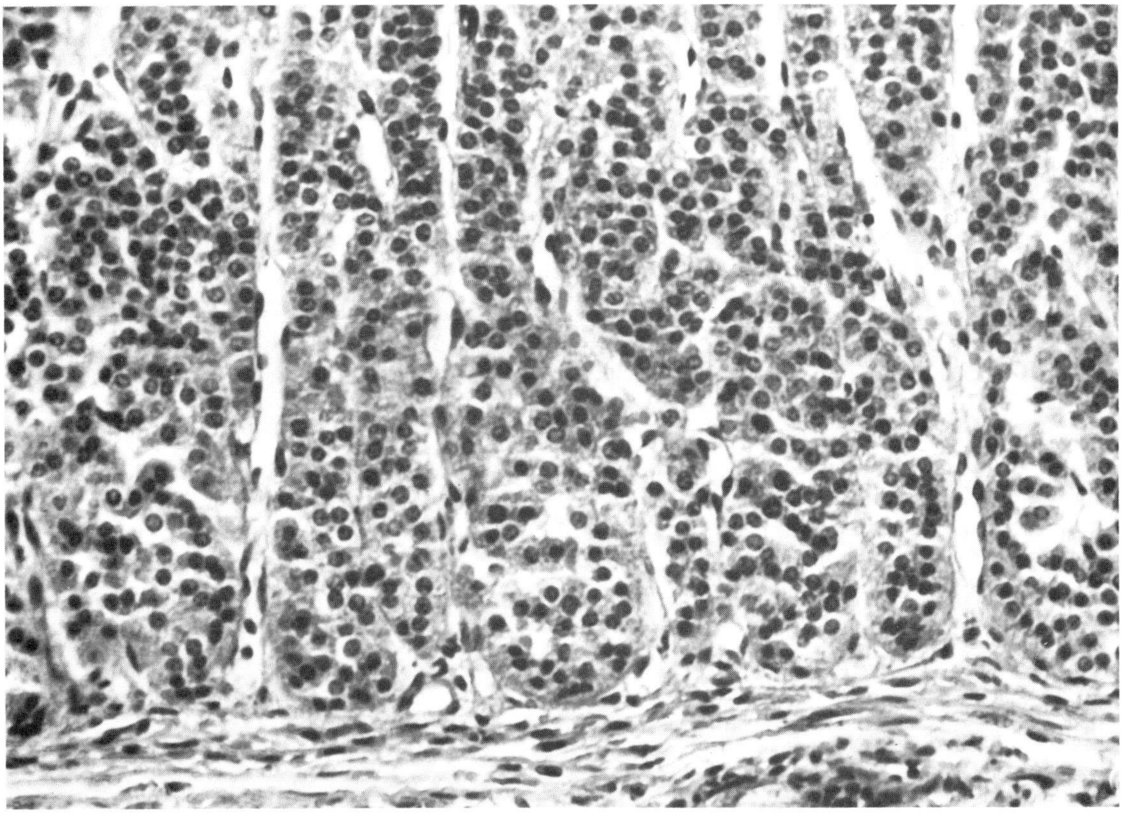

Figure 10-8

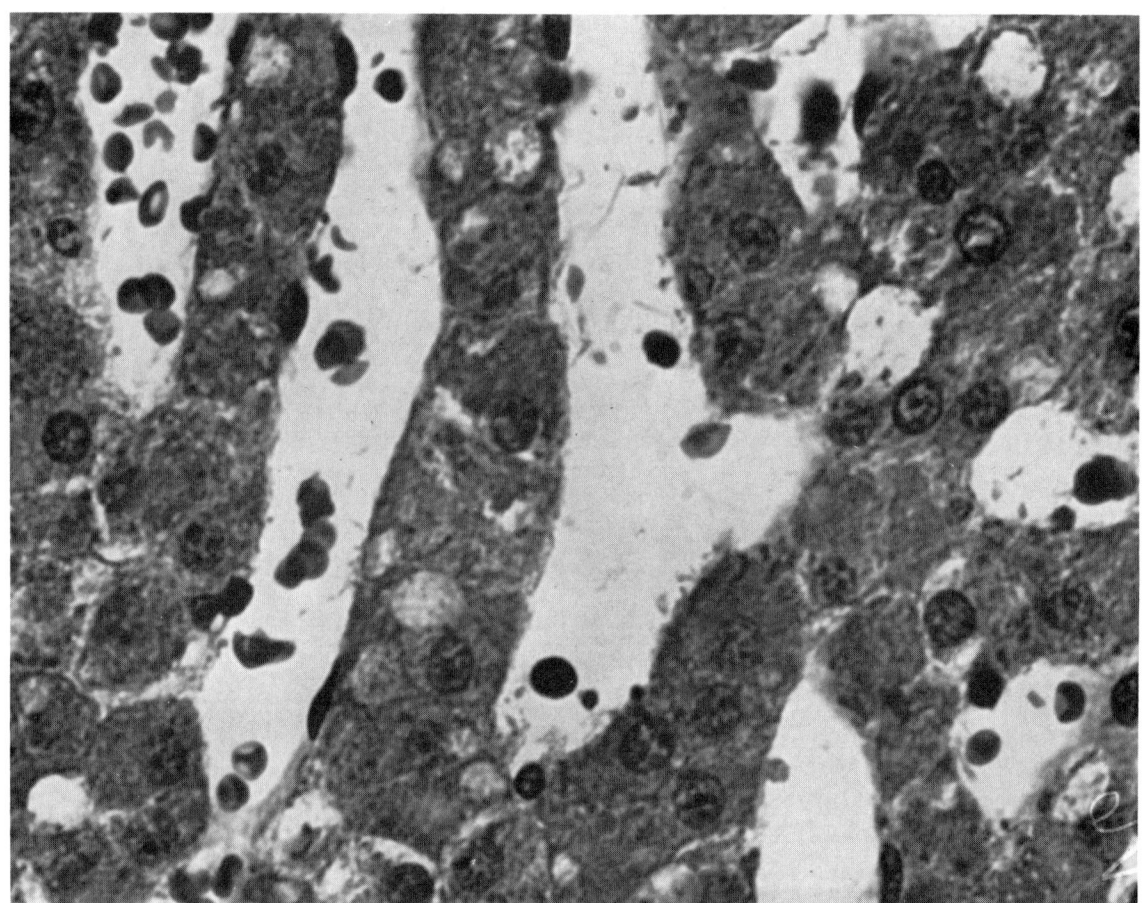

Figure 10–9

Figure 10–9. The columns of cells in the mid-cortex (fetal) of an immature infant are seen here in some detail. The columns are one to two cells in thickness and separated from each other by slender sinusoids, here abnormally dilated.

This is a section from the adrenal of 510 gram male infant born at 24 weeks of gestation, who died at 1 hour of age.

Hematoxylin and eosin stain. Mag. 660×.

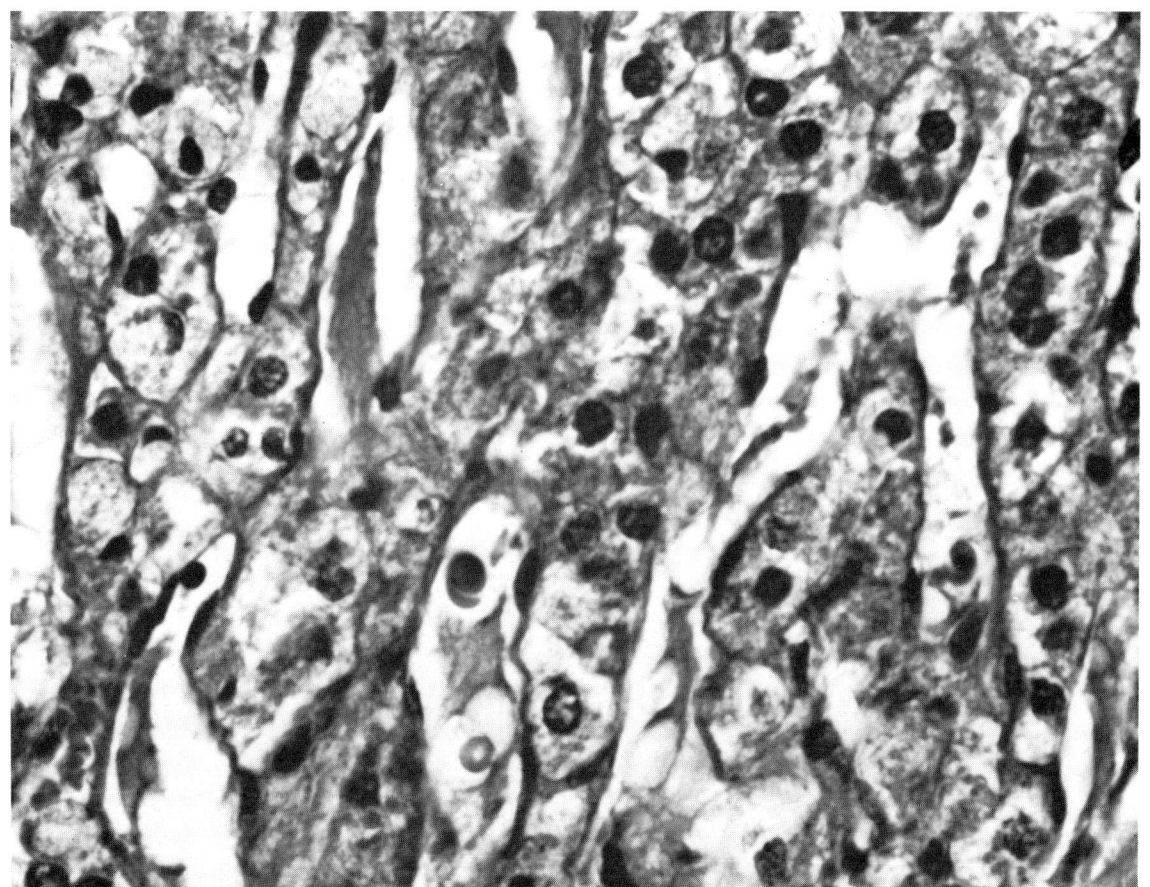

Figure 10–10

Figure 10–10. Frequently the cells of the fetal cortex, as seen at autopsy, have rather more clear or vacuolated cytoplasm than is seen in the cells of Fig. 10–9. This illustration depicts such an instance.

It is evident in both of these illustrations that the sinusoids are lined by very flat littoral cells.

This is representative of the adrenal cortex of a term infant. This male liveborn infant, whose body weight at necropsy was 3,100 grams, lived for 5 days and died as the result of multiple congenital anomalies.

Hematoxylin and eosin stain. Mag. 660×.

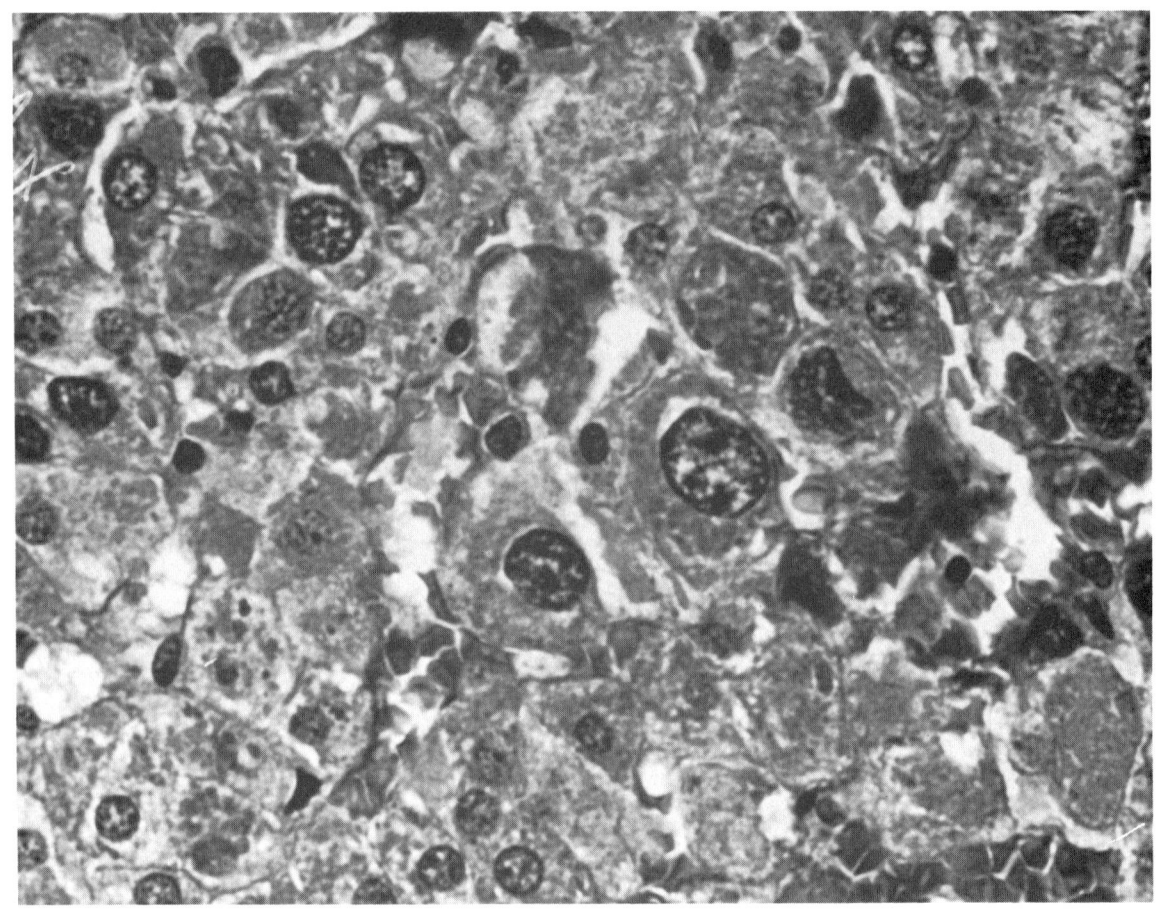

Figure 10–11

Figure 10–11. Disproportionately large cells are encountered fairly commonly in the adrenal cortex during late fetal life and early infancy; the more immature the fetus, as a matter of fact, the more frequently they are apt to be seen. They tend to be more numerous centrally. They are apparently part of the normal maturation process, but fail to disappear at times and especially in certain pathologic states, e.g., congenital adrenal hypoplasia. (They are not related to cytomegalic inclusion disease.)

Near the center of this photomicrograph are seen two such large cells with prominent nuclei. Identification of the infant from whom this section was taken has proved to be impossible. Hematoxylin and eosin stain. Mag. 660×.

ADRENAL GLAND 145

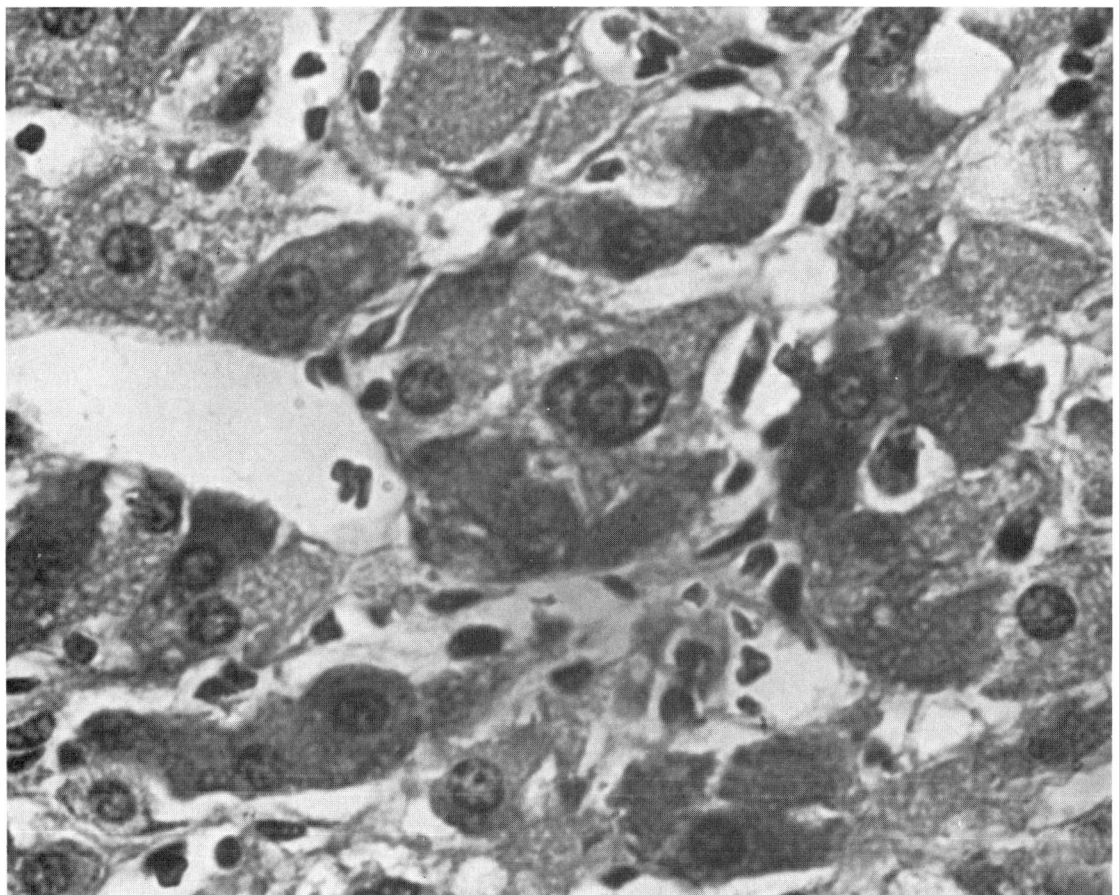

Figure 10–12

Figure 10–12. Again, near the center of this photograph is one large cortical cell, its nucleus being about three times the size of any of the neighboring nuclei.

This section is from the adrenal of a black male infant born at term, who weighed 2,850 grams at postmortem examination. He lived for 1 day, 1 hour and 30 minutes and died of massive pulmonary hemorrhage.

Hematoxylin and eosin stain. Mag. 660×.

ADRENAL GLAND

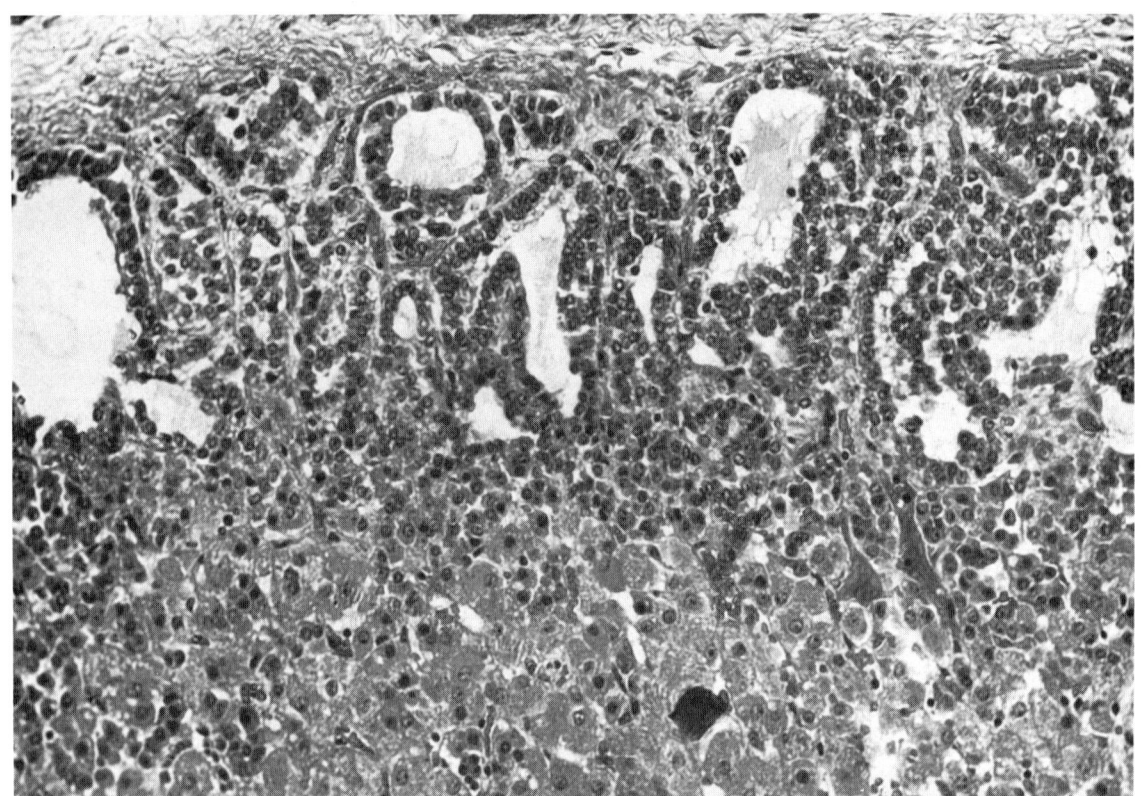

Figure 10–13

Figures 10–13 and 10–14. In the subcapsular portion of the cortex of the infant's adrenal there is apt to be an opening up of spaces which appear to contain lightly proteinaceous fluid and which seem to be completely encircled by a single layer of cuboidal cortical epithelial cells. The phenomenon, sometimes referred to as an "adenoid" change, is usually generalized, encompassing the entire gland. A number of investigators have attempted to determine the cause for this alteration but its genesis is not yet clearly understood.

Figure 10–13. This is a section of the definitive, subcapsular portion of the adrenal cortex of a two hour old black female infant whose body weight at autopsy was only 660 grams. (The stated gestational age was 5 months.) This infant died with early bronchopneumonia.
Hematoxylin and eosin stain. Mag. 219×.

ADRENAL GLAND 147

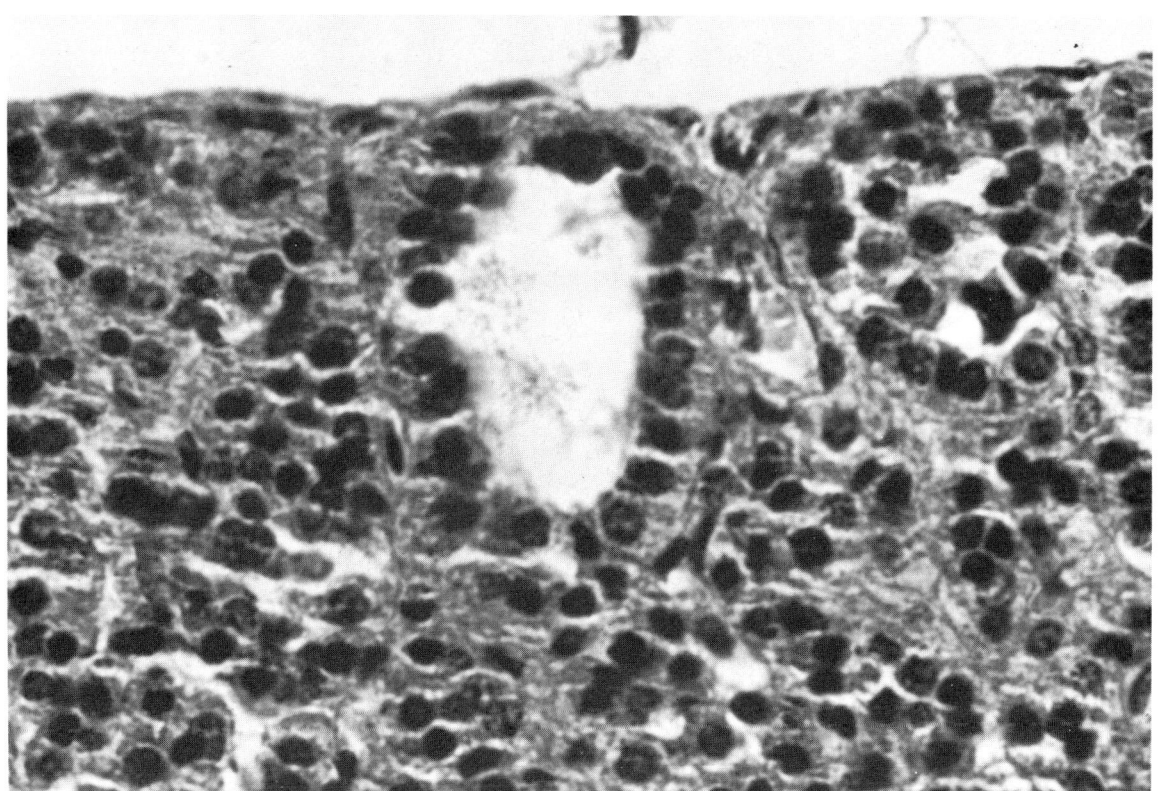

Figure 10-14

Figure 10-14. One such "adenoid" space is seen here at higher magnification. This is from a section of the adrenal of a 7 day old black male infant whose estimated gestational age was 27 weeks, and who weighed 1,100 grams at autopsy.
Hematoxylin and eosin stain. Mag. 639×.

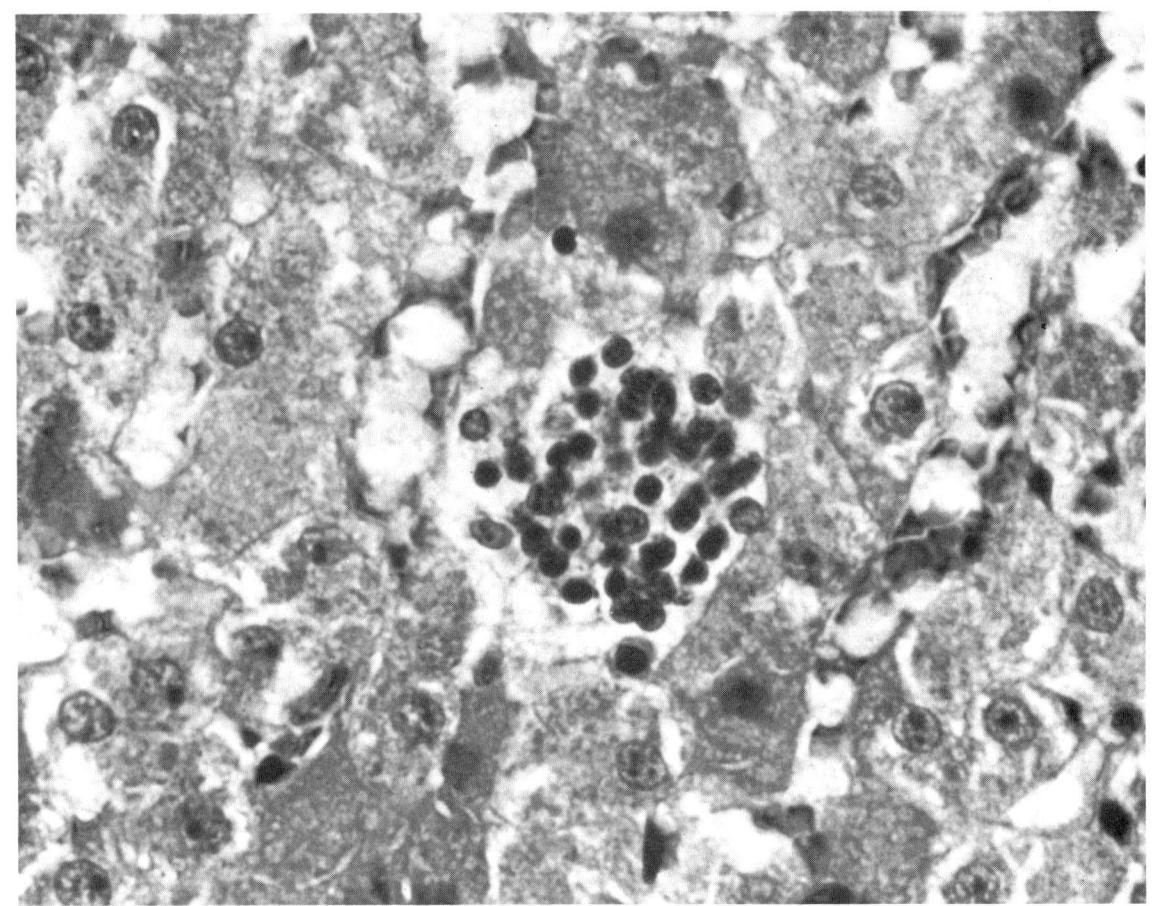

Figure 10–15

Figure 10–15. Especially in the premature infant, there is apt to be extramedullary hematopoiesis, occurring in focal nests between columns of cortical cells. One such cluster of hematopoietic elements is depicted in the center of this photograph.

This section was taken from the adrenal of a newborn infant, the product of a 29 week gestation, who lived for 18 hours and whose body weight at postmortem examination was 1,895 grams.

Hematoxylin and eosin stain. Mag. 660×.

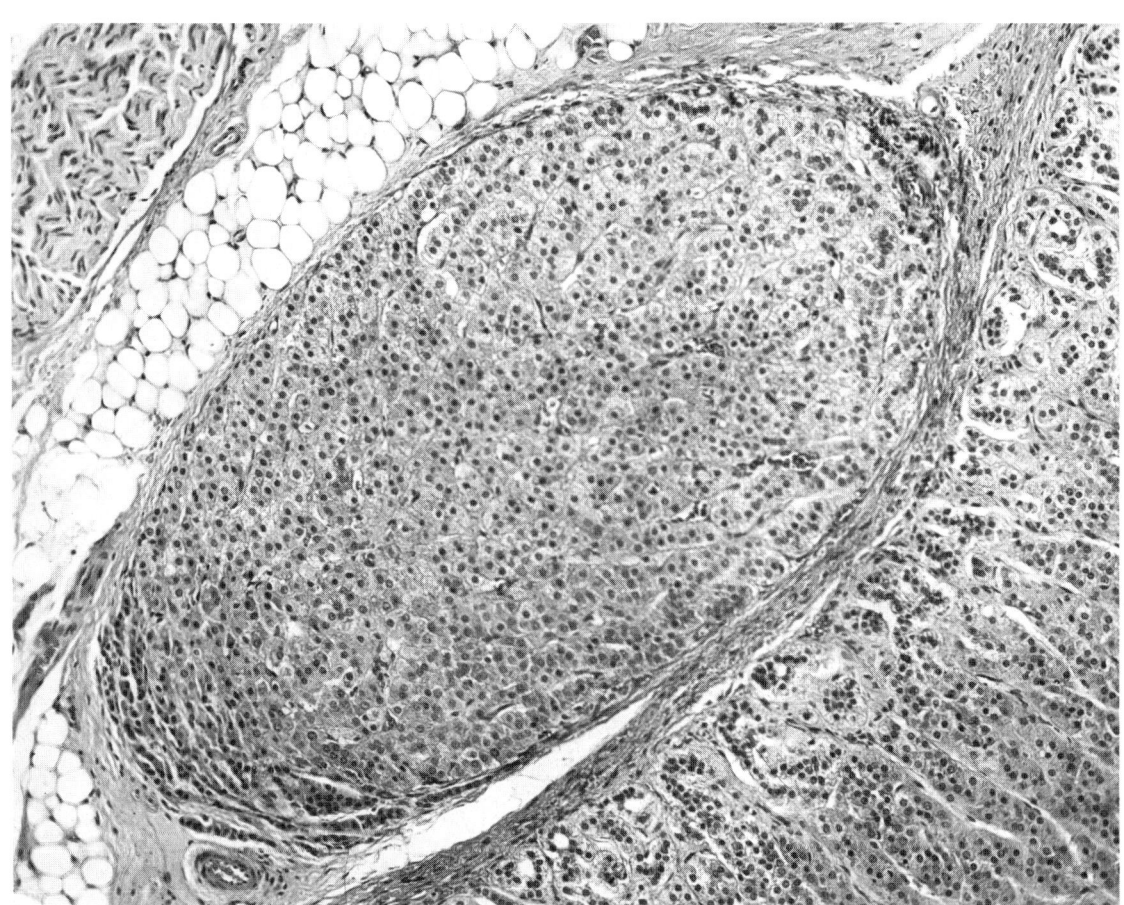

Figure 10–16

Figure 10–16. Even at the autopsy table, careful inspection of the neonatal adrenal gland at times reveals tiny, yellow, oval to spherical nodules of cortical tissue apparently attached to the capsule of the gland proper. Each nodule seems to have its own delicate capsule, and each is approximately 1 mm. or less in diameter. One has the impression that they are rather loosely attached or could easily be dissected away, leaving the major gland intact.

This photomicrograph illustrates one such pericapsular adrenal cortical nodule, from a three year old child.

Hematoxylin and eosin stain. Mag. 142×.

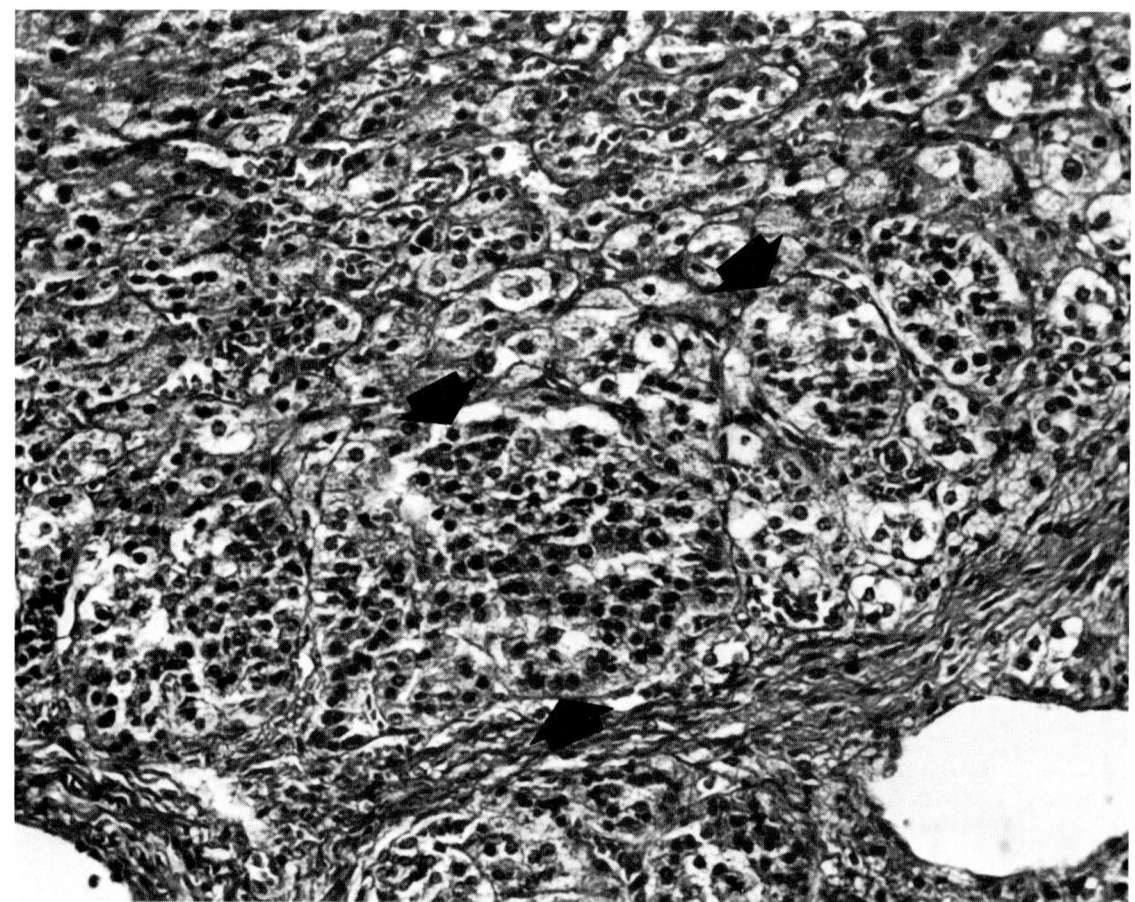

Figure 10-17

Figure 10-17. The adrenal medulla is relatively inconspicuous in the neonate and particularly in the premature infant. It appears as little sharply circumscribed clumps of tiny, darkly stained cells scattered at irregular intervals immediately adjacent to the central vein. In several sections of any given gland no such clumps of cells may be represented. In this illustration the three black arrows indicate two of the clusters (at least four are apparent). Portions of the central vein are seen in the right and left lower corners, and the larger paler staining cells of the cortex along the top.

This section is from the adrenal of a 9 month old white female whose weight at autopsy was 8,000 grams.

Hematoxylin and eosin stain. Mag. 225×.

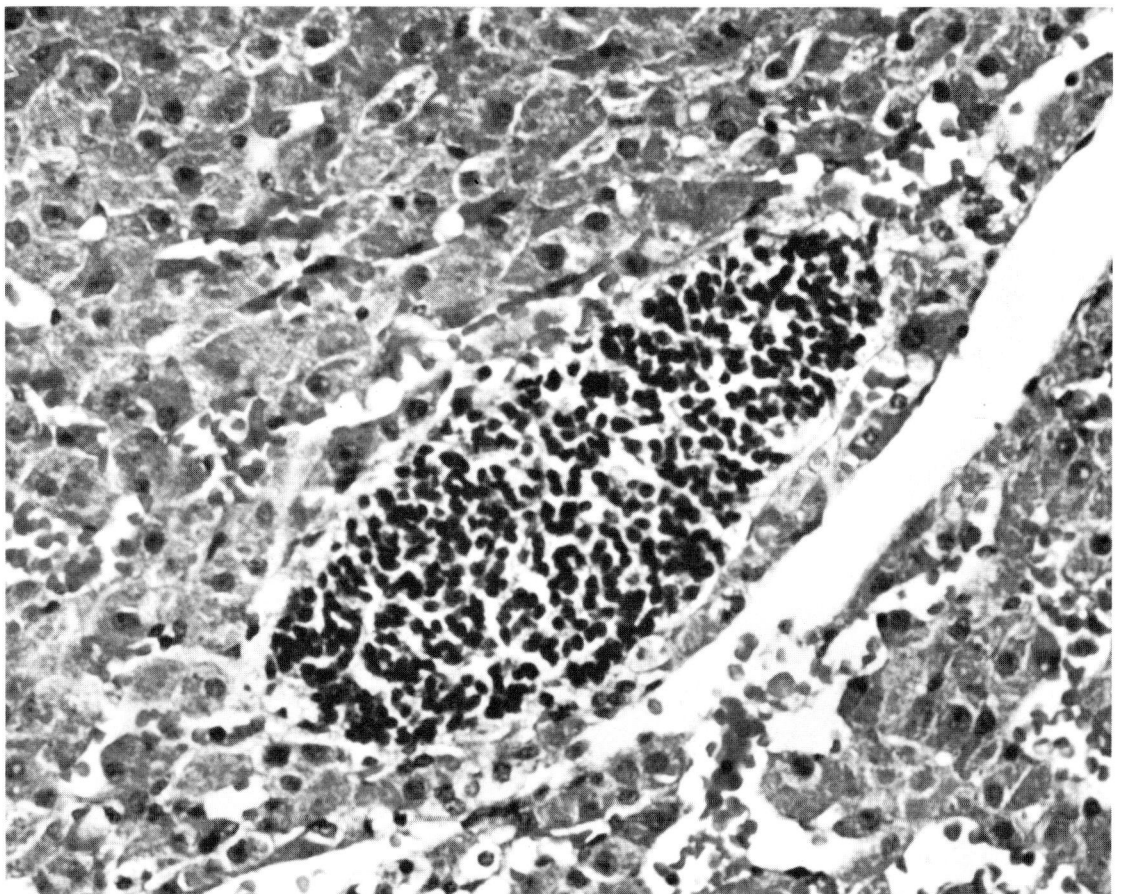

Figure 10–18

Figure 10–18. Sympathochromaffin cells, the predecessors of the adrenal medulla, actually migrate through the cortex during late fetal life. At autopsy one can occasionally see a cluster of them, such as is depicted here. Their histologic appearance is reminiscent of that of the neuroblastoma, and in the past they have occasionally been so misdiagnosed (neuroblastoma-in-situ) when in fact they are a morphologic feature of the normally developing gland.

Unfortunately, the label for this microscopic slide was lost, so its identification is impossible. Hematoxylin and eosin stain. Mag. 369×.

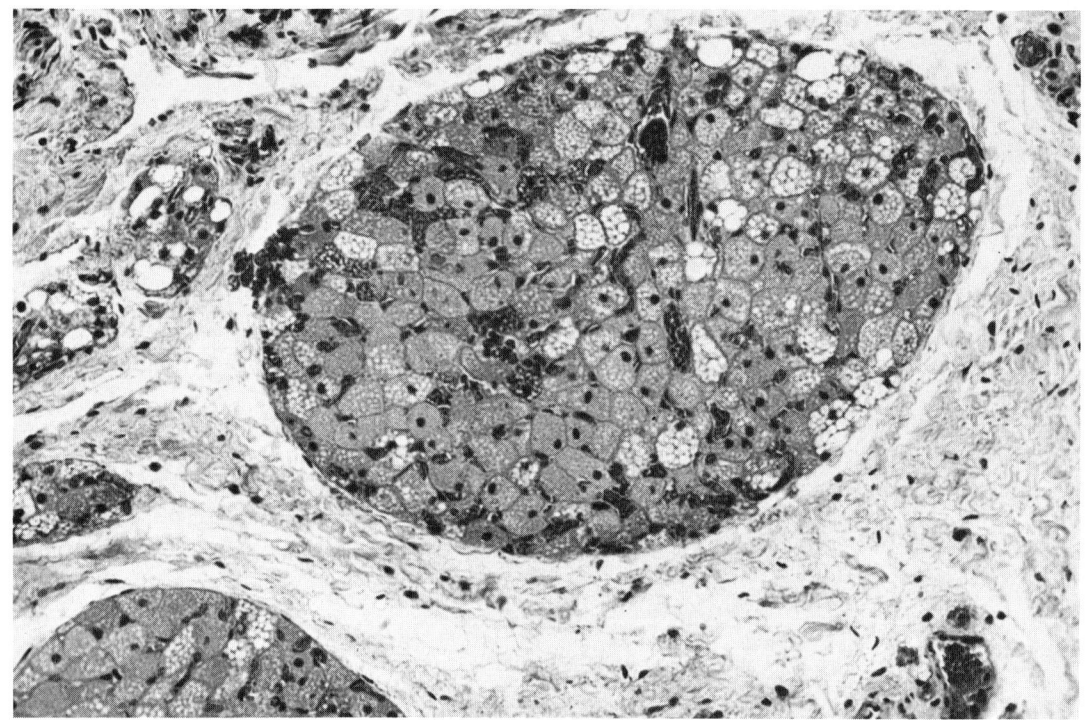

Figure 10–19

Figures 10–19 to 10–21. As is apparent in Fig. 10–1 and 10–2, the neonatal adrenal is usually surrounded by adipose tissue. In the premature infant, and to a lesser degree in the term infant, that adipose tissue is largely of the brown type. (In normal infants, this brown fat gives way—progressively—during the first year of life to white or adult fat.)

Nodules of brown fat such as that depicted in Fig. 10–19 are, at times, mistakenly considered to be accessory adrenal cortical nodules because their cells are of approximately the same size and their cytoplasm is apt to be pale staining and/or diffusely finely vacuolated.

Figure 10–19. This is a section of the periadrenal brown fat from a 3,940 gram female infant, born at 40 weeks of gestation, who died at 25 days of age.
Hematoxylin and eosin stain. Mag. 197×.

Figure 10-20

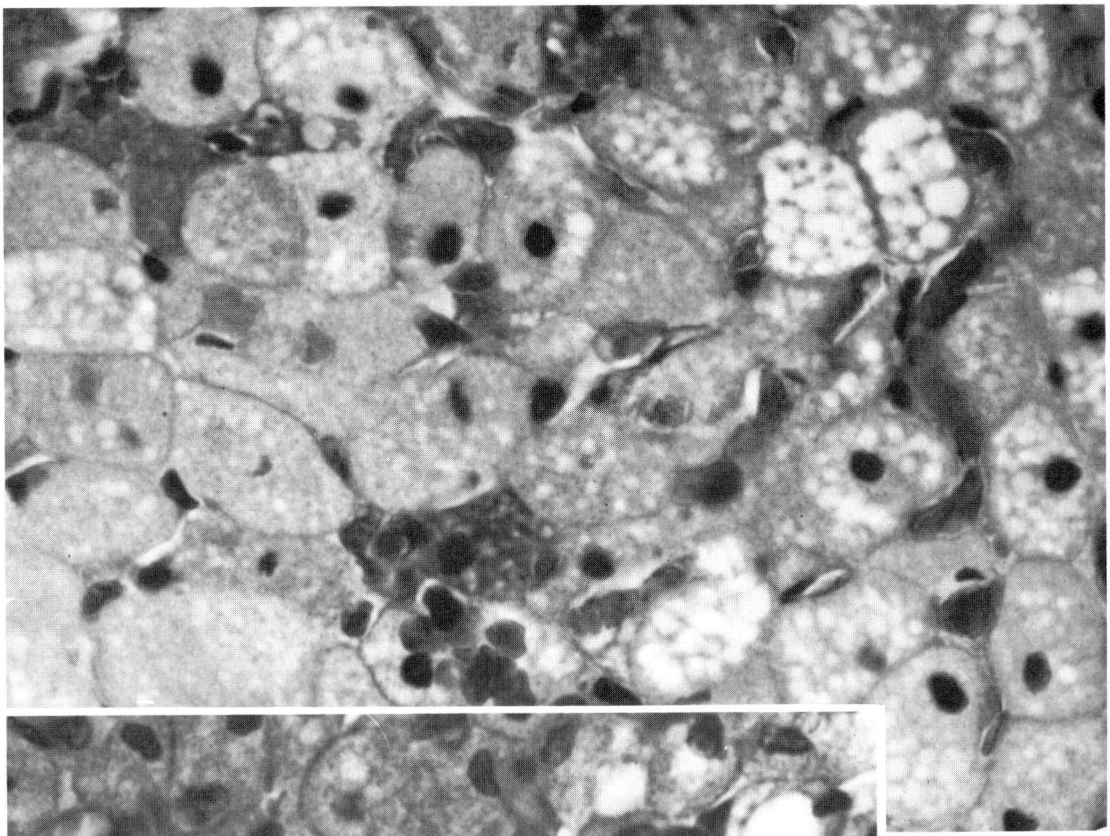

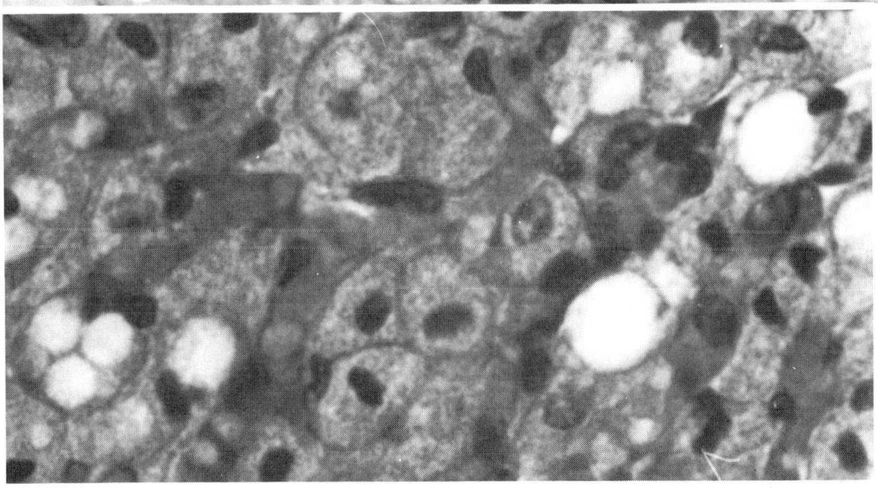

Figure 10-21

Figure 10-20. This photomicrograph is from the same histologic section as Fig. 10-19. Hematoxylin and eosin stain. Mag. 660×.

Figure 10-21. As the infant matures, brown fat cells with fine vacuolization diminish in number and are gradually replaced by cells with larger vacuoles, such as are seen here, until ultimately all of the fat at this site is of the adult type.

This is a section from a 6 day old white female neonate whose weight at autopsy was 2,800 grams. (Estimated gestational age: 35 weeks.)
Hematoxylin and eosin stain. Mag. 660×.

Part 5

SKIN

Chapter 11

SKIN

EMBRYOLOGY

The skin and subcutaneous adipose tissue increase in thickness and in weight throughout gestation up to the time of a term birth, at which point they compose 26 per cent of body weight. They show little change thereafter.[1]

The skin is of double embryonic origin. The stratified squamous epithelium, or epidermis, is derived from the general ectoderm (as distinct from that involved in the development of the nervous system). The fibrous layer, or dermis, is usually considered to have evolved from cells proliferated from the lateral walls of the paired somites. (As a consequence, the name dermatome is used for each successive region.) However, it is likely that much of the dermis must differentiate from non-specific mesenchyme subjacent to the epidermis, most of which comes from lateral sheets of somatic mesoderm.[1]

The epidermis first appears as embryonic ectoderm in the form of a single sheet of cuboidal cells. In the fifth week, a second layer is added. The outer layer is distinct but transitory and is referred to as the periderm. Its cells flatten, cornify, and eventually spread to several times the diameter of the deeper cells. The basal cells remain cuboidal. During the third and fourth months, the epidermis is typically three-layered, an intermediate stratum being gradually interposed between the basal and periderm cells.

After the fourth month the epidermis becomes increasingly stratified and specialized. The lower layers consist of living cells and the upper layers constitute the "dead skin." The basal cells and their immediate descendents in the layer just above, the stratum germinativum, are the actively dividing elements.

Pigment granules appear in the cells of the stratum germinativum of all races. They are obtained by transfer from the processes of the melanocytes. These cells migrate from the primitive neural crest tissue, invade the basal layer of the epidermis, and specialize in pigment formation. Pigment development is incomplete at birth; hence there is marked darkening of the skin of the black infant during the six or eight weeks after delivery.

When the hairs emerge, at about the sixth month of fetal life, they do not penetrate the periderm but loosen or break it. Desquamated superficial epidermal cells mingle with cast-off lanugo hairs and sebaceous secretions to form the pasty vernix caseosa which adheres, in a waxy white coat, to fetal skin. This material is said to protect the epidermis from the macerating influence that would normally be exerted by the amniotic fluid. As a lubricant, it also prevents chafing injuries from the amnion as the growing fetus becomes progressively confined in its fluid-filled sac.

The plane of union between the epidermis and dermis is smooth until early in the fourth month, when epidermal thickenings grow down into the dermis of the palms and soles. About two months later, in the sixth month, corresponding elevations first appear on the skin surface. These epidermal ridges complete their permanent, individual surfaces (e.g., fingerprints) in the second half of fetal life.[1]

Collagenous fibers of the dermis appear in the third month, and elastic fibers in the fifth month. The differentiation of collagenous fibers occurs in two phases; the first is marked by the appearance of thin fibrils resembling those of reticular tissue. In the third month those fibrils become arranged parallel to one another, and aggregate into wavy bundles with the physical and chemical characteristics of collagen. Elastic fibers differentiate later, in the fifth month, but in the same general manner. Typically, they remain as solitary, coarse fibers which branch and anastomose. They consist of elastin, which is different from collagen both chemically and physically.[1]

Only gradually does distinction between the compact dermis and the looser, subcutaneous tissue become recognizable. Columnar papillae project upward from the dermis into the stratum germinativum; some contain blood vessels, and others contain nerve endings. Some of the dermal cells acquire pigment granules. In the lower sacral region, deep-lying pigment tends to give local areas a bluish to brownish color. This is most common among infants of the dark-skinned races, and these areas are known as "Mongolian spots."

Fat develops in the subcutaneous layer, but does not become abundant until the later months of fetal life.

ANATOMY

As mentioned above, the skin consists of two layers, the epidermis and the dermis, each with distinctive structure, properties, and embryologic origin. Deep to the dermis lies a layer of loose, irregular connective tissue, forming the superficial fascia, hypodermis or subcutaneous layer. This in turn is bound to the underlying tissues by a dense, fibrous deep fascia (e.g., epimysium over muscle or periosteum over bone).

The interface between the epidermis and the dermis presents a complex topology, marked by peg-and-socket or ridge-groove interdigitations between the two.

Associated with the epidermis are the appendages it generates: the hair, nails, and sweat and sebaceous glands. The vascular supply of the skin is confined to the dermis; therefore, the epidermis relies for its supply of nutrients and metabolic exchange on diffusion to and from the capillaries of the most superficial regions of the dermis. The innervation of the skin, however, serves both the epidermis and the dermis.

The external surface of the epidermis is marked by various furrows, ridges, and other irregularities. Three principal varieties exist: tension lines, flexure lines, and papillary ridges. The tension lines form a network of linear furrows of variable size which divide the surface into a large number of polygonal or lozenge-shaped areas. Flexure lines correspond to folds in the dermis associated with habitual joint movements, and to the lines of attachment to the underlying deep fascia; they are conspicuous opposite the flexure of joints, particularly on the surfaces of the palms, soles, and digits. Papillary ridges or friction ridges are confined to the palmar surfaces of the hands and to the soles of the feet, including the digits of each, where they form narrow raised ridges separated by fine but distinct parallel grooves, disposed in curved arrays; the precise forms and positions of these ridges are related to the arrangement and size of the underlying dermal papillae interlocking with the base of the epidermis.[2] Sweat glands, which open in a row along the midline of each ridge, grow down during development into the gaps between papillae, dimpling the basal surface of the epithelium to form secondary epidermal pegs or rete pegs, which protrude into the dermis.

The pattern of papillary ridges, and particularly those of the fingers and thumbs, are morphologically stable throughout life and are slightly different in every individual. It is now clear that only three major patterns occur in human fingerprints: loops, whorls, and arches. There are, in addition, minor variations in orientation, distortion, ridge width and number, and continuity; minor features are determined genetically by multifactorial inheritance of Mendelian type, although prenatal disturbances of metabolism may also alter their character to some extent. Certain genetic disorders may also be reflected in fingerprints and palmar markings, as, in addition, they are in the pattern of flexure lines in some cases; thus, these markings may form a useful diagnostic tool in certain circumstances.[3]

The dermis or corium is strong, flexible, and highly elastic. It is very thick in the palms of the hands and soles of the feet, thicker on the posterior than on the anterior aspect of the body, and thicker on the lateral than on the medial aspects of the limbs. It is exceedingly thin and delicate in the eyelids, scrotum, and penis.

Skin appendages include the nails of the fingers and toes, the hairs, the sebaceous glands, and the sweat glands. The nail is analogous to the horny zone of thick skin.

Hairs are found on nearly every part of the surface of the body, but are absent from the palms of the hands, the soles of the feet, the dorsal surfaces of the distal phalanges, the umbilicus, the glans penis, the inner surface of the prepuce, and the inner surfaces of the clitoris, the labia majora, and the labia minora. The individual hair consists of a root (the part implanted in the skin) and a shaft (the portion projecting from the surface). The root has a proximal enlargement, the hair bulb, which is set in an invagination of the epidermis and superficial corium called the hair follicle. Follicles may extend all the way down into the subcutaneous tissue.

From the funnel-shaped opening of the follicle on the surface, the shaft courses inward in an oblique direction (Figs. 11–3 and 11–4). The ducts of one or more sebaceous glands open into the follicle near the surface of the skin.

Almost the entire skin of the human in the middle of fetal life is covered by fine hairs called lanugo or primary hairs. These are mostly shed by birth, and are replaced by fine hairs called vellus or secondary hairs during the early months of postnatal life. These are retained in most regions, but are replaced by terminal hairs on the scalp and eyebrows; they are also replaced by the axillary and pubic hairs, and by those on the face and front of the chest which appear at puberty in the male.[2]

Minute bundles of involuntary muscular fibers, termed arrectores pilorum, are connected with the hair follicles (Fig. 11–2). They arise from the superficial layer of the corium and are inserted into the outer coat of the hair follicle below the entrance of the duct of the sebaceous gland. They are located on the side toward which the hair slopes, and by their action diminish the obliquity of the follicle and elevate the hair.

Sebaceous glands are small, sacculated, and lodged in the substance of the dermis. They are especially abundant in the scalp and face (Figs. 11–2 to 11–4).

The *sweat glands* occur in almost every part of the skin and have been divided into two types, the eccrine and apocrine. The former are the more numerous and are found over every part of the body. The apocrine sweat glands occur in the axilla, eyelids, areola and nipple of the breast, and perianal region, and in association with the external genitalia.[2]

HISTOLOGY

The histology of the skin is probably best studied where it attains its greatest degree of development, the palm of the hand and the sole of the foot. There, in sections taken at right angles to the surface, four layers can be distinguished. The deepest of these is the stratum germinativum (also called stratum malpighii) which, as previously mentioned, consists of a layer of basal cells (the stratum basale) and, above that, a layer of prickle cells (the stratum spinosum). The second is the stratum granulosum or granular layer. That is followed by the stratum lucidum or clear layer and, on the surface, the stratum corneum or horny layer. The superficial keratinized part includes the last two.

Cells of the stratum basale are cuboidal to columnar and are arranged perpendicular to the basal lamina. In the stratum spinosum, cells have a flattened polyhedral form and lie parallel to the surface, the nucleus being elongated in that direction. All of these cells bear spines that are attached to similar projections from adjacent cells. (They are not properly termed "bridges" because they do not represent open communications between epidermal cells.)

Cells of the stratum granulosum lie in three to five layers; the cells contain conspicuous granules of irregular shape, the keratohyalin granules, which stain deeply with hematoxylin.

The stratum lucidum is a thin layer that appears as a wavy thin stripe interposed between the stratum granulosum and stratum corneum. Its nuclei have disappeared.

The stratum corneum consists of cornified cells lacking nuclei, the cytoplasm of which has been replaced by keratin. Processes of cells are no longer visible (Fig. 11–5).

The dermis is difficult to delineate inferiorly because it shades over into subcutaneous tissue without a sharp boundary. The sculptured upper surface fitting into the deep surface of the epidermis is called the papillary layer; the deeper portion is referred to as the reticular layer, but the two cannot be clearly separated.

The papillary layer consists of loose connective tissue with thin collagenous bundles. The reticular layer consists of dense connective tissue. Most of its collagenous fibers are arranged more or less parallel to the surface, with occasional bundles oriented perpendicularly. Elastic fibers form an abundant thick network between collagenous bundles.[4]

Each sebaceous gland consists of a single duct that emerges from a cluster of alveoli, usually two to five in number (Fig. 11–3). Each alveolus is composed of a basement membrane, enclosing a number of epithelial cells. The outer or marginal cells are small and polyhedral, and are continuous with the lining cells of the duct. The remainder of the alveolus is filled with larger cells containing fat. In its center the cells are broken up, leaving a cavity filled with their debris and a mass of fatty matter, the sebum cutaneum. As the sebaceous glands produce their secretion by complete fatty degeneration of their central cells, they are classed as holocrine glands. As the central cells disintegrate, they are replaced by proliferation of marginal cells. The ducts open most often into hair follicles but occasionally on the general surface.

Each eccrine sweat gland consists of a single tube, the deep part of which is coiled into a ball located in the deeper layers of the corium or in the subcutaneous tissue (Fig. 11–2). Superficially, the duct is straight and opens onto the surface of the skin. These glands are merocrine in nature, producing their thin watery secretion without demonstrable epithelial cell disintegration.

Apocrine sweat glands are larger than eccrine ones, and produce a thicker secretion.

References

1. Arey, L. B.: Developmental Anatomy, rev. 7th ed. Philadelphia, W. B. Saunders Co., 1974, pp. 18 and 439–443.
2. Warwick, R., and Williams, P. L.: Gray's Anatomy, 35th British ed. Philadelphia, W. B. Saunders Co., 1973, pp. 1159–1169.
3. Valentine, G. H.: The Chromosome Disorders. London, Heinemann, 1966.
4. Bloom, W., and Fawcett, D. W.: A Textbook of Histology. Philadelphia, W. B. Saunders Co., 1975, pp. 563–597.

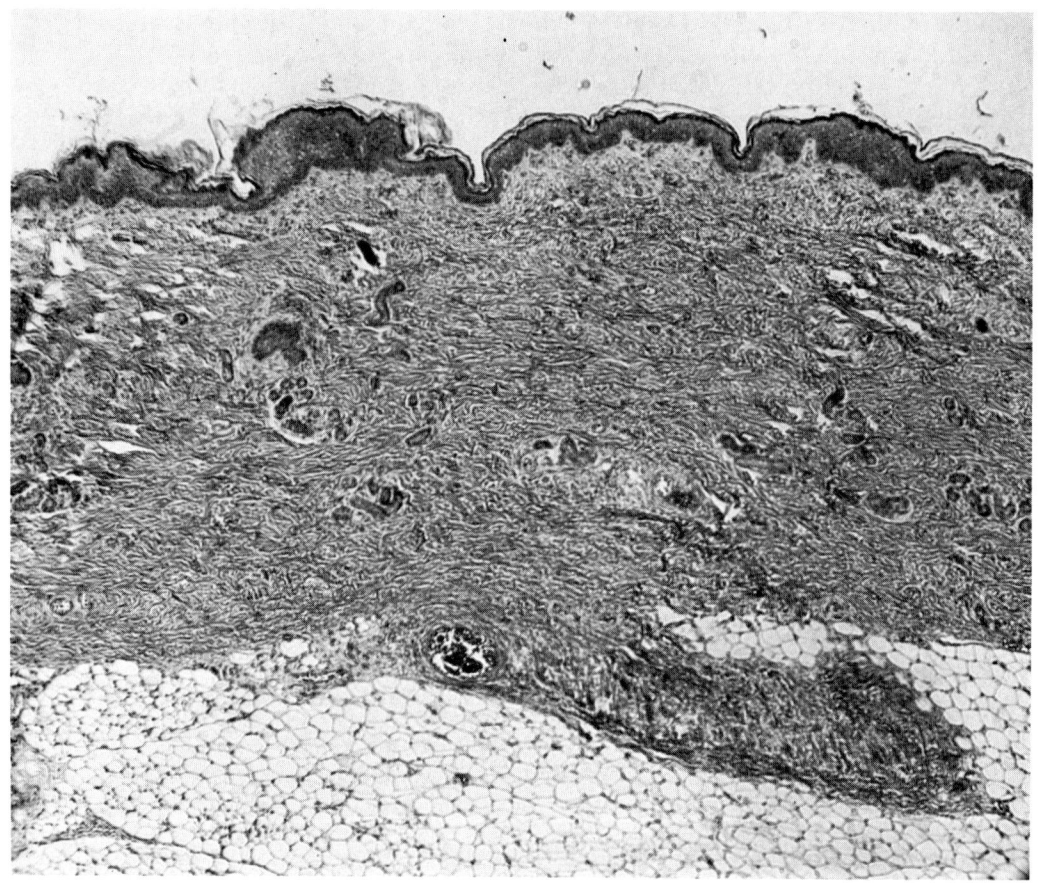

Figure 11–1

Figure 11–1. This is a photograph of the skin from the anterior abdominal wall of a 2,501 gram black male infant, born at the 37th week of gestation. The baby survived for 11 hours. A moderate amount of keratin lies superficial to the epidermis. Sweat glands and their ducts appear in moderate numbers in the dermis. Adipose tissue of the subcutaneous layer (mostly of the adult or white type) is visible along the inferior margin of the picture.

Hematoxylin and eosin stain. Mag. 55×.

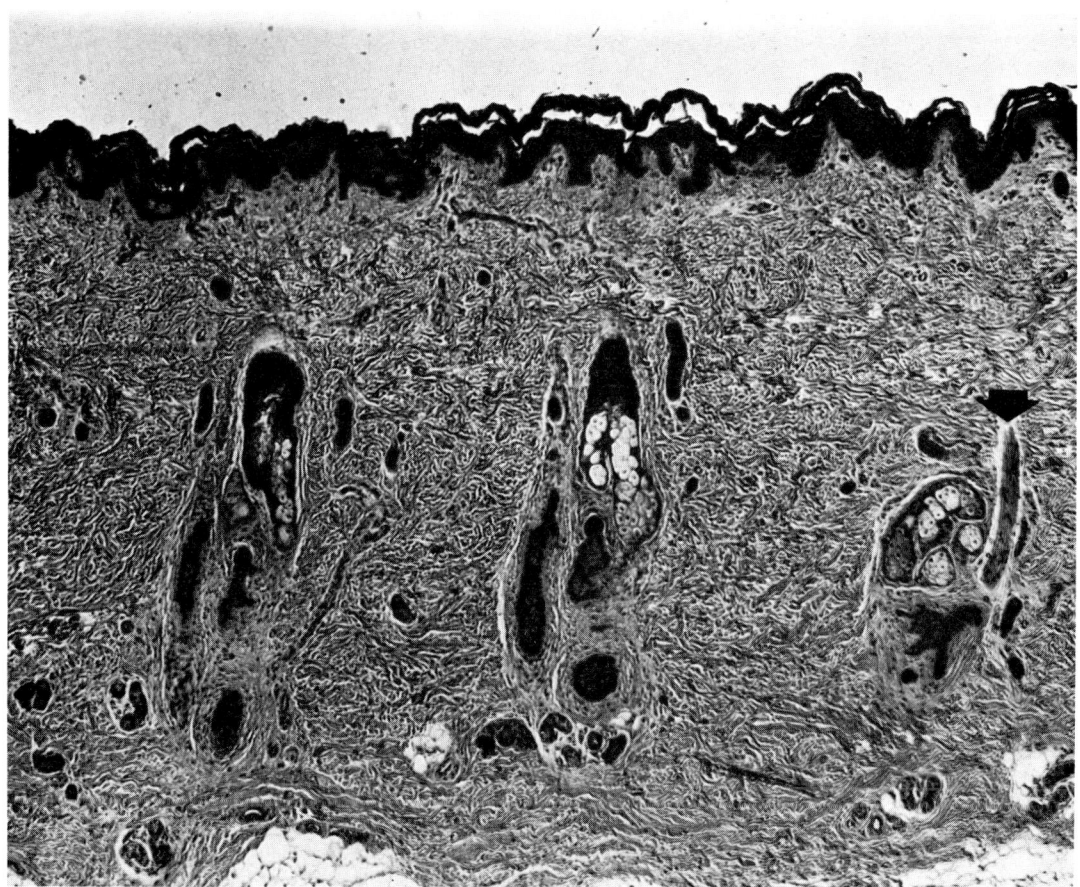

Figure 11-2

Figure 11-2. This figure illustrates hair-bearing skin. The epidermis is fairly heavily keratinized. Portions of three hair follicles appear. The associated sebaceous glands of all three can be seen; in addition, the arrector pili muscle of the follicle on the right is clearly delineated (arrow).

The patient was a 4,600 gram infant, born in the 37th week of gestation, who lived for three weeks.

Hematoxylin and eosin stain. Mag. 60×.

164 SKIN

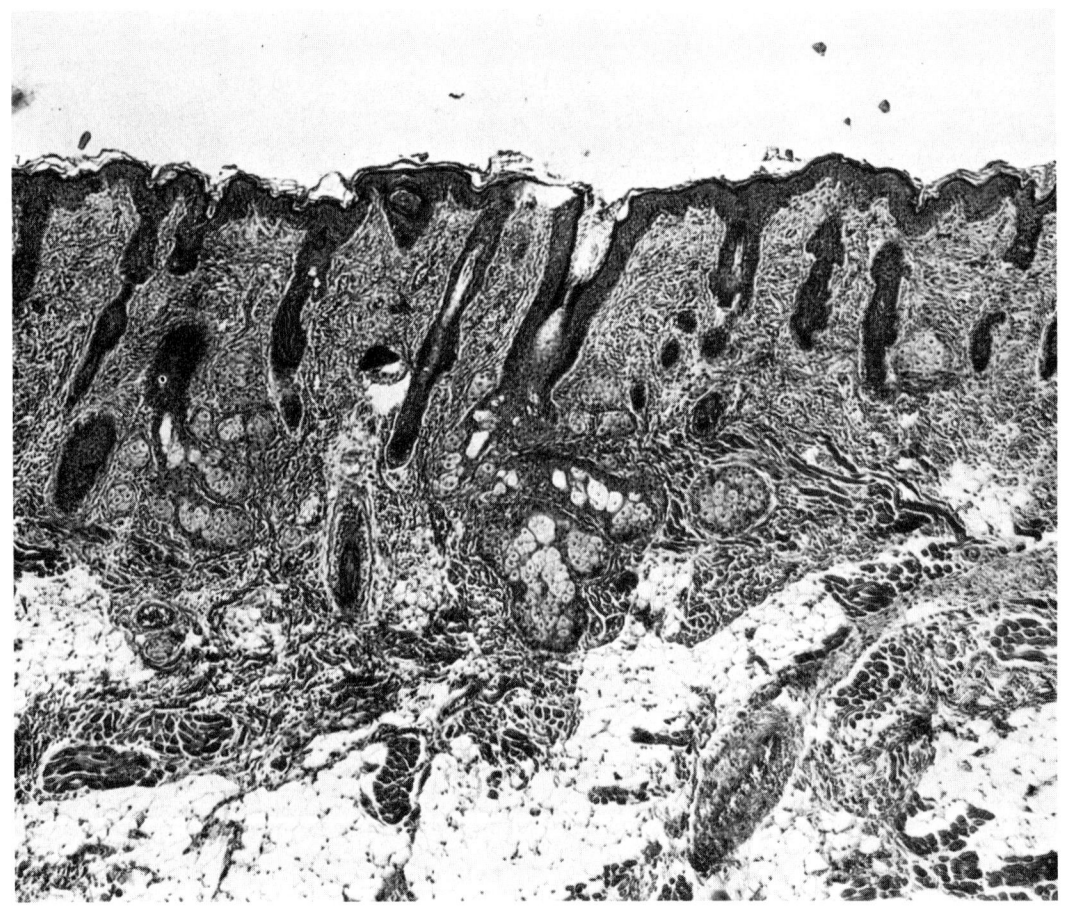

Figure 11–3

Figure 11–3. This is a section of skin from the lip; it bears many hair follicles. The related sebaceous glands of several of them are scattered across the breadth of the photograph. Prominent, darkly stained ribbons of skeletal muscle can be seen in the lower half on the left and extending up into the dermis on the right.

Details regarding this infant are no longer available to us.

Hematoxylin and eosin stain. Mag. 60×.

SKIN   165

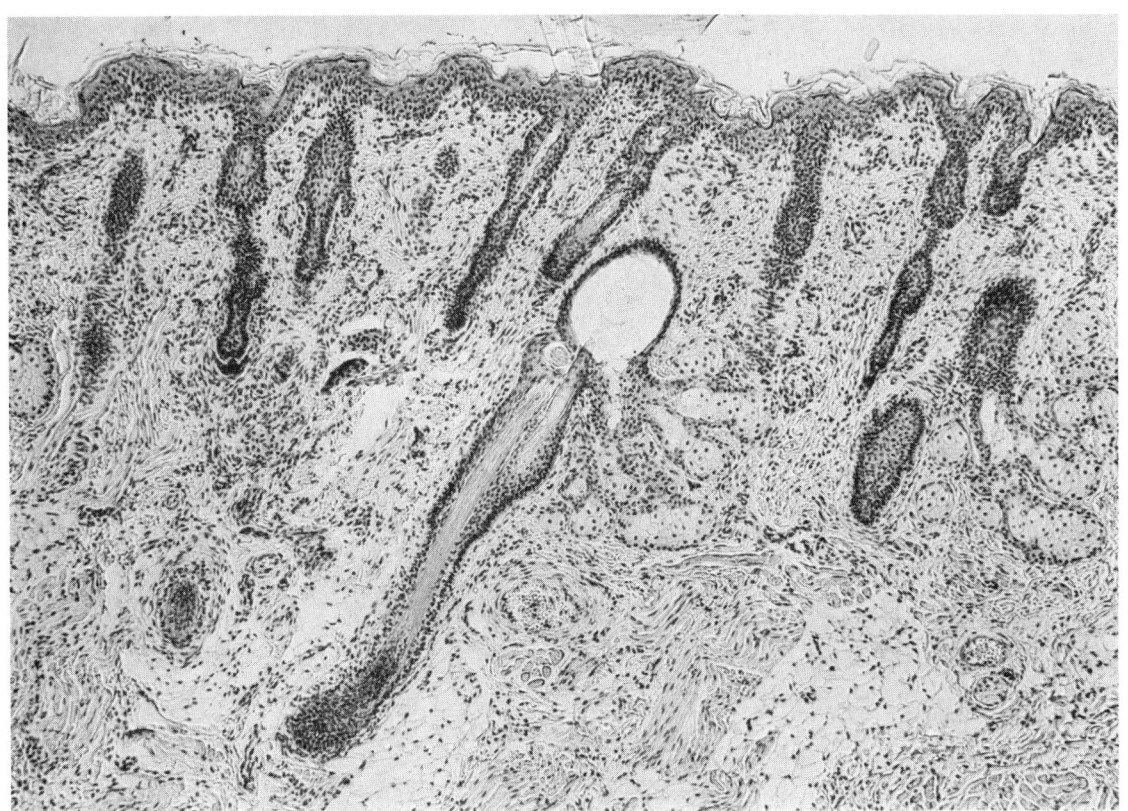

Figure 11–4

Figure 11–4. This is another section of skin from the lip and, once more, of an unknown infant. The centrally placed hair follicle shows up particularly well. Within it the hair shaft is visible. The duct for the associated sebaceous gland appears to be abnormally dilated.

As is characteristic of the lip, there are bundles of skeletal muscle in the lower portion of the dermis.

Hematoxylin and eosin stain. Mag. 88.5×.

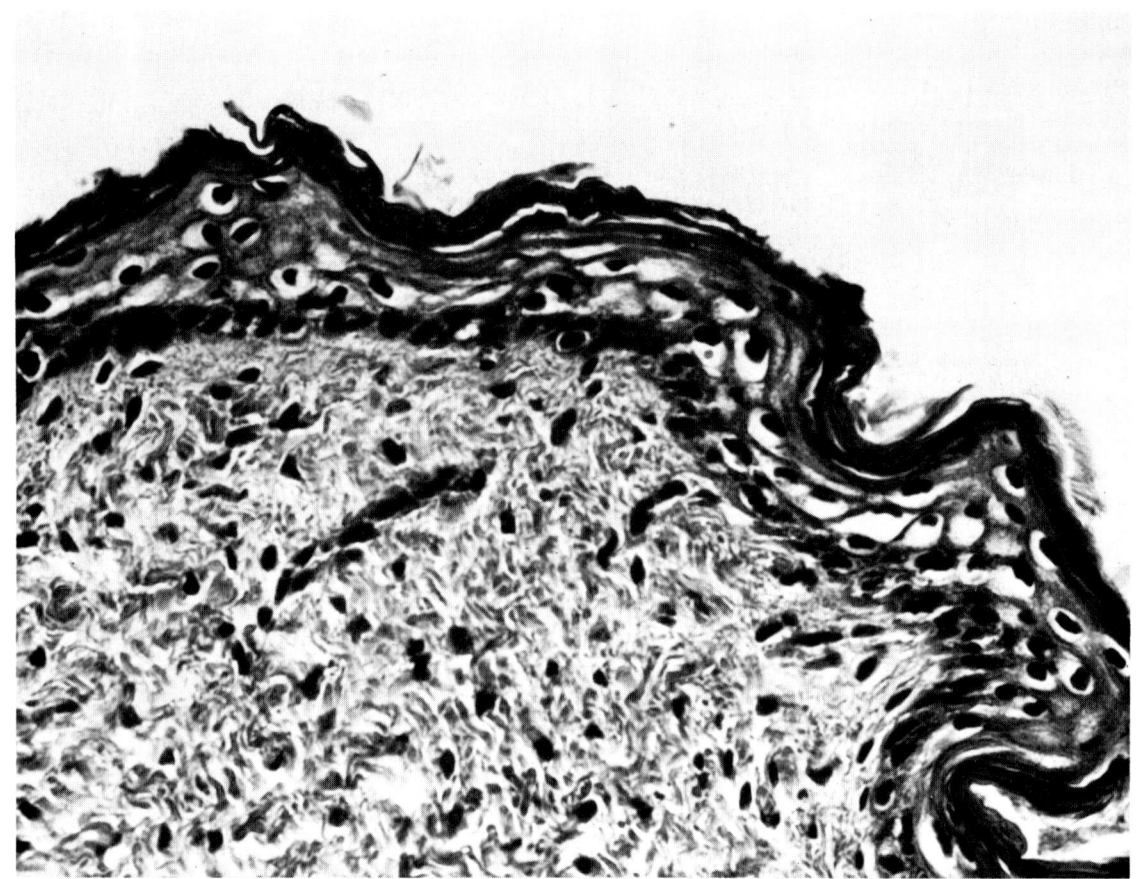

Figure 11–5

Figure 11–5. This photograph was taken at very high magnification to illustrate the nature of the epidermis of an infant in the perinatal period.

Surface layers of the stratified squamous epithelium are keratinized. There is some vacuolation of cells in the prickle-cell layer. No skin appendages are included. The dermis here is dense and moderately cellular.

The infant was prematurely born and weighed 1,100 grams at postmortem examination. He was a black male who lived for 20 hours. This section of skin was taken from the trunk.

Hematoxylin and eosin stain. Mag. 471×.

Part 6

GASTROINTESTINAL TRACT

Chapter 12

TONGUE

EMBRYOLOGY

All four branchial arches contribute to the embryologic development of the tongue but, in fact, it seems to evolve in two distinct regions — an anterior two thirds and a posterior one third. Around the end of the fourth week of gestation, the very first evidence of its appearance is manifest, directly *anterior* to the foramen cecum, in the form of a midline mound called the tuberculum impar. Shortly thereafter, the other two anterior contributions become apparent, one on either side of the midline just in front of the tuberculum. These are the oval lateral lingual swellings, which, like the tuberculum, are derived from the first branchial arch. The two lateral swellings fuse (the line of their fusion is evident in the adult as the median sulcus) and become the anterior two thirds of the tongue; the tuberculum impar contributes virtually nothing.

The posterior third (ultimately the root) of the tongue is initially heralded by the appearance just *behind* the foramen cecum of another small midline mound, called the copula, from the second branchial arch, as well as a somewhat larger one posterior to it, known as the hypobranchial eminence, derived from mesoderm of the third and fourth branchial arches. Like its predecessor, the tuberculum impar, the copula later disappears from the scene while the larger hypobranchial eminence gives rise to the entire posterior one third of the tongue.[1] Lingual muscle appears to arise in situ from mesenchyme of the arches.[2]

The line of demarcation between the anterior two thirds and the posterior third is finally indicated by the V-shaped groove on the dorsal surface, called the terminal sulcus.

Early in development, the covering of the tongue consists of cuboidal epithelium; at two months that is replaced with epithelium of a stratified squamous character.[2] In fetuses of nine and eleven weeks, respectively, the fungiform and filiform papillae become apparent grossly. The vallate papillae, along the V-shaped ridge just in front of the terminal sulcus, appear at intervals between two and five months of gestation, and the foliate papillae appear during the third month.[2]

Taste buds (Figs. 12–7 and 12–8) arise at about eight weeks; one precedes the appearance of each fungiform papilla and then occupies its top surface. Several occur also on the domes of the vallate papillae, but these disappear before birth at term and are replaced by buds on the sides.[2]

ANATOMY

The tongue consists chiefly of striated muscle, and much of it is clothed in mucous membrane (Figs. 12–1 and 12–2). Part of it lies in the mouth and part in the so-called oropharynx. The latter is referred to as the root. At the anterior extremity is the tip. The dorsal surface has a convex curve, as does the inferior surface (Figs. 12–1 and 12–2). Normally the covering epithelium is pink.

The root of the tongue is attached to the hyoid bone and the mandible. The dorsum is divided into an anterior portion, which faces superiorly, and a posterior part, which faces posteriorly. These two are separated, as previously mentioned, by a V-shaped furrow, the sulcus terminalis, the limbs of which run laterally and forward from a midline pit called the foramen cecum to the palatoglossal arches.

The oral part of the tongue rests on the floor of the mouth. Its entire peripheral margin is in contact with the gingival ridge; its superior surface is applied against the hard and soft palates. The mucous membrane of the superior surface is covered with papillae (Figs. 12–1 and 12–2). The inferior surface is smooth. In the median plane, the tongue is connected to the floor of the mouth by the frenulum linguae.

The pharyngeal part of the tongue lies behind the palatoglossal folds. Its posterior surface forms the anterior wall of the oropharynx. Its surface is devoid of papillae. Although there are superficial collections of lymphoid tissue located superficially in this part of the tongue in older individuals, the so-called lingual tonsils, none are ordinarily seen here in the perinatal period.

The papillae of the tongue are projections of the corium covered by stratified squamous epithelium. On the dorsal surface they are of three types: the vallate, fungiform, and filiform (Figs. 12–3 through 12–6). The vallate are large, eight to twelve in number, and situated so as to form a V-shaped row immediately in front of and parallel to the sulcus terminalis. Each is shaped like a truncated cone, the smaller end of which is attached to the tongue (Figs. 12–5 and 12–6).

The fungiform papillae are more numerous than the vallate and are located chiefly at the sides and apex of the tongue. Each is rather large and round.

The filiform papillae (Figs. 12–3 and 12–4) are minute, conical or cylindrical, and cover the presulcal part of the dorsum of the tongue. They are arranged in rows that run parallel with the vallate papillae except at the apex of the tongue, where their direction is transverse. The taste buds are microscopic specialized clumps of cells about the endings of the nerves of taste. They are much more widespread than the papillae (Fig. 12–7). They are scattered over the entire dorsal surface of the tongue, the sides of the tongue, the epiglottis, and the lingual surface of the soft palate.

The musculature of the tongue is divided into right and left halves by a median fibrous septum which is fixed below to the body of the hyoid bone. In each half there are two sets of muscles, the extrinsic, with attachments outside the tongue, and intrinsic, contained within it.

The mucous membrane on the oral part of the dorsum of the tongue is thin and intimately adherent to the muscle beneath it. The lingual corium consists of a dense network of fibrous connective tissue firmly attached to the muscle bundles (Figs. 12–3 through 12–6). It contains the vessels and nerves supplying the papillae, the plexuses of lymph vessels, and the glands (Figs. 12–9 through 12–11).

The lingual glands are of both the mucous and serous varieties (Fig. 12–10). The mucous glands are similar in structure to the labial glands (Fig. 12–11). Lingual glands are numerous in the pharyngeal portion of the tongue but are also present at the tip and margins. The anterior lingual glands are particularly prominent (Figs. 12–8 to 12–10). They are situated on the ventral surface of the apex, one on each side of the frenulum; each consists of both mucous and serous alveoli. They open by three or four ducts on the inferior surface of the lingual apex (Fig. 12–10).

The serous glands appear near the taste buds.[3]

HISTOLOGY

The tongue consists of interlacing bundles of striated muscle that run in three planes and cross one another at right angles (Figs. 12–1 and 12–2). The muscular mass is covered by a tightly adherent mucous membrane. The fibrous lamina propria is continuous with the interstitial connective tissue within the muscle. A submucous layer is apparent only on the undersurface (Fig. 12–8).

The dorsal surface is covered with countless papillae in the anterior two thirds. A dimple, sometimes quite deep, known as the foramen cecum, is located at the posteriorly projecting apex of a V-shaped line of demarcation between the anterior two thirds and posterior third. (It is a remnant of the thyroglossal duct.)

Four types of papillae are present: the filiform, fungiform, vallate, and foliate. The filiform are depicted in Figs. 12–3 and 12–4. The connective tissue core of each is beset with secondary papillae with pointed ends, which show to good advantage in Fig. 12–3 in the last papilla on the right. The epithelium covering those outgrowths may also taper into pointed processes. The superficial squamous cells are hard scales with shrunken nuclei (Fig. 12–3).

The fungiform papillae have short, slightly constricted stalks and slightly flattened hemispherical upper portions. Their connective tissue cores also bear secondary papillae projecting into the recesses of the overlying stratified squamous epithelium, which has a smooth free surface. Taste buds may be located within the covering epithelium of many of these (Fig. 12–7).

The vallate papillae are almost sunken into the surface of the mucous membrane. Each is surrounded by a deep circular furrow. The covering epithelium is smooth (Fig. 12–6). Lateral surfaces may contain many taste buds. Related to the vallate papillae are glands of the serous type, whose bodies are embedded deep in the underlying muscular tissue and whose excretory ducts open into the bottom of the furrow.

The foliate papillae, which look like parallel folds of the mucosa, are rudimentary in man and are located laterally and posteriorly just anterior to the palatine tonsils. They bear many taste receptors.

The taste buds are pale oval bodies located within darker-staining epithelium, as depicted in Figs. 12–6 and 12–7. They extend from the basal lamina almost to the surface. The epithelium over each is said to be pierced by a tiny opening.[4]

On either side of the midline near the tip of the tongue are the anterior lingual glands, depicted in Figs. 12–8, 12–9, and 12–10. The anterior portion of this gland contains secretory tubules with seromucinous cells only. Its posterior part consists of mixed branching tubules, which contain mucous cells and, on their blind ends, demilunes of seromucinous cells. (This mix is well illustrated in Figs. 12–9 and 12–10.)

Scattered about the oral cavity are numerous other salivary glands. Many of them are small and located in either the mucosa or submucosa; they are named according to their location. They seem to secrete continuously and furnish the saliva which moistens oral mucous membranes. This is in contrast to the major salivary glands, which secrete only upon special stimulation. Lobules of a labial group of glands are depicted in Fig. 12–11. Labial glands are of the mixed type, including both serous and mucous cells.

References

All references for Part Six appear on page 271.

TONGUE

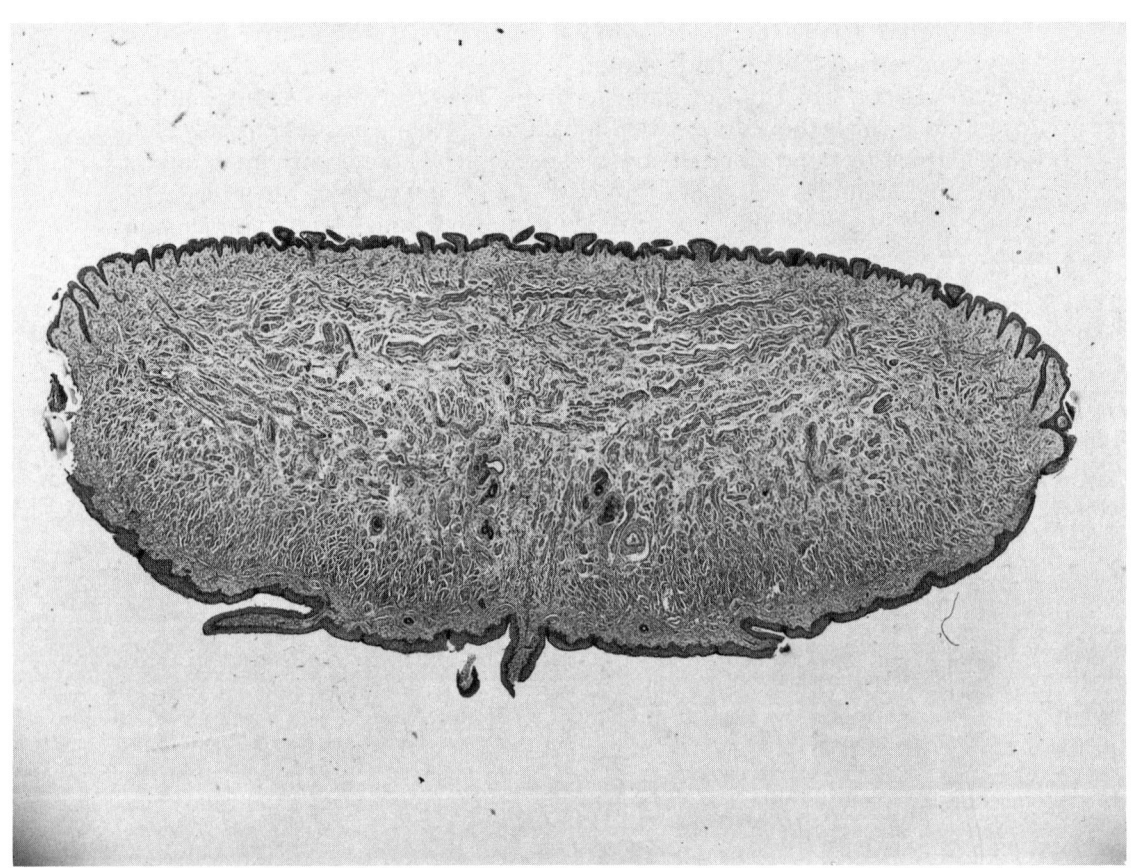

Figure 12–1

Figure 12–1. This is a survey view of a sagittal section of the oral part of the tongue of a female infant, weighing 200 grams, who was stillborn at 18 weeks gestation.

Note the intricate interdigitation of the skeletal muscle bundles throughout the body of the tongue, and the frenulum at the inferior margin.

Hematoxylin and eosin stain. Mag. 19.6×.

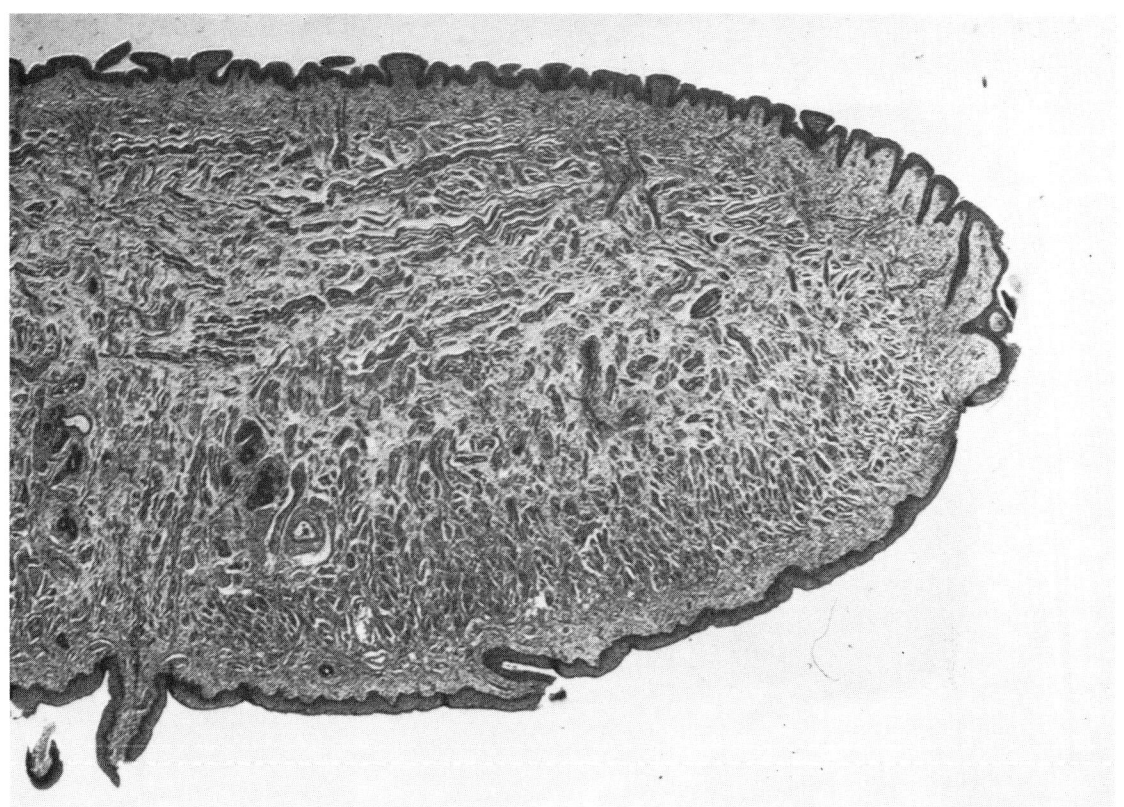

Figure 12–2

Figure 12–2. This is an enlargement of the section shown in Fig. 12–1.
Arranged along the dorsal surface are numerous filiform (conical) and fungiform (round) papillae and, at the right-hand margin, several of the foliate papillae.
The frenulum linguae projects downward from the inferior surface near the left edge of the picture.
The intricate interdigitation of skeletal muscle within the body of the tongue is easily apparent here.
Hematoxylin and eosin stain. Mag. 31×.

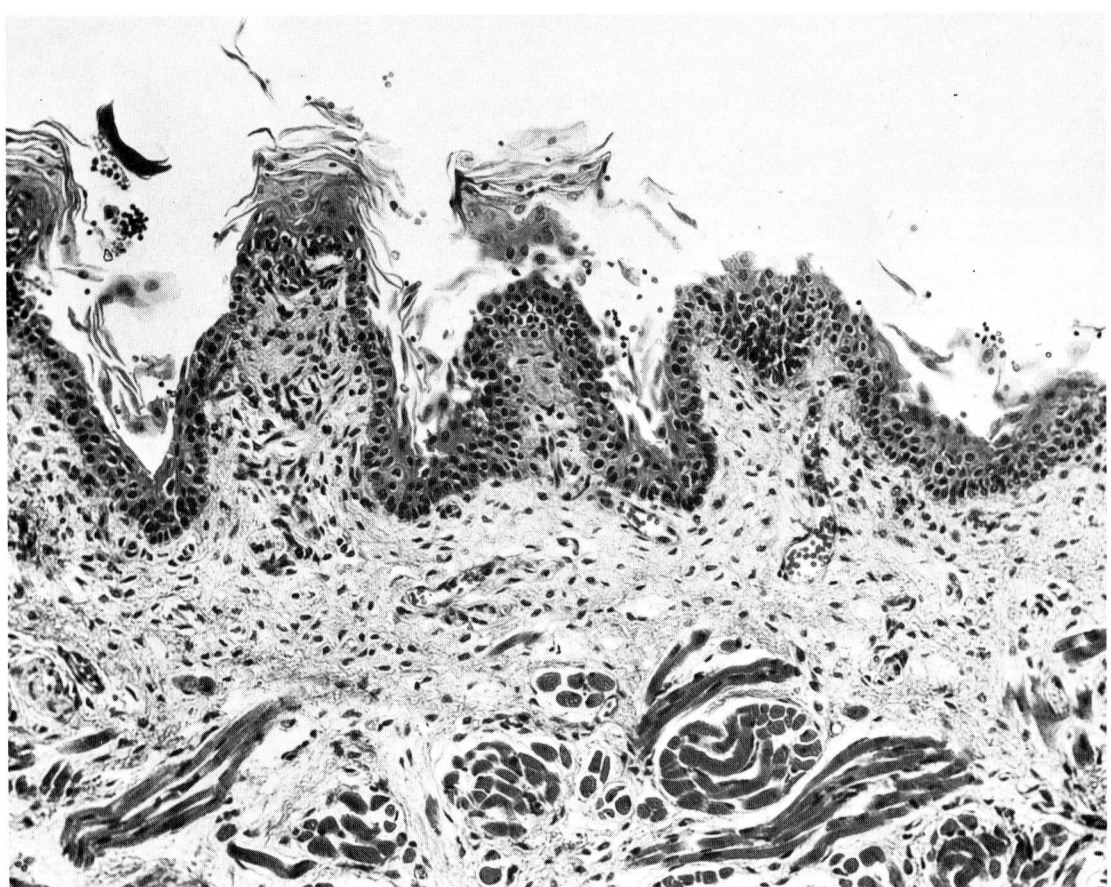

Figure 12-3

Figure 12-3. Seen here, at higher magnification, is a cross section of the dorsal surface of the oral portion of the tongue of a somewhat more mature infant, stillborn at 34 weeks of gestation; the patient was a 1,900 gram female.

Two clear-cut conical filiform papillae appear on the left. Note the two secondary papillae beneath the epithelial covering of the papilla on the right.

Intertwined skeletal muscle bundles appear at the lower border.

Hematoxylin and eosin stain. Mag. 186×.

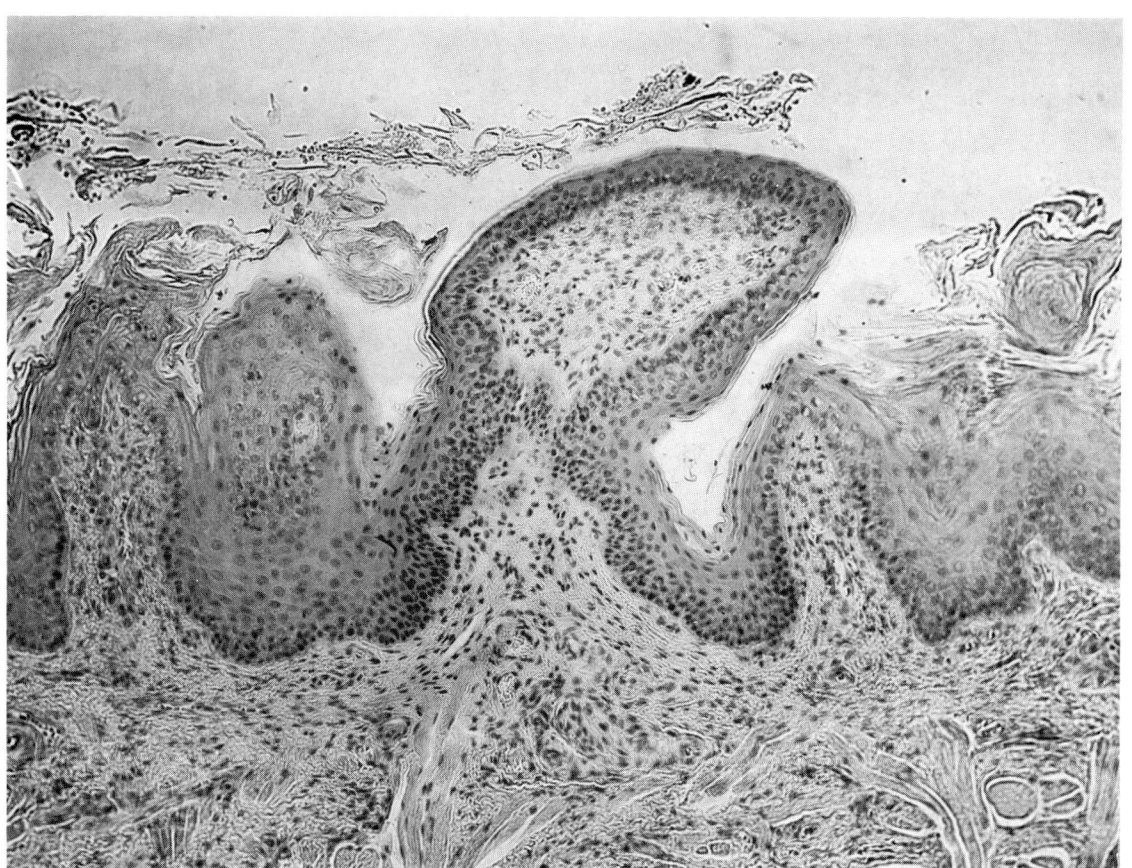

Figure 12–4

Figure 12–4. Here, at about three-fourths of the magnification employed in Fig. 12–3, is the dorsal surface of the oral portion of the tongue of a term infant, a female weighing 2,850 grams, who lived for 14 hours.

A prominent filiform papilla appears centrally.

Hematoxylin and eosin stain. Mag. 142×.

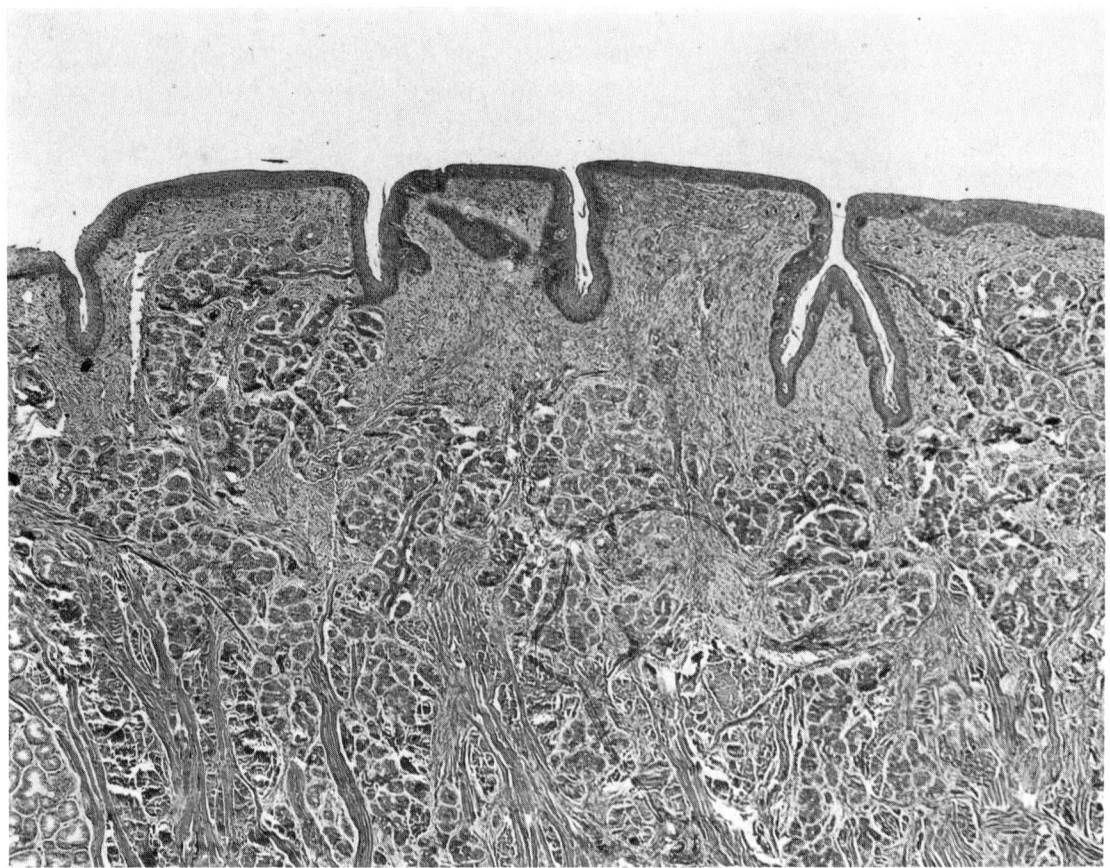

Figure 12–5

Figures 12–5 and 12–6. This pair of photographs illustrates the appearance of the more posterior portion of the oral part of the tongue.

Figure 12–5. These are the vallate papillae characteristic of the area. The patient, born at 40 weeks of gestation, was a white male weighing 4,100 grams, who died at 16 days of age.
Hematoxylin and eosin stain. Mag. 45×.

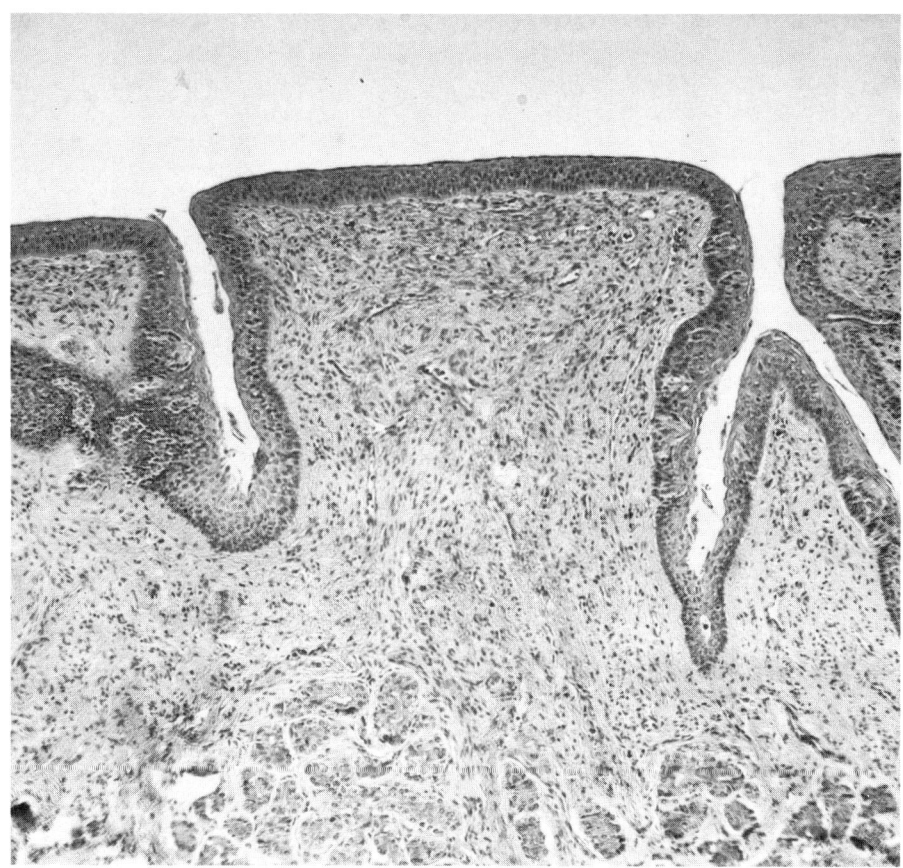

Figure 12–6

Figure 12–6. A single vallate papilla, just to the right of center in Fig. 12–5, is shown here at higher magnification. Note the rounded taste buds within the epithelium of the lateral aspects and the underlying glands.
Hematoxylin and eosin stain. Mag. 108×.

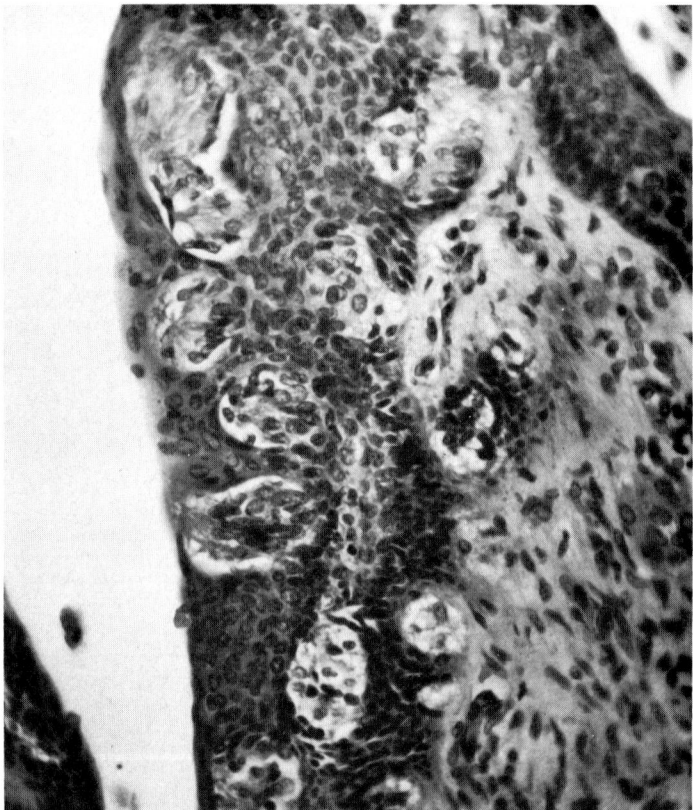

Figure 12–7

Figure 12–7. Located within the stratified squamous epithelium on the surface of a single papilla, at least six taste buds are seen here at rather high magnification.
This infant was a black male, of 29 to 30 weeks gestation, who was stillborn.
Hematoxylin and eosin stain. Mag. 267×.

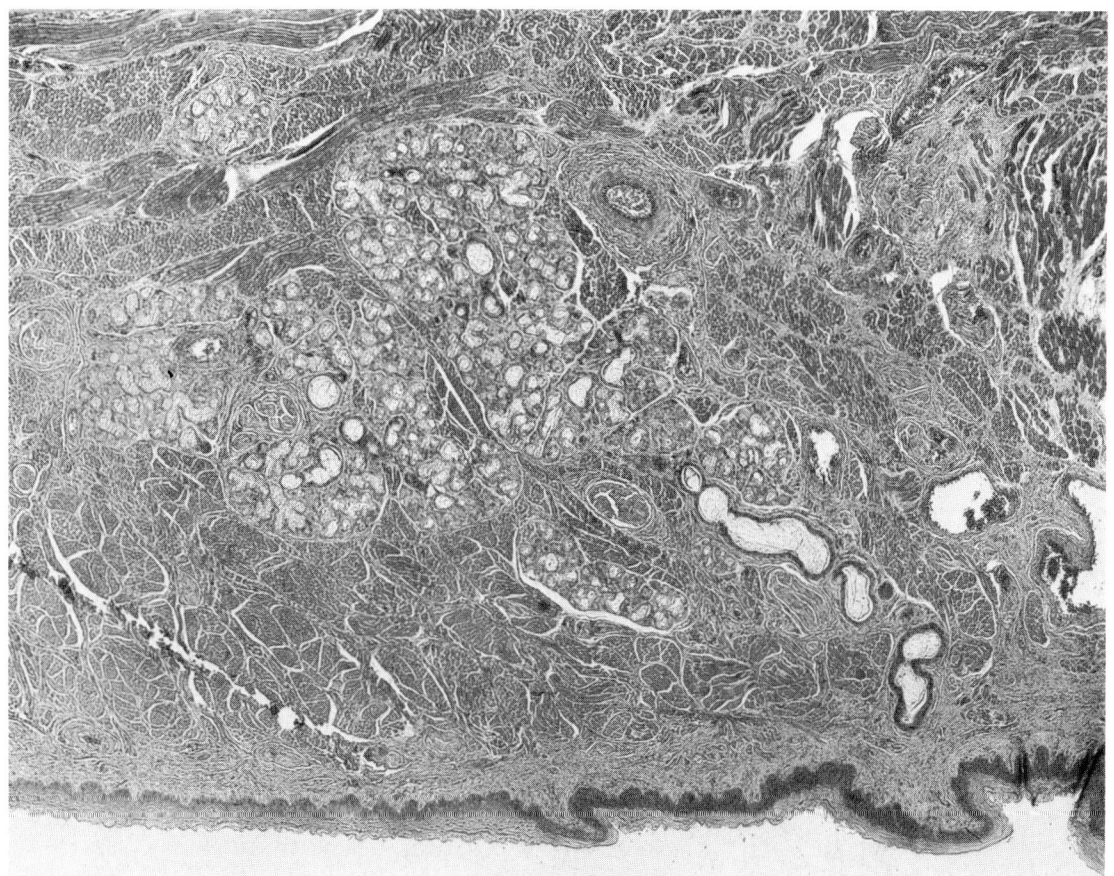

Figure 12–8

Figure 12–8. Illustrated here are the anterior lingual glands, of mixed serous and mucous types. They are situated on the ventral surface of the apex of the tongue, one on each side of the frenulum. They are covered by a mucous membrane and a fasciculus of muscle fibers. They open by 3 or 4 ducts on the inferior surface of the lingual apex.

The patient was a 14 hour old female, born at term, whose body at postmortem examination weighed 2,850 grams.

Hematoxylin and eosin stain. Mag. 43.5×.

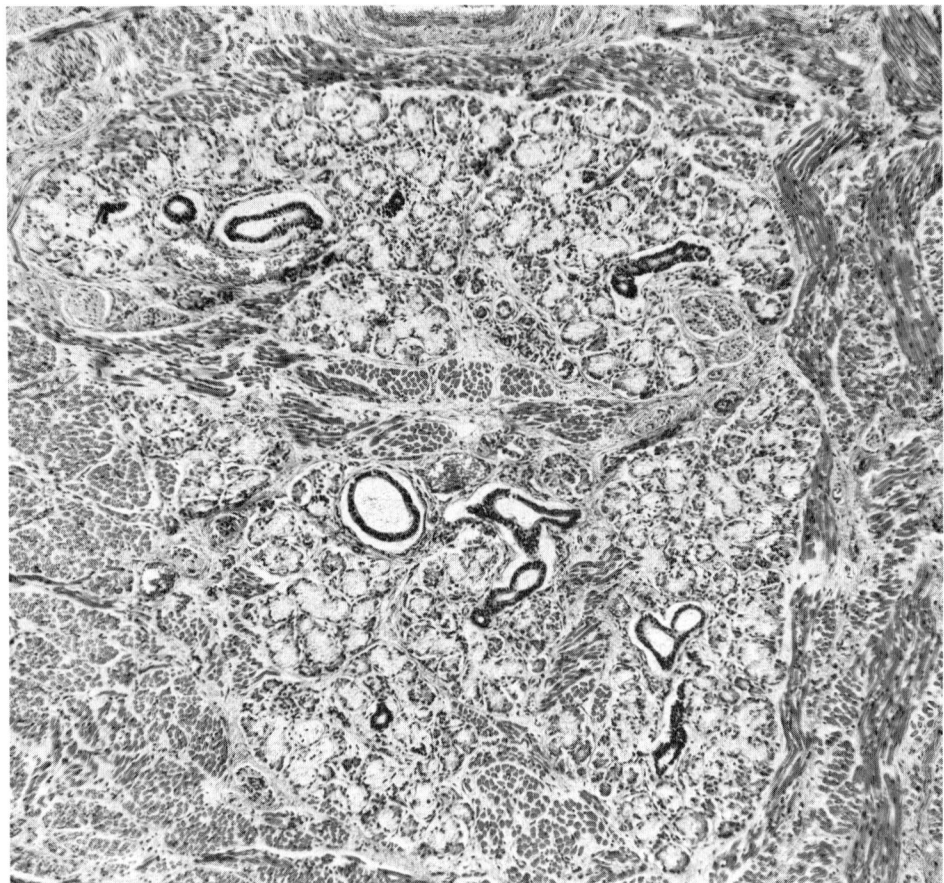

Figure 12–9

Figure 12–9. Seen here at somewhat higher magnification are the mixed serous and mucous elements of the anterior lingual gland and some of its ducts.

This patient was a 1,900 gram stillborn female who was born at 34 weeks of gestation. Hematoxylin and eosin stain. Mag. 76×.

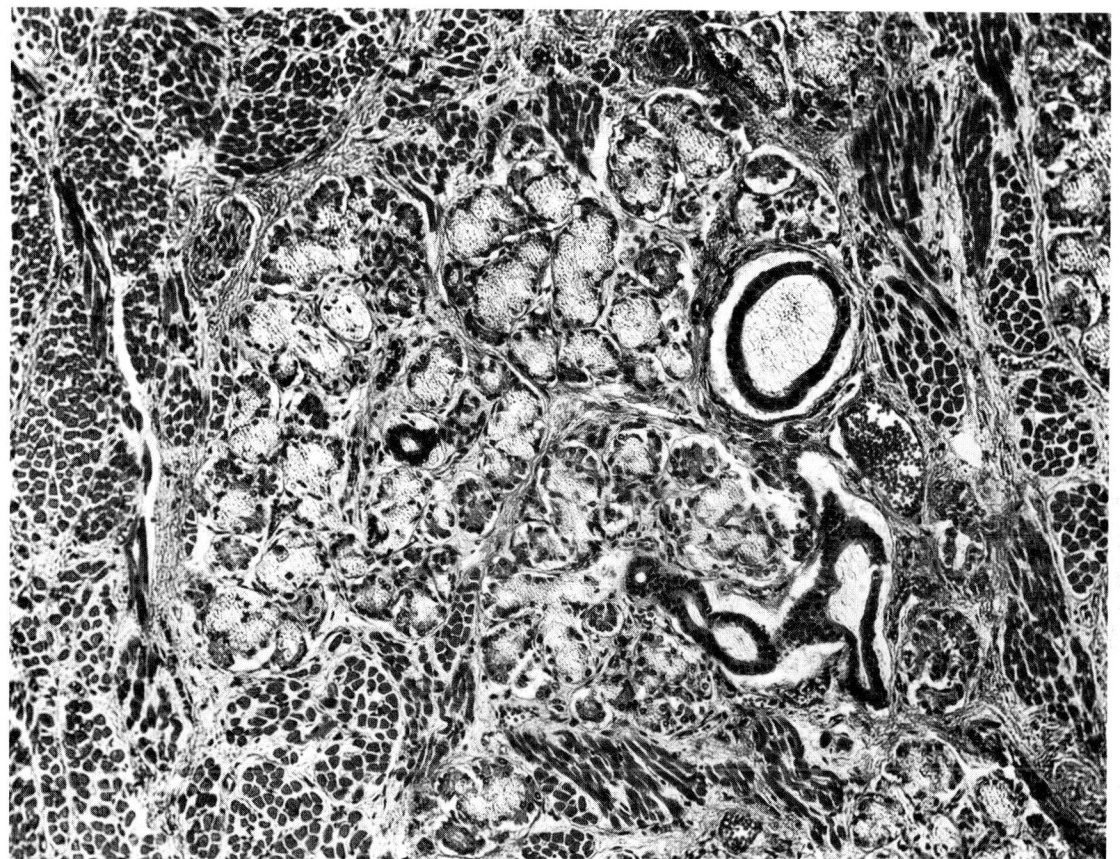

Figure 12–10

Figure 12–10. In this photomicrograph one can see the nature of the mixed serous and mucous elements in the glands on the inferior aspect of the tongue of the infant. On the right are seen two ducts with a prominent lining of cuboidal to low columnar epithelium. All of these elements are embedded in bundles of striated muscle.

This patient was a female infant, born dead at 28 weeks of gestation. Her body weight at postmortem examination was 1,900 grams.

Hematoxylin and eosin stain. Mag. 142×.

182 TONGUE

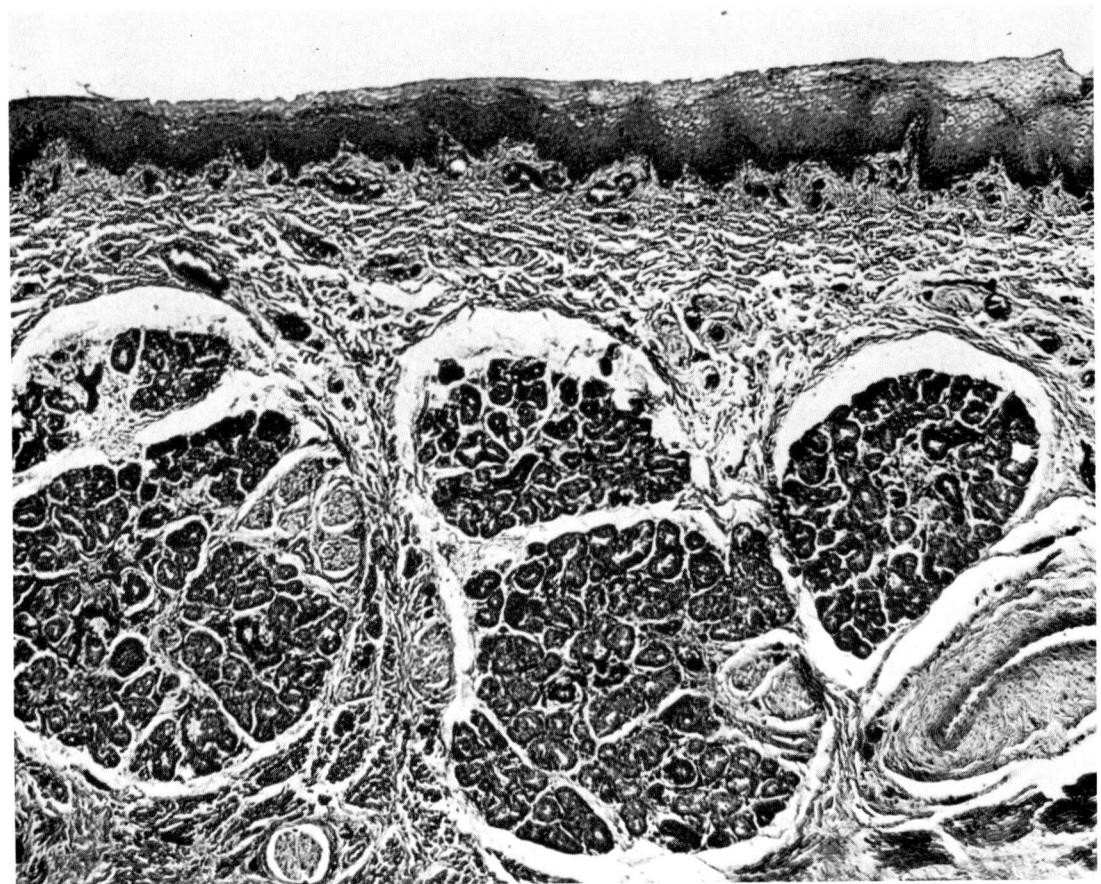

Figure 12–11

Figure 12–11. These are salivary glands, lying in clusters within the submucosa on the inner aspect of the lip of an infant.

Note the numerous nerve bundles nearby, and the covering of non-keratinized, rather thick stratified squamous epithelium.

The infant is unidentified.

Hematoxylin and eosin stain. Mag. 60×.

Chapter 13

SALIVARY GLANDS

EMBRYOLOGY

The major salivary glands begin as solid clusters of cells derived from the epithelium of the mouth during the sixth and seventh weeks.[1]

The *parotid* develops from buds that originate in the ectodermal lining of the primitive mouth. The buds branch to form solid shafts with rounded ends. They develop lumina later, and the rounded ends give rise to acini. Surrounding mesenchyme gives rise to interstitial connective tissue, which divides the gland into lobules, and to the capsule.

The *submandibular glands* develop from endoderm in the floor of the mouth.[1] The solid bud grows backward beside the tongue; it branches and differentiates like the developing parotid.

The *sublingual glands* appear last, and arise as multiple buds of the endoderm and in the paralingual sulcus.

The smaller, or minor, salivary glands in the lips, cheeks, and palate arise at about three months from multiple epithelial buds in their respective locations.[2]

ANATOMY

There are three main salivary glands, the parotid, the submandibular, and the sublingual, each of which is paired. The minor salivary glands include the anterior lingual glands, mentioned in Chapter 12, the many small glands in the mucous membranes of the tongue, and the numerous small glands in the lips, the cheeks, and the roof of the mouth.

The parotid gland is the largest of the three major glands. It is irregular and lobulated, and lies between the mandible and the sternocleidomastoid muscle below the external acoustic meatus. It is shaped like a flattened three-sided pyramid, and is enclosed within a fibrous capsule. The facial nerve traverses it. The duct opens upon a small papilla on the oral surface of the cheek.

The submandibular gland (Fig. 13–1) is also irregular. In the infant it is roughly button-shaped. Its inferior surface is covered by skin and deep fascia. The lateral surface lies against the inner surface of the body of the mandible. The gland is palpable, especially in dissection, from below. The wall of its duct is thinner than that of the parotid gland. It opens through a narrow orifice in the floor of the mouth, on the summit of a papilla at the side of the frenulum of the tongue.[3]

The sublingual gland is the smallest of the three. It is situated beneath the mucous membrane of the floor of the mouth, on the lingual surface of the mandible near the symphysis. It is narrow, flat, and almond-shaped. Its ducts are numerous, and most open separately into the floor of the mouth on the summit of the sublingual fold.

The salivary glands are compound racemose glands consisting of numerous lobes, which are made up of lobules connected to one another by dense areolar tissue bearing vessels and ducts (Fig. 13–1).

HISTOLOGY

Of the major salivary glands, by far the largest are the two parotid glands that are situated subcutaneously on either side of the face just in front of the ears. Each is connected to the oral cavity by a long parotid duct known as Stensen's duct, which opens into the mouth through an ostium in the cheek. Although in the adult this gland is nearly a pure serous gland, in the newborn the glandular cells are often mucous in type.[4]

The submandibular gland lies between the mandible and the muscles forming the floor of the mouth (Fig. 13–1). Its duct, Wharton's duct, opens into the floor of the mouth adjacent to the frenulum of the tongue. The secretory portion of this gland in the term infant comprises both mucous and serous cells, but there is a predominance of the former. In Fig. 13–4 one can see mucoid cells associated with serous demilunes.

The sublingual glands are located deep to the mucous membrane beneath the tongue, on either side of the frenulum. In these glands the mucous cells are more numerous than they are in the submandibular glands. Serous cells are in the minority, and many of them are mucoserous.

The small ducts of these glands are lined by cuboidal to low columnar epithelium (Figs. 13–4 and 13–5). Larger ducts (Fig. 13–6) are lined by columnar pseudostratified epithelium in which there are scattered goblet cells.

References

All references for Part Six appear on page 271.

186 SALIVARY GLANDS

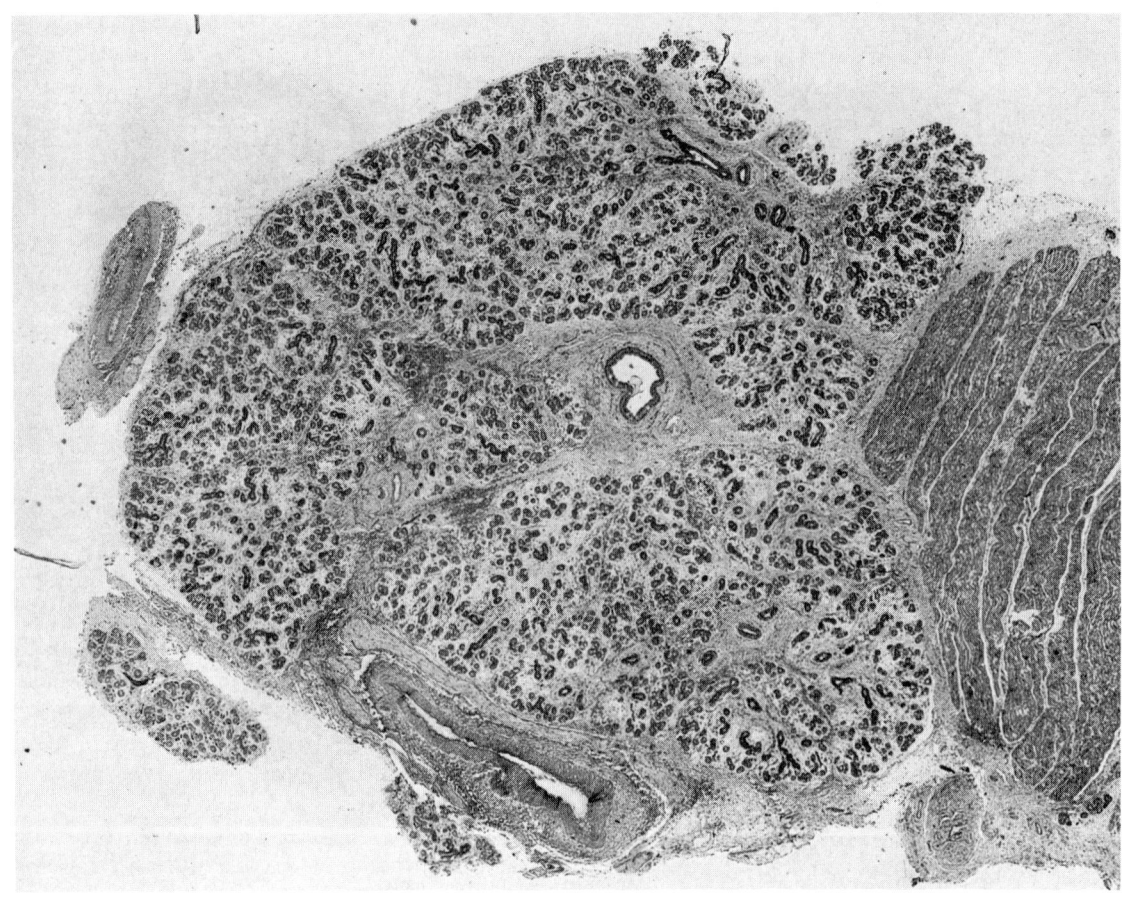

Figure 13–1

Figure 13–1. Section through the submandibular gland, seen at very low magnification.
 The patient was a very immature infant, a female born at 23 to 25 weeks of gestation. At necropsy her body weighed 450 grams.
 Note the single large duct seen in cross section in the center of the section.
 Hematoxylin and eosin stain. Mag. 29×.

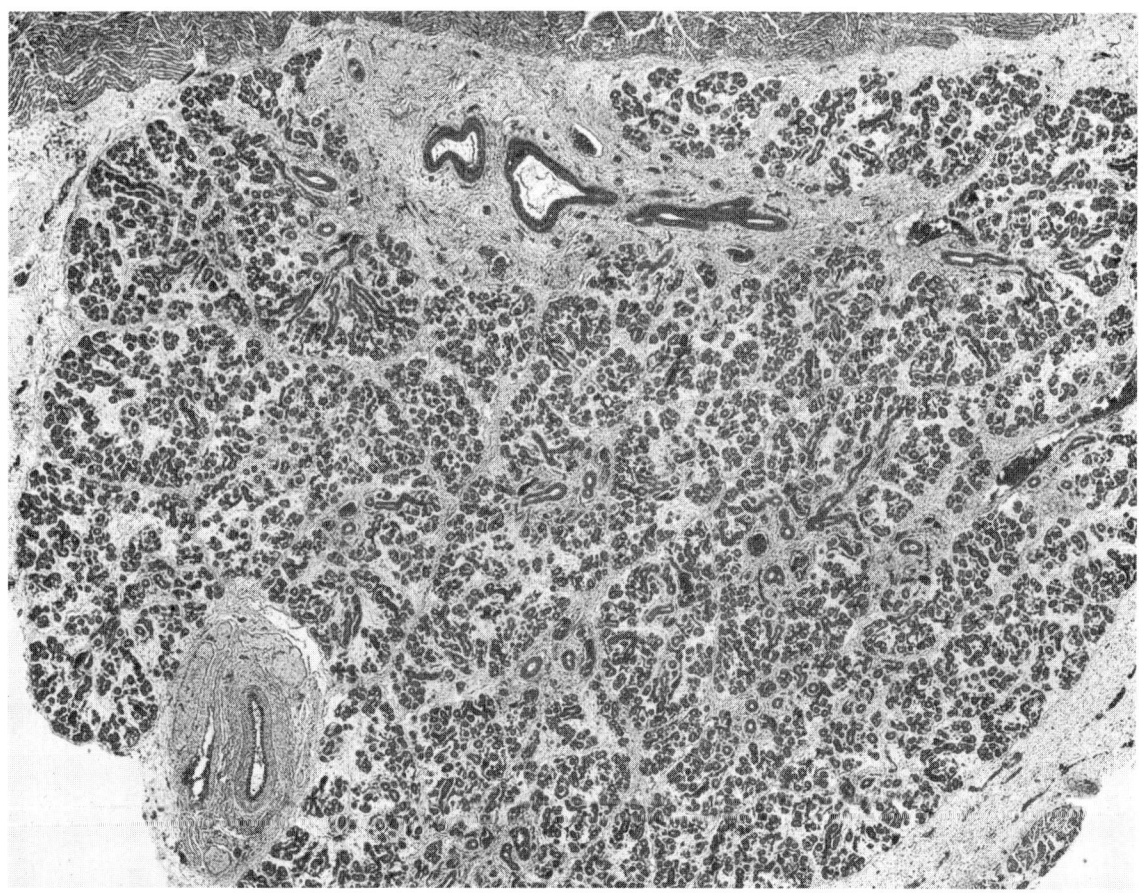

Figure 13–2

Figure 13–2. Seen here, at the same magnification as Fig. 13–1, is a section of the submandibular gland of a considerably more mature infant.

The patient was a male of 26 weeks gestation who survived for 6½ hours. Body weight at autopsy was 760 grams.

Note the considerable increase in the numbers of acini and the apparent diminution of fibrous stroma with advancing age and development.

Hematoxylin and eosin stain. Mag. 29×.

188 SALIVARY GLANDS

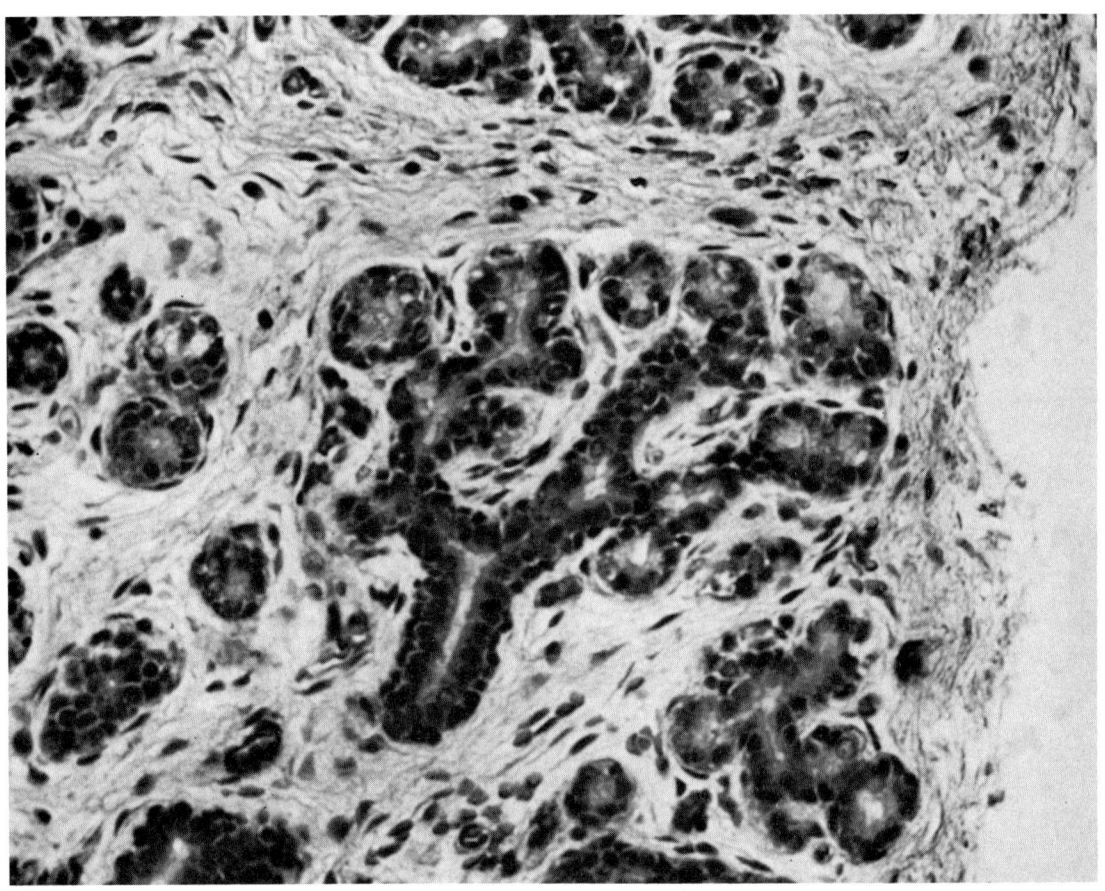

Figure 13–3

Figures 13–3 and 13–4. These are two photographs taken at the same magnification to illustrate the change that takes place in the histologic appearance of the submandibular salivary gland during the latter half of gestation. Both represent lobules at the very perimeter of the gland (capsule to the right). Each includes a ductule located centrally, in longitudinal section in Fig. 13–3, and in cross section in Fig. 13–4.

Hematoxylin and eosin stain. Mag. 382×.

Figure 13–3. Represented here is an entire simple peripheral lobule of the submandibular gland of a female infant of 23 to 25 weeks gestation. The infant survived for 48 hours, and her body weight at postmortem examination was 450 grams.

Note the abundant intra- and interlobular connective tissue characteristic of this stage of development.

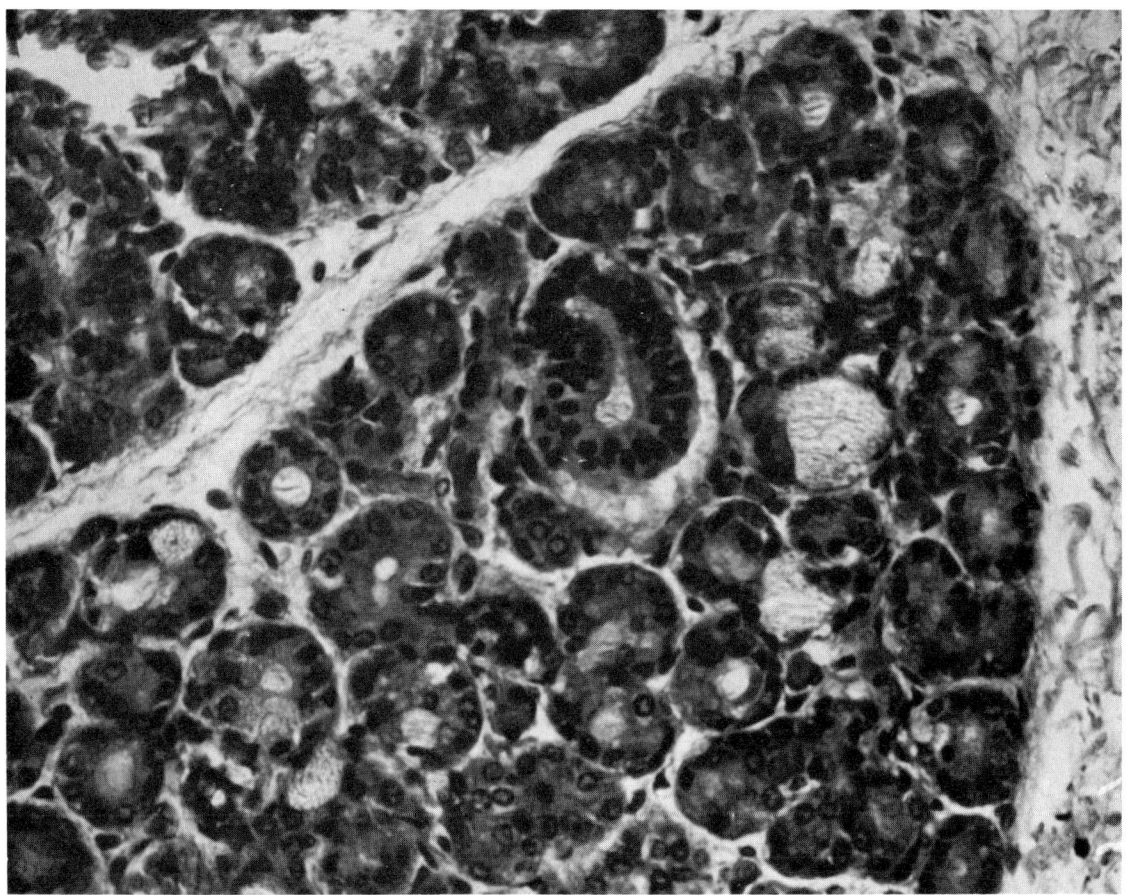

Figure 13-4

Figure 13-4. By comparison, this photomicrograph, at the same magnification, includes only a portion of a single peripheral lobule. This infant was a female born at 40 weeks of gestation, whose body weight at autopsy was 2,850 grams; she lived for 14 hours.

To the right of the centrally located ductule there is one clear mucoid alveolus with its associated serous demilune, toward the left. Serous acini, on the other hand, line the right-hand margin beneath the capsule.

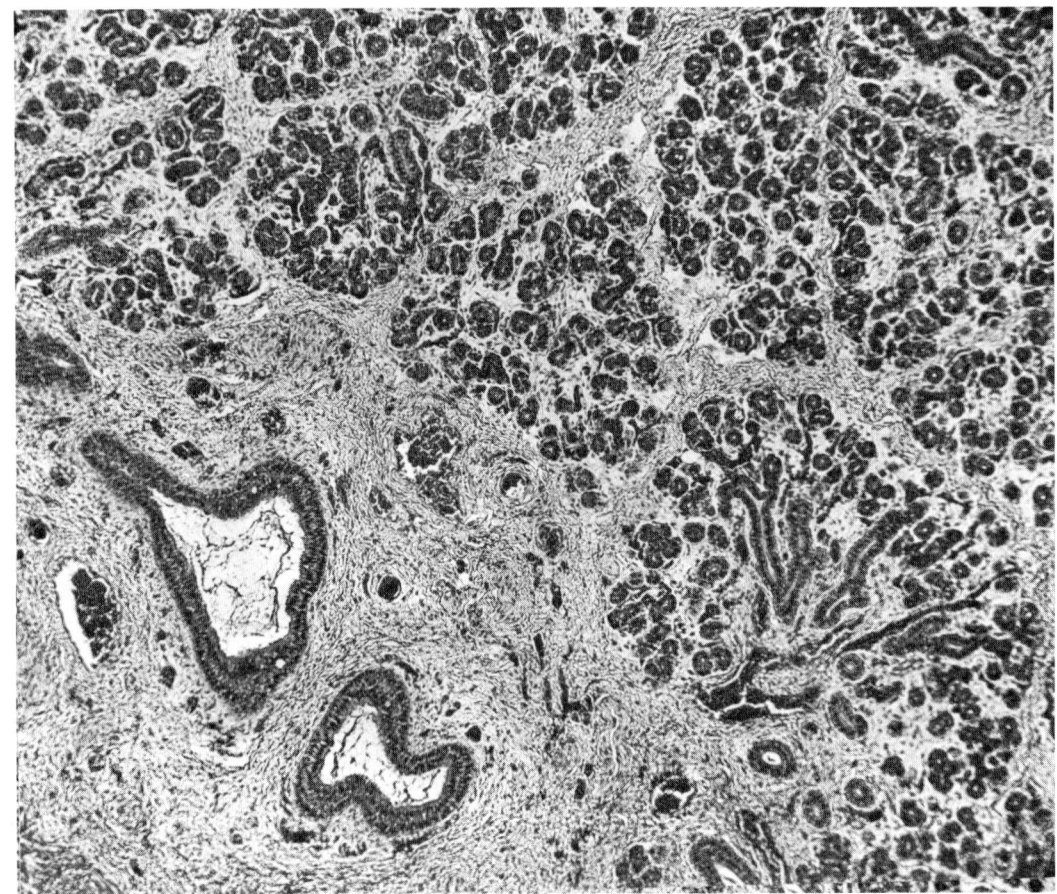

Figure 13-5

Figure 13-5. The submandibular gland of a term infant seen at medium magnification. The lobular arrangement of the acini is quite apparent, as is the tree-like branching of small ducts in the right lower corner.

This infant weighed 2,850 grams at postmortem examination. She was born at 40 weeks of gestation and lived for 14 hours.

Hematoxylin and eosin stain. Mag. 179×.

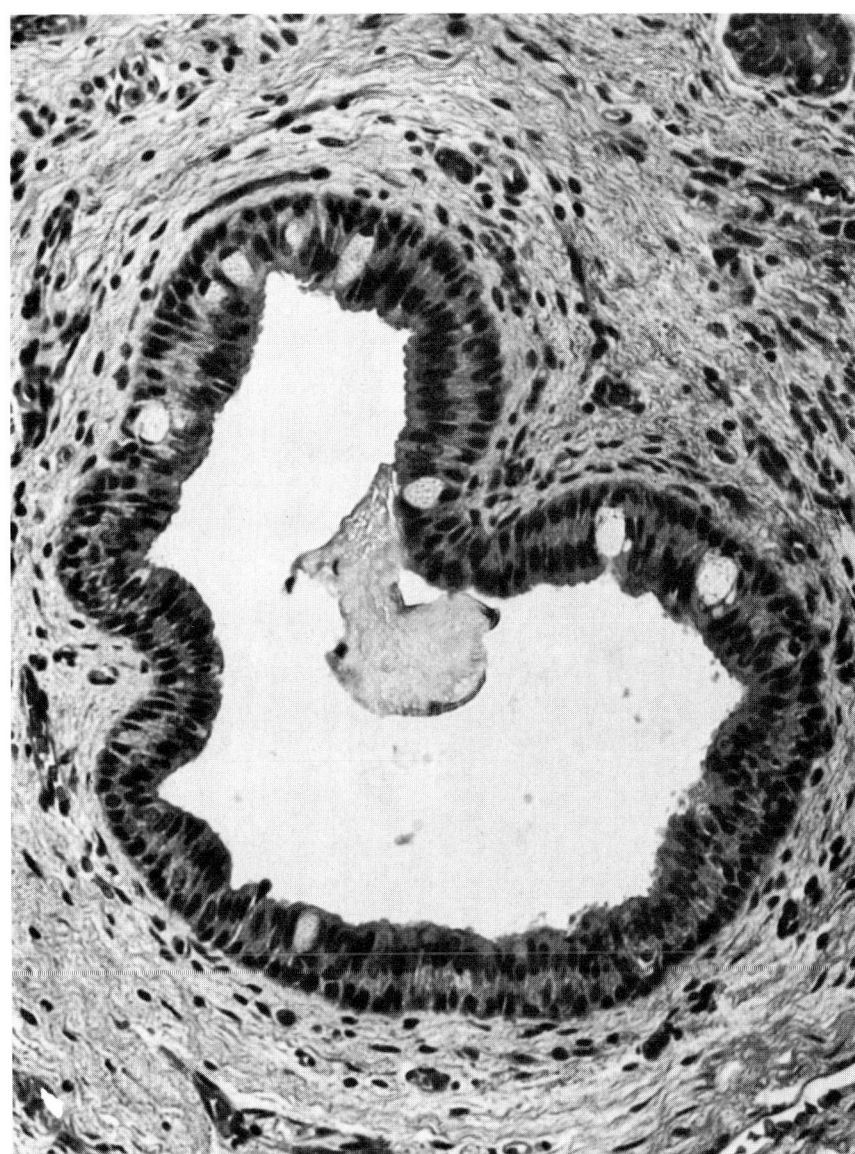

Figure 13-6

Figure 13-6. This illustration depicts the character of the epithelial lining of a large duct within the submandibular gland shown in Fig. 13-3. A single serous acinus appears in the upper left corner.

The epithelial lining is columnar pseudostratified at this point, and it contains scattered individual goblet cells. The nature of this epithelium does not change with time.

This section is from the same patient as Fig. 13-3.

Hematoxylin and eosin stain. Mag. 317×.

Chapter 14

ESOPHAGUS

EMBRYOLOGY

In the four millimeter human embryo during the fourth week of development, the esophagus is a short tube connecting the caudal end of the pharynx with the minimal dilation of the endodermal tract or foregut distally, representing the primitive stomach.[2] Early on, the esophagus is incompletely divided longitudinally from the trachea, which is developing ventral to it. This separation, in the form of a tracheoesophageal septum, begins caudally and proceeds cranially. (The two, of course, remain permanently united at the level of the pharynx.)

The esophagus elongates rapidly, keeping pace with the differentiating neck and growing heart and lungs adjacent to it.[2] Most of this is the result of cranial body growth or "ascent" of the pharynx. The endoderm of the esophagus proliferates, almost obliterating the lumen; then it recanalizes by the end of the embryonic period, at about seven weeks. At no time is the lumen totally occluded. The epithelium begins to acquire cilia at ten weeks, and it is not until the fifth month that a stratified squamous epithelium starts replacing it. At birth, the lining epithelium is multilayered but, especially in the premature infant, it may still include surface patches of ciliated cells, particularly near the cardioesophageal junction (Figs. 14–6 and 14–7).

The striated muscle of the upper end (Figure 14–11a) is derived from the caudal branchial arches;[1] the smooth muscle of the lower end (Fig. 14–11b) develops from surrounding splanchnic mesenchyme.

Superficial glands develop in the fifth month (Figs. 14–8 to 14–10). Deep glands arise mostly after birth.[2]

ANATOMY

The esophagus is a muscular tube connecting the pharynx to the stomach. It descends anterior to the vertebral column, through the superior and posterior parts of the mediastinum, pierces the diaphragm, and ends at the cardiac orifice of the stomach.[3]

The general direction of the esophagus is vertical, but it deviates slightly to the left as far as the root of the neck. There are also anteroposterior flexures corresponding to the curvatures of the cervical and thoracic parts of the vertebral column.

The esophagus is the narrowest part of the alimentary canal except for the vermiform appendix. It is slightly constricted at four sites: at its commencement, where it is crossed by the aortic arch, where it is crossed by the left main stem bronchus, and where it pierces the diaphragm.

Immediately anterior to the cervical part lies the trachea, the posterior membranous wall of which is attached to the esophagus by loose connective tissue. The recurrent laryngeal nerves are located one on each side.

The thoracic part of the esophagus is situated at first in the superior mediastinum between the trachea and the vertebral column, a little to the left of the midline. It passes behind and to the right of the aortic arch and descends in the posterior mediastinum along the right side of the descending thoracic aorta. In the lower part of the posterior mediastinum, the thoracic portion of the esophagus, bending forward and to the left, passes in front and to the right of the descending aorta.

The abdominal part of the esophagus below the diaphragm is slightly to the left of the midline. It is curved a little to the left. The right border continues evenly into the lesser curvature of the stomach; its left border is separated from the fundus by the cardiac notch. Peritoneum covers it anteriorly and on the left side only.

HISTOLOGY

The esophagus is lined by stratified squamous epithelium that is not keratinized. The lamina propria consists of loose connective tissue with thin collagenous fibers and networks of fine elastic fibers (Figs. 14–5 and 14–8). At the level of the cricoid cartilage, the elastic layer of the pharynx is succeeded by a lamina muscularis mucosae, which consists of longitudinal smooth muscle fibers and some elastic fibers as well (Figs. 14–3, 14–4, and 14–8).

The connective tissue of the tela submucosa, which is collagenous and elastic, may contain some lymphocytes, especially around glands (Figs. 14–8 and 14–9).

The muscular coat in the upper third of the esophagus consists of striated muscle in both the inner and outer layers (Fig. 14–11a). In the middle third it is gradually replaced by smooth muscle, and in the lower third it is exclusively smooth muscle (Figs. 14–4 and 14–11b). In both the internal and external layers there may be spiral, oblique, or other irregularly oriented bundles of muscle.[4]

The outer surface of the esophagus is connected with surrounding structures by a layer of loose connective tissue composing the tunica adventitia (Fig. 14–1).

There are true glands in the tela submucosa of the esophagus of the newborn (Figs. 14–8 to 14–10). They are unevenly distributed, small, compound glands with branched tubuloalveolar secretory portions containing only mucous cells. The branches fuse into main ducts, which pierce the lamina muscularis mucosae and open into the lumen by way of small orifices (Fig. 14–10). The epithelium of the smallest ducts is low columnar, and that of the main ducts is stratified squamous. Especially in prematurely born infants, in the lowest portion of the esophagus, there are patches of epithelium that, at least superficially, are columnar and ciliated (Fig. 14–6). Such patches are presumably remnants of the embryonic condition. They are larger and more numerous in more prematurely born babies, but are scarce to nonexistent in infants born at term.

Islets of gastric mucosa, appearing to the naked eye as minute, pale pink, ovoid, slightly elevated, discrete patches, can be seen at autopsy in the mucosa of the upper third of the esophagus. They occur invariably at the level of the larynx, usually anteriorly, and are oriented in the long axis of the esophagus.

References

All references for Part Six appear on page 271.

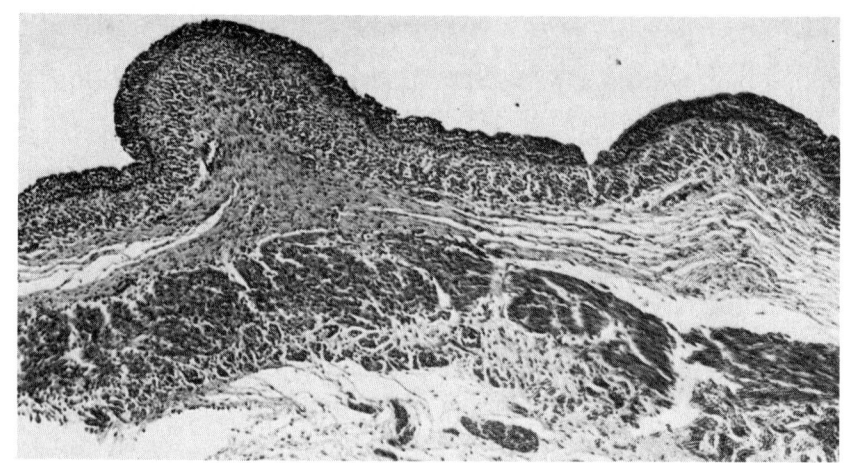

Figure 14–1

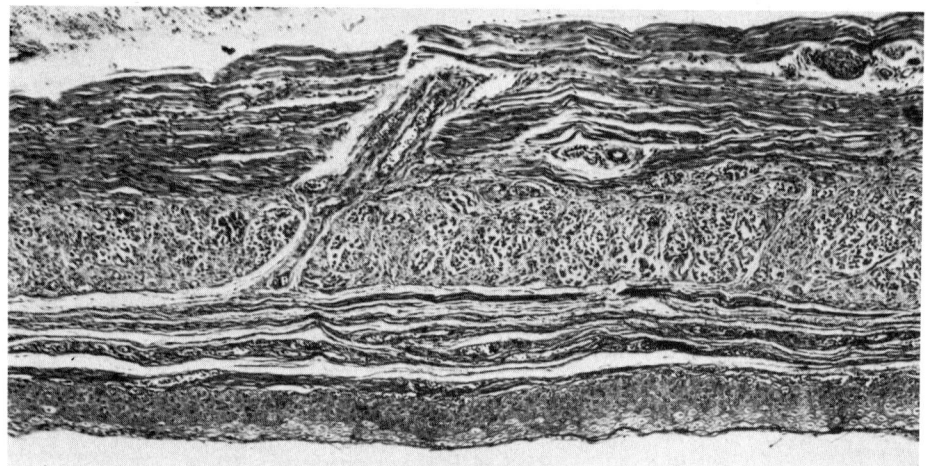

Figure 14–2

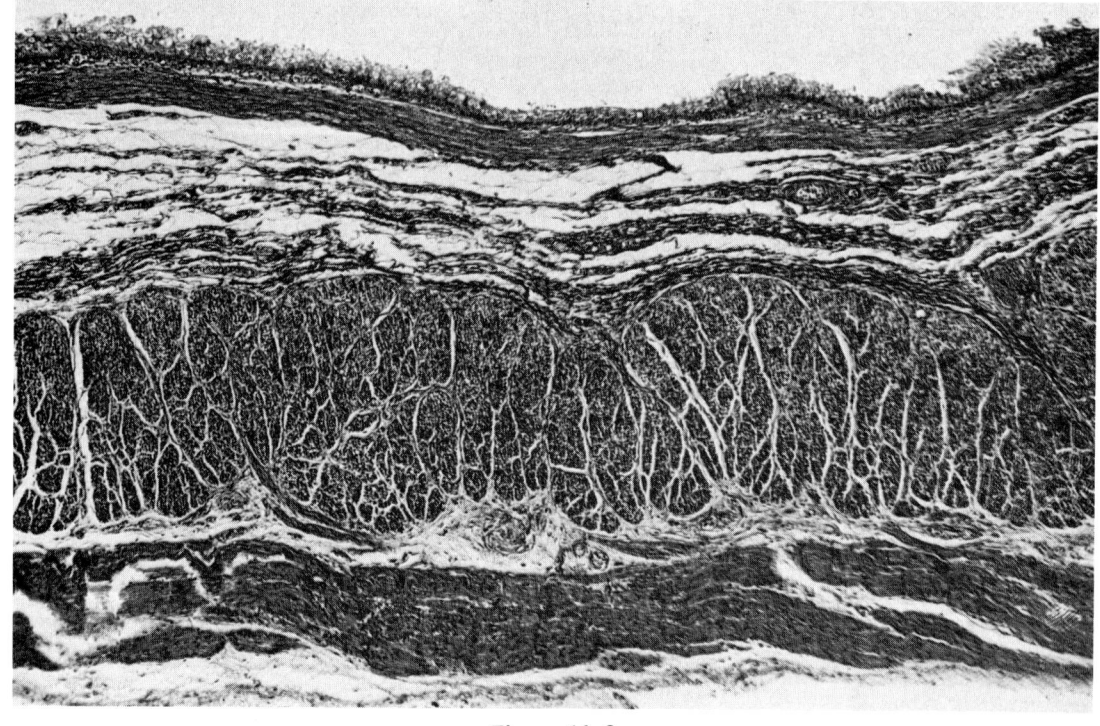

Figure 14–3

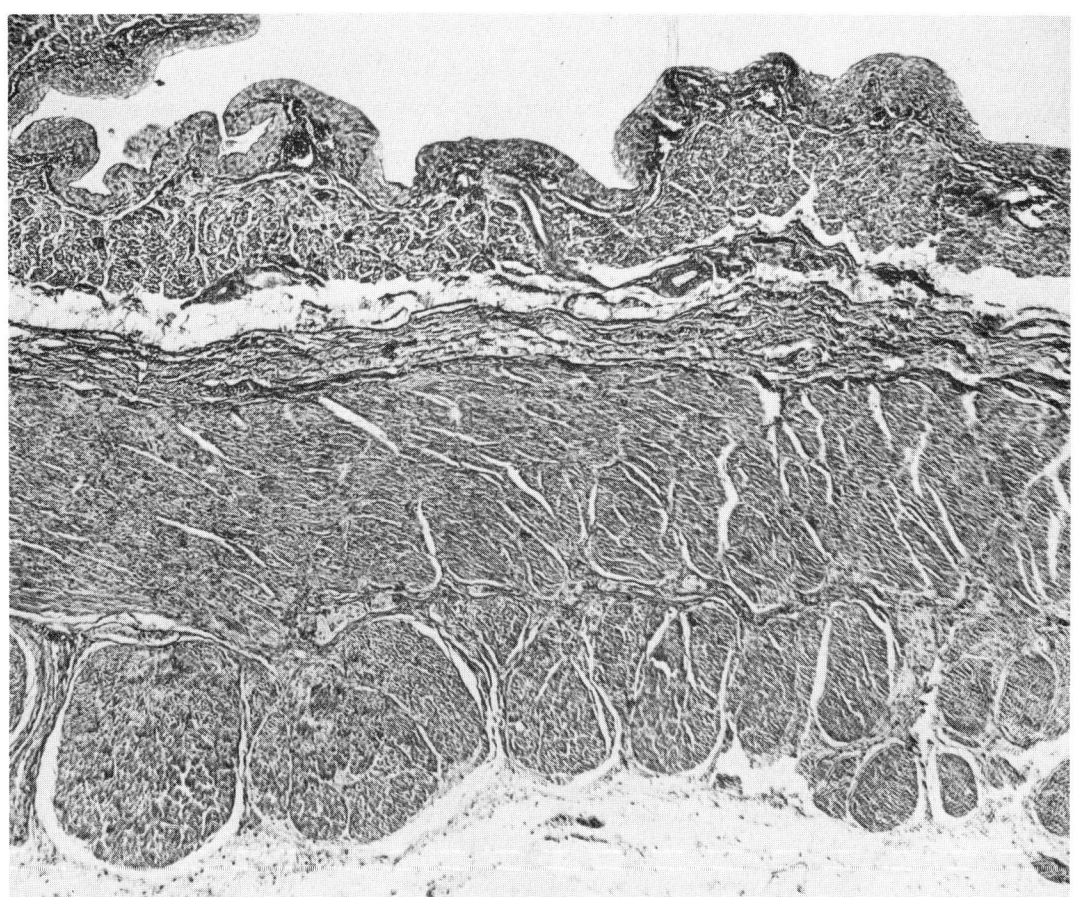

Figure 14–4

Figures 14–1 to 14–4. This set of four photomicrographs, taken at the same magnification, illustrates the changes that take place in the histologic appearance of the esophagus during the latter half of gestation and the first weeks of extrauterine life.

Hematoxylin and eosin stain. Mag. 55×.

Fig.	Wt.	Race	Sex	Gestation	Age
14–1	308 gm. (twin)	B	F	17 wk.	2 hr.
14–2	1,240 gm.	W	F	27 wk.	15 days
14–3	2,000 gm.	W	F	32 wk.	13 hr. 18 min.
14–4	3,800 gm.	?	M	40 wk.	21 days

198 ESOPHAGUS

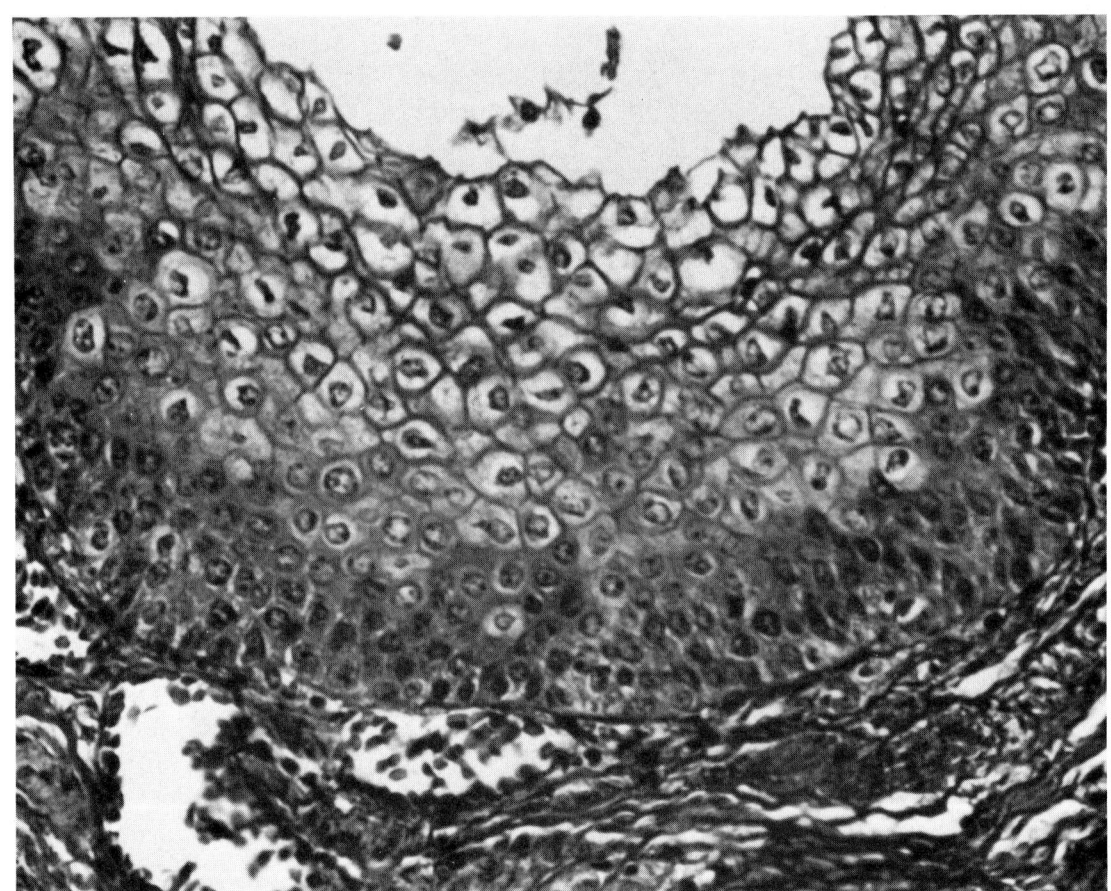

Figure 14–5

Figure 14–5. This illustration shows, in some detail, the nature of the lining of the esophagus in the fetus and the newborn. It is orderly, nonkeratinized, stratified squamous epithelium.

The patient was a 6 day old female infant who died of pneumonia and whose body weighed 3,090 grams at autopsy.

Hematoxylin and eosin stain. Mag. 369×.

ESOPHAGUS

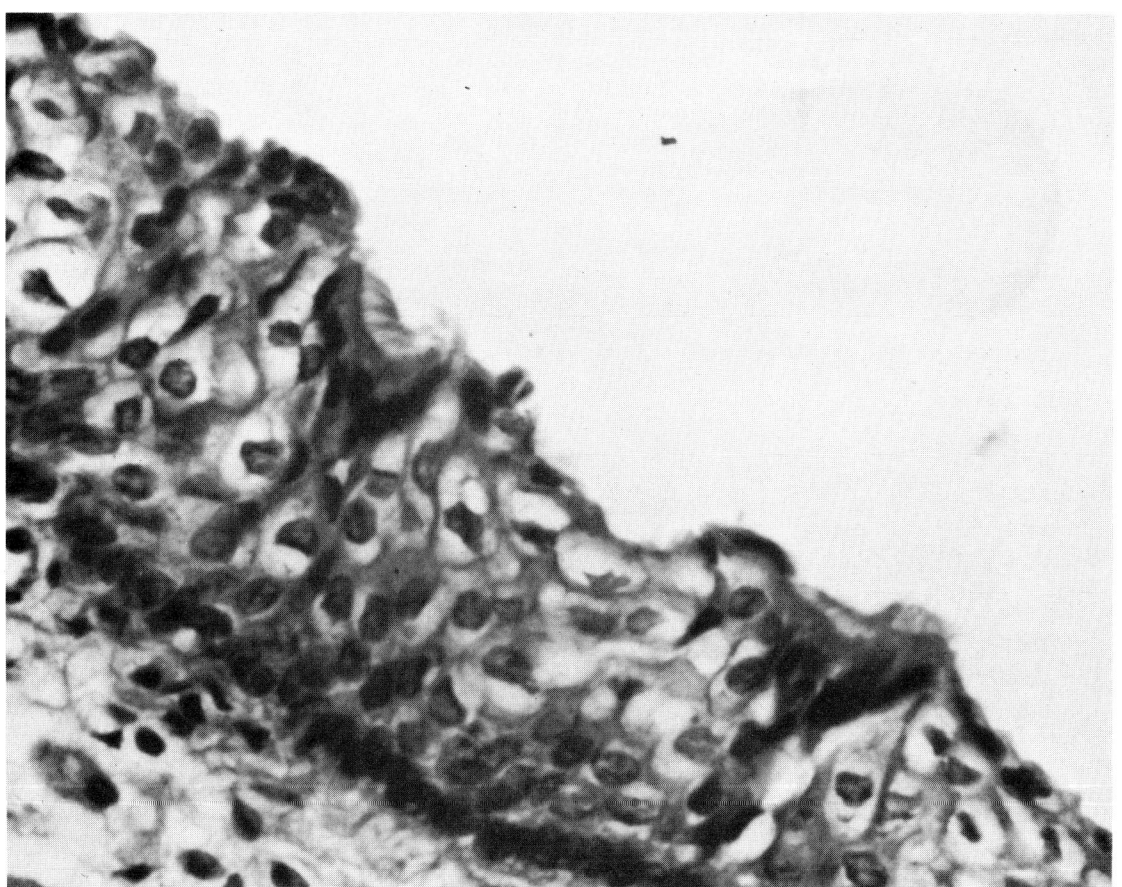

Figure 14-6

Figure 14-6. Relatively commonly, particularly among premature infants, the epithelial lining of the lower end of the esophagus harbors an island or two of superficially placed, ciliated columnar epithelium. These are said to be remnants of the foregut, which, during the fourth week of embryonic life, divides into the trachea ventrally and the esophagus dorsally.

The patient was a male infant who died at 13 hours of age of pulmonary hyaline membrane disease. His body weighed 1,360 grams at necropsy. (Estimated gestational age: 28 weeks.)

Hematoxylin and eosin stain. Mag. 660×.

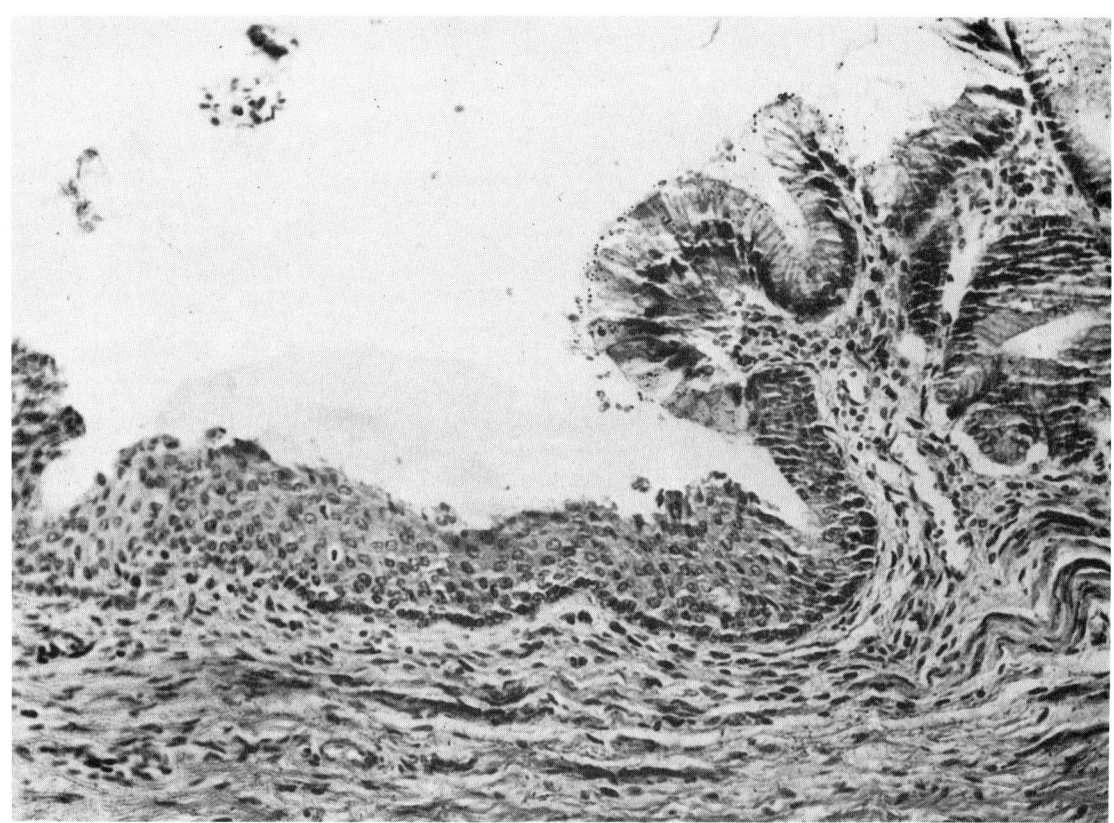

Figure 14–7

Figure 14–7. This represents the junction of stratified squamous and tall columnar mucus-producing epithelium at the level where the lower portion of the esophagus joins the cardia.

The patient was a 2,850 gram black male infant who lived for 1 day, 1½ hours. (Estimated gestational age: 36 weeks.)

Hematoxylin and eosin stain. Mag. 208×.

Figure 14–8. The entrance of a duct into the lumen of the esophagus; acini of the related mucous gland appear along the lower border.

The subject was a 2,120 gram white male, 4 days and 8 hours of age, whose gestation was said to have been of 35 weeks' duration.

Hematoxylin and eosin stain. Mag. 153×.

Figure 14–9. Several acini of an esophageal gland from a 12 day old male infant weighing 2,820 grams. (Estimated gestational age: 37 weeks.)

Hematoxylin and eosin stain. Mag. 270×.

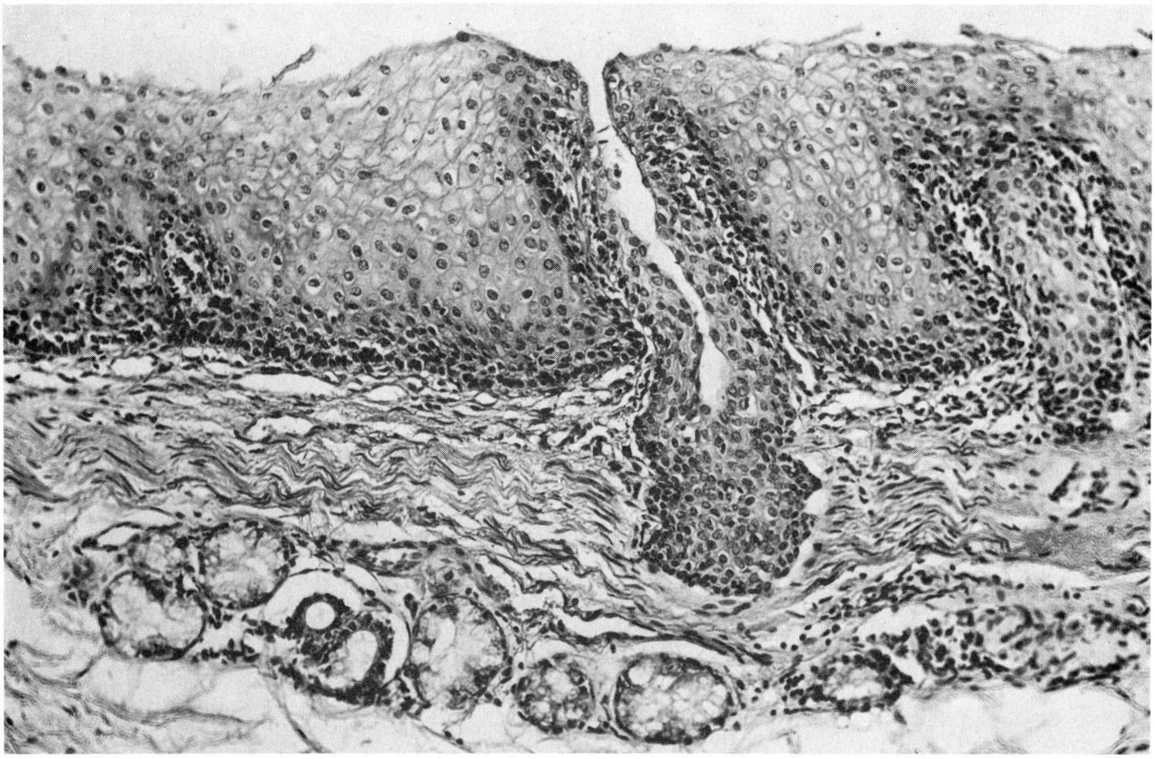

ESOPHAGUS 201

Figure 14–8

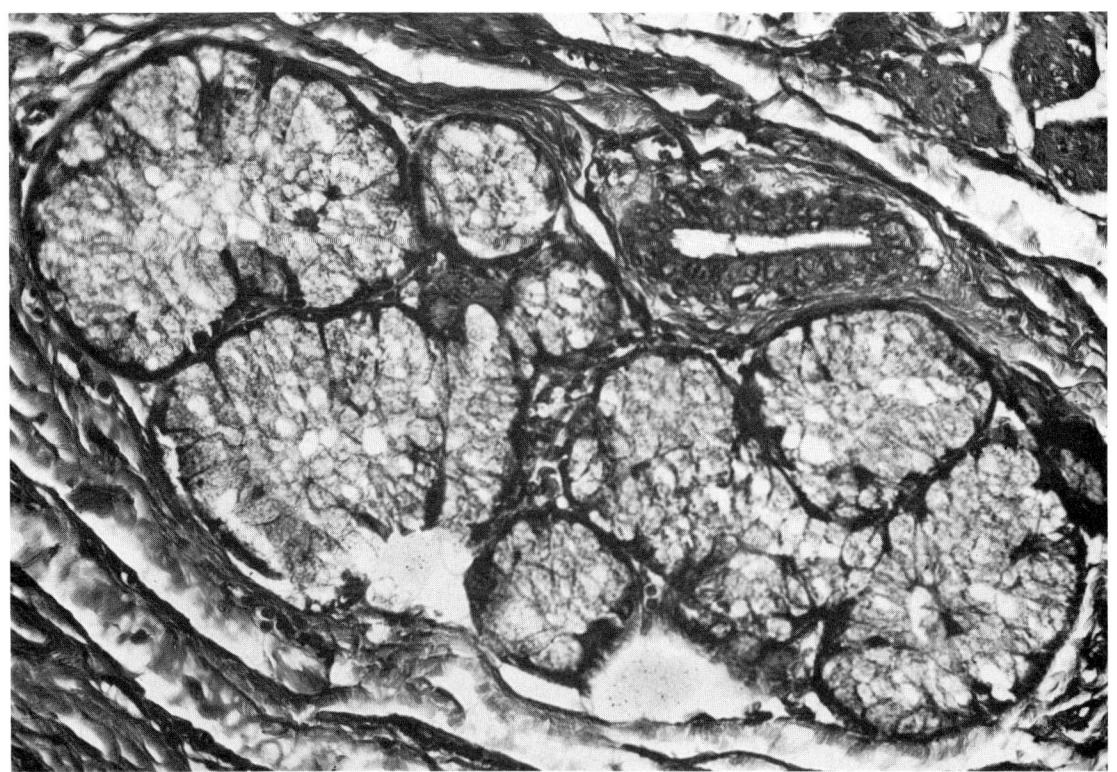

Figure 14–9

Figure 14–10. These are ducts of esophageal glands from a rather mature infant, a female who died at 9 days of age. Her body weighed 2,420 grams at postmortem examination. (Estimated gestational age: 34 weeks.)
Hematoxylin and eosin stain.

Figure 14–10a. Longitudinal section, moderate magnification. Mag. 153×.

Figure 14–10b. Cross section of one of the larger ducts from the same esophagus. Mag. 555×.

Figure 14–10c. Enlargement of a portion of Fig. 14–10a. Mag. 370×.

See illustrations on the opposite page

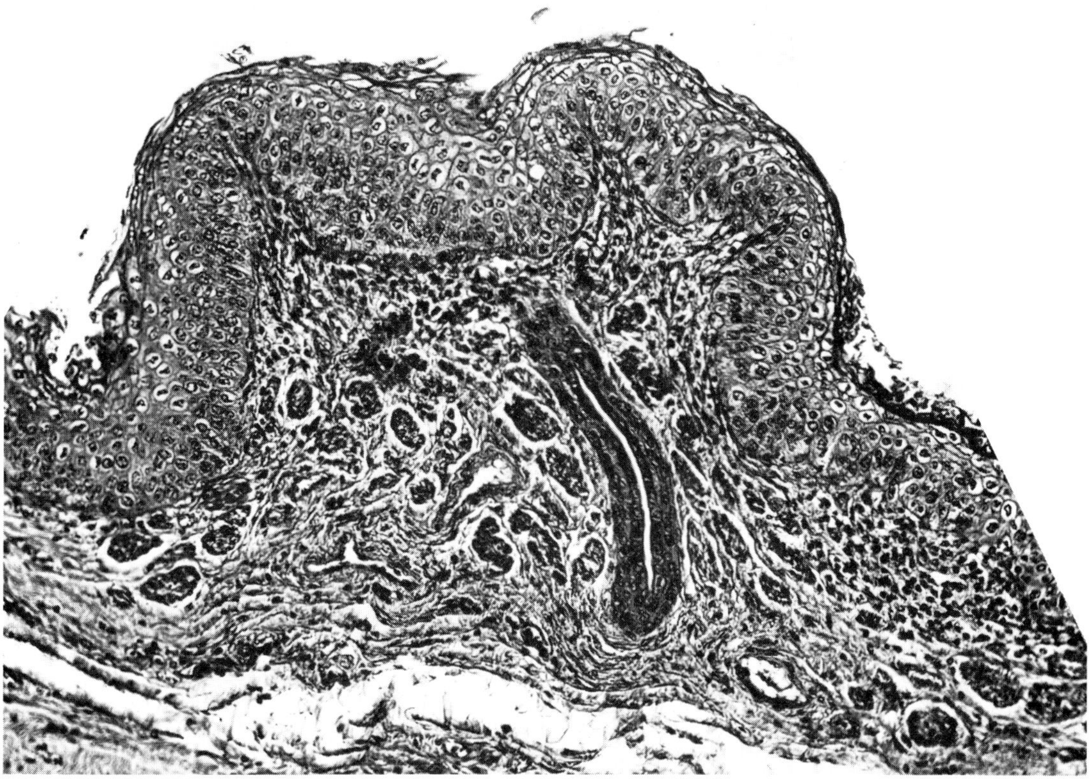

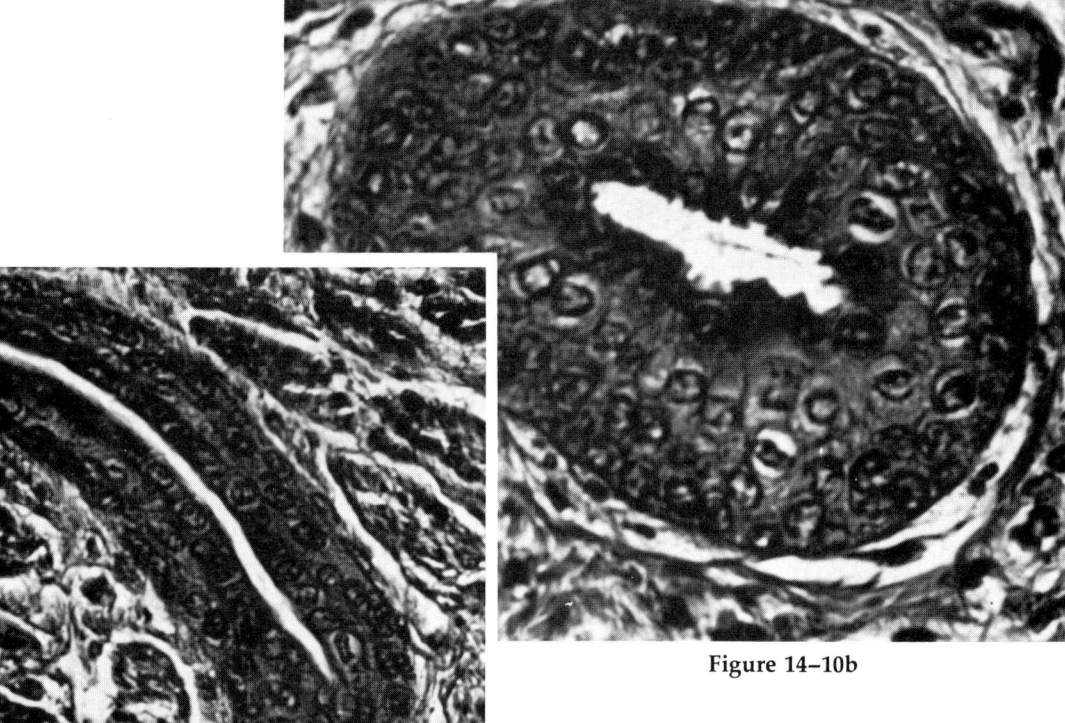

Figure 14–10a

Figure 14–10b

Figure 14–10c

See legend on the opposite page

204 ESOPHAGUS

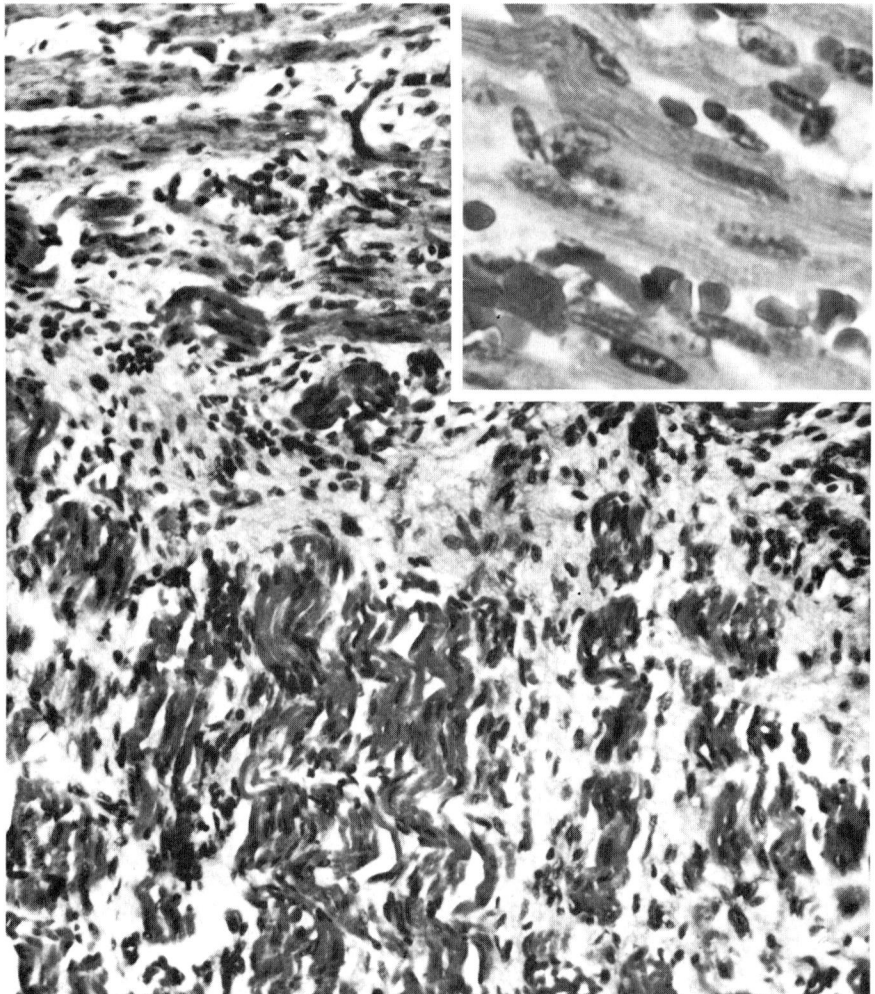

Figure 14–11a

Figures 14–11a and 14–11b. These two photomicrographs, taken at the same magnification (220.8×), show the two types of muscle in the esophagus, the skeletal muscle of the upper portion (Fig. 14–11a) and the smooth muscle of the lower (Fig. 14–11b). Notice that in each instance the muscular coat is arranged in two layers, an inner circular (above) and an outer longitudinal (below).

In the inset, upper right (mag. 771.7×), several individual fibers show quite clearly the identifying cross striations.

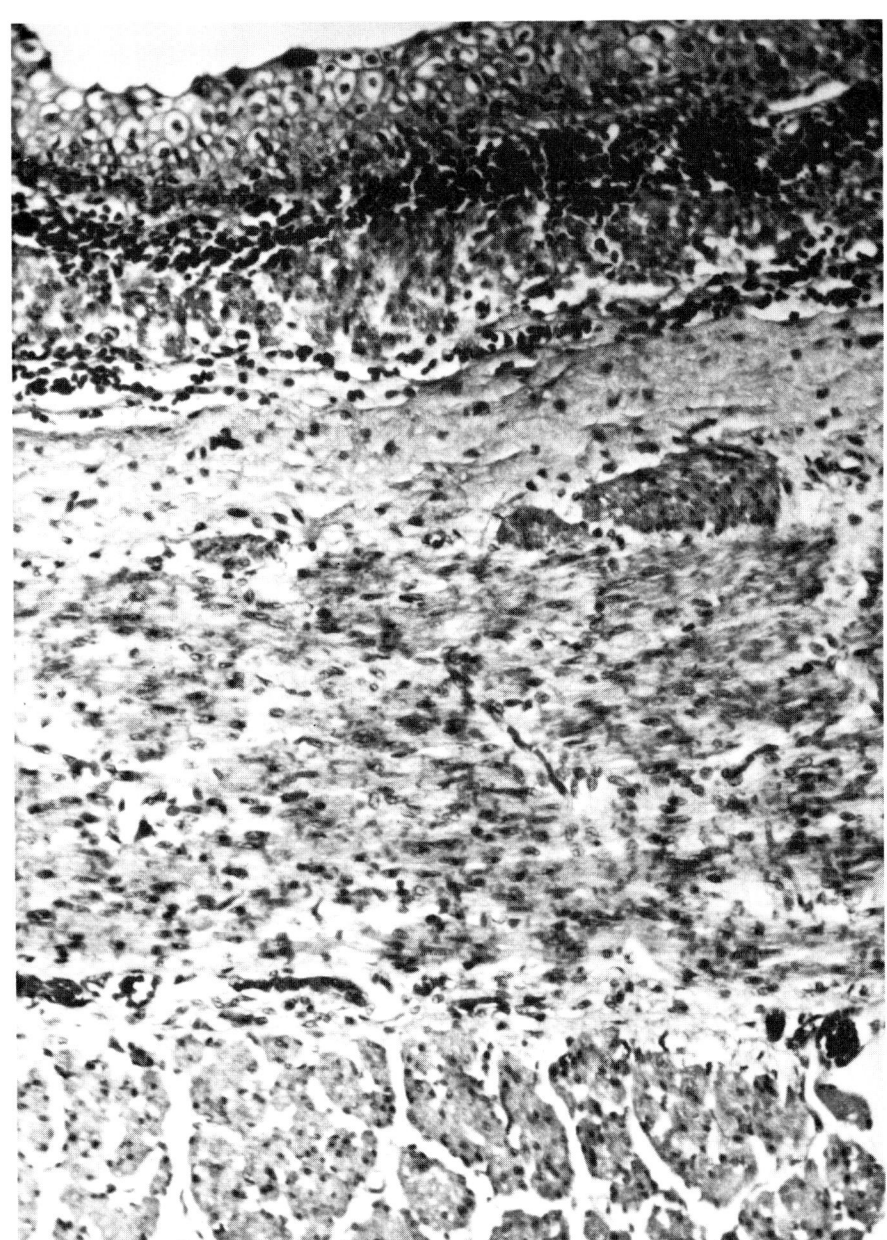

Figure 14–11b

Figures 14–11a and 14–11b Continued. Both of these sections were taken from the same infant. The baby was a one day old black male, born after 30 weeks of gestation. His body weight at autopsy was 1,500 grams.

Hematoxylin and eosin stain. Mag. 220.8×.

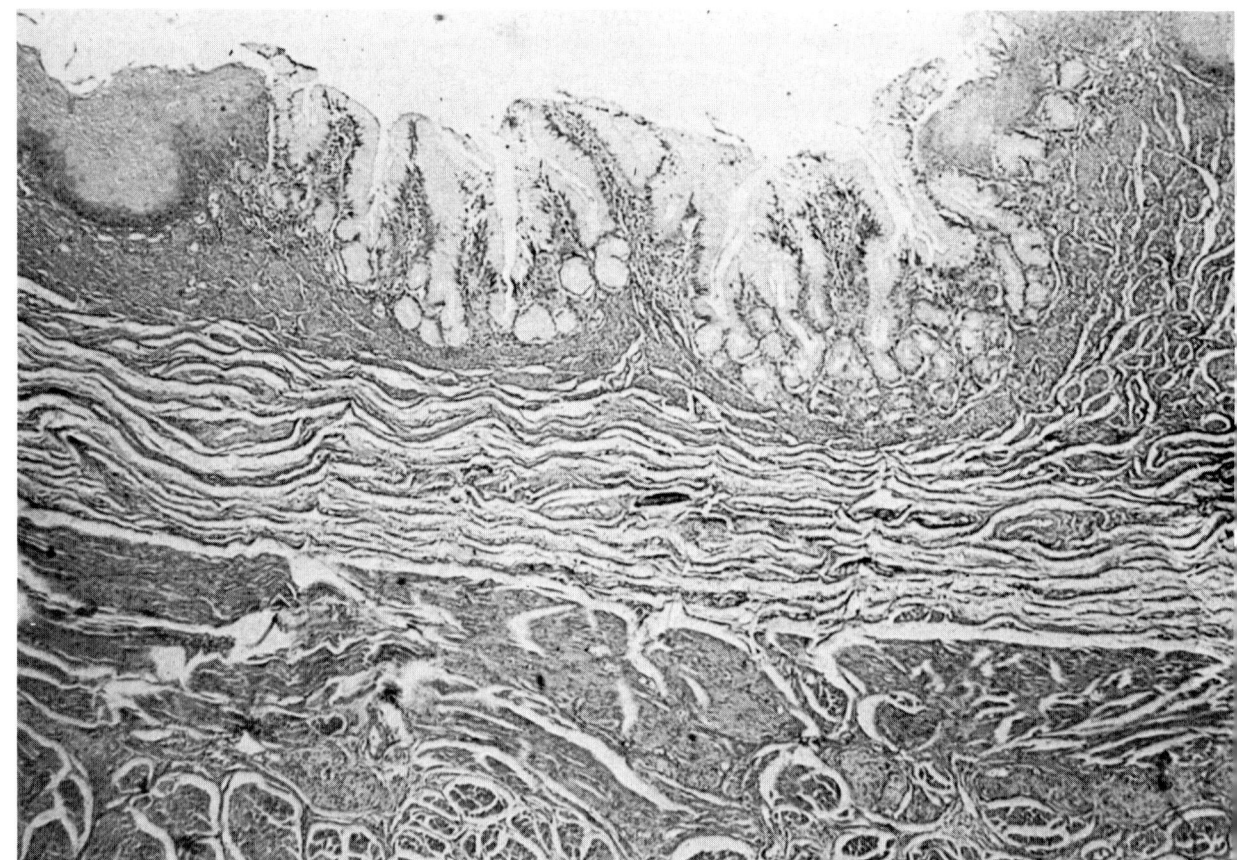

Figure 14–12

Figure 14–12. This is a cross section taken from the upper third of the esophagus of a newborn infant, through the very center of a sharply demarcated patch about 7 mm. in greatest dimension, elliptical, with its long axis vertically oriented, pointed at each end, pink against a grey background, and ever so slightly depressed. Grossly and microscopically this is typical of an island of aberrant gastric mucosa, a relatively common feature of the esophagus in newborns. Most are located at the level of the larynx and in close proximity to it, near the midline and on the anterior wall.

The identity of the infant from whom this section was taken has been lost to us. Hematoxylin and eosin stain.

Chapter 15

STOMACH

EMBRYOLOGY

The stomach first manifests itself at about four weeks as a gradual spindle-shaped dilatation of the caudal part of the foregut, somewhat flattened on its lateral surfaces. Originally it lies in the future neck region, but by the end of the seventh week it is permanently located in the abdomen. During this "descent" the dorsal border grows faster than the ventral, producing the greater curvature.[1] As the organ acquires its ultimate shape, it also rotates clockwise 90 degrees around its longitudinal axis so that the lesser curvature moves to the right, the greater to the left; the original left side becomes the ventral aspect and the right side becomes the dorsal aspect.[1] Meanwhile, the fundus arises as a local bulge near the cranial end, and the stomach is somewhat displaced by the enlarging liver until it extends obliquely from left (above) to center (below).[2]

The epithelium differentiates into distinctive gastric glands, first as pits at seven weeks and finally as budding glands at fourteen weeks. The mesenchyme produces three incomplete layers of the muscular coat, and the pylorus becomes distinguishable in the third month.

ANATOMY

The stomach is the most dilated part of the digestive tract, and it is situated between the lower end of the esophagus and the upper end of the small bowel. Its mean capacity is said, at the time of a term birth, to be 30 ml.

The stomach has two openings and, in a rough way, two curvatures or borders, and two surfaces. In fact, its external surface is a continuum and has no definable borders. However, the peritoneal surface is interrupted by the attachments of the greater and lesser omenta along its profiles, so that these "borders" may be considered as separating the surfaces.

The opening by which the esophagus communicates with the stomach is called the cardiac orifice, and it is situated just to the left of the midline.

That part of the stomach to the left of and above the cardiac orifice is called the fundus, which really is not a very appropriate term. The opening into the duodenum is the pyloric orifice; externally it is made apparent, though just slightly in the perinatal period, by a broad groove on the surface of the organ which corresponds to the pyloric muscle. The pyloric orifice is located to the right of the midline.

The lesser curvature extends between the cardiac and pyloric orifices, forming the right or posterosuperior border of the stomach. It descends as a continuation of the right margin of the esophagus. The most dependent part of the curve is referred to as the angular incisure. The lesser curvature of the stomach serves as the site of attachment of the lesser omentum.

The greater curvature is directed anteroinferiorly and is several times longer than the lesser curvature. Starting from the cardiac orifice at the cardiac notch, it forms an arc bending backward, upward, and to the left; the highest point of the convexity represents the apex of the fundus. From this level it proceeds downward and forward with a slight convexity to the left; then it turns to the right to end in the pylorus.

The two surfaces are the anterosuperior and the posteroinferior.

HISTOLOGY

The entire thickness of the mucous membrane of the stomach is occupied by a multitude of glands that open into the bottoms of the gastric pits. The epithelium that lines the gastric pits and covers the entire free surface of the mucosa between them is of the same structure throughout the entire stomach (Figs. 15–5, 15–7, 15–8b, 15–9, and 15–10). This epithelium is tall columnar, and it begins abruptly at the cardioesophageal junction. It is mucus-producing and highly vacuolated.

On the basis of the cell population of the gastric glands, the stomach has been divided into three regions: (1) the cardiac area, which contains only cardiac glands (Fig. 15–11), (2) the corpus, containing gastric glands (Fig. 15–12), and (3) the pyloric region in the distal third, characterized by the presence of pyloric glands (Fig. 15–13). These zones are not sharply demarcated.

Of the three types of glands, the gastric are the most important and are found over the entire corpus. They are closely packed and oriented perpendicular to the surface of the mucosa, extending through its entire thickness. From one to several glands open through a narrow neck into a single gastric pit. Their blind ends are slightly expanded and coiled, and sometimes divide into two or three branches (Figs. 15–3, 15–7, 15–9, 15–10, and 15–12). The gastric glands are composed of four types of cells: (1) chief cells, (2) parietal cells, (3) neck mucous cells, and (4) argentaffin cells.

By contrast, the pyloric glands are lined by only one type of cell, having pale cytoplasm (Figs. 15–2, 15–5, 15–6, 15–8a, and 15–13). The nucleus of the cell is often flattened against the base of the cell. The gastric pits in the pyloric area are deeper than those in the gastric area (Fig. 15–8b). The pyloric glands are simple and branched tubular glands (Figs. 15–8a and 15–13).

The cardiac glands in the immediate vicinity of the esophageal orifice are composed of mucous cells that are indistinguishable from those of the pyloric glands (Figs. 15–11 and 15–13).

The lamina propria is narrow between the glands and the muscularis mucosae; it forms larger masses in the vicinity of the necks of the glands and about the gastric pits (Figs. 15–5, 15–7, 15–8a, and 15–9). It consists of a delicate network of collagenous and reticular fibers.[4] In the newborn, it contains a moderate number of lymphoid cells.

The submucosa in the newborn infant consists of dense connective tissue only. It may contain a few lymphoid and wandering cells; it also contains blood vessels, lymph vessels, and venous plexuses.

The muscular coat is said to consist of three layers, but these are often difficult or impossible to distinguish in the newborn (Figs. 15–1, 15–3, 15–4, 15–14, 15–15, and 15–16). They are the outer longitudinal, the middle circular, and the inner oblique layers. The middle is said to be the most continuous and the most regularly organized of the three. It is this one that forms the thick, circular sphincter of the pylorus (Fig. 15–2). As the stomach of the newborn infant becomes distended, there are often prominent gaps between bundles within individual layers; this is apparently physiologic and does not represent congenital absence at the site (Fig. 15–16).

The serosa or outermost coat of the stomach is a thin layer of loose connective tissue overlying the muscular coat, covered on its external aspect with mesothelium (Figs. 15–14, 15–15, and 15–16).

References

All references for Part Six appear on page 271.

STOMACH

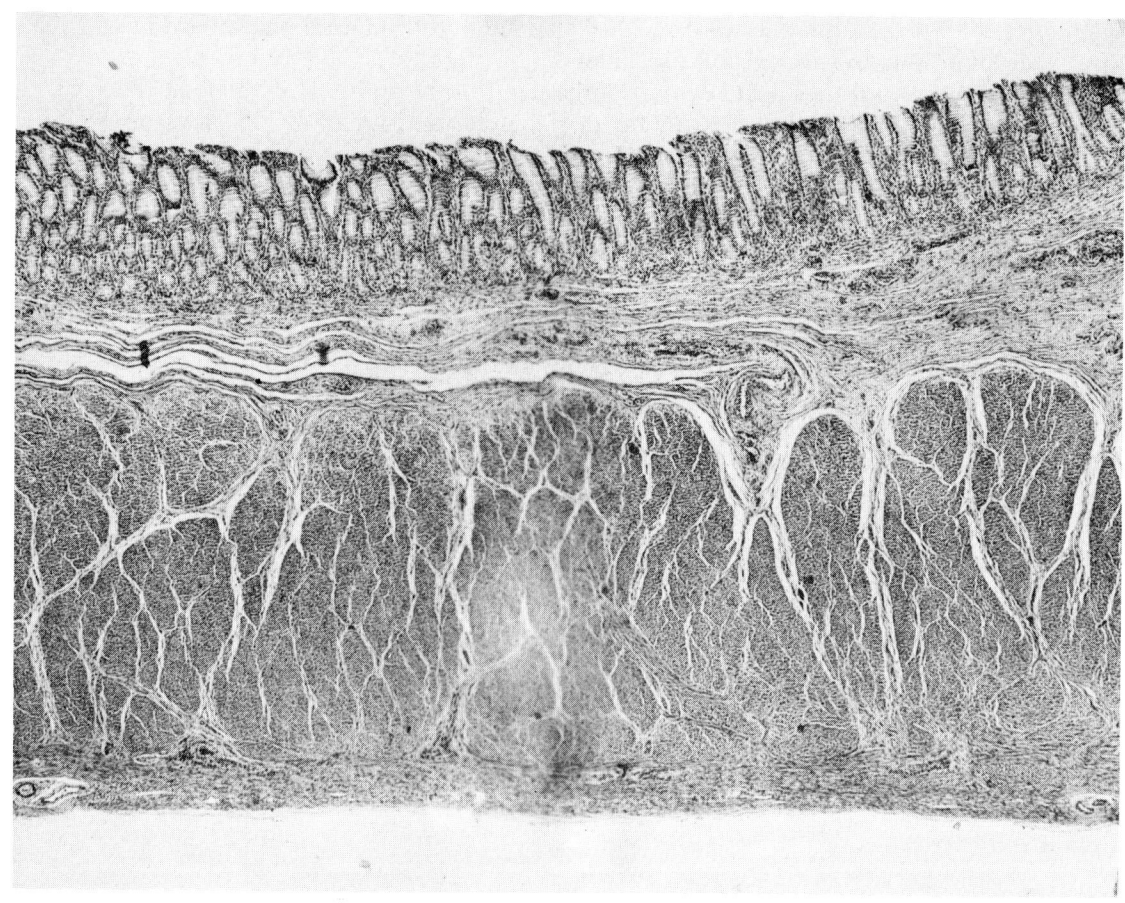

Figure 15–1

Figure 15–1. This is a survey view of the wall of the stomach of a male infant who died at 42 hours of age of pulmonary hyaline membrane disease and bronchopneumonia. His body weight at necropsy was 2,615 grams. (Estimated gestational age: 34 weeks.)
Hematoxylin and eosin stain. Mag. 45×.

STOMACH 211

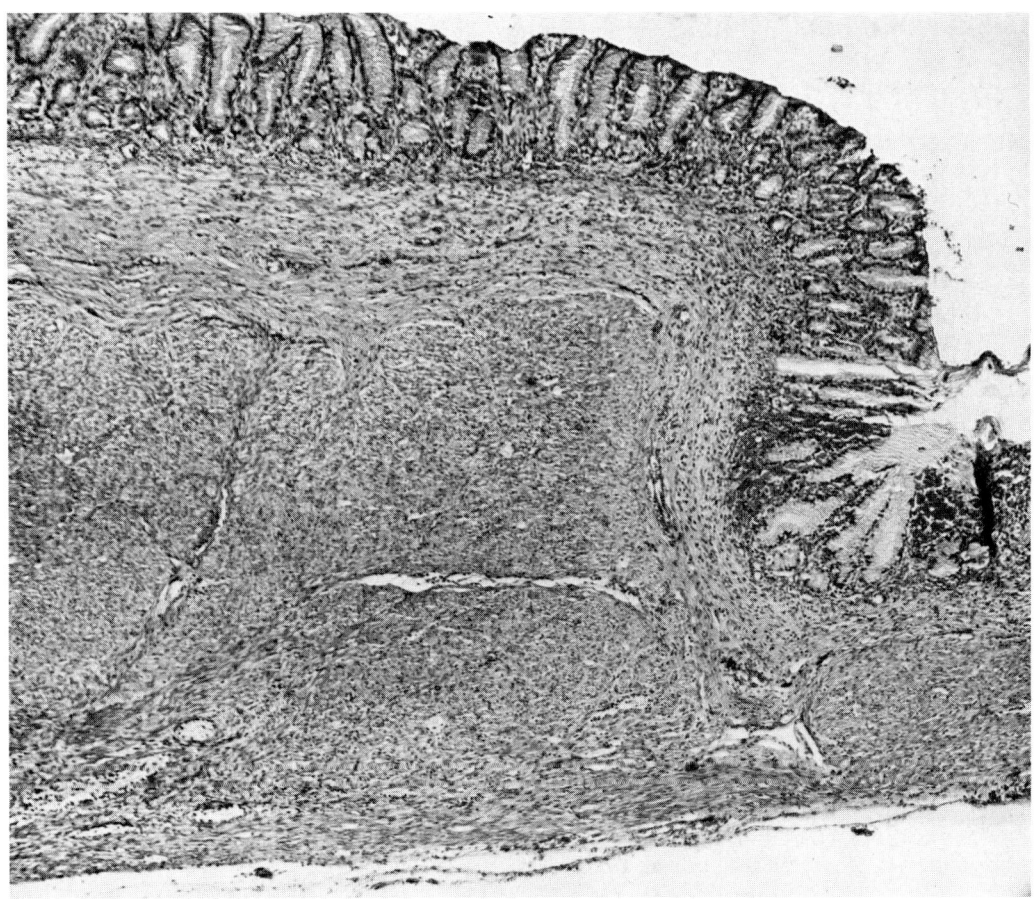

Figure 15-2

Figure 15-2. This is a longitudinal section through the pylorus of a 15 hour old white infant whose body weighed 1,250 grams at postmortem examination. (Estimated gestational age: 27 weeks.)
Hematoxylin and eosin stain. Mag. 55×.

212   STOMACH

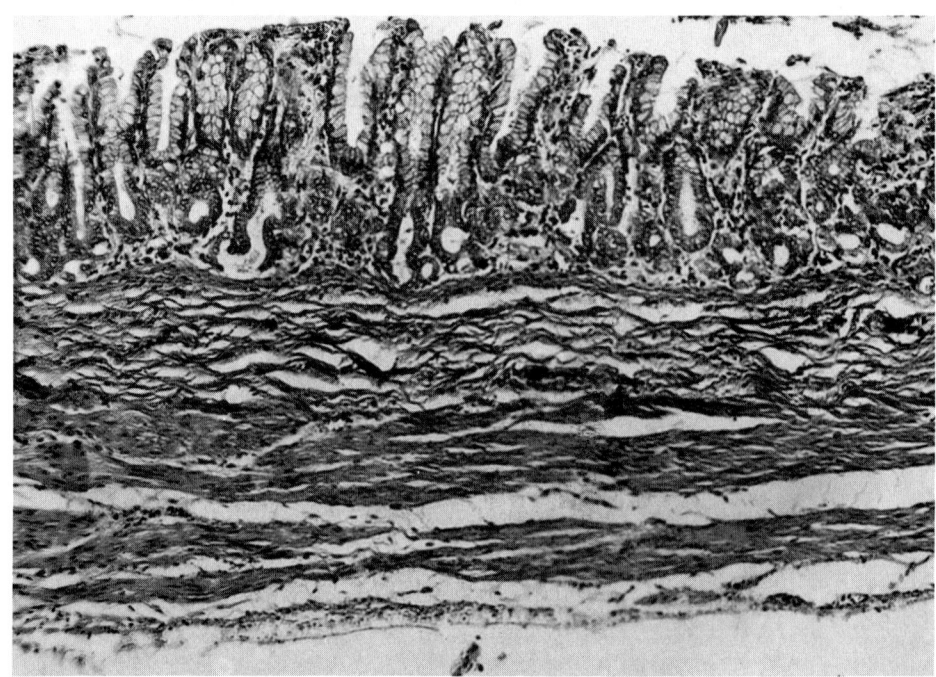

Figure 15–3

Figure 15–3. This photograph provides a view, at higher magnification, of the entire thickness of the wall of the stomach of a premature infant.

This female newborn died at the age of 7 days. Body weight at autopsy was 2,045 grams. (Estimated gestational age: 31 weeks.)

Hematoxylin and eosin stain. Mag. 124×.

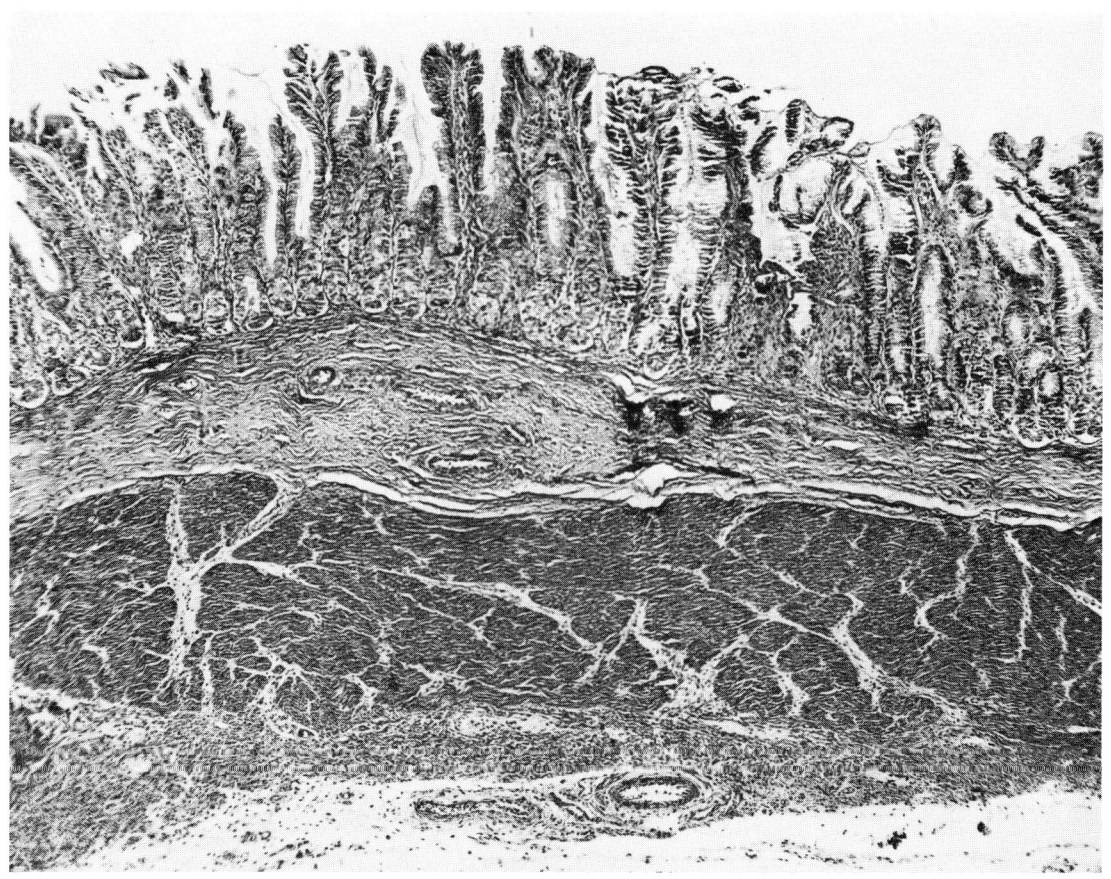

Figure 15-4

Figure 15-4. This is a section through the thickness of the wall of the stomach of a somewhat more mature infant, a female who survived for 6 days. Her body weighed slightly more than 3,000 grams. (Estimated gestational age: 33 weeks.)
Hematoxylin and eosin stain. Mag. 76×.

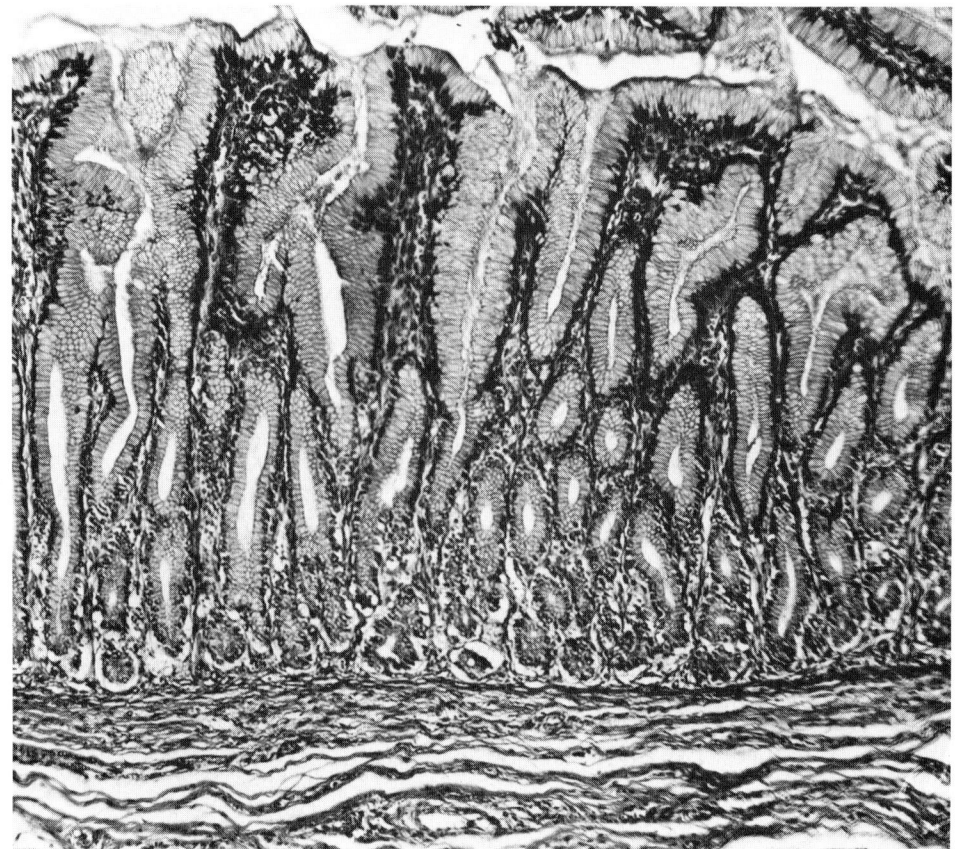

Figure 15–5

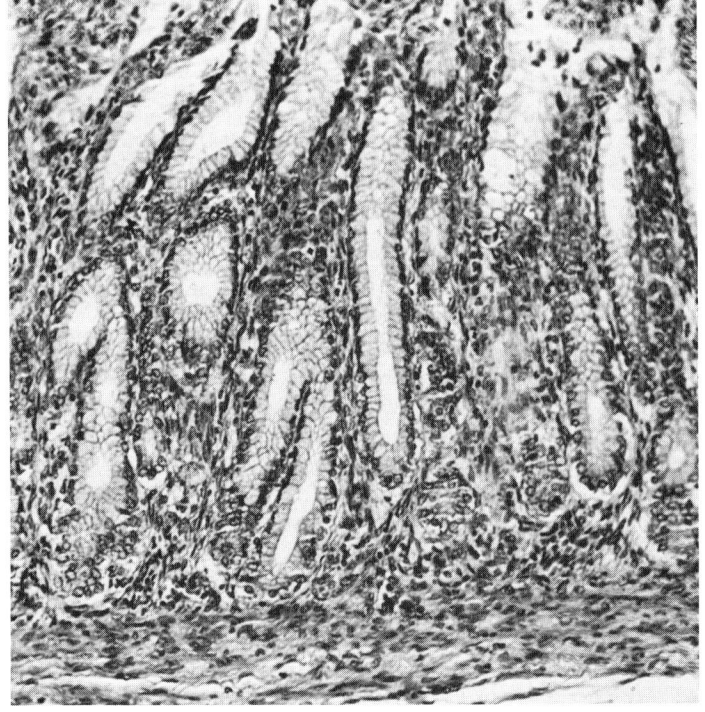

Figure 15–6

See legend on the opposite page

STOMACH 215

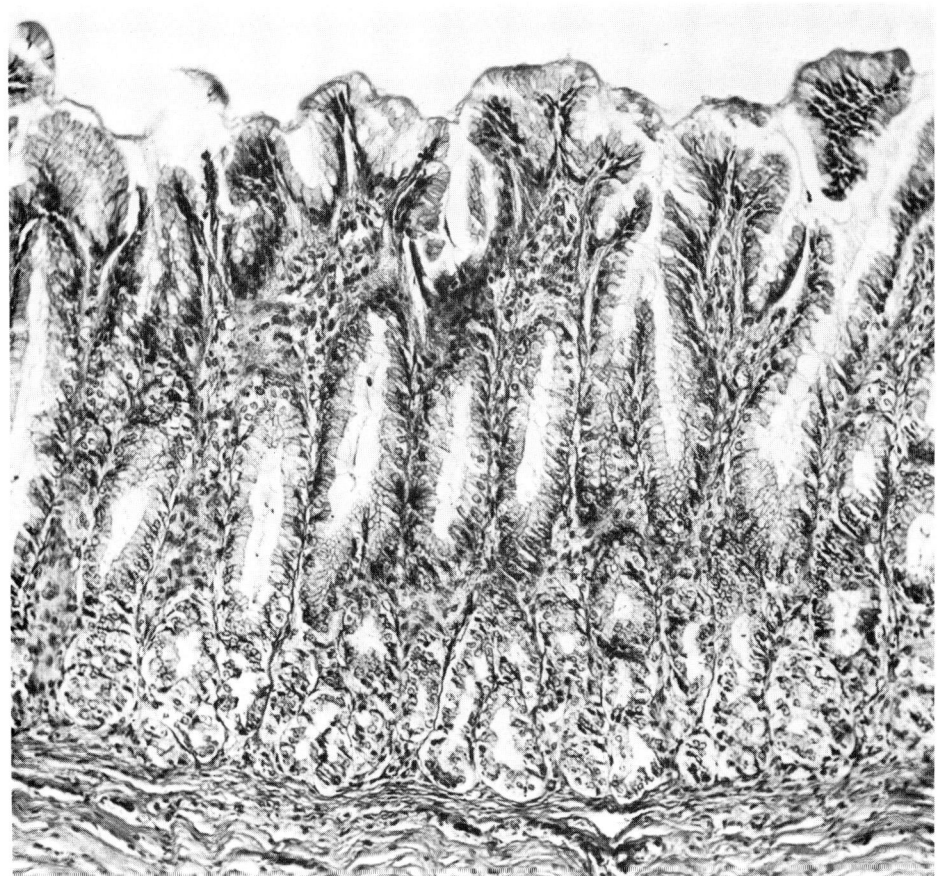

Figure 15–7

Figures 15–5, 15–6, and 15–7. These three photographs represent a detailed view of the mucosa of the stomach in the premature and mature newborn infant.
Hematoxylin and eosin stain.

Figure 15–5. A section of the pyloric glands of a stillborn white female whose body weight at autopsy was 2,270 grams. (Estimated gestational age: 33 wks.) Mag. 124×.

Figure 15–6. The gastric mucosa of a black male infant (pyloric glands represented here). The patient was born at 37 weeks of gestation and the body weight at necropsy was 2,501 grams. Mag. 175×.

Figure 15–7. Gastric glands of a 6 day old white female whose weight slightly exceeded 3,000 grams. (Estimated gestational age: 37 weeks.) Mag. 142×.

See illustrations on the opposite page

Figure 15-8b

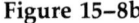

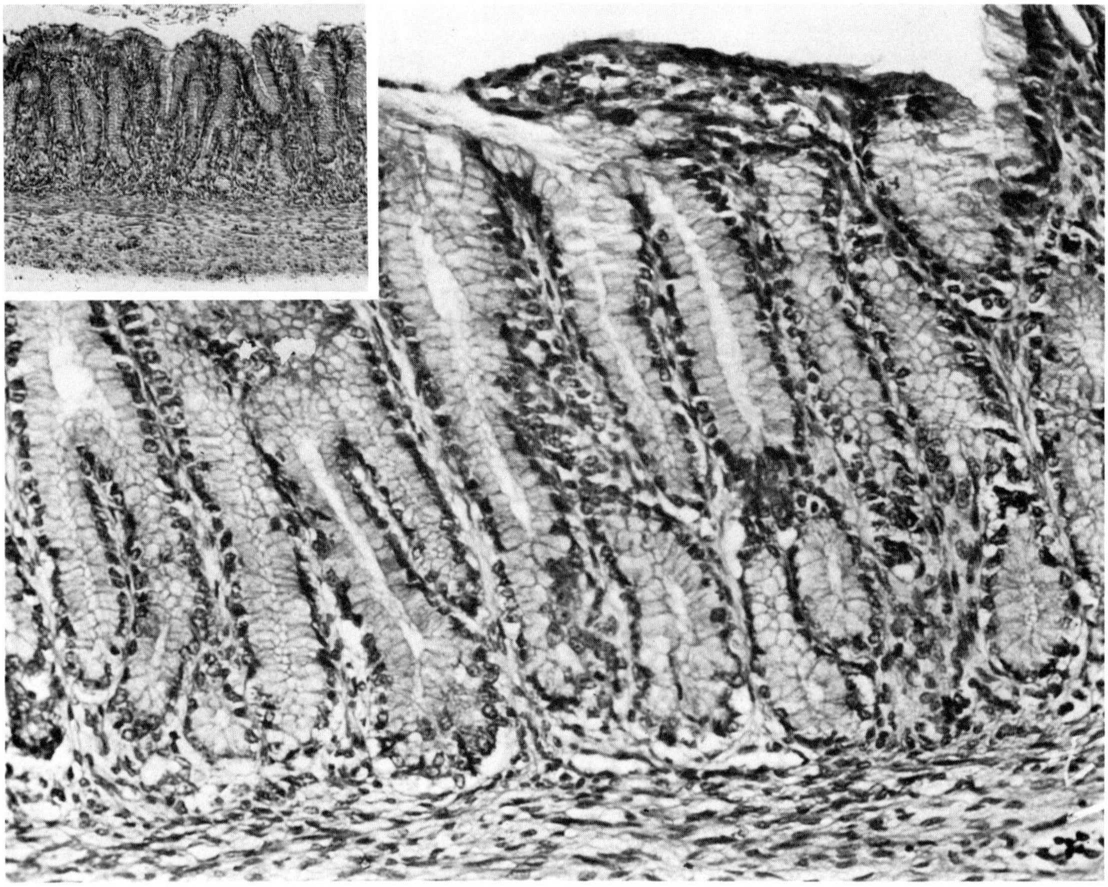

Figure 15-8a

Figures 15-8, 15-9, and 15-10. Higher magnification of gastric glands of different types at different ages.
Hematoxylin and eosin stains, all figures.

Figure 15-8a. These are the pyloric glands of a very small, premature infant of 5 months gestation. The subject was a black female who died at 8½ hours of age and whose body weight at autopsy was only 865 grams. Mag. 219×.

Figure 15-8b. Here, at lower magnification, are the pyloric glands of a more mature infant weighing 1,165 grams, a black male, whose age at death was 2 hours and 3 minutes. Mag. 64×.

Figure 15-9. These represent gastric glands in the body of the stomach of a 7 day old female infant who died with multiple anomalies. Body weight was 2,045 grams. (Estimated gestational age: 31 weeks.) Mag. 219×.

Figure 15-10. Gastric glands in the body of the stomach of a female infant whose body weighed 2,760 grams at postmortem examination. The infant died of pulmonary hyaline membrane disease at 34 hours of age. (Estimated gestational age: 35 weeks.) Mag. 219×.

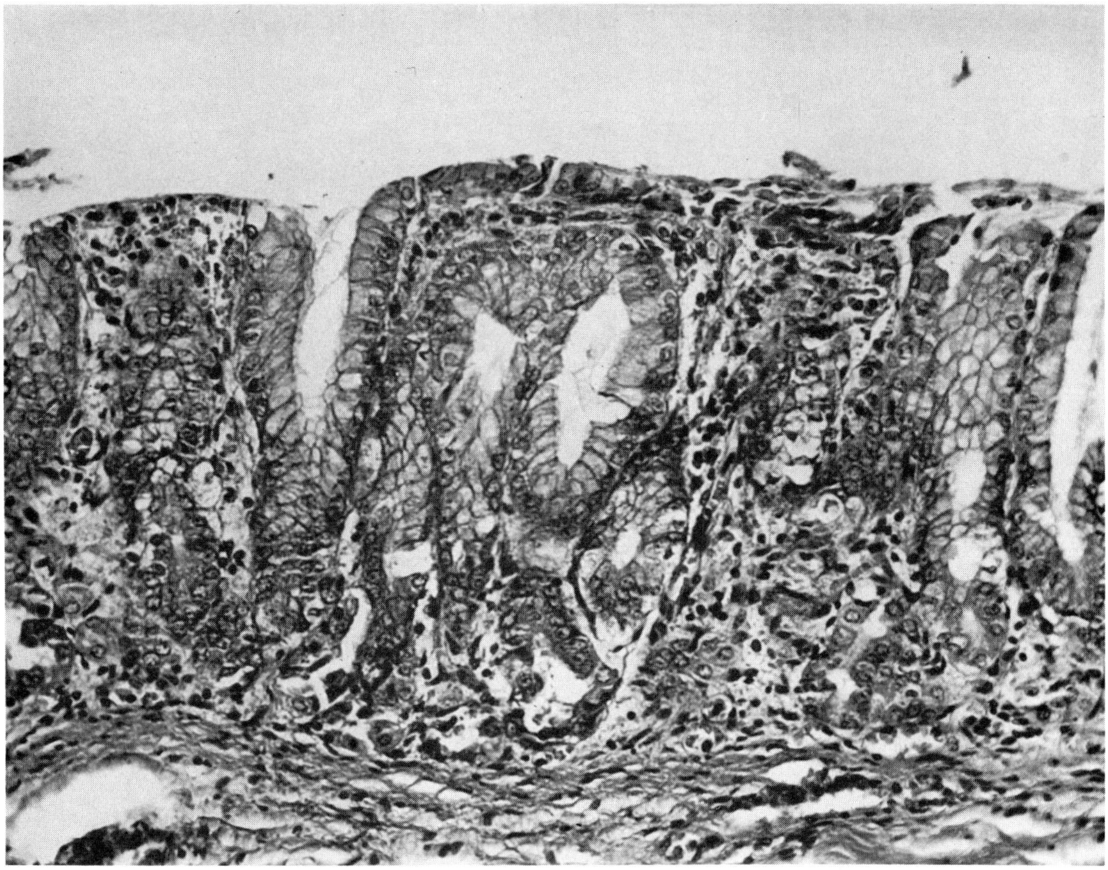

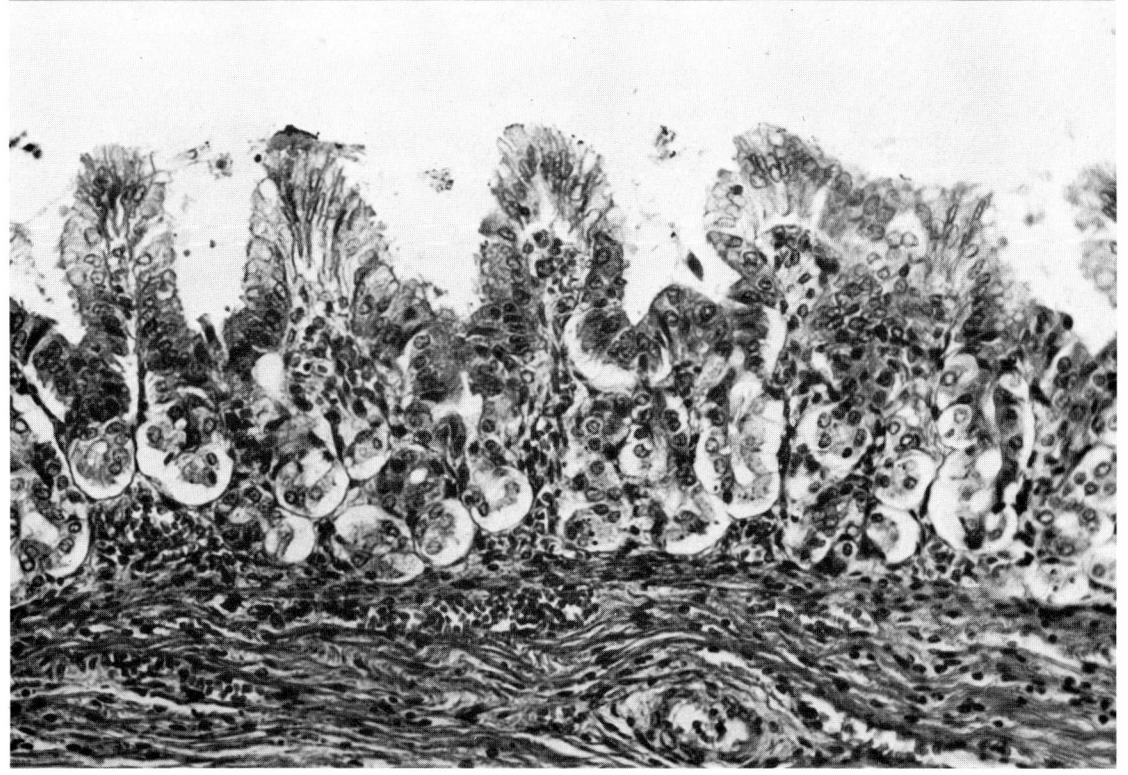

Figure 15–9

Figure 15–10

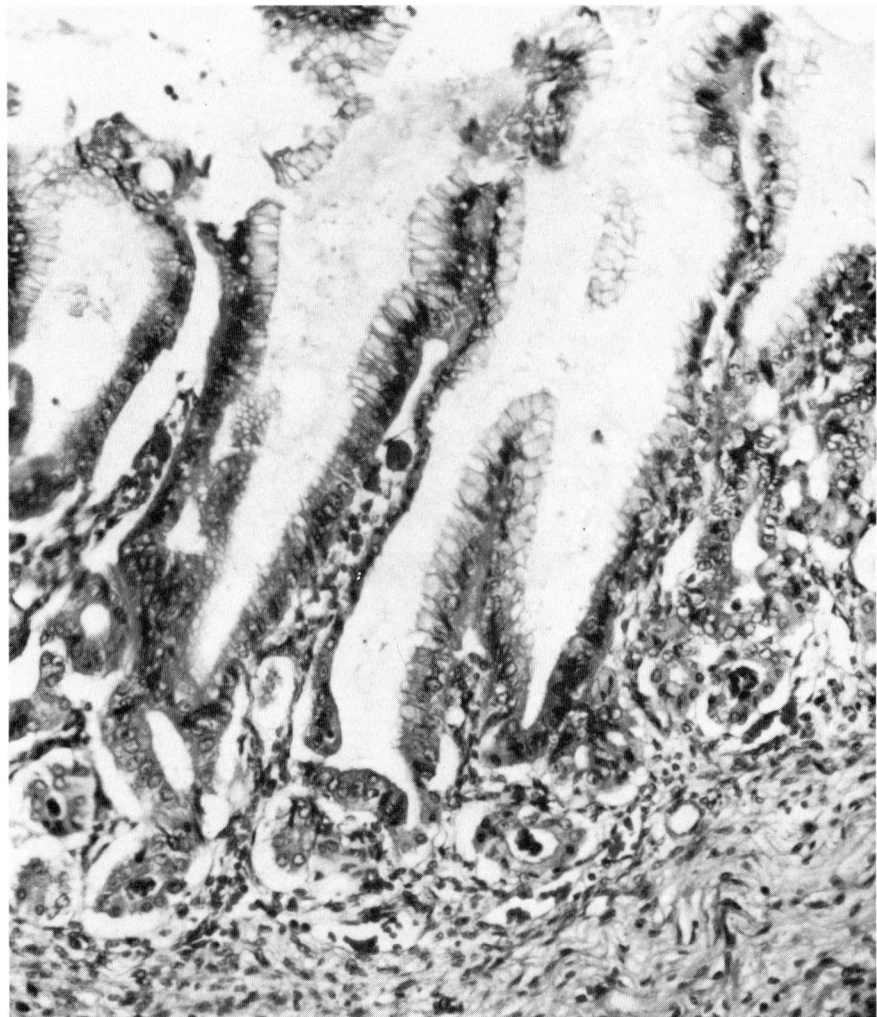

Figure 15–11

Figures 15–11, 15–12, and 15–13. This set of pictures, all taken at the same magnification from different segments of the stomach of the same infant, shows the different types of glands to be seen in the fundus (Fig. 15–11), body (Fig. 15–12), and pyloric region (Fig. 15–13).

The infant was a black male weighing 1,500 grams at postmortem examination. He was delivered after 30 weeks of gestation and survived for one day.

Hematoxylin and eosin stain. Mag. 220.8×.

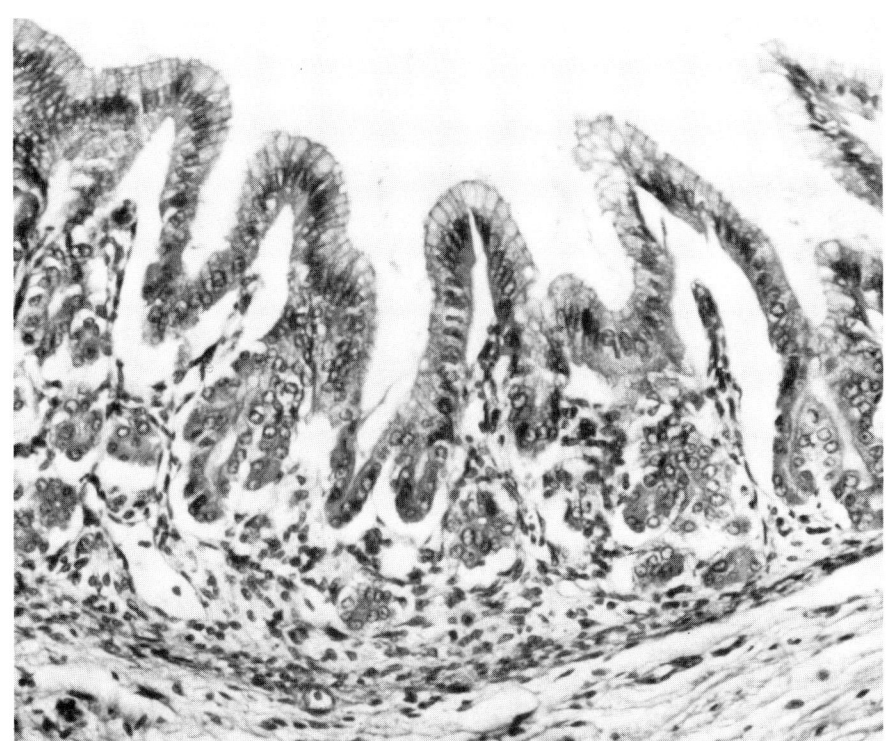

Figure 15–12

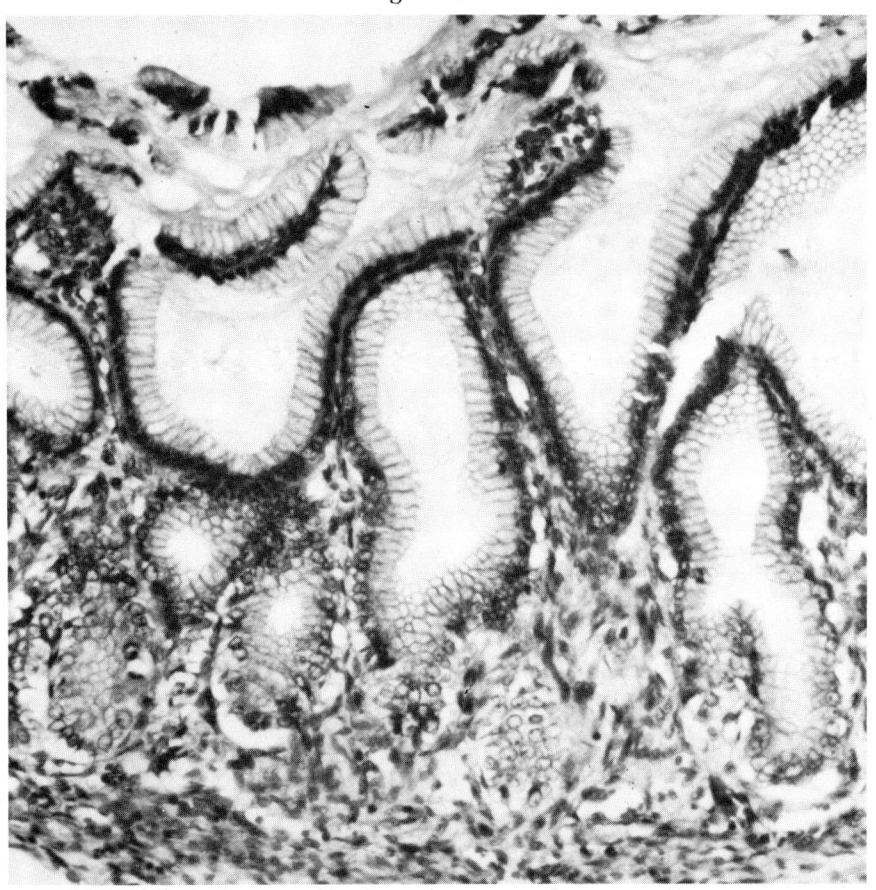

Figure 15–13

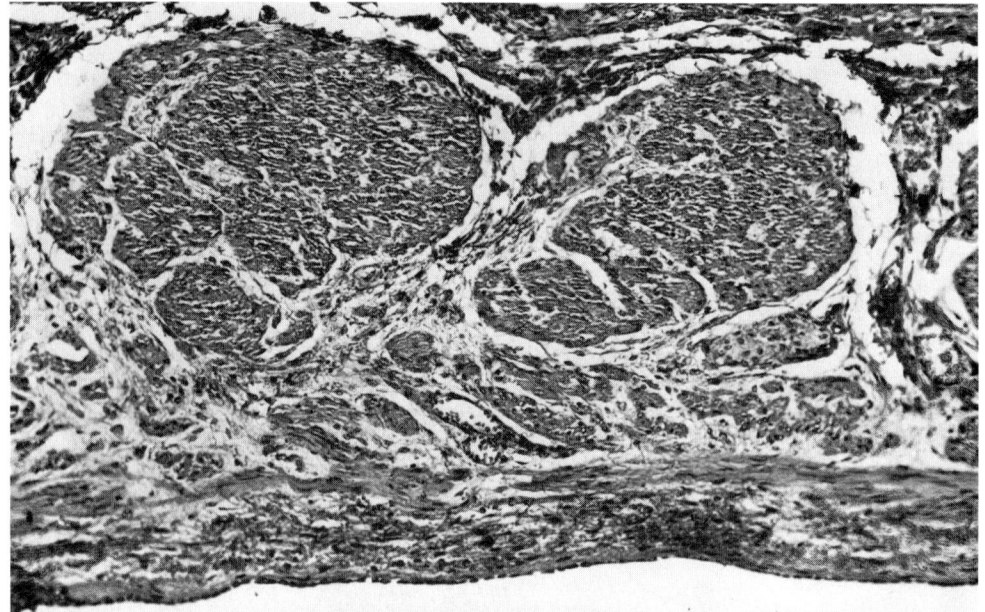

Figure 15-14

Figures 15-14, 15-15, and 15-16. A fairly common accident, involving infants in the newborn period, is spontaneous gastric perforation. For some years there has been dispute among pathologists concerning the fundamental mechanisms for that event. One group maintains that the perforation occurs because of deficiency or absence of gastric musculature at the site. The other group contends that what appears to be absence is simply the retraction of muscle bundles from the edges of the defect. These muscle bundles are intertwined and normally exhibit spaces where they would seem to be deficient (Fig. 15-16).

Figure 15-14. Three layers of smooth muscle in the muscular coat of the stomach wall of a 12 day old male infant. Body weight 3,350 grams. (Estimated gestational age: 38 weeks.) Death due to congenital heart disease.

Figure 15-15. Muscular coat of a 1 day old black male infant whose body weighed 1,750 grams at autopsy. (Estimated gestational age: 30 weeks.)

Figure 15-16. This is the entire thickness of the muscular coat of a 2 day old black female infant whose body weight at necropsy was similar to that of the subject in Fig. 15-15, 1,740 grams. (Estimated gestational age: 30 weeks.) Note the separation of muscle bundles internally.

Hematoxylin and eosin stain. Mag. 142×.

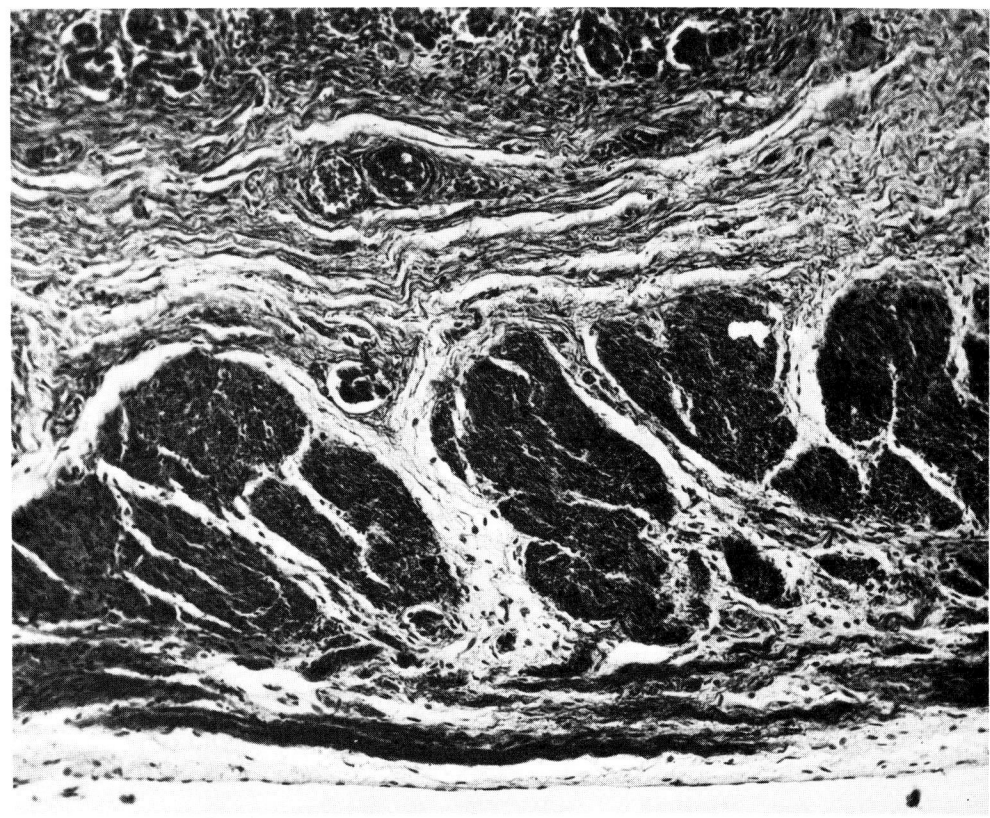

Figure 15–15

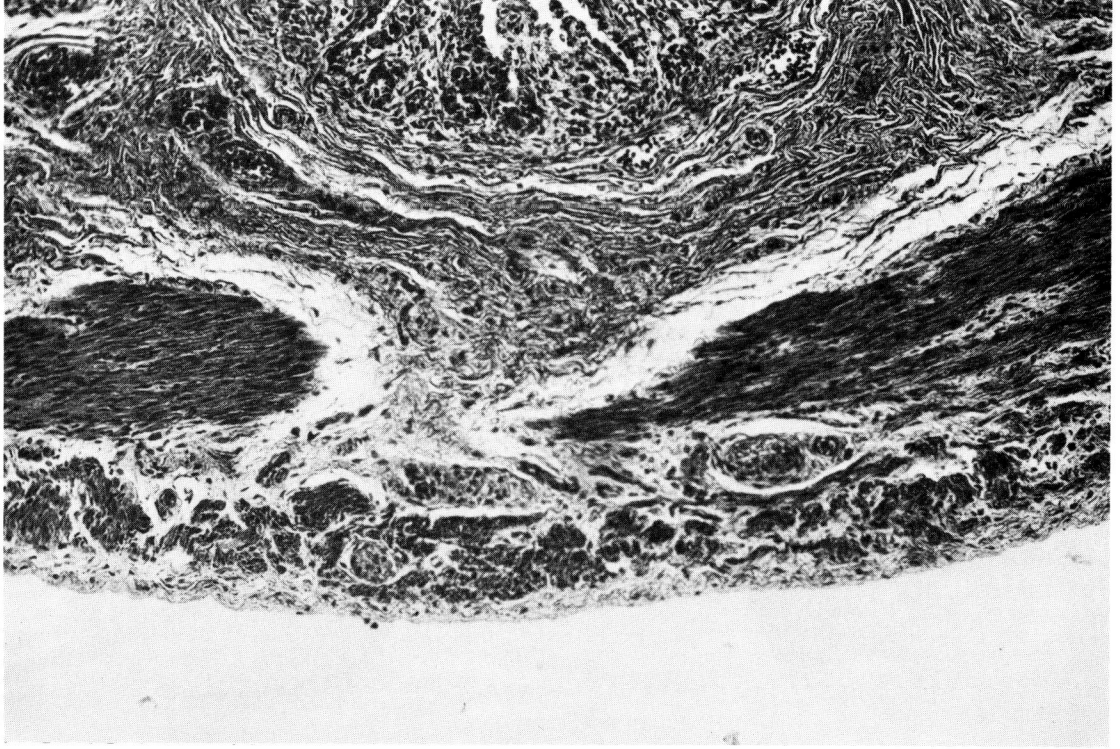

Figure 15–16

Chapter 16

SMALL INTESTINE

EMBRYOLOGY

The duodenum develops from the most caudal part of the so-called foregut and the most cranial part of the midgut. These two segments grow rapidly to form a C-shaped loop that projects ventrally. (The junction of the two parts is located at the apex of the loop.) During the second month the lumen is temporarily obliterated by proliferation of the lining epithelial cells; however, it is recanalized by the end of the second month.

The remainder of the small intestine is derived (together with the cecum, appendix, ascending colon, and right "half" of the transverse colon) from the midgut, that segment of primitive gut immediately distal to the foregut.

Initially the midgut is suspended from the dorsal abdominal wall by a short mesentery, and the midgut communicates widely with the yolk sac. As time passes, the mesentery elongates and the open communication with the yolk sac narrows to become the yolk stalk or vitelline duct.[1]

As the midgut elongates, it forms a ventral V-shaped intestinal loop, which projects out into the base of the umbilical cord because there is not enough room in the abdomen on account of the relatively large size of the developing liver and kidneys. The loop has two limbs, an upper or cranial and a lower or caudal. The yolk stalk is attached at the apex. The upper or proximal loop elongates rapidly, forming the coils of the small intestine, while the caudal does little except develop the cecal diverticulum. Inside the umbilical cord, the midgut then revolves 90 degrees counterclockwise around the axis of the superior mesenteric artery so that the upper or proximal limb is on the right and the lower limb is on the left.[1]

During the tenth week, the intestines return rapidly to the abdomen. The small bowel returns first, passing behind the superior mesenteric artery. As the intestines return, they rotate another 180 degrees counterclockwise, making the total 270 degrees.[1]

Between the fifth week and term, the small intestine becomes six times as long as the large intestine.

Just as the lumen of the duodenum is temporarily occluded by proliferation of its own lining epithelial cells, so also is that of the remainder of the small bowel during the sixth and seventh weeks, after which, by a process of vacuolation of cells, the lumen is restored and the entire tract relined by a single layer of epithelium.[2]

Villi begin to appear at eight weeks as independent rounded elevations of the lining membrane. Intestinal glands arise as tubular ingrowths of the epithelium about the bases of the villi; they first appear toward the end of the third month, closely followed by the Brunner's glands of the duodenum. Lymph nodules and Peyer's patches are present at five months.

ANATOMY

The small intestine is a convoluted tubular structure extending from the pylorus to the ileocecal valve. In an infant born at term, it is approximately 200 to 250 cm. in length. It lies in the left upper, central, and lower parts of the abdomen. It is, in a rough way, encircled by the large intestine. It consists of (1) the duodenum, which is short, curved, and devoid of mesentery, and (2) the jejunum and ileum, which are long, greatly coiled, and attached to the posterior abdominal wall by the dorsal mesentery. It is said that the proximal two fifths represent jejunum and the distal three fifths constitute the ileum.[3]

The duodenum is the shortest of the three segments and the most fixed. It is only partially covered (anteriorly) with peritoneum. Its course is remarkably constant and more or less in the shape of an incomplete circle, enclosing the head of the pancreas. The first part, called the superior, begins at the pylorus and passes backward, upward, and to the right. It then makes a sharp curve and descends as the second or descending portion. Then it makes a second bend and passes almost horizontally as the third part, from right to left across the vertebral column with a slight inclination upward. The fourth part (the ascending part) then ascends in front of and to the left of the abdominal aorta. At its union with the jejunum, it turns abruptly forward, forming the duodenojejunal flexure which is located to the left of the midline.

The remainder of the small intestine extends from that flexure to the ileocecal valve. It is arranged in a series of coils attached to the mesentery. This part of the gut is completely covered with peritoneum, except for a narrow strip along its mesenteric border where the two layers of mesentery diverge from each other to embrace it. There is no sharp line of distinction between the jejunum and ileum, and the division is arbitrary; nevertheless, the character of the intestine changes gradually from the beginning of the jejunum to the end of the ileum.[4]

The wall of the jejunum is a bit thicker than that of the ileum. The folds of its mucous membrane are prominent. Aggregates of lymphoid tissue are not present in the upper part and are virtually absent in the lower part.

The ileum, by contrast, has a thinner wall; the circular folds, although present in the upper part, are small and disappear almost completely from the distal end. Here the aggregated lymphoid follicles, Peyer's patches (Fig. 16–3), are prominent.

HISTOLOGY

As in the other parts of the gastrointestinal tract, the wall of the small intestine is made up of four concentric coats: the mucosa, the submucosa, the muscular coat, and the serosa.

The mucosa is arranged in grossly visible crescentic folds that extend half to two thirds of the way around the lumen (Fig. 16–3). They are permanent structures involving the mucosa and the submucosa. They are absent from the first portion of the duodenum, and are most prominent in the last part of the duodenum and first part of the jejunum. From there on they diminish in size and number, and are seldom seen beyond the middle of the ileum.

The surface area of the small bowel is also augmented by the presence of villi, minute finger-like projections of the mucosa, which cover the entire mucosa and lend it a characteristic velvety appearance grossly. They are most numerous in the duodenum and proximal jejunum.[4]

The surface of the epithelium is increased not only by elevation of the villi but also by invagination to form tubular glands that open into the lumen between the bases of the villi. These are simple tubular glands, which extend down into the lamina propria nearly to the muscularis mucosae. The spaces between the glands are occupied by loose connective tissue of the lamina propria (Figs. 16–3 to 16–7).

The epithelium covering the free surface of the mucosa is simple columnar (Fig. 16–3). In the prematurely born infant, they all appear to be the same; but in the infant born at term, scattered goblet cells can be seen among them (Figs. 16–5 to 16–7). The epithelium covering the villi continues into the intestinal glands. The upper portions of the glands are lined with low columnar cells resembling the surface cells, and these include goblet cells. The lower portions contain cells that are less well differentiated. (It is here that new cells are formed to move upward and replace those that are exfoliated at the tips of the villi.[4]) Here one encounters a distinctive type of cell seen only in the depths of those crypts, the Paneth cell (Fig. 16–6). These cells are pyramidal, with their nuclei near the base. They contain conspicuous secretory granules, which stain bright pink with eosin, in their apical cytoplasm. (They are said to occur in the glands of the colon, but we have seen them there only rarely, and then in the mucosa of the most proximal portion of the cecum.)

The lamina propria fills the spaces between the glands. It is highly cellular (Figs. 16–5 to 16–7). In the newborn, most of the cells contained there, besides fibroblasts, are small lymphocytes and occasional plasma cells.

The lamina propria also contains isolated aggregates of lymphoid tissue (Fig. 16–3). They are most prominent and numerous in the terminal ileum, where they are referred to as Peyer's patches. Small aggregates occupy only the mucosa; larger ones extend down into the submucosa through the muscularis mucosae. Peyer's patches always occur on the side of the intestinal wall opposite the mesenteric attachment.

The muscularis mucosae is very thin in the newborn infant (Figs. 16–3 and 16–5). The submucosa consists of rather dense connective tissue with an elastic component. It contains no adipose tissue in the neonate. In the duodenum it is occupied by a thick layer of duodenal or Brunner's glands. The secretory parts of these glands are richly coiled and branched tubules arranged in lobules. The ducts penetrate the muscularis mucosae to open into the lumens of intestinal glands (Figs. 16–1 and 16–2).

The two layers of the muscular coat are well developed in the small intestine. They are the external longitudinal and inner circular. Between them is the myenteric nerve plexus. Some strands of smooth muscle cells pass between the two[4] (Fig. 16–5).

The external serous coat consists of a single layer of mesothelial cells resting on loose connective tissue (Figs. 16–3 to 16–5).

References

All references for Part Six appear on page 271.

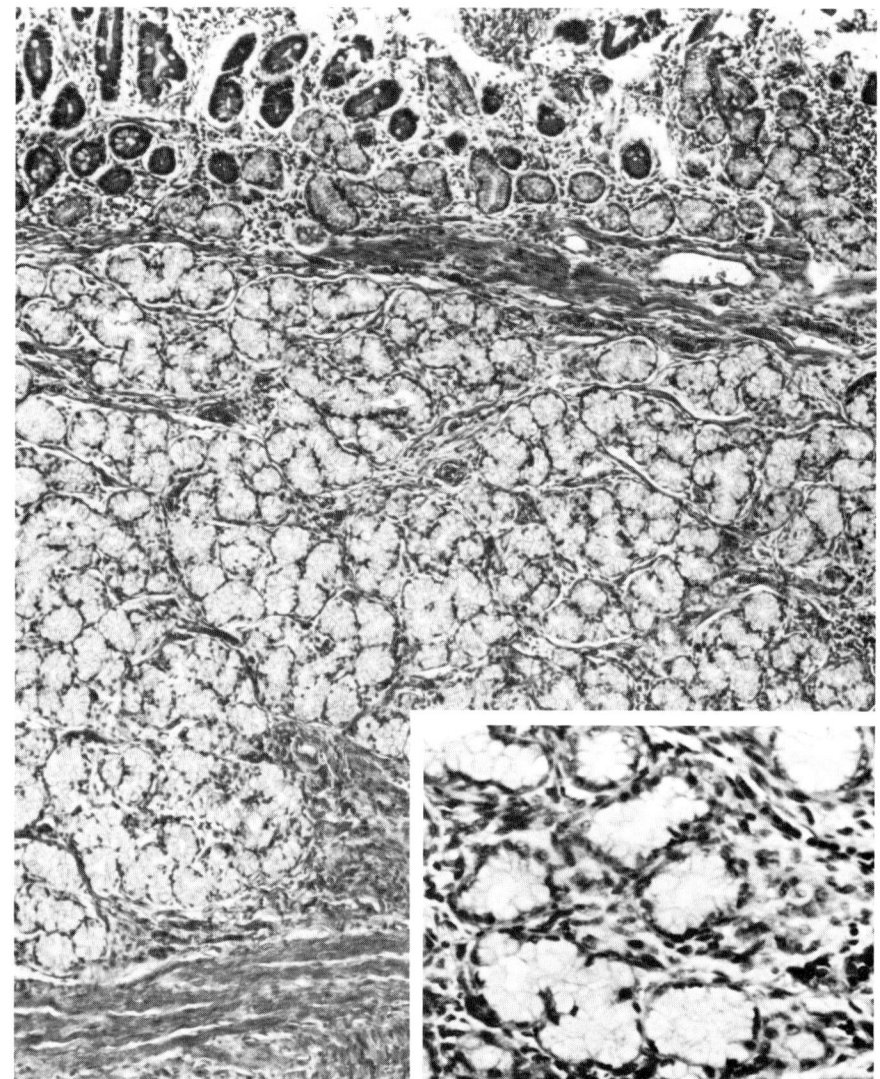

Figure 16-1

Figures 16-1 and 16-2. These two photographs of the duodenum were taken principally to illustrate the nature of Brunner's glands in the infant.
This infant was a two month old black male who, at autopsy, weighed 2,830 grams.
Hematoxylin and eosin stain.

Figure 16-1. Mag. 87.5×.

Inset: From a black male infant, weighing 1,320 grams, who lived for 2 hours. Gestational age: 32 weeks. Mag. 125×.

Figure 16-2. Mag. 774×.

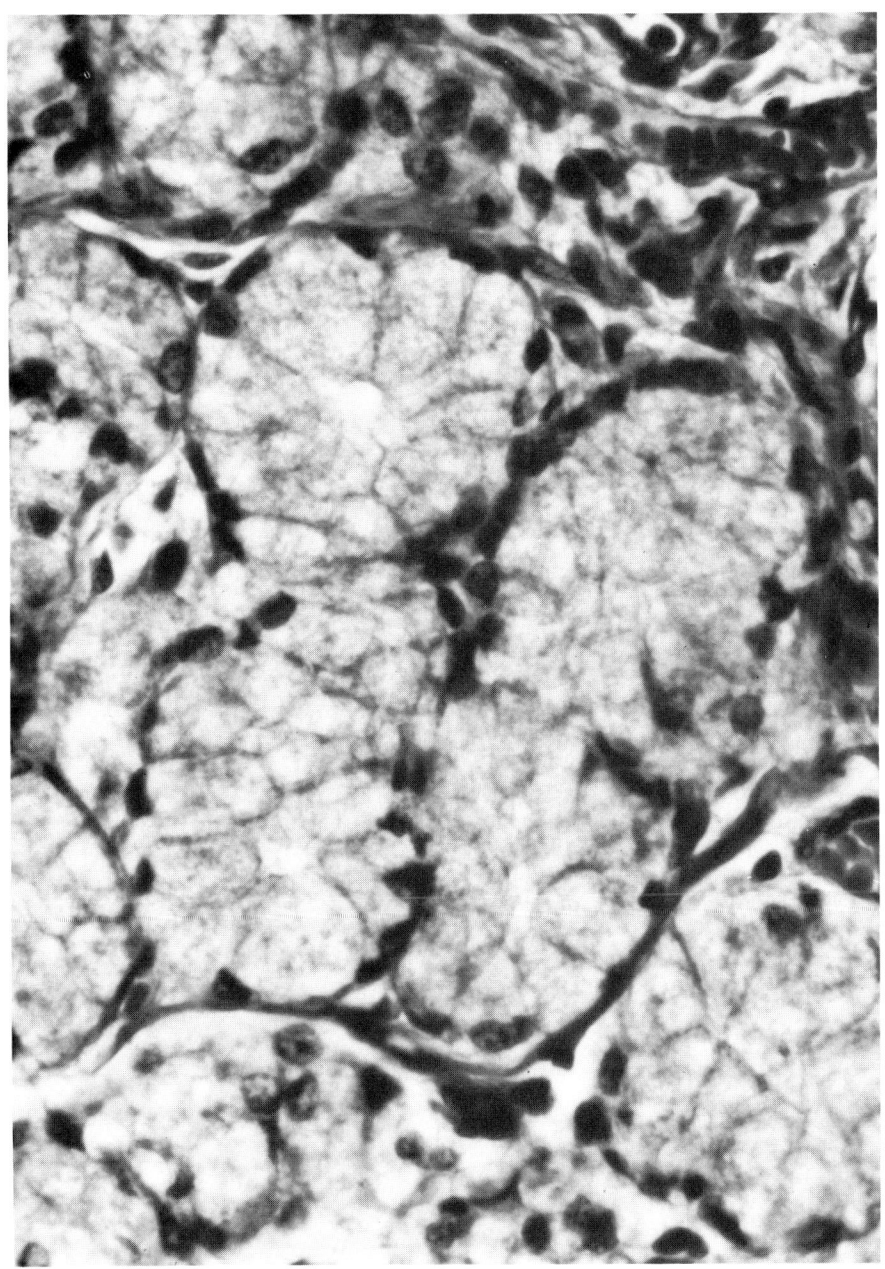

Figure 16–2

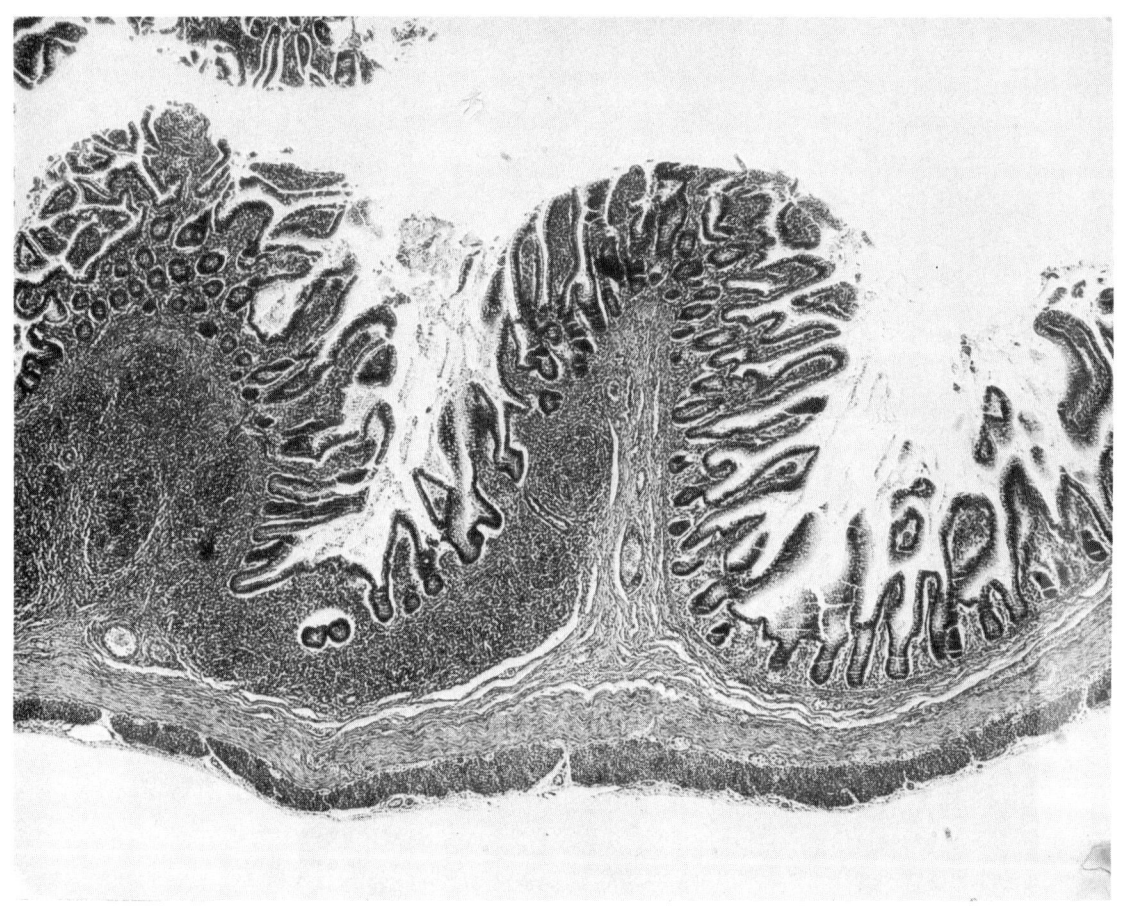

Figure 16-3

Figure 16-3. This is a survey view of the ileum, showing a single Peyer's patch on the left. Mucosal folds are quite apparent, as are the long delicate villi.

This patient was an 18 day old white male born at term, whose body weighed 4,150 grams at postmortem examination.

Hematoxylin and eosin stain. Mag. 45×.

SMALL INTESTINE 229

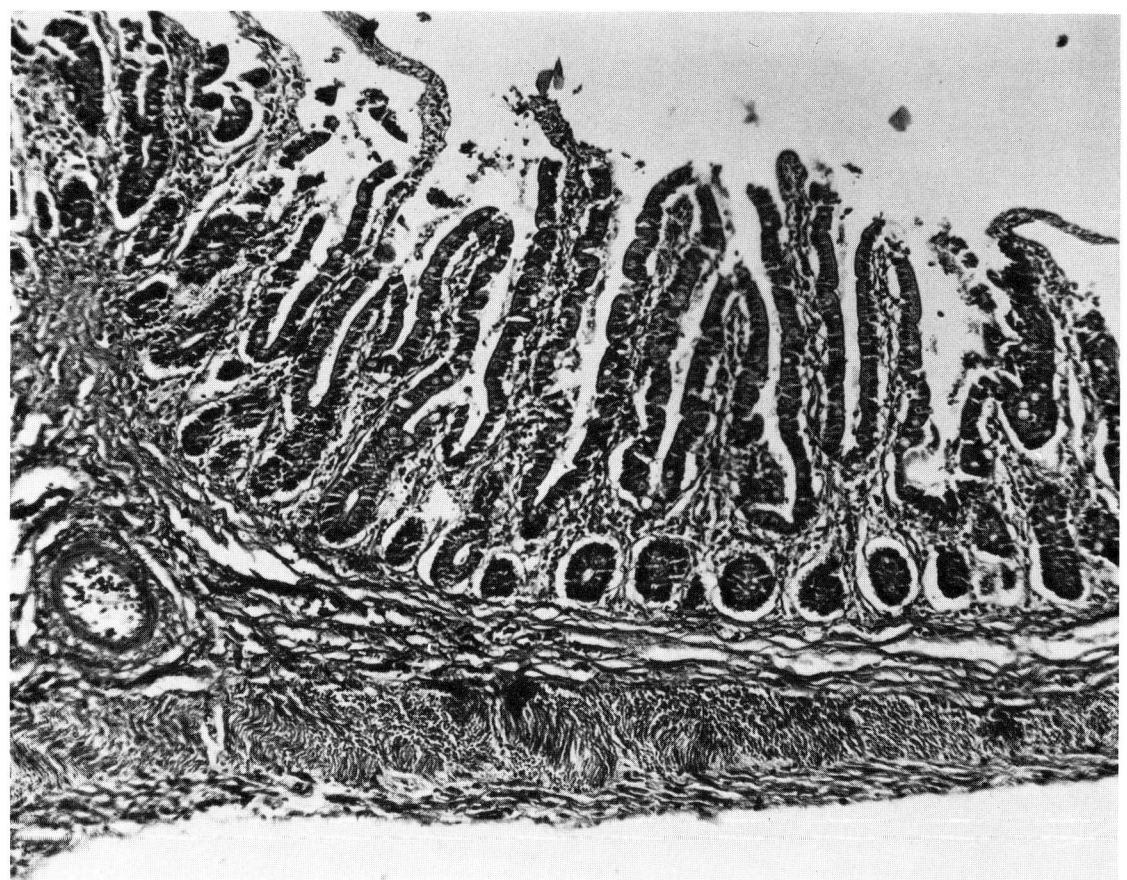

Figure 16-4

Figure 16-4. Small bowel of a newborn infant, seen at somewhat higher magnification than in Fig. 16-3.

The subject was a male infant, 21 days of age. (Estimated gestational age: 38 weeks.) The baby's weight at autopsy was 3,320 grams. He died of congenital heart disease.

Hematoxylin and eosin stain. Mag. 116×.

230 SMALL INTESTINE

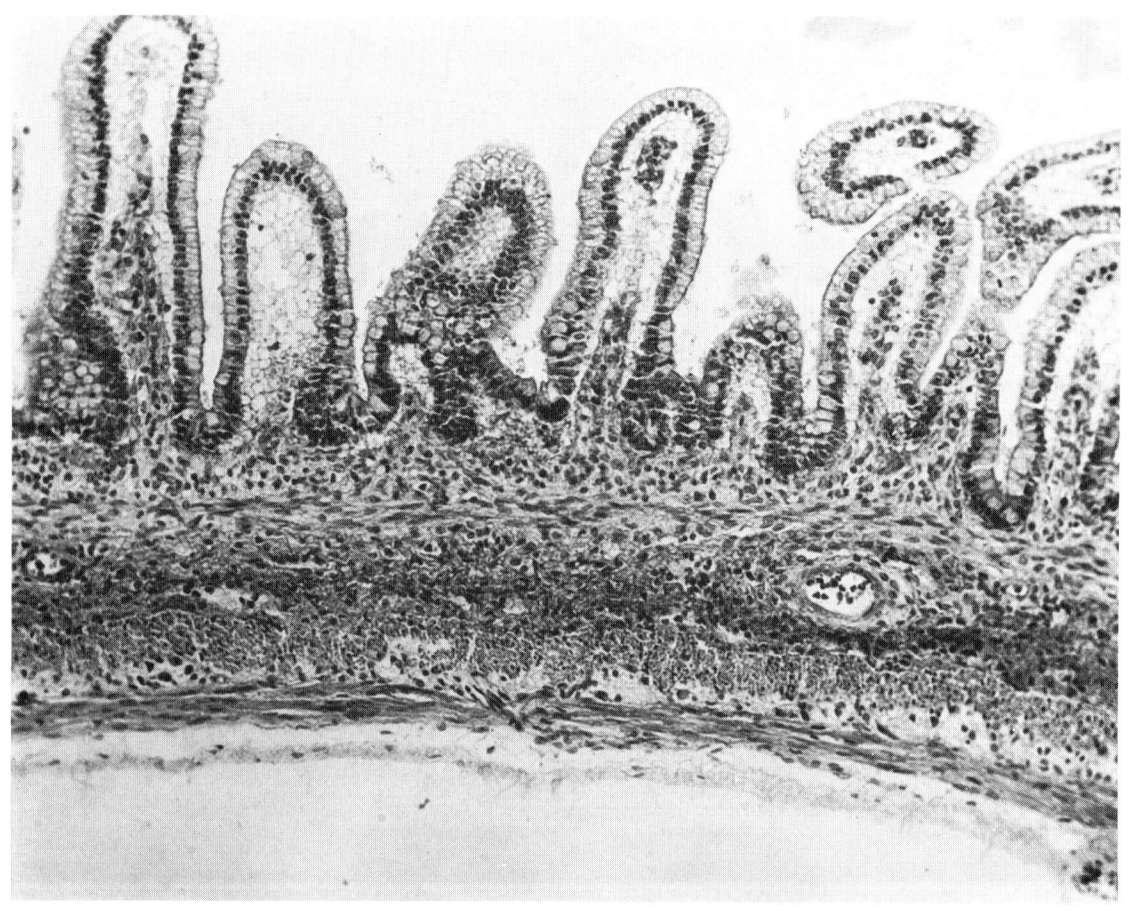

Figure 16–5

Figures 16–5, 16–6, and 16–7. These three photomicrographs were all taken at the same magnification to illustrate the changes that take place in the histologic appearance of the wall of the small bowel during the latter half of gestation.

Figure 16–5. The entire thickness of the wall of the small bowel is visualized here, including the inner and outer muscle layers and the plexus of Auerbach between them.

Figure 16–6. Because the wall of the bowel is thicker at this stage of development, only the mucosa is seen. (The arrow indicates a single Paneth cell.)

Figure 16–7. Again, only the mucosa with villi is visible in this field.

Fig.	Wt.	Race	Sex	Gestation	Age
16–5	512 gm.	B	F	21 wk. (est.)	27 hr.
16–6	2,501 gm.	B	M	37 wk.	17 hr.
16–7	2,850 gm.	B	M	37 wk. (est.)	$25^{1}/_{2}$ hr.

Hematoxylin and eosin stain. Mag. 186×.

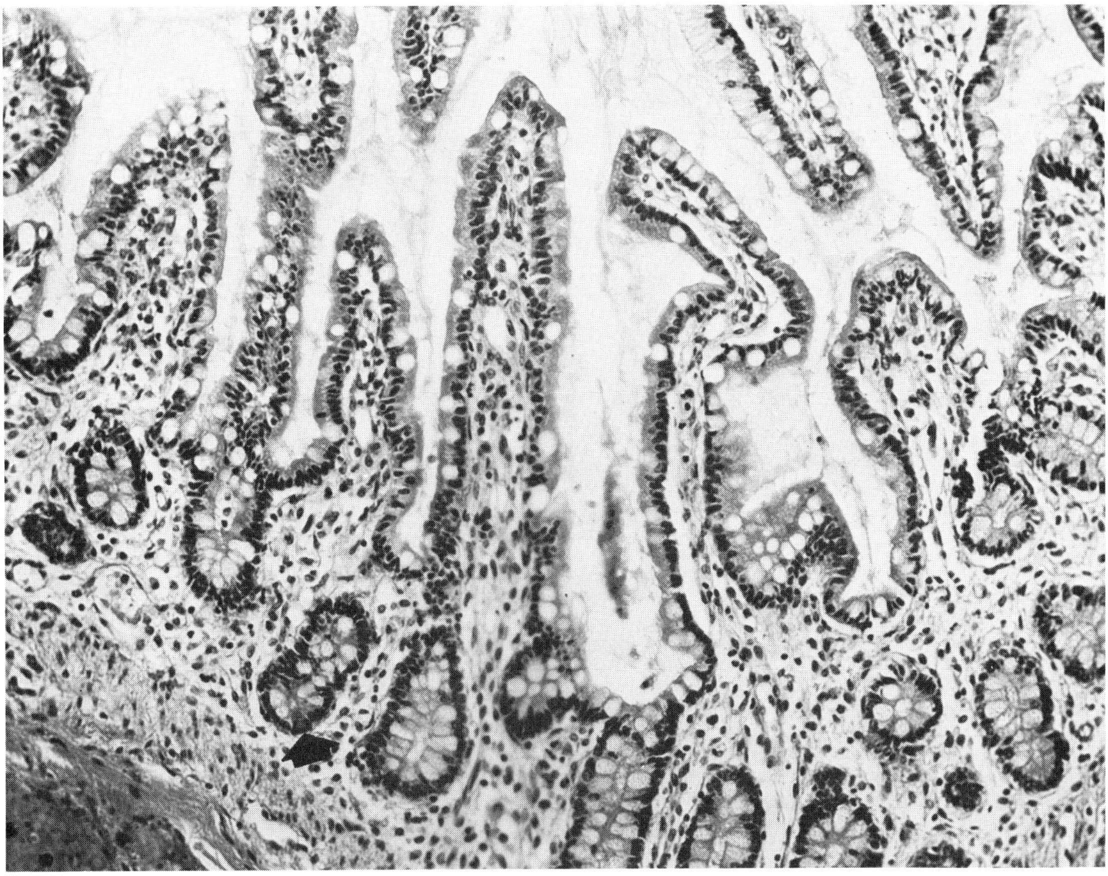

Figure 16-6

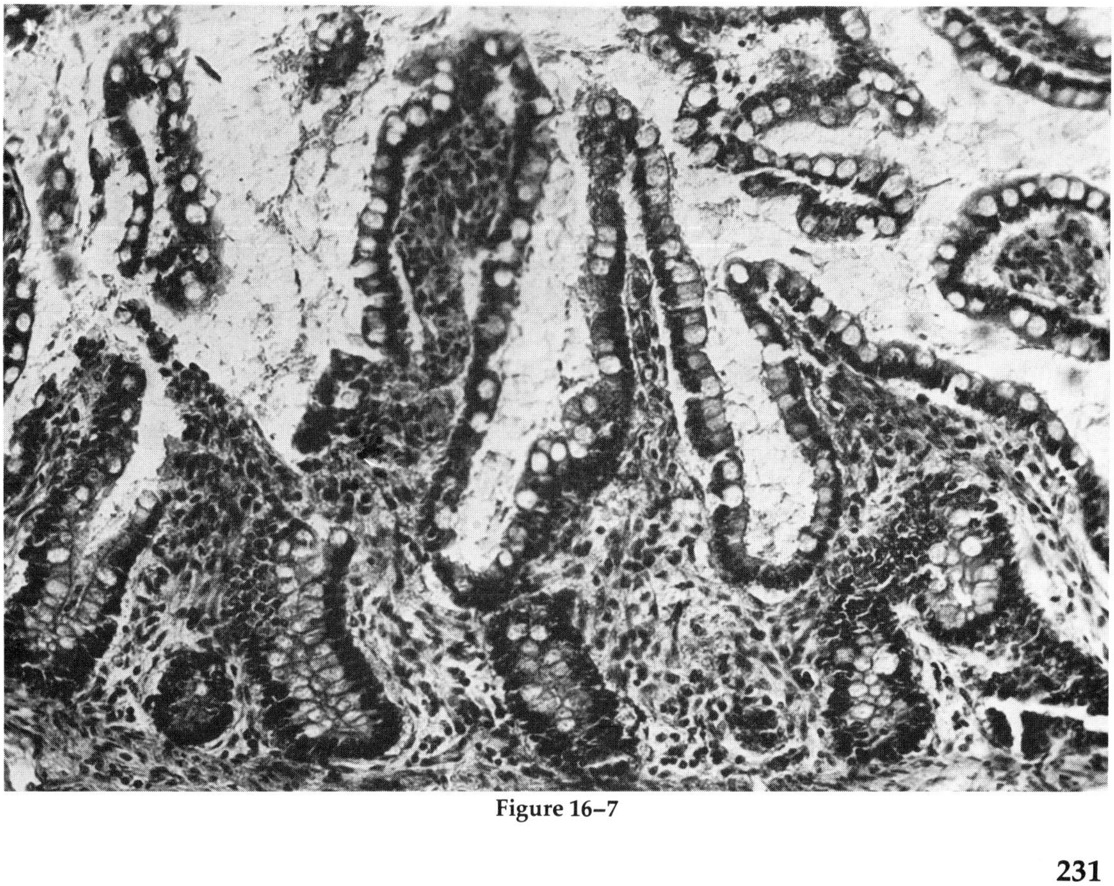

Figure 16-7

Chapter 17

LARGE INTESTINE

EMBRYOLOGY

As mentioned in Chapter 16, the cecum, appendix, ascending colon, and first portion of the transverse colon are derived from the so-called midgut and participate (together with the small bowel) in "herniation" outside the abdominal cavity into the base of the umbilical cord, and in rotation. The left half of the transverse colon, the descending colon, the sigmoid, the rectum, and the upper portion of the anal canal are derivatives of the hindgut, supplied by the inferior mesenteric artery. The distal end of the hindgut is represented by the cloacal membrane, composed of the endoderm of the cloaca internally and the ectoderm of the proctodeum or anal pit externally.[1]

The original cecal bulge enlarges and makes a definite blind sac, which extends the large intestine caudally beyond its junction with the ileum. The distal end of the sac lengthens for a time, and at the site arises the vermiform appendix.

The ascending colon begins to elongate in the middle of fetal life, a process not completed until early childhood.

A relatively early and pronounced elongation of the most caudal portion of the colon becomes the sigmoid colon. The expanded terminal part of the hindgut, the cloaca, also receives the allantois (later to be the urogenital sinus) ventrally and the mesonephric ducts (ducts of the transitory mesonephric kidneys) laterally. This cloaca is divided in two by a coronally oriented sheet of mesenchyme, the urorectal septum. As the septum extends caudally toward the cloacal membrane, it separates the rectum and upper anal canal dorsally from the urogenital sinus ventrally; by the end of the sixth week this septum has fused with the cloacal membrane.[1] The site of fusion becomes the perineal body. Mesenchyme proliferates around the anal membrane, elevating the surface of the ectoderm and forming a shallow anal pit. The anal membrane, at the bottom of that pit, ruptures at the end of the seventh week, so that the digestive tract caudally then communicates with the amniotic cavity.

The upper two thirds of the anal canal is derived from the hindgut, the lower third from the anal pit. The junction of the epithelium derived from the ectoderm and the endoderm is at the level of the pectinate or dentate line, or at the level of the anal valves.

The lumen of the colon, like that of the small bowel, is temporarily occluded by epithelial proliferation but is shortly thereafter re-established. The colonic glands or crypts of Lieberkühn appear near the end of the third month.[2] The colon bears temporary villi in the middle of the third month.

Meconium begins to collect in the intestine after the third month. It is a pasty mixture of mucus, bile, and cast-off epithelial cells, to which are added lanugo hairs, desquamated epidermal cells, and sebaceous secretion swallowed with amniotic fluid. Its color is dark green. At birth the intestinal contents are sterile.

ANATOMY

The large intestine extends from the end of the ileum to the anus. In the term infant it may be up to 30 cm. in length. In the newborn infant its diameter is not very different from that of the small bowel. Its color, however, is more often grey-green externally, reflecting the color of the meconium within it, whereas that of the small intestine tends to be pale pink. For the most part, it is more fixed in its position than is the small bowel. Its longitudinal muscle fibers, unlike those of the small intestine, are arranged in three longitudinally oriented bands known as the taeniae coli, which, even in the newborn infant, create at least suggestions of sacculations known as haustrations. There are no appendices epiploicae attached to the large intestine of the premature or newborn infant.

The large intestine, as previously mentioned, encircles the small intestine in a general way, beginning in the right lower quadrant of the abdomen. It then ascends to a flexure, the hepatic flexure, in the right upper quadrant (where it is, in the infant, often tightly adherent to the gallbladder or structures in that vicinity by means of dense fibrous adhesions). It traverses the midline, as the transverse portion, to the splenic flexure in the left upper quadrant. It then descends to the left lower quadrant, where it suddenly loops upward, in the infant, in the form of a large, usually green and fairly tense sigmoid. This is probably the most prominent loop in the entire abdomen of a neonate. Finally, it descends by way of the rectum to the anus.

The cecum of the newborn, especially the prematurely born, is often conical with its apex directed downward. Frequently the vermiform appendix arises at its apex.

The vermiform appendix of the neonate, again especially in the prematurely born infant, is usually surprisingly large and long, and often of grey-green color. The two most common positions for it are caudal to the cecum and retrocecal. Sometimes it is completely hidden behind the cecum and ascends posterior to the ascending colon for a surprising distance; not uncommonly, its distal tip may be posterior to the lower border of the liver.

Also not uncommonly in the newborn, the cecum is on quite a long mesentery, permitting considerable mobility. In such situations the cecum and appendix may be located in the right upper quadrant, but this is not to be misconstrued as malrotation of the gut.

HISTOLOGY

Appendix. The lumen of the appendix in the newborn infant never has the angular outline it so often has in the adult. Instead, it is quite round; of course, the lumen is never obliterated in any portion of the organ, as it so often is distally in the adult. The mucosa is exactly like that of the colon, with regularly radiating crypts of Lieberkühn; these are typically test-tube shaped and all of the same length, extending down through the lamina propria toward a delicate muscularis mucosae.

The lamina propria contains mostly lymphocytes and usually has no follicles at all. The epithelium of the surface and that lining the glands consists of pale-staining, tall columnar cells.

The submucosa is moderately thick and contains blood vessels and nerves, but no adipose tissue.

The muscularis is thin, but is made up of the usual two layers. The serosa resembles that seen throughout the rest of the intestinal tract.

Large Intestine. The mucosa of the large intestine is flat and, except in the rectum, bears no folds such as are seen in the upper portion of the small bowel (Fig. 17–1). It is also rather thin, especially compared with the mucosa of the stomach (Fig. 17–2). Furthermore, it bears no villi.

The lining epithelium is uniform, being composed entirely of a single layer of pale-staining columnar cells with many scattered goblet cells (Figs. 17–1 to 17–3). The crypts of Lieberkühn are straight tubules, lined by the same type of cells as those on the surface. (The only Paneth cells I have ever seen in the large intestine of infants were in the fundi of glands within the mucosa of the cecum, quite near the ileocecal valve.)

The lamina propria is quite like that of the small intestine, being populated principally by lymphocytes (Figs. 17–2 and 17–3). The muscularis mucosae is very delicate.

Of particular interest in the infant, because of the possibility of aganglionosis,[5,6,7] are the ganglion cells in the submucosa and in the plexus of Auerbach, between the two muscle layers of the muscularis externa. In both of these sites, particularly in the prematurely born baby, the cells may be small and not at all generously endowed with cytoplasm as they are in older children and adults; as a consequence, they may be difficult to identify without some practice. Most helpful, especially in the submucosa, is the fact that they occur in clusters and fairly often have prominent nucleoli (Figs. 17–4 and 17–5). In the submucosa they often appear in little oval rings and are larger than any of the nuclei in surrounding connective tissue (Figs. 17–8 and 17–9).

The taeniae coli are not nearly so clear in their configuration in the infant as they are in the adult, and there are no appendices epiploicae.

In the rectum (Fig. 17–10) the crypts of Lieberkühn become short and disappear, and there is then an abrupt transition from simple columnar to stratified squamous epithelium. In that zone of transition there occurs a very distinctive sort of columnar epithelium, not quite like any other, which is depicted in Fig. 17–12.

References

All references for Part Six appear on page 271.

236 LARGE INTESTINE

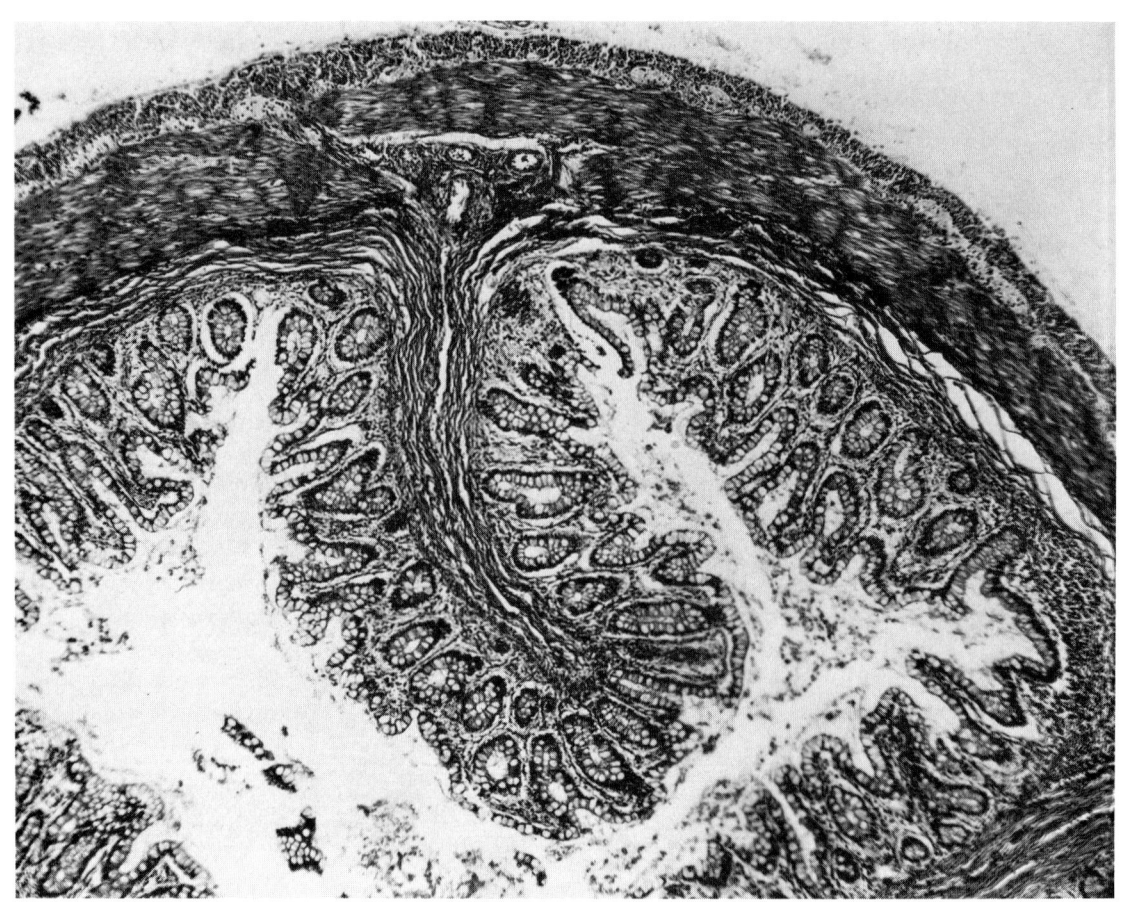

Figure 17–1

Figures 17–1, 17–2, and 17–3. This series of three photomicrographs, a survey view, middle power, and high power, illustrate the principal histologic features of the colon. The four coats, the typical mucosa, and mucosal fold are well seen in Fig. 17–1. The arrangement of the crypts of Lieberkühn is apparent in Fig. 17–2, and the mucus-producing character of the lining epithelium of a crypt is clear in Fig. 17–3.

The normal distribution of the elements of the plexus of Auerbach, between the two muscle layers, is easily visible in Fig. 17–1.

Hematoxylin and eosin stain.

Fig.	Wt.	Race	Sex	Gestation	Age	Mag.
17–1	2,270 gm.	W	F	33 wk. (est.)	Stillborn	85×
17–2	1,060 gm.	?	F	26 wk. (est.)	5½ hr.	186×
17–3	2,600 gm.	W	M	34 wk.	1½ days	370×

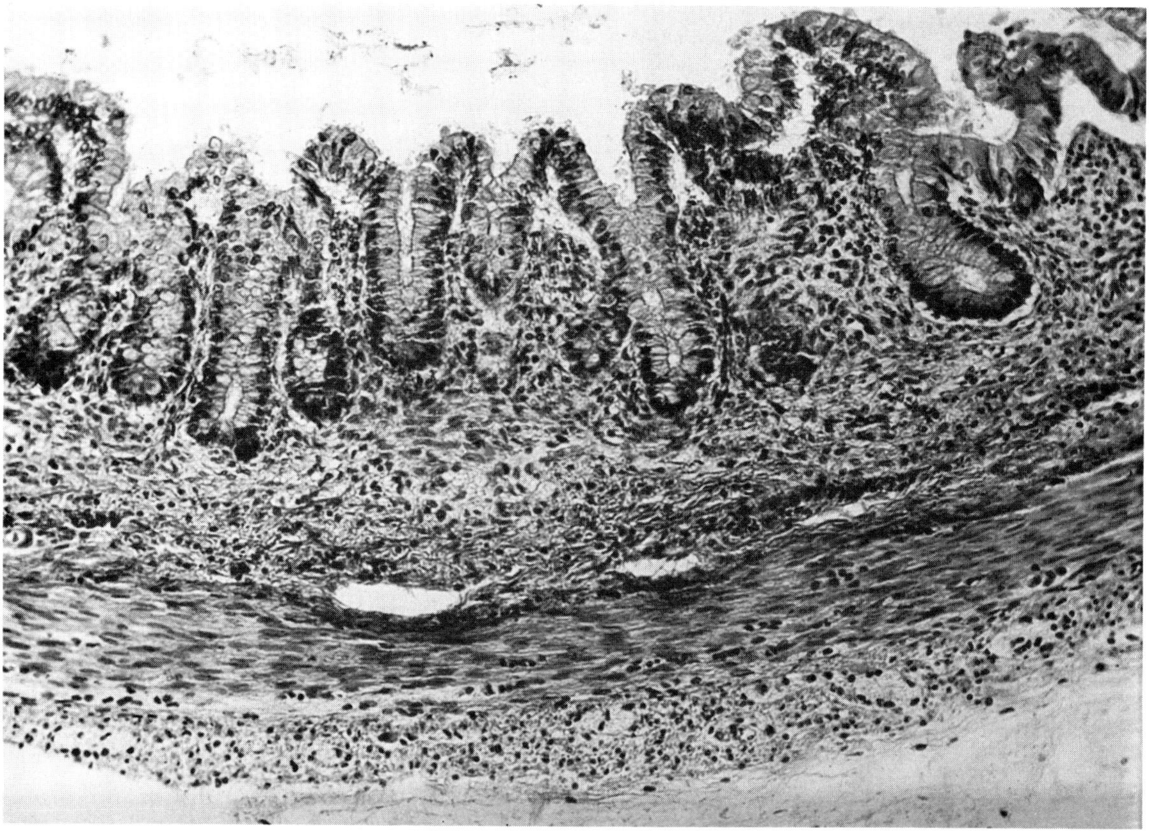

Figure 17-2

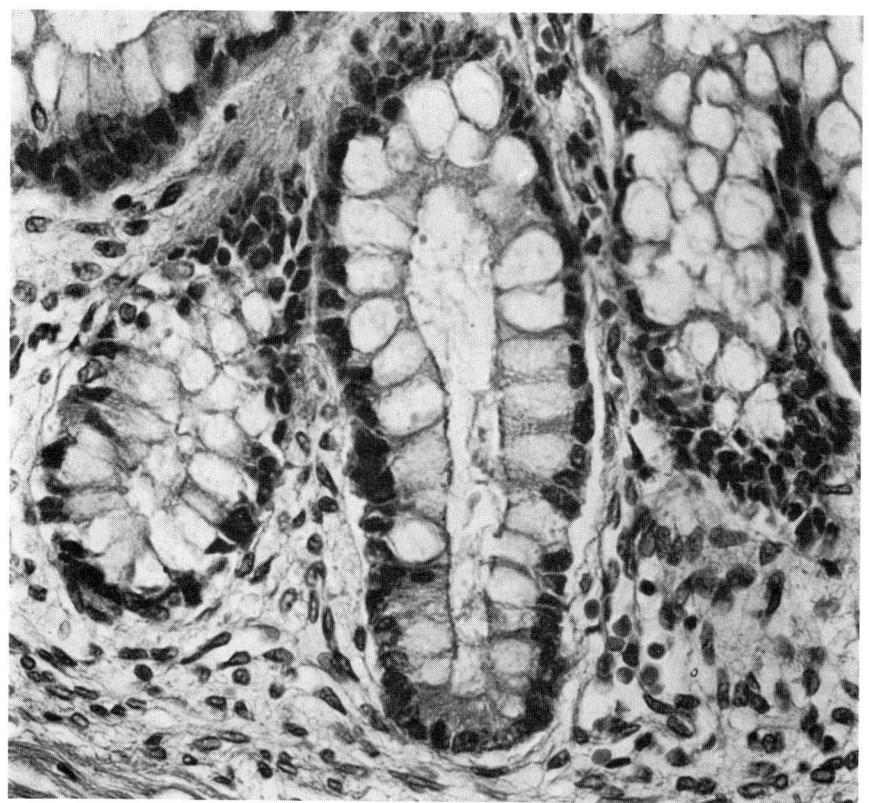

Figure 17-3

238 LARGE INTESTINE

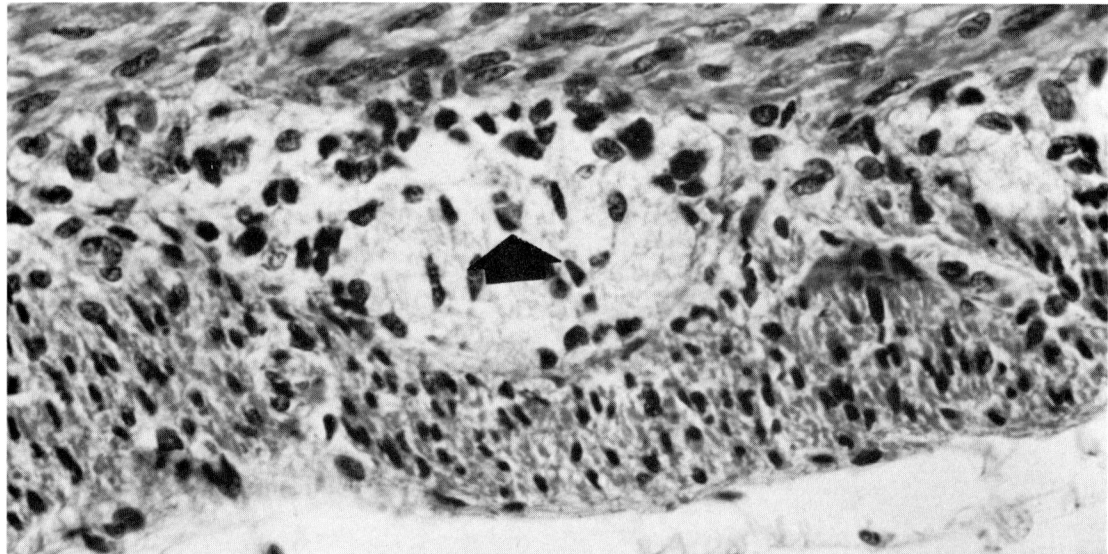

Figure 17–4

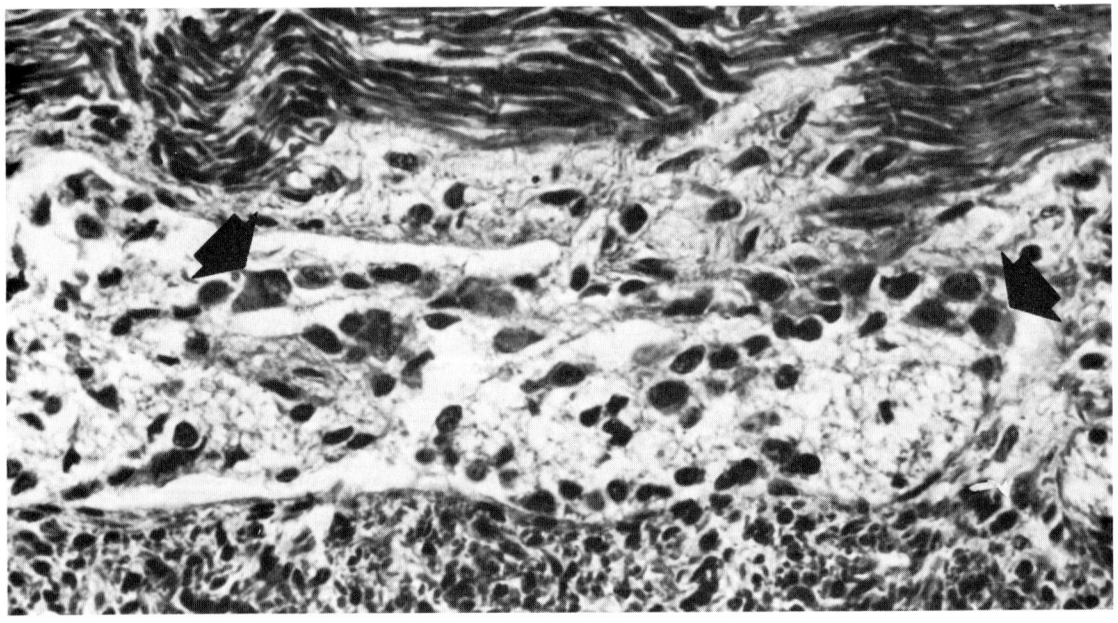

Figure 17–5

Figures 17–4 to 17–7. Ganglion cells in the plexus of Auerbach are not easily seen in the infant, particularly in one born prematurely. This set of photographs, taken at the same magnification, illustrates ganglion cells in premature and term infants.
Hematoxylin and eosin stain. Mag. 471×.

LARGE INTESTINE 239

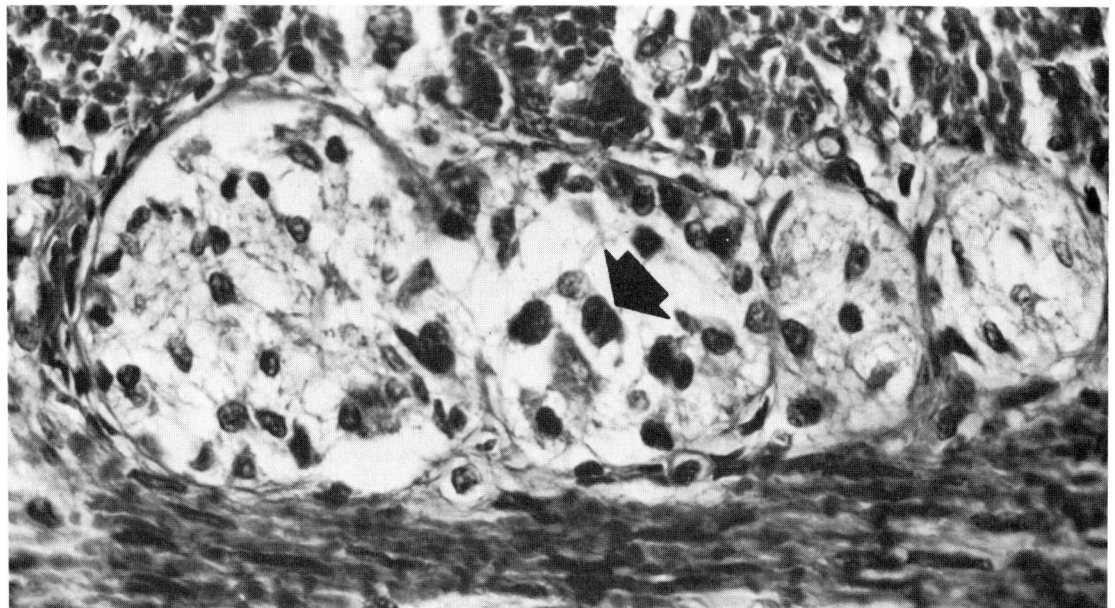

Figure 17–6

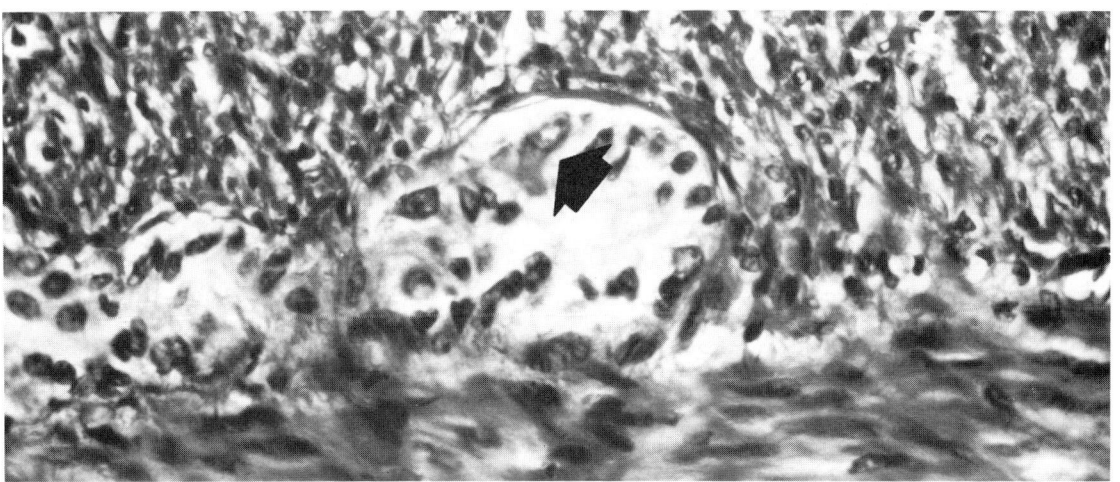

Figure 17–7

Fig.	Wt.	Race	Sex	Gestation	Age
17–4	510 gm.	B	F	21 wk. (est.)	1 hr. 26 min.
17–5	800 gm.	B	F	23 wk. (est.)	19 min.
17–6	3,400 gm.	?	F	38 wk. (est.)	55 hr.
17–7	?	B	F	40 wk. (est.)	14 days

Note: In each photograph, arrows indicate the more obvious and typical ganglion cells.

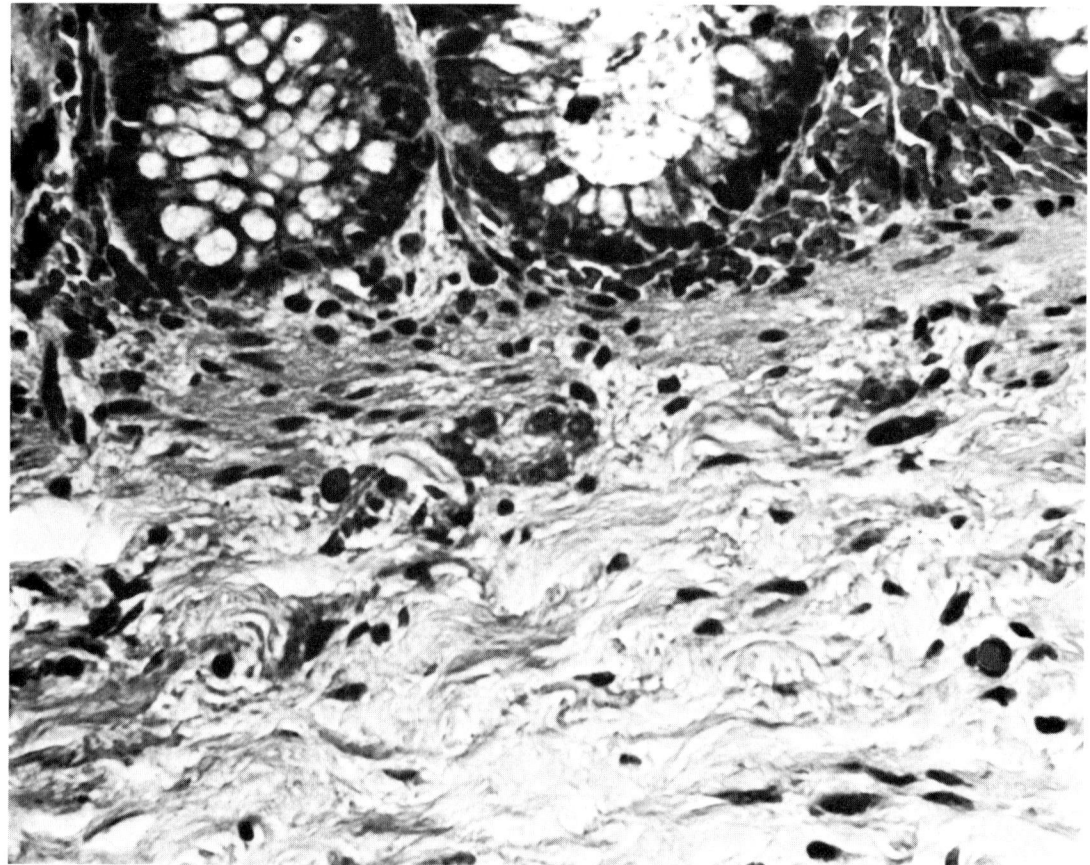

Figure 17–8

Figures 17–8 and 17–9. Now that suction biopsy of the mucosa and submucosa has become more popular as a means of establishing the diagnosis of aganglionic megacolon, the pathologist has had to become more familiar with the appearances of ganglion cells, and especially immature ganglion cells, in the submucosa. Two clusters are depicted here to illustrate their characteristic ovoid clumping, which is a very helpful feature in surveying sections; the size of their nuclei, which is greater than that of any cells in the vicinity; the relatively obscure cytoplasmic mass; and the very occasional prominent nucleolus, seen in the upper right portion of the cluster depicted in Fig. 17–9.

Figure 17–8. This is a portion of a section from a four day old female. Note the incomplete oval configuration of the group of cells and the tendency to "hug" the lower edge of the muscularis mucosae, a rather common characteristic.

Hematoxylin and eosin stain. Mag. 617.4×.

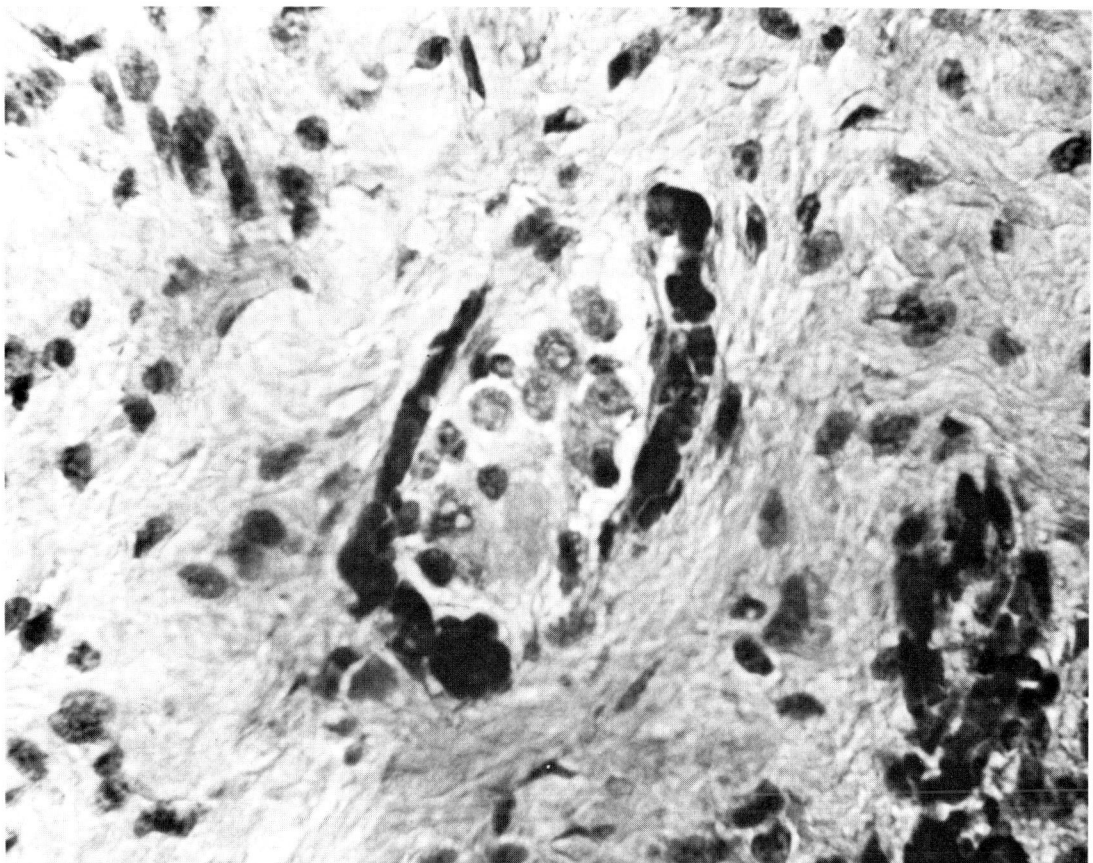

Figure 17–9

Figure 17–9. This ovoid clump of ganglion cells in the submucosa is accentuated by two capillaries that embrace it, one on the left and one higher on the right.

One can see very easily here a single prominent nucleolus near the apex of the group on the right side. Seeing such a nucleolus assists the pathologist in deciding that the cluster of cells in question truly represents a group of ganglion cells.

The patient was a one month old black female.

Hematoxylin and eosin stain. Mag. 621.6×.

242 LARGE INTESTINE

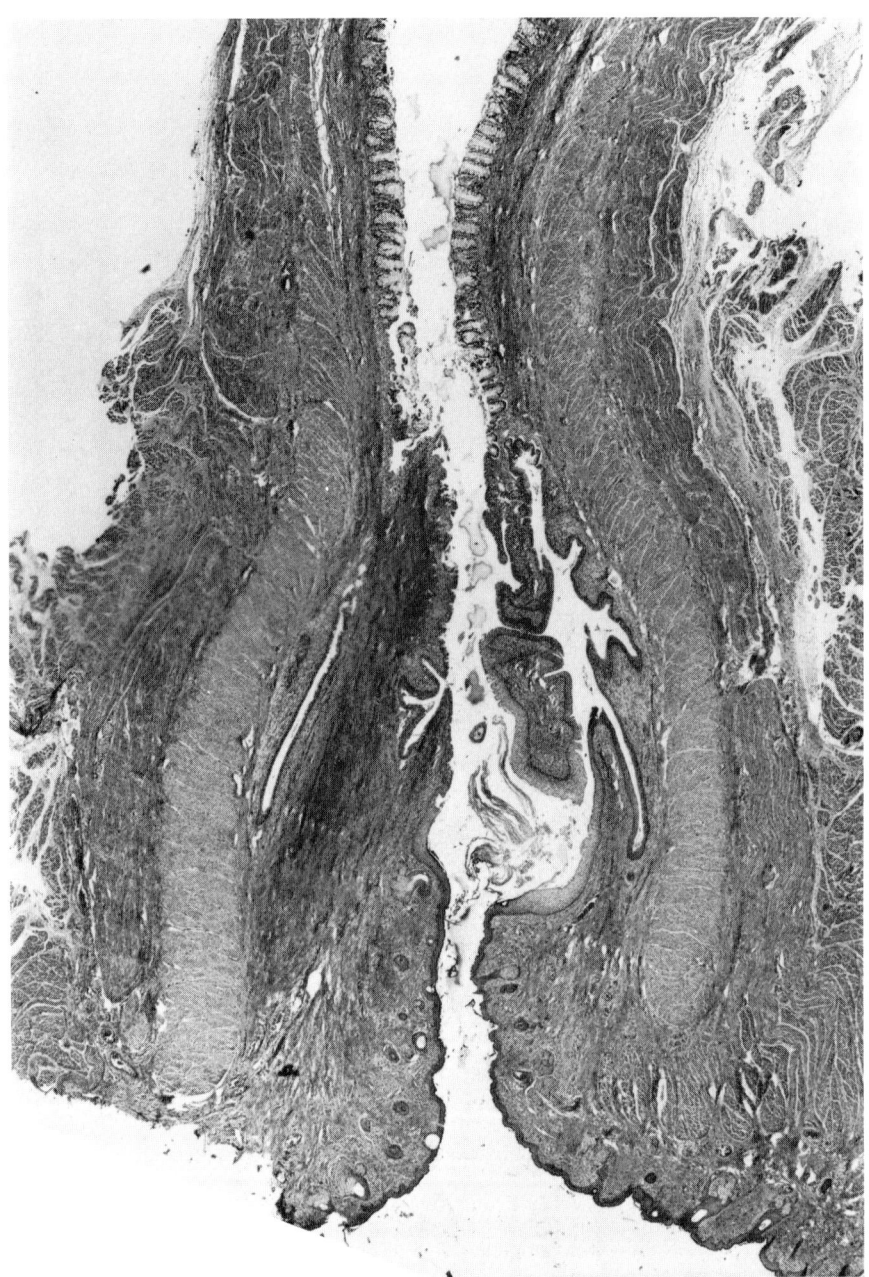

Figure 17–10

Figure 17–10. This photomicrograph, taken at very low magnification, shows the entire length of the anorectal canal of an infant.

The mucosa at the top is typical of the colon. Folds in the lining and a transitional kind of epithelium are found in the mid-portion, followed by non-keratinized stratified squamous epithelium, which, in the anal canal itself, gives way to hair-bearing skin.

The pale-staining smooth muscle layers of the colonic muscularis can be seen on both sides; they end blindly just below the level of transition of mucosa to skin.

This subject was a black female infant, the same one described in the legend for Fig. 17–9.
Hematoxylin and eosin stain. Mag. 20.2×.

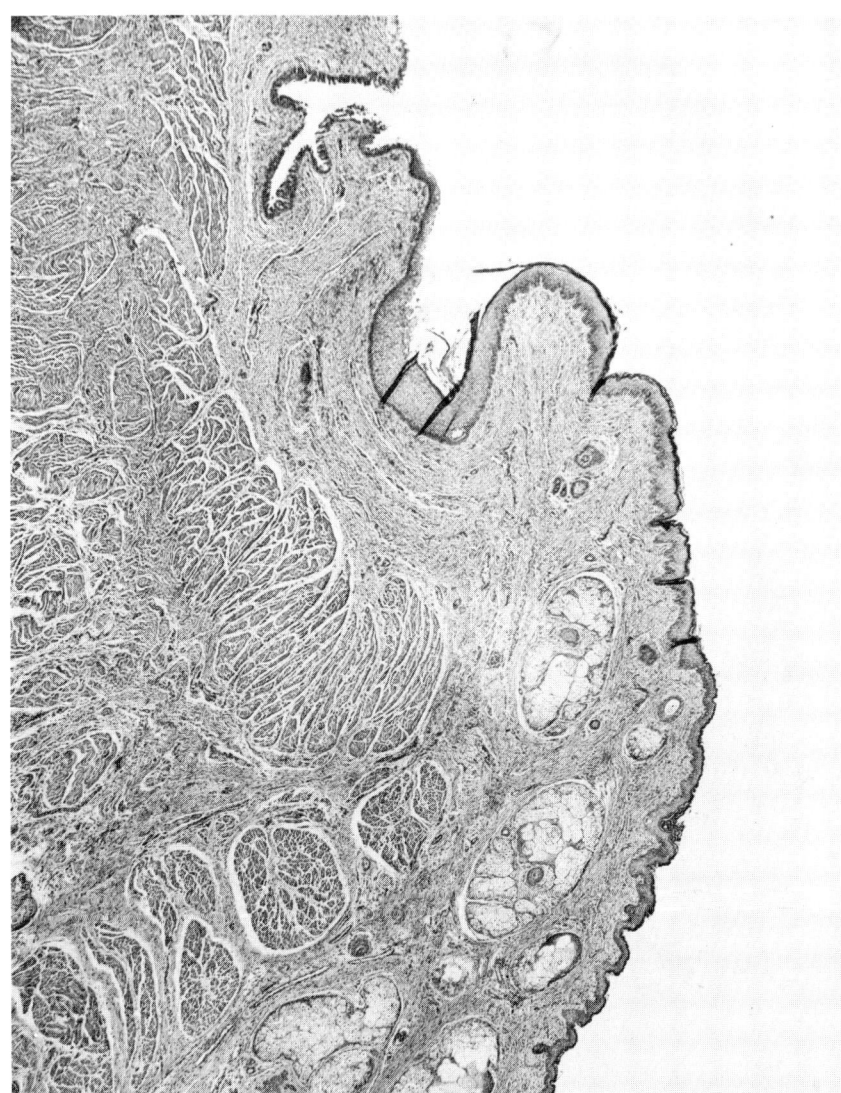

Figure 17–11

Figure 17–11. Here, at slightly higher magnification but in the same orientation as Fig. 17–10, is the anal canal of an infant. Notice the arrangement of the muscle bundles and the prominence of skin appendages.

The patient was a black male infant weighing 2,460 grams, who lived for 7 hours and 30 minutes.

Hematoxylin and eosin stain. Mag. 34×.

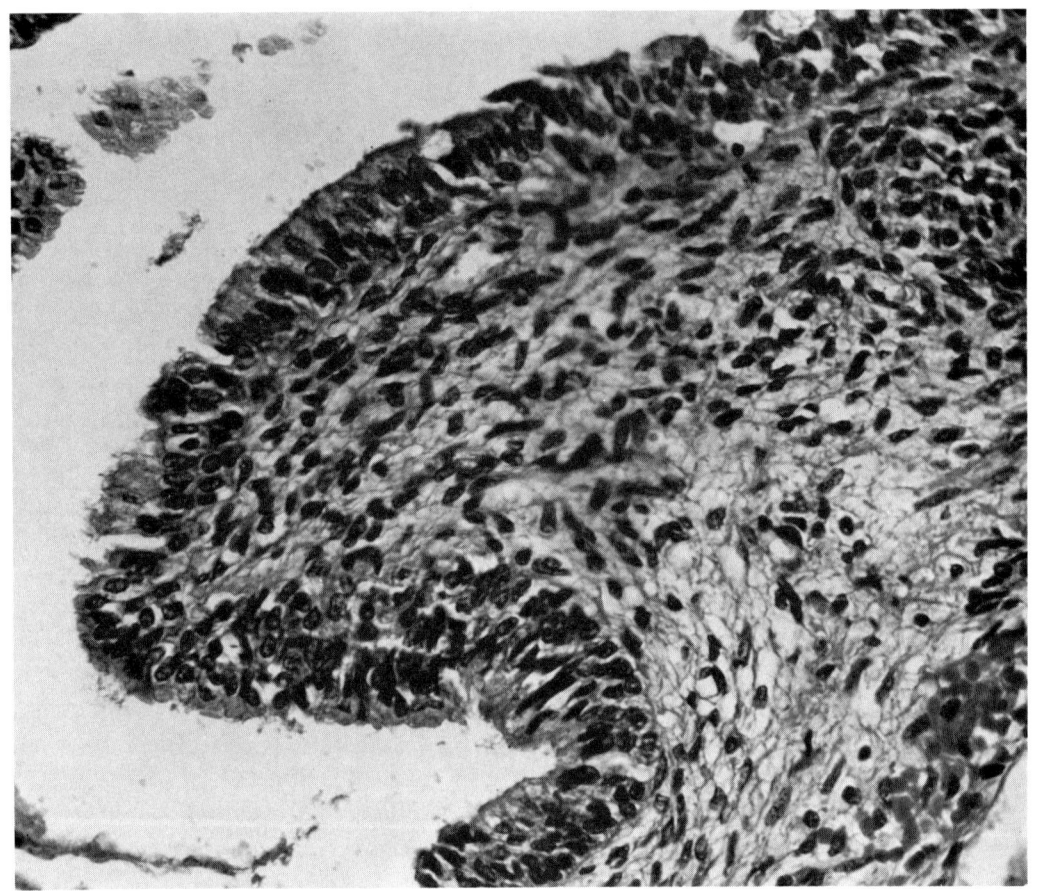

Figure 17–12

Figure 17–12. This is the unique, rather transitional type of epithelial lining encountered in the transition zone between colonic mucosa and the non-keratinized stratified squamous epithelium in the mid-portion of the anal canal. It is quite distinctive and may, at times, be confusing.

This patient lived for 8½ hours. She was a black female weighing only 865 grams at autopsy. (Estimated gestational age: 24 weeks.)

Hematoxylin and eosin stain. Mag. 350×.

Chapter 18

LIVER AND GALLBLADDER

Liver

EMBRYOLOGY

The liver arises as a bud from the most caudal part of the foregut at its junction with the yolk sac.[1] This hepatic diverticulum extends into the septum transversum, where it enlarges rapidly and divides into two parts; the larger cranial part is the primordium of the liver. The proliferating endodermal cells therein give rise to interlacing cords or cribriform sheets of liver cells, which come into close relationship with the vitelline veins. The intrahepatic portion of the biliary duct system is of the same embryologic derivation.

As the liver enlarges, it projects from the undersurface of the septum transversum into the abdominal cavity and so becomes mainly intraperitoneal.[8] There is some evidence that liver cells may arise not only from this endodermal outgrowth but also from mesenchymal or mesothelial cells of the septum transversum.[8]

By the sixth week of gestation, trabeculae of liver cells are already recognizable in intimate relationship with the vitelline veins. During the second and third months the organ grows rapidly; at the end of the third month it has attained its largest size relative to the rest of the body, about 10 per cent of the body weight.[8]

During this period its trabecular pattern is characteristic but lobules are not yet distinct; they appear gradually during later fetal months.

Bile capillaries are present in the 10 mm. embryo of six weeks. Bile ducts begin to appear toward the end of the second month by means of an *in situ* metamorphosis of liver cell cords lying near branches of the portal vein.[8] Liver cells and bile ducts seem to differentiate independently.

The fibrous and hematopoietic tissue and Kupffer cells of the liver are derived from the splanchnic mesenchyme of the septum transversum. Hepatic hematopoiesis (Figs. 18–14 to 18–17) begins in the sixth week of gestation and attains its maximum in the fifth month.

ANATOMY

The liver consists of a very large number of polyhedral hepatic lobules, which may appear to be more or less hexagonal in histologic section (Figs. 18–1 to 18–4). Each is about 1 mm. in diameter, having a small central vein (Figs. 18–7 and 18–8), a tributary of the hepatic veins, as its central axis. Each lobule is surrounded at its edges by groups of portal triads (Figs. 18–9 to 18–11). Each triad or portal area bears a thin-walled branch of the portal vein, a branch of the hepatic artery, an interlobular bile duct, and, at times, a small lymphatic vessel; all of these are surrounded by a sheath of connective tissue, the perivascular fibrous capsule.[3]

HISTOLOGY

The bulk of the cells within the liver are the hepatocytes, derived (as previously mentioned) from the endodermal lining of the caudal foregut, with which they retain their connection by way of the biliary duct system. They are arranged in cords or plates one cell thick, radiating in almost spoke-like manner from the central vein (Figs. 18–7 and 18–8).

These laminae of hepatocytes form a "wall-work"[3] and are somewhat irregularly arranged, with interlaminar bridges of liver cells connecting adjacent laminae. (The columns of cells are not truly arranged like the spokes of a wheel but are actually rather irregular and branching.[3])

Each hepatocyte (Fig. 18–5) has from five to twelve sides.[3] The nucleus is spheroidal and the nucleolus is prominent. In all probability the normal liver cell has but one nucleus. Both glycogen and lipid vacuoles are encountered commonly in the cytoplasm of the liver cells of the neonate; glycogen vacuoles usually are very small (much smaller than the nucleus), whereas, generally speaking, lipid vacuoles tend to be larger than the nucleus.

Located between hepatic cells within the cords or columns there are very fine channels, the bile canaliculi, which conduct bile toward the periphery of the lobule where it enters the bile ducts (Figs. 18–12 and 18–13). These minute anastomosing canaliculi are difficult to visualize in the neonatal liver when not filled with bile, as in instances of bile duct obstruction. Bile canaliculi join one another to form thin intralobular bile ducts, which in turn enter the interlobular bile ducts.

The radiating columns of liver cells are separated from one another by spaces, the hepatic lacunae; these spaces contain slender vascular channels, the sinusoids, which are lined by endothelial cells. The sinusoids are wider than capillaries and anastomose with one another through perforations in the laminae.[3] Special reticuloendothelial cells in the walls of these sinusoids, known as Kupffer cells, are phagocytic. They, too, may be difficult to distinguish by light microscopy — especially when they bear no foreign particles — but are sometimes made visible by artifactual breaking away from adjacent hepatocytes (Fig. 18–6).

The sinusoids are separated from the liver plates by a layer of reticulin and by the perisinusoidal space of Disse, which is continuous at the periphery of the lobule with the space of Mall surrounding the portal canal, vessels, and bile ducts. On the exposed surface of the liver there is a thin connective tissue layer beneath peritoneal mesothelium. It is called Glisson's capsule (Fig. 18–18).

During fetal life, especially between the second and seventh months of gestation, the liver acts as one of the main hematopoietic organs. Both red and white blood cells are developed in the mesenchyme covering the endothelium of the sinusoids[3] (Figs. 18–16 and 18–17).

References

All references for Part Six appear on page 271.

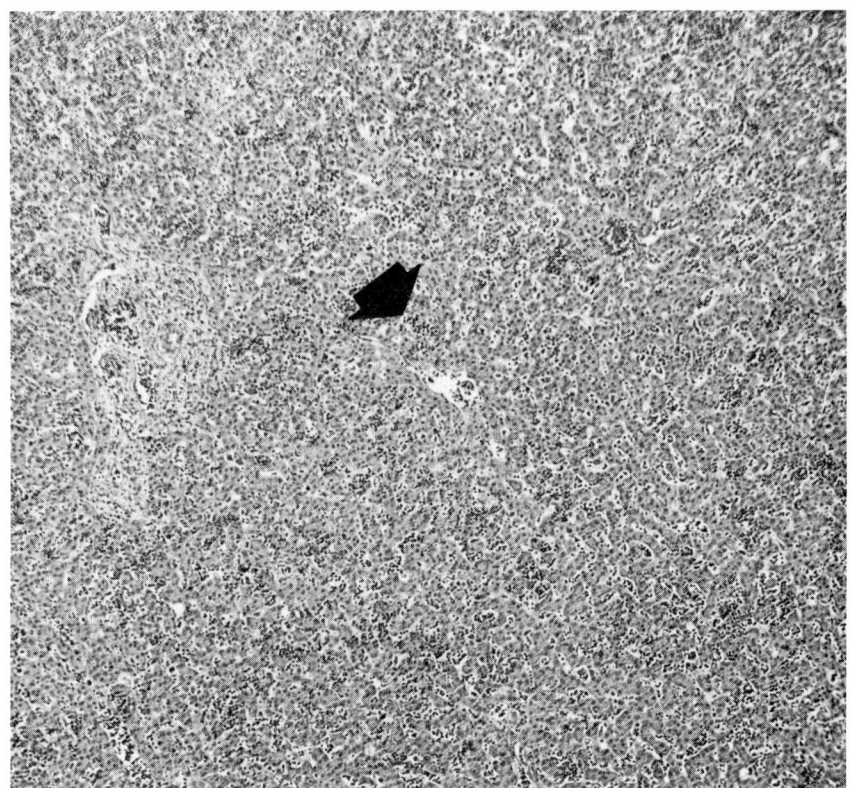

Figure 18–1

Figure 18–1. This is an illustration of the microscopic appearance of the liver of a prematurely born baby who died at 12 hours and 31 minutes of age and whose body weight at necropsy was 925 grams. (Estimated gestational age: 25 weeks.)

Even at this low magnification, clusters of hematopoietic cells are visible throughout, as is to be expected; one such nest is marked with an arrow. There is a central vein to the right of and above the arrow, and a large portal area to the left.

Hematoxylin and eosin stain. Mag. 55×.

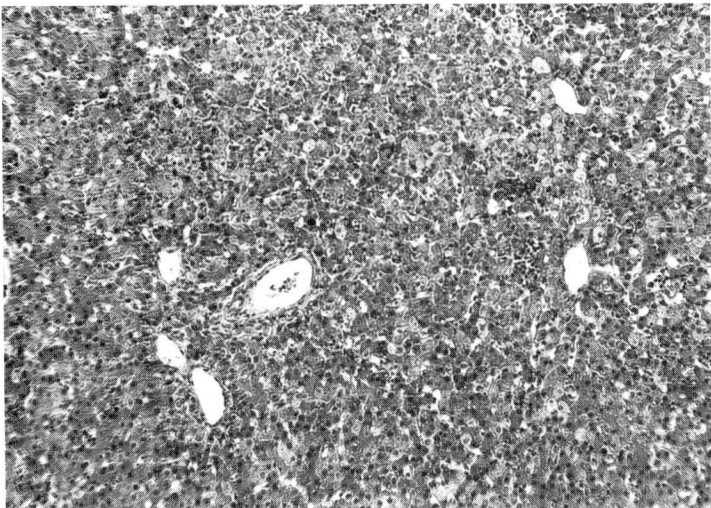

Figure 18–2a

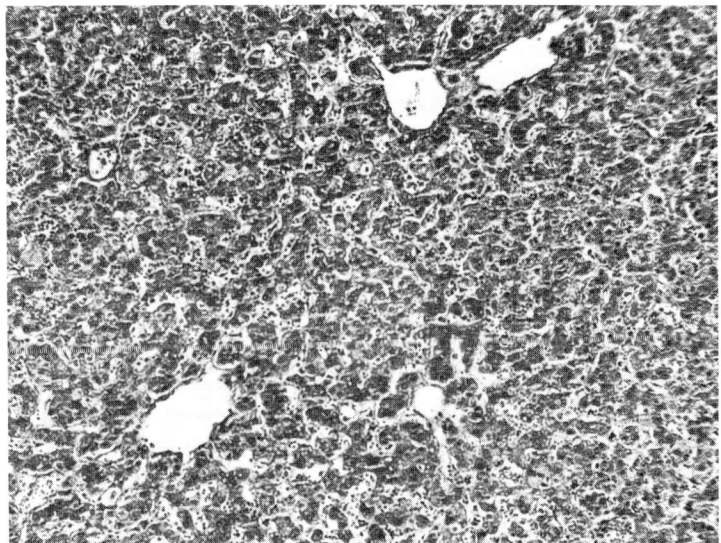

Figure 18–2b

Figures 18–2a and 18–2b. These two photographs show the almost adult histologic appearance of the fine architecture of the liver from early on.

Figure 18–2a is derived from a prematurely born white male infant who died of an intraventricular hemorrhage at the age of 4 days, weighing 1,175 grams.

Figure 18–2b is taken from a 16 hour and 40 minute old term white female infant whose body weight at postmortem examination was 4,251 grams.

Hematoxylin and eosin stain. Mag. 108×.

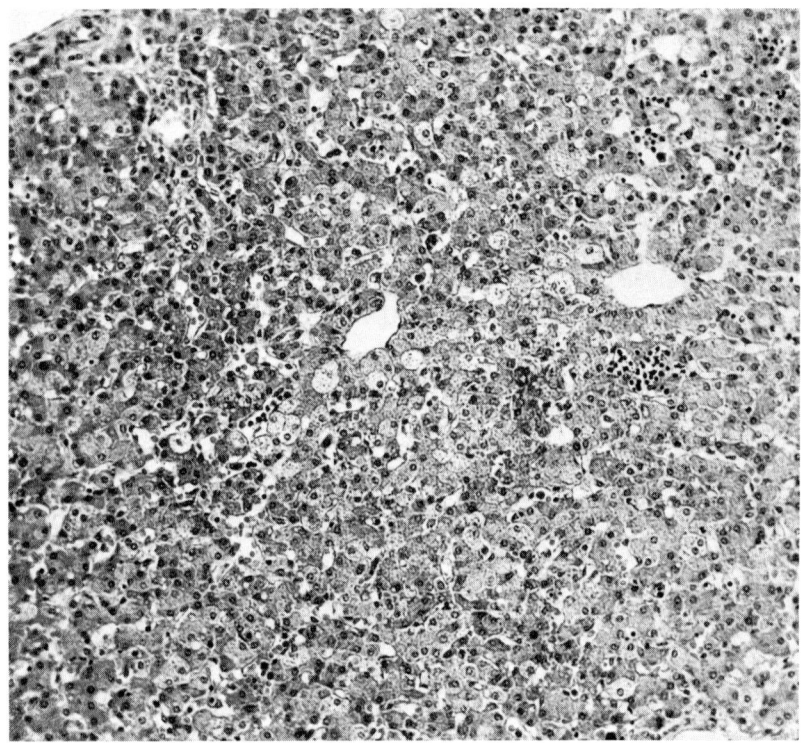

Figure 18-3

Figure 18-3. Depicted here is a single lobule of the liver of a prematurely born baby. There is a central vein to the right side of the photograph, just above a cluster of hematopoietic cells; its corresponding portal area is in the upper left corner.

The infant is the same as that described for Fig. 18-2a.

Hematoxylin and eosin stain. Mag. 152×.

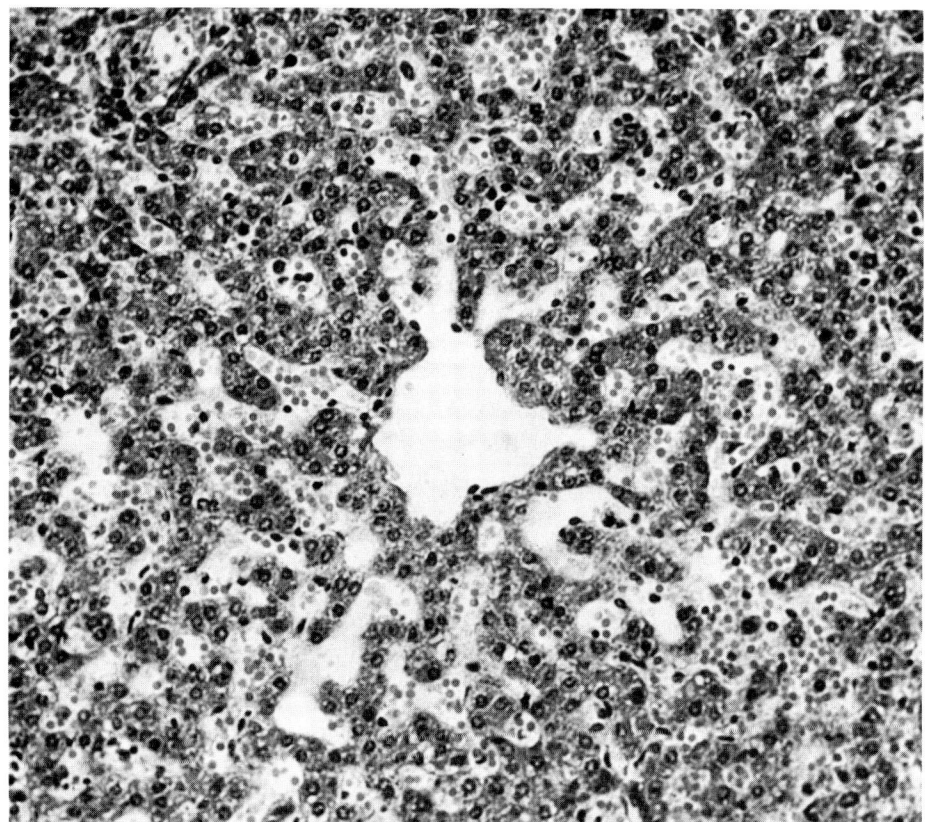

Figure 18–4

Figure 18–4. This photograph illustrates the general tendency for plates of liver cells, within a lobule, to radiate away from the central vein.

The subject was a prematurely born black male infant (gestational age: 28 weeks) who survived for 5 days and 20 hours and whose weight at autopsy was 880 grams.

Hematoxylin and eosin stain. Mag. 231×.

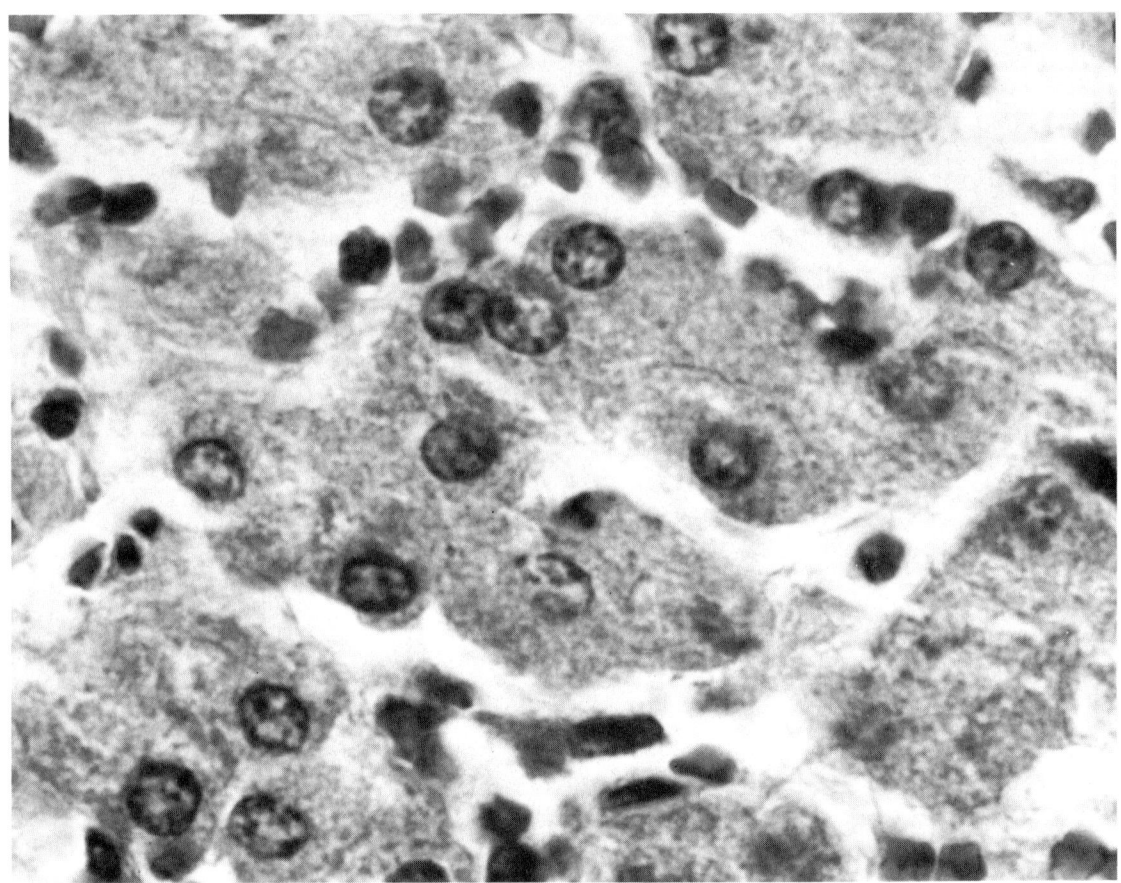

Figure 18–5

Figure 18-5. In this illustration, the morphology of individual liver cells, as seen by light microscopy, is readily apparent. The individual cell, of polyhedral shape, has a prominent nucleus and nucleolus. The sinusoids, in this instance, contain many red blood cells.

This section was taken from a one month old black male infant who, at autopsy, weighed 4,005 grams.

Hematoxylin and eosin stain. Mag. 1,211×.

LIVER 253

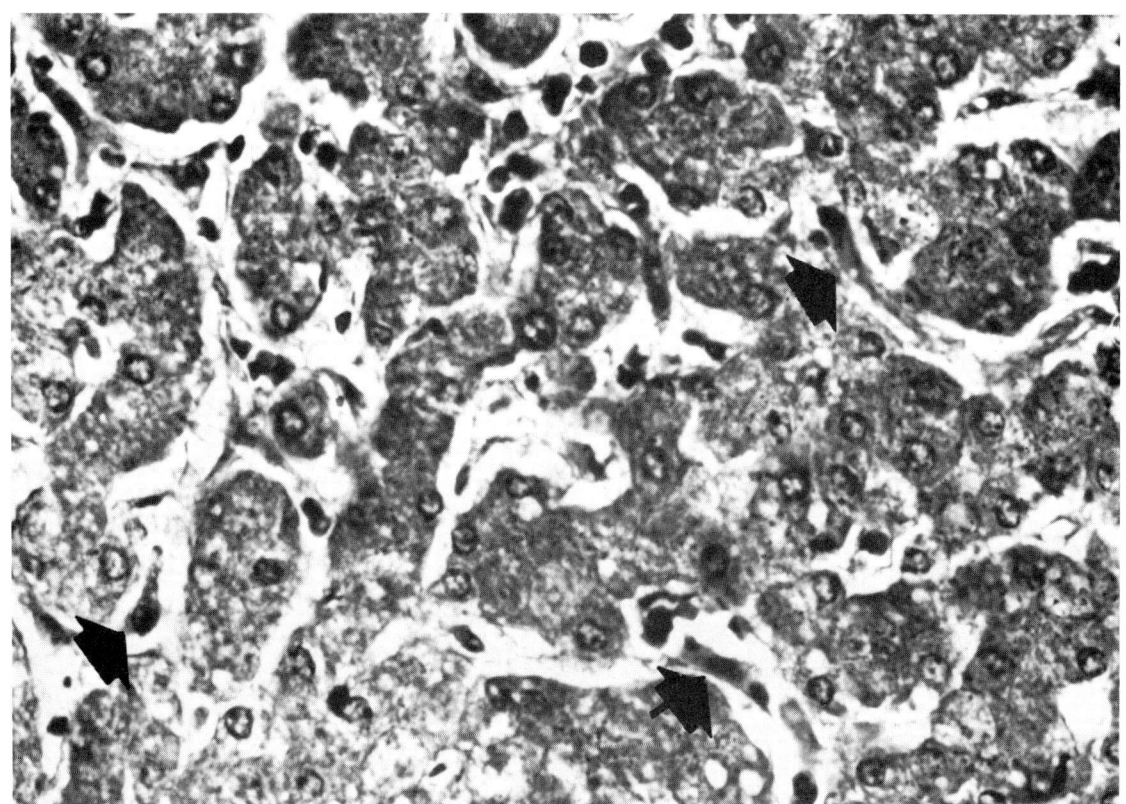

Figure 18-6

Figure 18-6. Kupffer cells, artifactually separated in this section from adjacent liver cells, appear as elongate, spindle-shaped cells with obviously pointed ends. (Three are marked with arrows, one in the lower left corner, one in the upper right, and one just to the right of center near the inferior margin of the photograph.)

This is from a 21 day old white male infant who weighed 3,320 grams at necropsy.

Hematoxylin and eosin stain. Mag. 513×.

254 LIVER AND GALLBLADDER

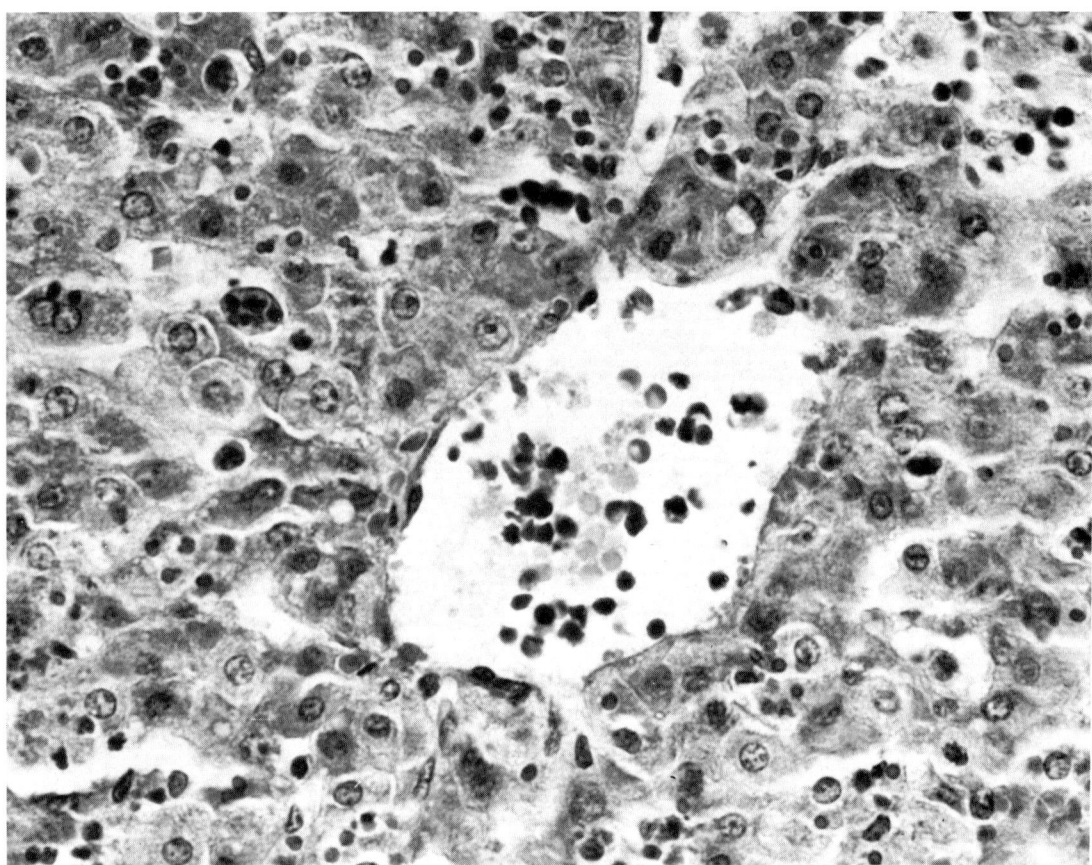

Figure 18–7

Figure 18–7. This photomicrograph illustrates details of a central vein from the liver of a small prematurely born infant, a black female, who died at the age of 27 hours. The baby's weight at autopsy was 512 grams. (Estimated gestational age: 21 weeks.)

At least two endothelial cell nuclei can be identified in cells lining this central vein. The lumen contains both red and white cells. At least four sinusoids are seen entering at this level.

Hematoxylin and eosin stain. Mag. 471×.

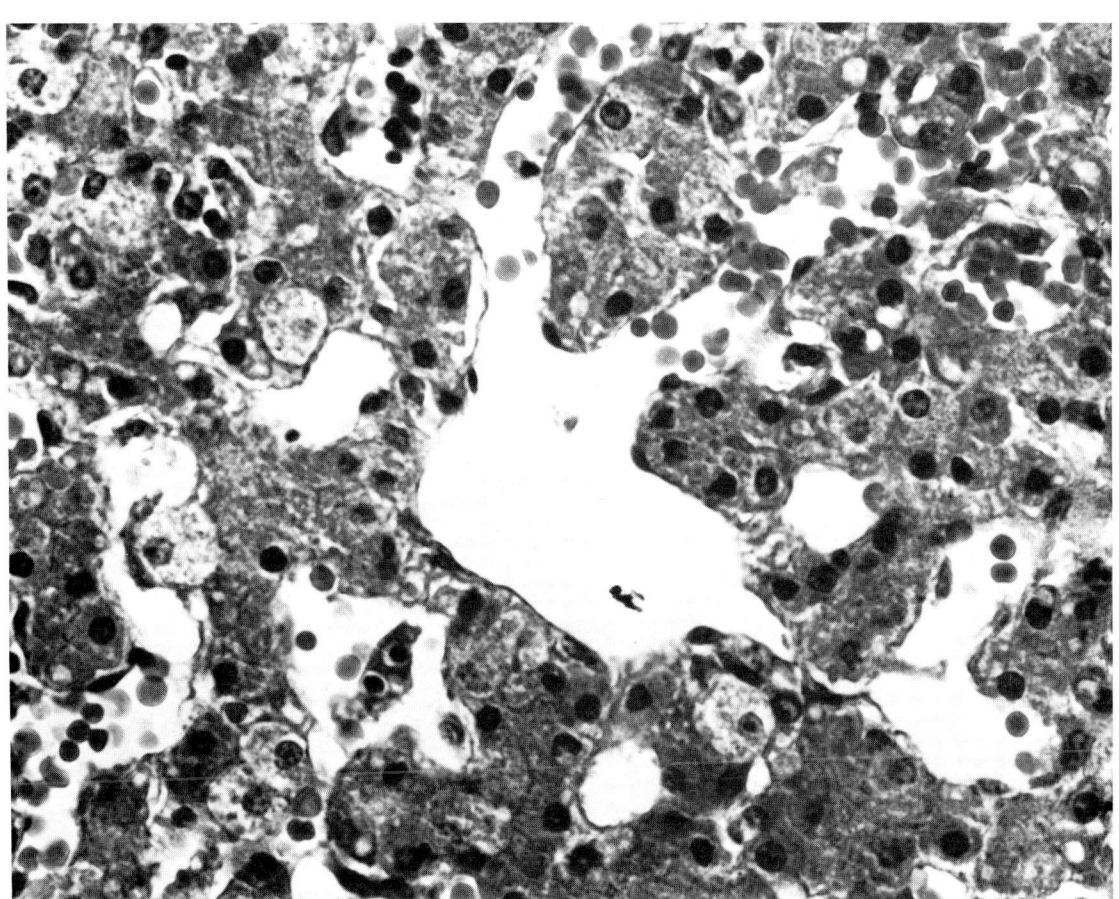

Figure 18-8

Figure 18-8. This is the central vein of a much larger infant, a four day old white male weighing 1,175 grams. (Estimated gestational age: 27 weeks.)

Two sinusoids clearly open into this vein from above.

Hematoxylin and eosin stain. Mag. 513×.

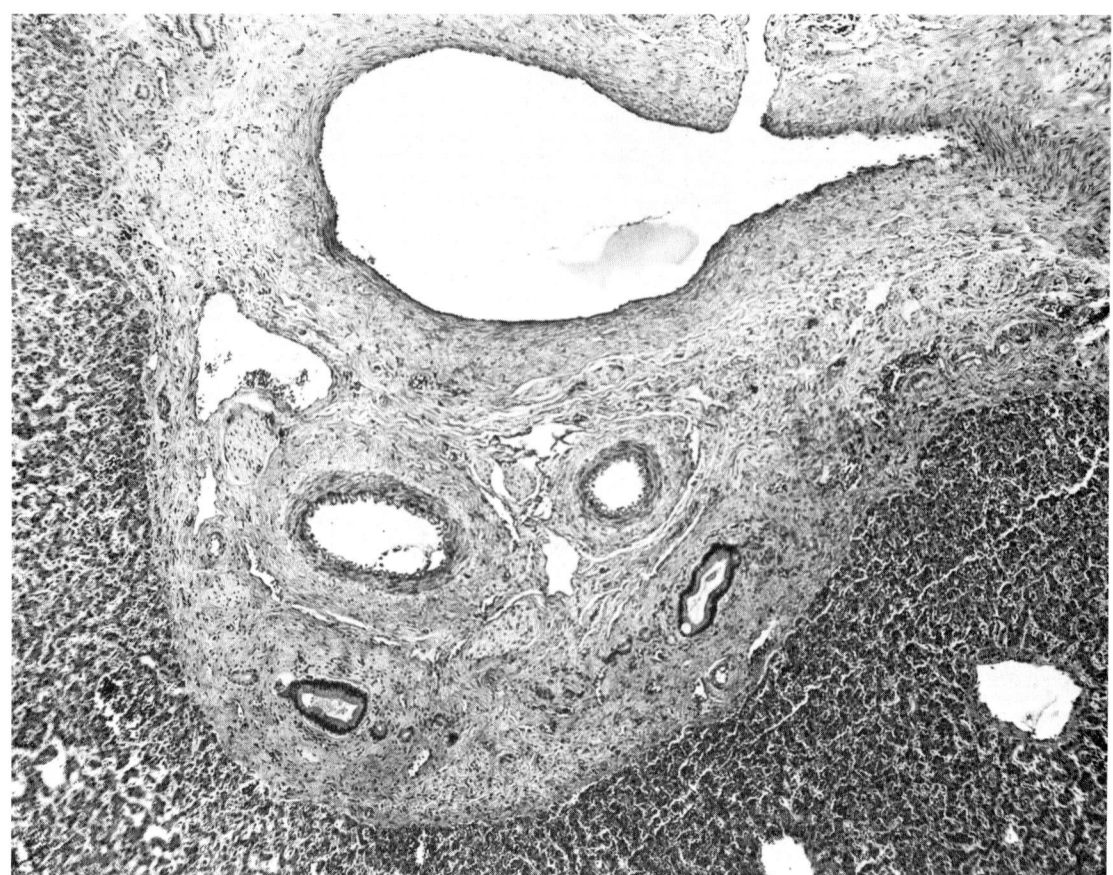

Figure 18-9

Figures 18-9, 18-10, and 18-11. This set of three photomicrographs, each taken at progressively higher magnification (76×, 219×, and 390×), illustrates typical portal areas from those of largest size to the smallest ramification.

In Fig. 18-9, two arteries, two veins, and two bile ducts appear; connective tissue is abundant. In Fig. 18-11, a large centrally placed vein is flanked on the upper left by an arteriole and a very small bile duct, marked by two black arrows.

Figs. 18-9 and 18-10 are taken from a section of the liver of an 11 hour old black male who, at postmortem examination, weighed 2,560 grams; he was born post-term. Fig. 18-11 is from a white male infant, 16 hours and 40 minutes of age, who weighed 4,251 grams at autopsy.

Hematoxylin and eosin stain.

Figure 18-10

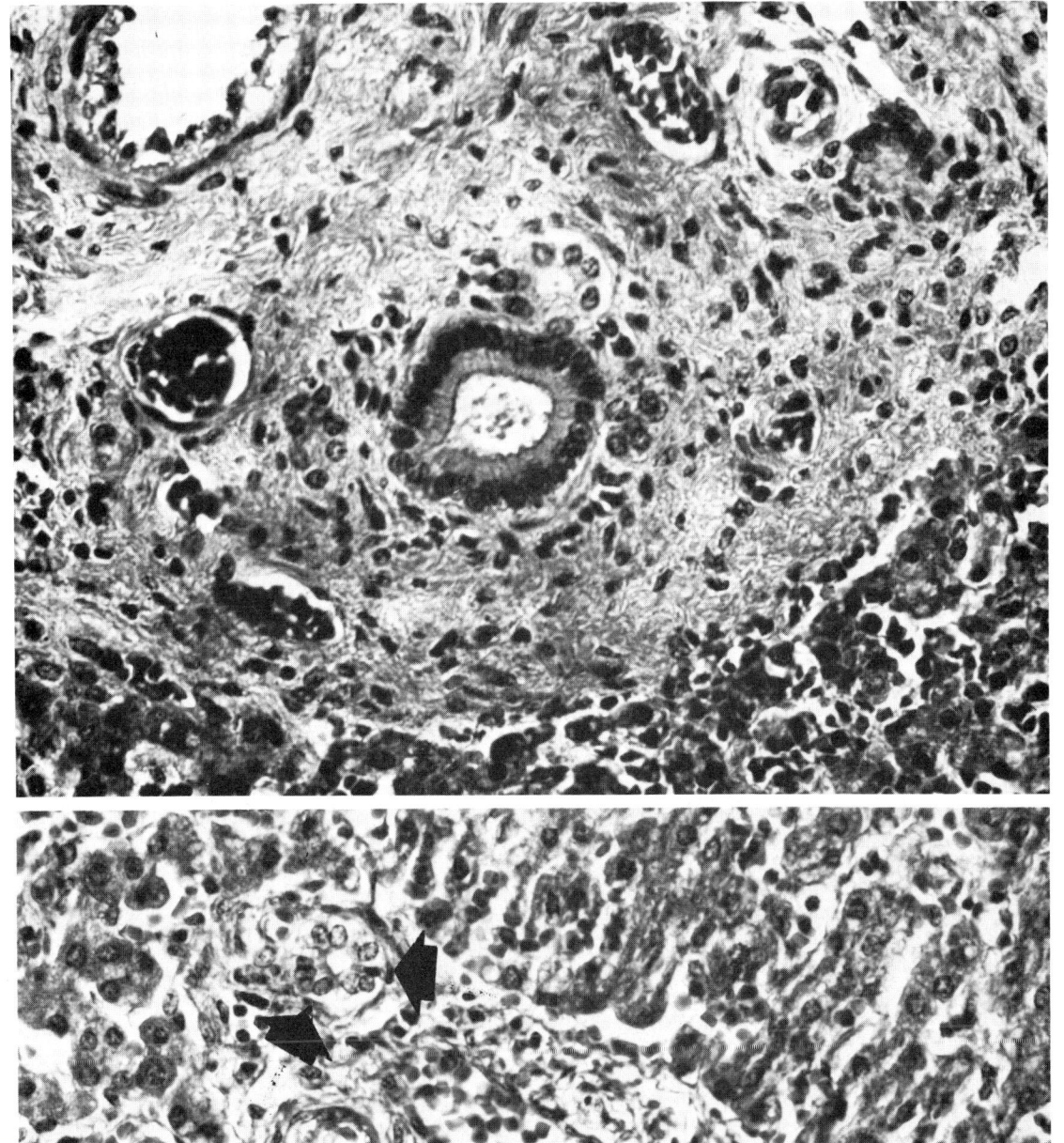

Figure 18-11

258 LIVER AND GALLBLADDER

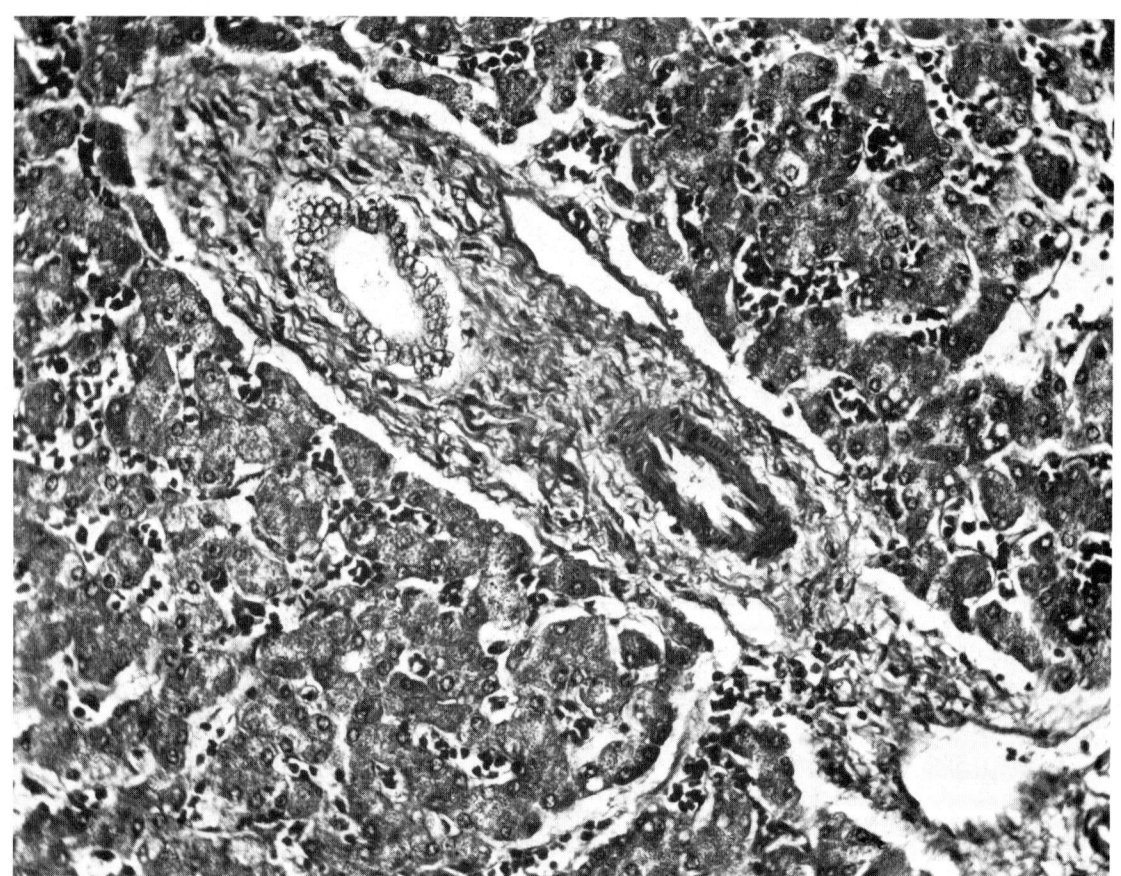

Figure 18–12

Figure 18–12. In this portal area, of medium size, a bile duct is illustrated. It is cut somewhat tangentially. The duct is lined by a single layer of cuboidal to low columnar epithelial cells.

This section was taken from a 21 day old white female infant, born at term, whose weight at autopsy was 3,230 grams.

Hematoxylin and eosin stain. Mag. 250×.

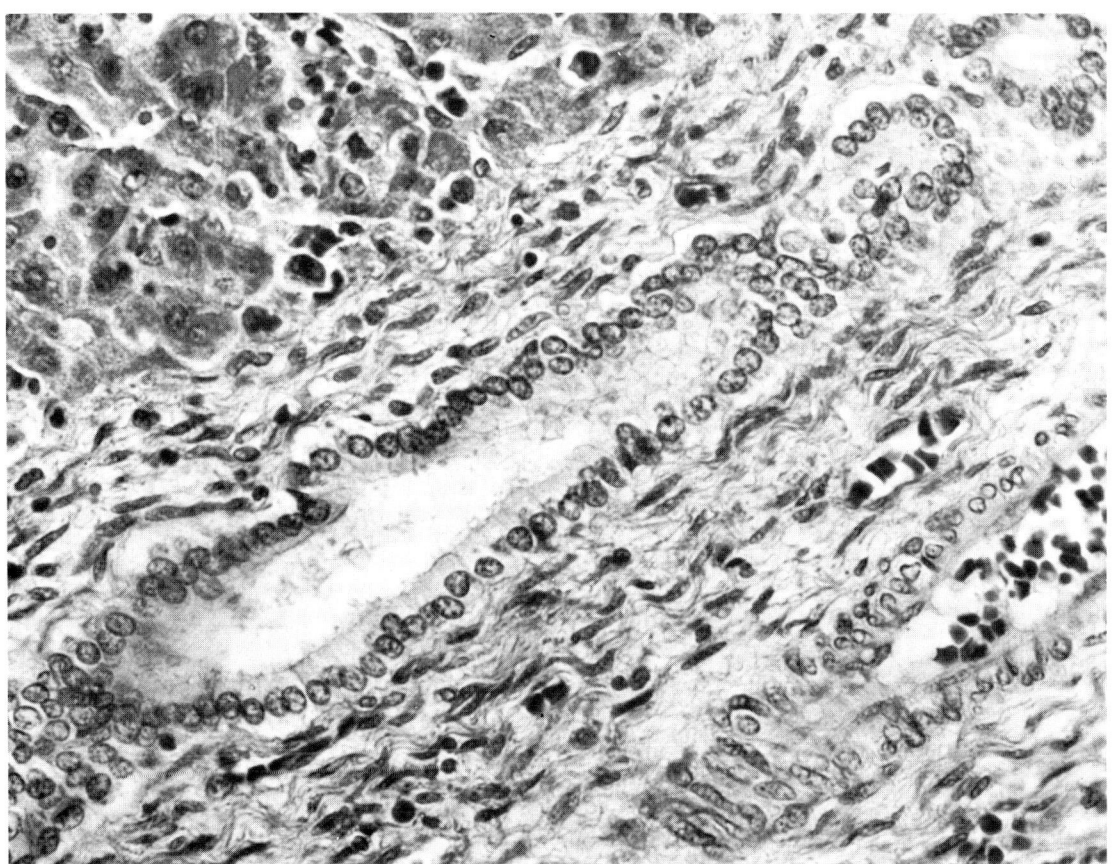

Figure 18–13

Figure 18-13. At somewhat higher magnification, a bile duct of comparable order is seen here, this from a prematurely born black female infant whose body weight at necropsy was 512 grams. (Estimated gestational age: 21 weeks.) The infant survived for 27 hours.

Note that the single layer of columnar cells is uniformly rather tall.

Hematoxylin and eosin stain. Mag. 440×.

260 LIVER AND GALLBLADDER

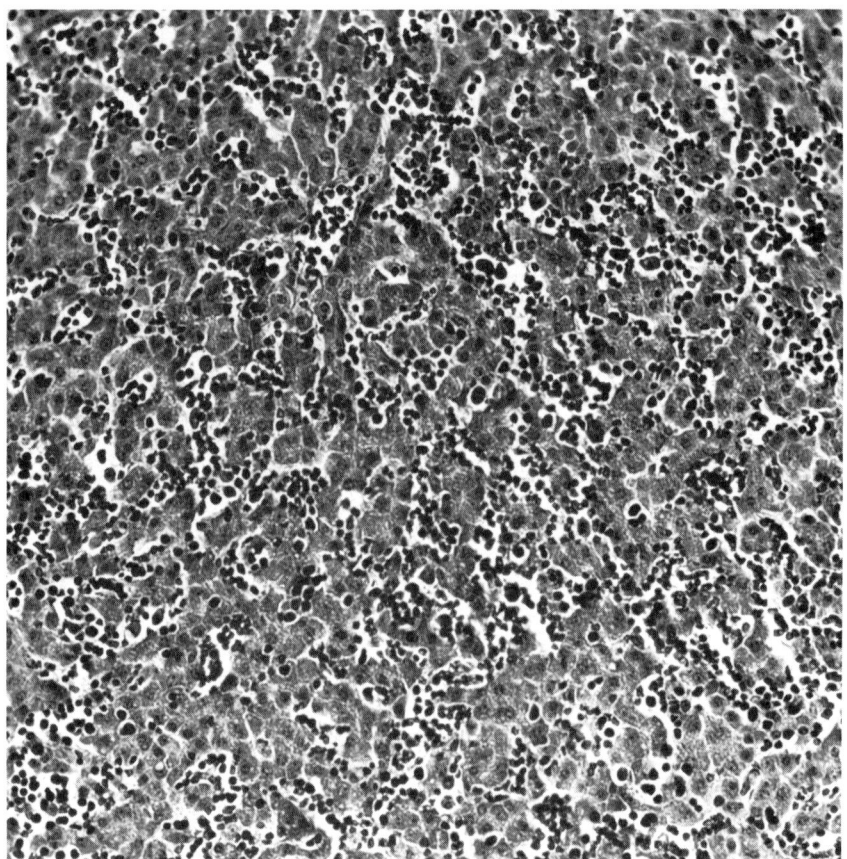

Figure 18–14

Figure 18–14. One of the unique features of the histology of the liver in the perinatal period is the relatively common appearance of extramedullary hematopoiesis within both the lobules and portal areas. Naturally it diminishes in amount and extent as the infant approaches the time of a term birth, at which point it would be expected to have disappeared for practical purposes.

In this instance, hepatic parenchyma is seen from the liver of a 650 gram, 7 hour old black male infant. Most of the tiny round black nuclei crowded in sinusoids represent hematopoietic elements. The degree and extent are compatible with the gestational age, estimated to be about 22 weeks.

Hematoxylin and eosin stain. Mag. 186×.

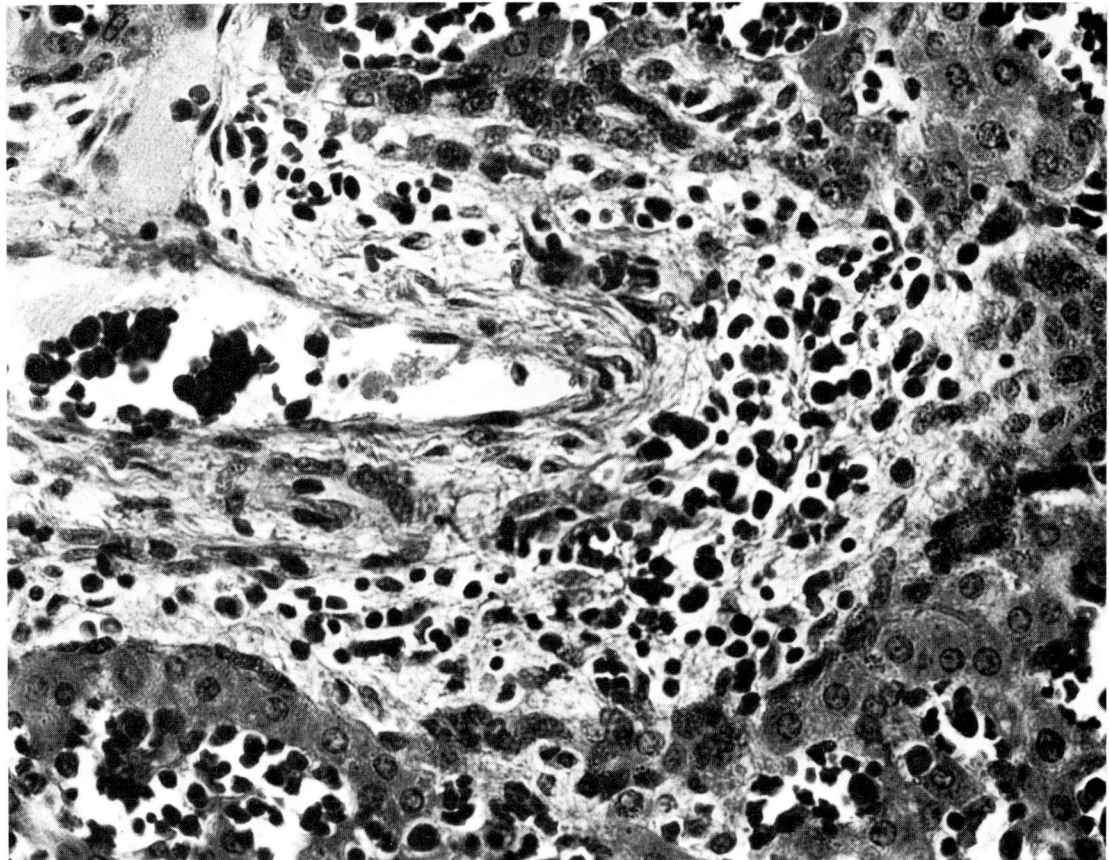

Figure 18–15

Figure 18–15. In this illustration, at higher magnification than the preceding illustration, a segment of a single portal triad is depicted. This is from an 830 gram white male infant who lived for 7 hours. (Estimated gestational age: 24 weeks.) This much hematopoiesis is also compatible with the gestational age of this infant.

Hematoxylin and eosin stain. Mag. 219×.

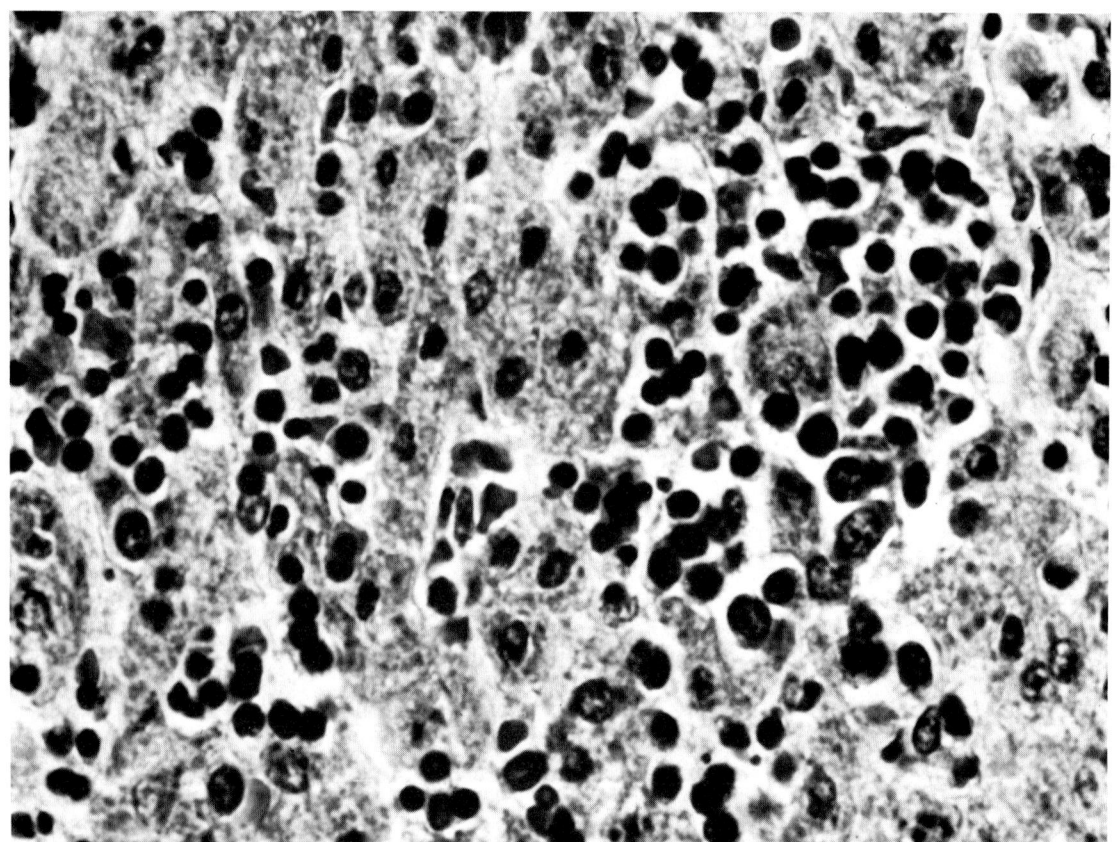

Figure 18–16

Figure 18–16. Here, at still higher magnification, extramedullary hematopoiesis is seen within the sinusoids of the liver of a premature infant. The numbers of hematopoietic cells here are clearly greater than those in Fig. 18–17 (at the same magnification). Both are within limits of normal for their respective gestational ages.

This section was taken from the liver of a 470 gram white female infant who died at 3 hours of age. (Estimated gestational age: 20 weeks.)

Hematoxylin and eosin stain. Mag. 660×.

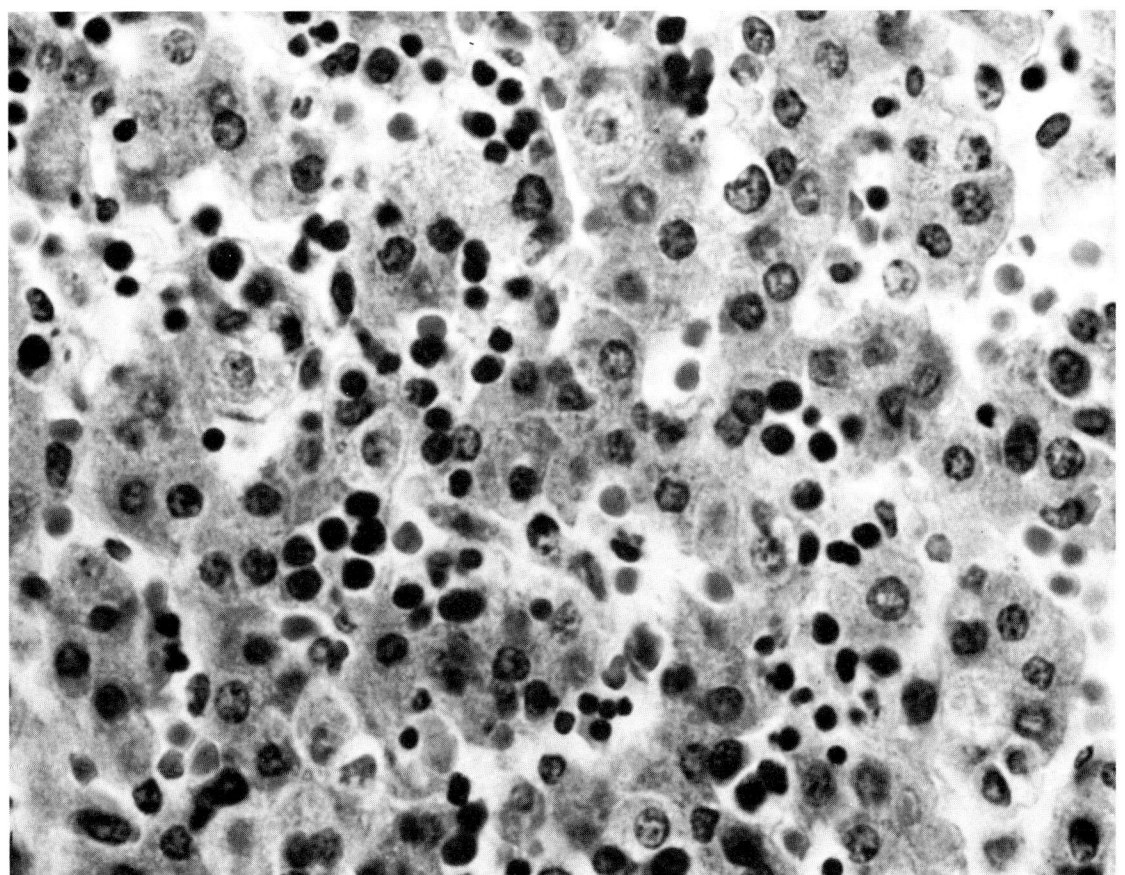

Figure 18–17

Figure 18–17. By comparison with Fig. 18–16, this is typical of the extent of hematopoiesis that may be seen in the liver at 32 weeks of gestation.

This is a section from the liver of a 1,125 gram black female twin who survived for 10 hours and 30 minutes.

Hematoxylin and eosin stain. Mag. 660×.

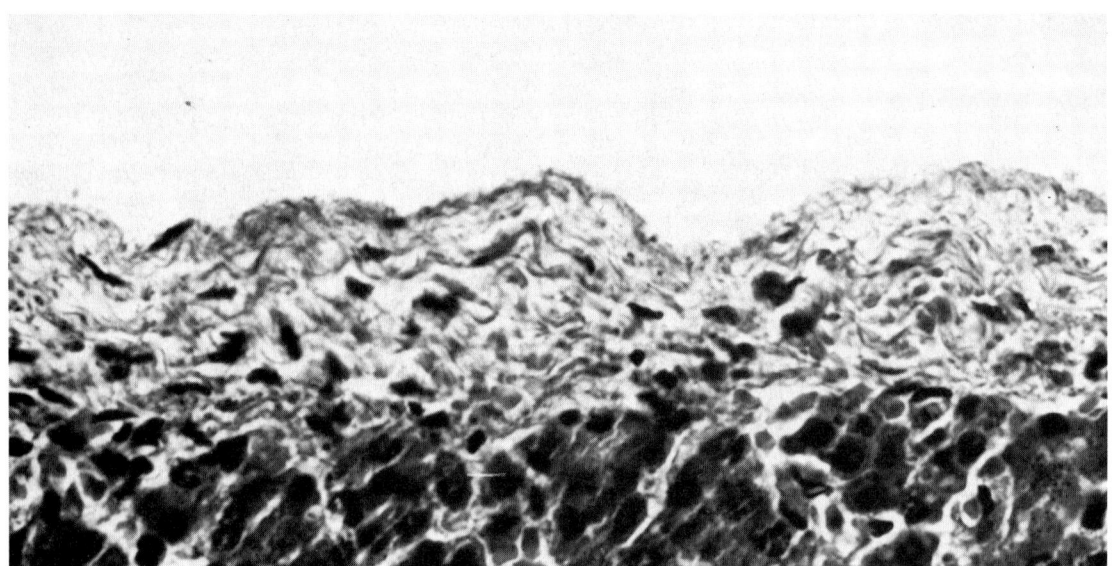

Figure 18–18

Figure 18-18. There is great variability in the thickness of the capsule of the liver, Glisson's capsule, during the perinatal period. Although it is often thinner than depicted here, it is commonly of breadth as great as this.

The patient was a 7 day old black male who weighed 1,100 grams at autopsy. (Estimated gestational age: 27 weeks.)

Hematoxylin and eosin stain. Mag. 534×.

Gallbladder

EMBRYOLOGY

The development of the gallbladder begins with a separate, caudal region of the shallow original hepatic diverticulum arising from the floor of the future duodenum. Early on, in the embryo, it is a solid epithelial cylinder carried away from the duodenum by elongation of the common duct. At about six weeks a distinct stem or cystic duct is recognizable; in the seventh week a lumen has been established throughout most of the tract that appears like an offshoot from the main biliary passage.[2]

ANATOMY

The gallbladder is a piriform, thin-walled sac located in a fossa on the undersurface of the right lobe of the liver. Its fundus or expanded end is directed downward, forward, and to the right. The body is directed upward, backward, and to the left; near the right end of the porta hepatis it is continuous with the neck. The neck is narrow; it curves upward and forward, and then, turning abruptly, backward and downward to become continuous with the cystic duct. At its point of continuity with the duct there is a constriction.[3]

The mucous membrane lining the gallbladder is arranged in anastomosing fine folds. That lining the neck projects into the lumen in the form of an oblique ridge creating a sort of spiral valve.

The cystic duct joins the common hepatic duct; it runs parallel to and adheres to the latter for a short distance before joining it. The mucous membrane of the cystic duct forms a series of crescentic folds like those in the neck of the gallbladder; the set is known as the spiral valve of Heister. The common duct enters the duodenum at the ampulla of Vater (Fig. 18–20).

HISTOLOGY

The wall of the gallbladder consists of the following: a mucosa consisting of a surface epithelium and a lamina propria; a true muscular coat; perimuscular connective tissue; and a serous layer clothing only that part of the organ not in contact with the liver.[4]

The mucosa is, as previously mentioned, thrown into many folds or rugae. The major folds are subdivided into many smaller folds. When the organ is distended, many of the folds disappear, but some of them can always be seen. The epithelium consists of a single layer of tall columnar cells (Fig. 18–19). They have an inconspicuous striated border; with electron microscopy they are seen to bear very large numbers of short microvilli.

In the lamina propria and in the perimuscular layer near the neck of the gallbladder are simple tubuloalveolar glands (Fig. 18–19). Their epithelium is cuboidal and clear. These glands are said to secrete mucus. The so-called Rokitansky-Aschoff sinuses or outpouchings of the mucosa are not seen in the gallbladder of the fetus or newborn.

Beneath the epithelium is an irregular network of variously oriented bundles of smooth muscle fibers. The spaces between them are occupied by collagenous, reticular, and some elastic fibers together with a few fibroblasts.

External to the muscle is a dense layer of connective tissue completely surrounding the gallbladder and, on the hepatic aspect, continuous with its interlobular connective tissue.

That portion of the gallbladder not attached to the liver is covered with peritoneum.

References

All references for Part Six appear on page 271.

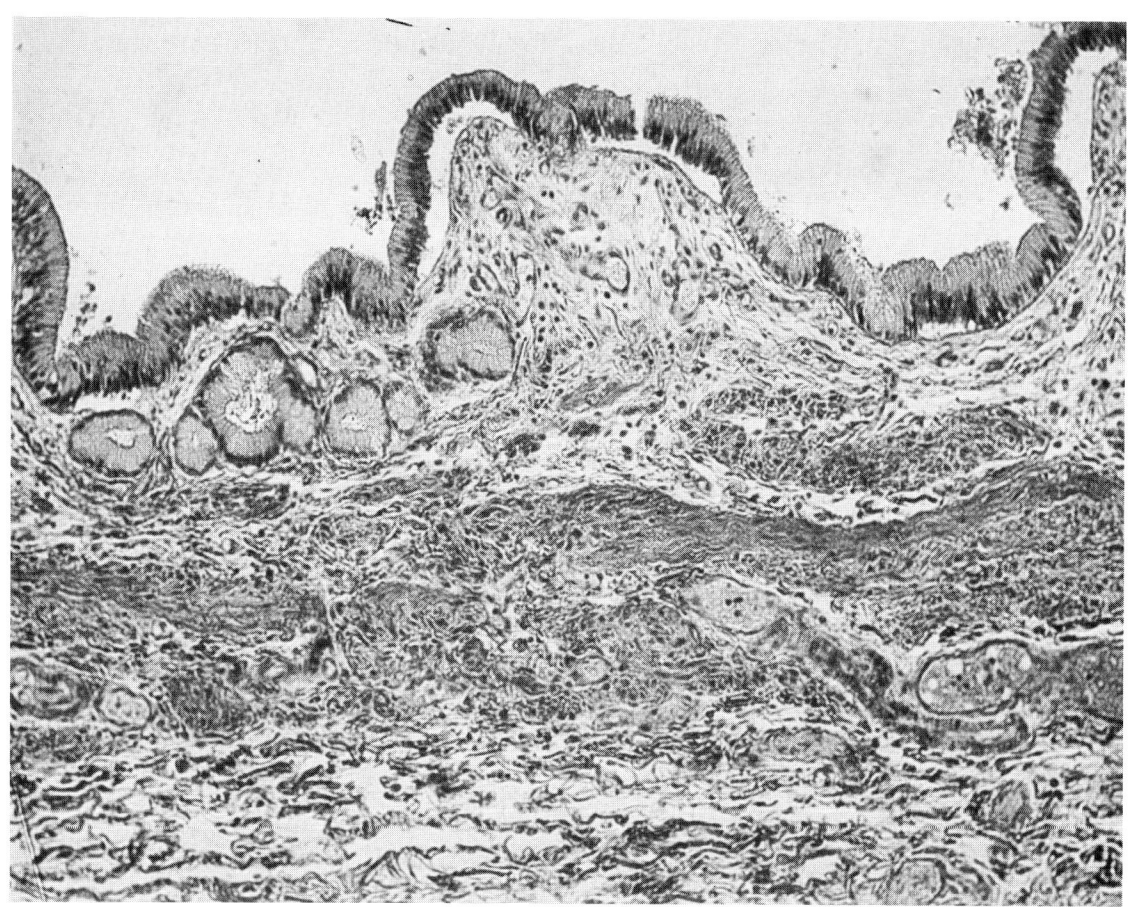

Figure 18–19

Figure 18–19. This is a section taken through the wall of the gallbladder near the neck.
  The mucosa consists of a surface layer of tall columnar epithelium and a lamina propria in which there are a few simple glands. A layer of smooth muscle is apparent in the middle of the photograph and, peripheral to that, connective tissue. Note the large and small folds into which the mucosa is thrown.
  This patient was a male infant, born at 33 weeks of gestation, who lived for three days. His body weight at autopsy was 2,860 grams.
  Hematoxylin and eosin stain. Mag. 142×.

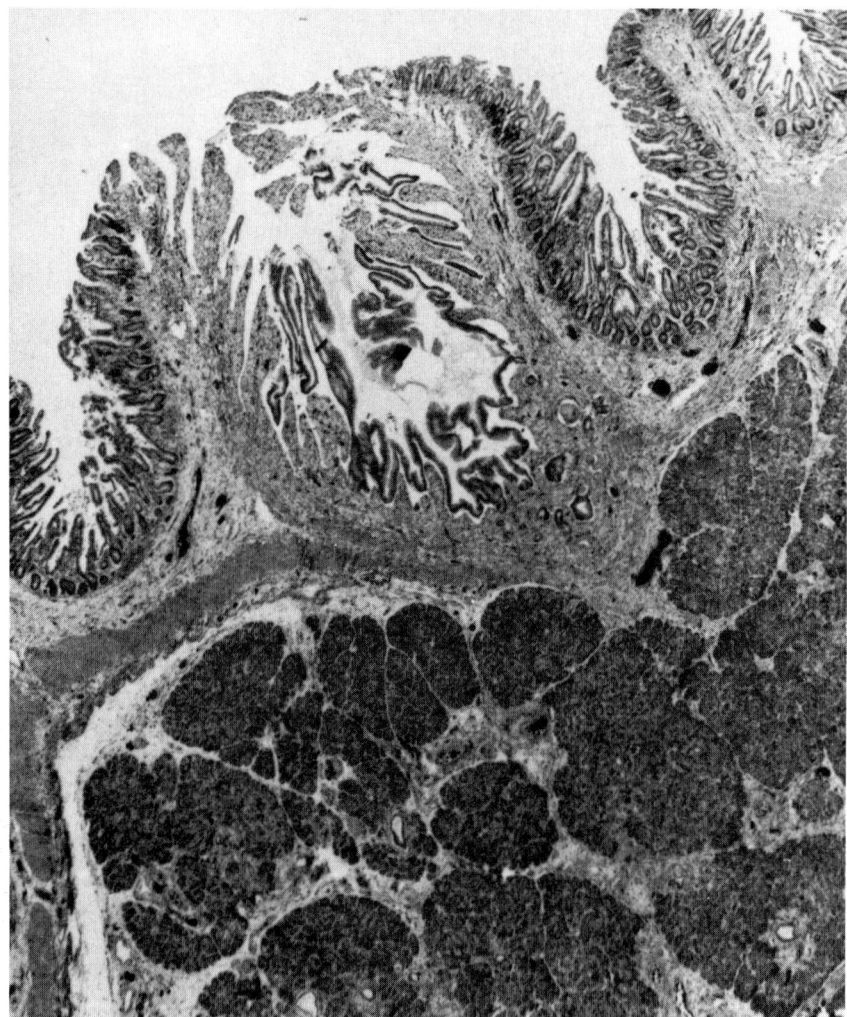

Figure 18–20

Figure 18–20. Depicted here is the ampulla of Vater, projecting somewhat into the lumen of the duodenum. The lining epithelium is mucus-producing and tall columnar.

This infant was a one day old black male, born at the 30th week of gestation. His body, at postmortem examination, weighed 1,500 grams.

Hematoxylin and eosin stain. Mag. 45×.

Chapter 19

PANCREAS

EMBRYOLOGY

The pancreas develops from two separate buds of endodermal cells, the dorsal and ventral pancreatic buds, which arise from the dorsal and ventral aspects, respectively, of the most caudal portion of the foregut. The larger dorsal bud appears first and grows rapidly into the dorsal mesentery. The ventral bud, which is much the smaller of the two, develops near the entry of the common bile duct into the duodenum.

As the duodenum grows and rotates to the right, it carries the ventral bud (together with the common bile duct) dorsally. The ventral bud lies eventually in the mesoduodenum, and it fuses with the dorsal bud to form a joint organ.

The dorsal pancreas forms all of the mature gland except most of the head and the uncinate process, which are derived from the ventral primordium.[1] Each pancreatic bud has an axial duct. The dorsal duct arises directly from the duodenal wall, but the base of the ventral duct shares a common stem with the common bile duct. As the pancreatic buds fuse, the ducts anastomose; the main pancreatic duct forms from the ducts of the ventral bud, and the distal part from those of the dorsal bud (this chief line of drainage is the duct of Wirsung). The proximal section of the duct of the dorsal bud may, in some instances, persist as an accessory pancreatic duct opening cranial to the main duct, the duct of Santorini. The two ducts often communicate with each other.

Secretory acini begin to appear in the third month as terminal and side buds from the primitive ducts. The islets of Langerhans also differentiate from ducts at about the same time.[2]

The connective tissue envelope and the septa of the pancreas are derived from surrounding splanchnic mesenchyme.

ANATOMY

The pancreas of the newborn infant is a relatively firm organ, light pink-tan and elongate, extending nearly transversely across the posterior abdominal wall, behind the stomach, from the duodenum to the spleen.

Its large rounded right extremity, securely embraced by a loop of the duodenum on its right, is the head; it blends imperceptibly with the main part of the gland, or body, on its left; the tapering left extremity of the gland is the tail. As previously mentioned, the tail is frequently tightly adherent to the hilus of the spleen; in fact, accessory nodules of splenic tissue are occasionally embedded in the tail of the pancreas and conversely, in some instances, the tail of the pancreas may be inextricably embedded in the hilus of the spleen.

HISTOLOGY

The lobules of which this branched gland is composed are still very clearly distinguishable from one another in histologic sections of the fetus at 20 weeks of gestation (Fig. 19–1). The connective tissue septa between lobules are prominent at this stage in the evolution of the gland. Furthermore, supportive reticular tissue within the lobule is also very much in evidence at this time (Fig. 19–6). It diminishes steadily in importance thereafter, until 40 weeks when it is quite obscure (Fig. 19–2).

The secretory cells of the exocrine part of the organ are pyramidal in shape and arranged in flask-shaped or tubular groups (Fig. 19–8).

The narrow, most distal segment of the duct system enters deep into the secretory lobule; it is into this ductule, lined by cuboidal cells, that the individual acini empty (Figs. 19–6 and 19–7).

As the ductules enter into small ducts coursing between lobules, their epithelial lining cells become slightly taller (Fig. 19–5b), and the duct is gradually invested in a thicker coat of concentric layers of collagenous tissue (Figs. 19–5a, 19–5c, and 19–4) until it reaches the neck of the pancreas, where the wall is exceedingly stout (Fig. 19–3). Glands of a mucoid character enter into the lumens of the larger ducts (Fig. 19–4), and fibers of smooth muscle and the autonomic nervous system are identifiable in the connective tissue sleeve of these larger ducts. The epithelial lining becomes increasingly taller as the duct system enlarges, coming nearer and nearer its "entry" into the duodenum (Figs. 19–3 and 19–4).

The islets of Langerhans are compact, spheroidal or ellipsoid clusters of cells randomly embedded in the exocrine part of the pancreas. Each islet is ultimately separated from surrounding acini by a delicate sheath of reticular tissue (Fig. 19–9). In the premature infant of 16 to 18 weeks, however, the islets, which are still in the process of formation, may be difficult to distinguish from surrounding small acini. Furthermore, in the premature infant and in infants during the perinatal period, islet cells may be scattered singly and in small groups about the exocrine elements. As such they are ordinarily difficult to distinguish with certainty in sections stained with hematoxylin and eosin.

Extramedullary hematopoiesis is commonly encountered in the fetal and neonatal pancreas (Fig. 19–10). The clusters of hematopoietic elements usually lie within interlobular septa.

Small and, at times, even large infiltrates of lymphocytes are commonly encountered within the fetal and neonatal pancreas. Participating lymphocytes are usually small and darkly stained; follicles are not ordinarily observed within such clusters. The lymphocytes are often rather insidiously intermingled with acini and ducts of the area (Fig. 19–11). Such focal infiltrates are probably part of the normal histology of the organ at this stage in its development, but are frequently a matter of some concern for the uninitiated.

References for Part Six

1. Moore, K. L.: The Developing Human. Clinically Oriented Embryology. Philadelphia, W. B. Saunders Co., 1973, pp. 146–148, 175–188.
2. Arey, L. B.: Developmental Anatomy. A Textbook and Laboratory Manual of Embryology. 7th ed., revised. Philadelphia, W. B. Saunders Co., 1974, pp. 257–262.
3. Warwick, R., and Williams, P. L.: Gray's Anatomy, 35th British ed. Philadelphia, W. B. Saunders Co., 1973, pp. 1237–1241, 1251–1252, 1270–1292, 1299–1302, 1306–1311.
4. Bloom, W., and Fawcett, D. W.: A Textbook of Histology. Philadelphia, W. B. Saunders Co., 1975, pp. 598–614, 639–675, 718–720.
5. Yunis, E. J., Dibbins, A. W., and Sherman, F. E.: Rectal suction biopsy in the diagnosis of Hirschsprung's disease in infants. Arch. Pathol. Lab. Med., *100*:329–333, (June) 1976.
6. Meier-Ruge, W., Lutterbeck, P. M., Herzog, B., Morger, R., Moser, R., and Schärli, A.: Acetylcholinesterase activity in suction biopsies of the rectum in the diagnosis of Hirschsprung's disease. J. Pediatr. Surg., 7:11–17, 1972.
7. Weinberg, A. G.: Hirschsprung's disease: A pathologist's view. Perspectives in Pediatric Pathology, 2:207–239, 1975.
8. Willis, R. A.: The Borderland of Embryology and Pathology. London, Butterworth and Co., Ltd., 1958, pp. 41, 86.

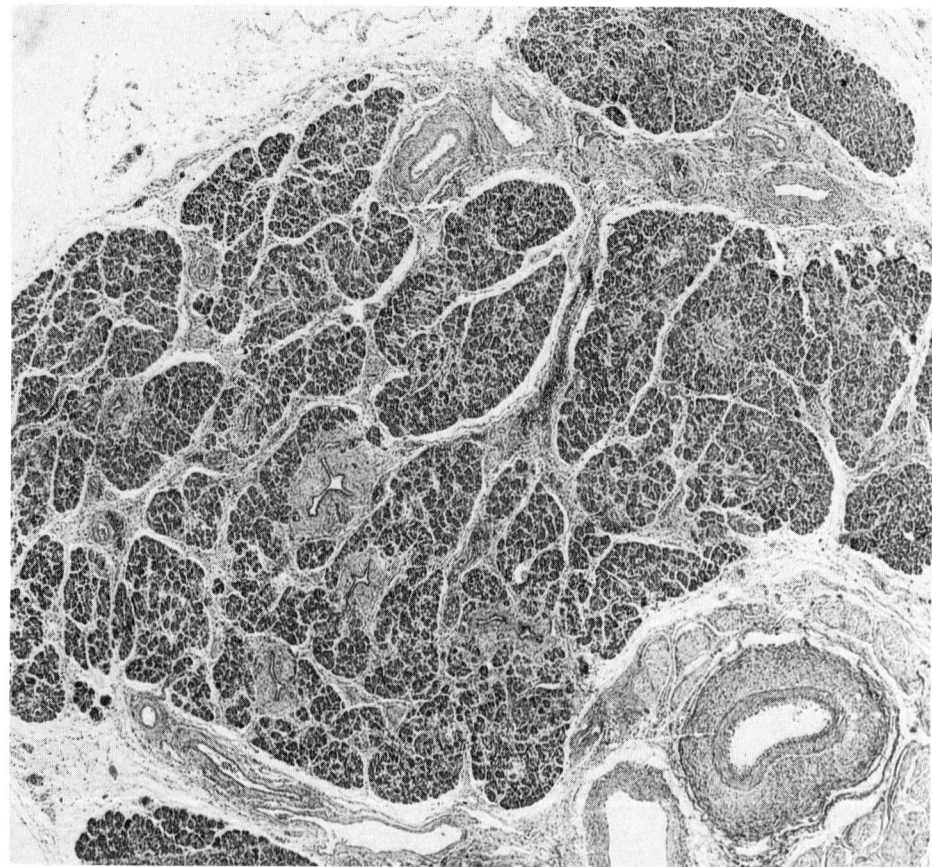

Figure 19–1

Figure 19–1. In Figs. 19–1 and 19–2, a marked contrast is immediately apparent between the histologic pattern of the pancreas—as it is seen at low magnification—in the immature infant and that in the mature infant.

This is a section of the pancreas of an eight day old black female whose body weight at autopsy was 540 grams. (Estimated gestational age: 22 weeks.)

Hematoxylin and eosin stain. Mag. 45×.

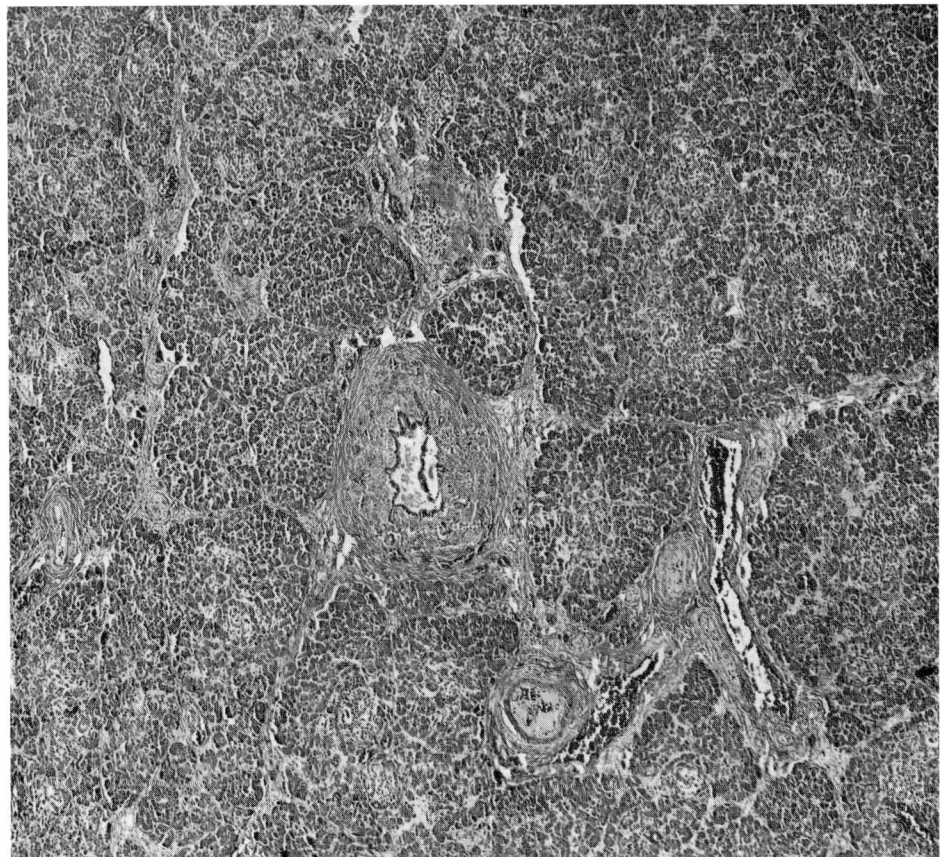

Figure 19-2

Figure 19-2. By contrast with Fig. 19-1, this is a section of the pancreas of an infant, a one month old black male, born at term. The patient's body weight at autopsy was 4,005 grams.

Note the larger size of individual lobules and the relative diminution in interlobular connective tissue (and perhaps intralobular, as well.)

The transition from the obvious, almost glaring, lobular pattern of the fetus at about five months of gestation (Fig. 19-1) to the almost adult appearance of the neonate at term (Fig. 19-2) is gradual but steadily progressive.

Hematoxylin and eosin stain. Mag. 45×.

Figure 19–3b

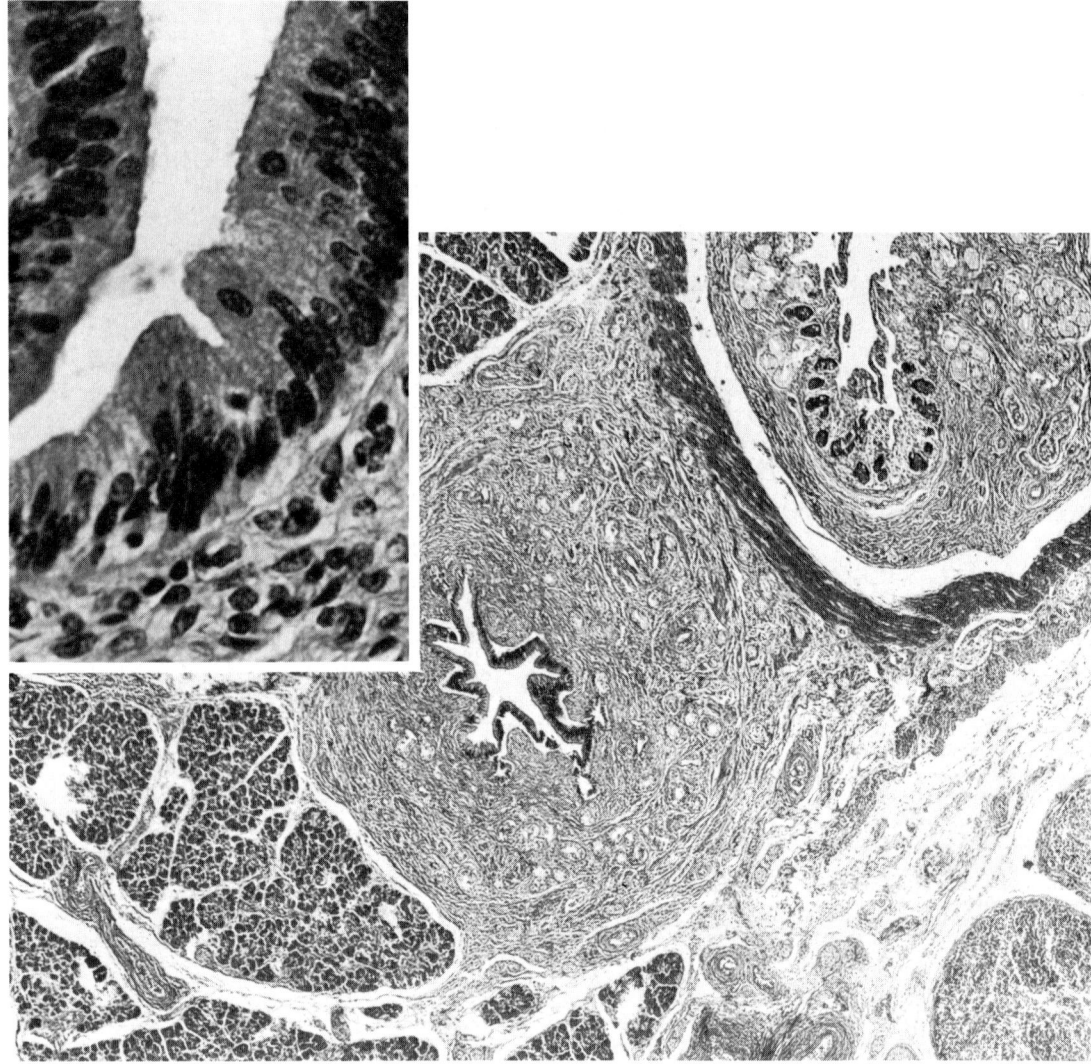

Figure 19–3a

Figure 19–3. In Fig. 19–3a is depicted, at very low magnification, the histologic appearance of the main duct of the pancreas, in cross section, immediately adjacent to its entrance into the duodenum (upper right corner). Note the broad band of connective tissue embracing it.

In Fig. 19–3b the tall columnar epithelial lining of the main and major ducts is clearly illustrated.

Fig. 19–3a is from a stillborn white female infant, born at term and weighing 3,115 grams.
Fig. 19–3b is from an 855 gram female infant who lived for 4½ hours.
Hematoxylin and eosin stain. Fig. 19–3a, mag. 45×; Fig. 19–3b, mag. 492×.

PANCREAS 275

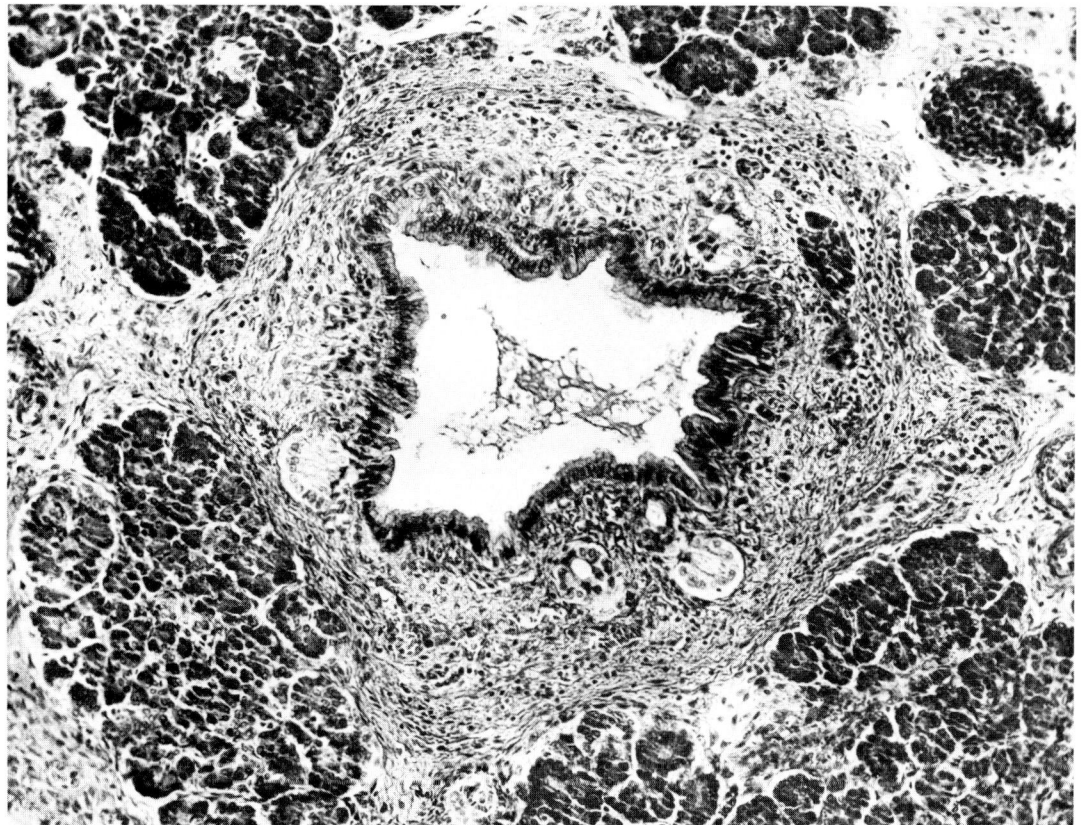

Figure 19–4

Figure 19–4. This photomicrograph illustrates the microscopic appearance of one of the larger ducts within the pancreas. The lining epithelium, although not quite so tall as that in Fig. 19–3b, is still of the columnar type. The duct lies in interlobular connective tissue that contains some smooth muscle and autonomic nerve fibers. Mucous glands are related to the lining epithelium.

The section is from a 13 day old black male who weighed 1,770 grams at autopsy. (Estimated gestational age: 8 months.)

Hematoxylin and eosin stain. Mag. 153×.

Figure 19-5. The more peripheral segments of the pancreatic duct system are lined by low columnar (as seen in some portions of Fig. 19–5c) to frankly cuboidal epithelial cells (as in Figs. 19–5a and 19–5b). The cuff of interlobular connective tissue still visible in c is somewhat less prominent in a. In b the details of the lining cells are more distinct.
Hematoxylin and eosin stain.

Fig.	Wt.	Race	Sex	Gestation	Age	Mag.
19–5a	1,060 gm.	?	F	7 mo. (est.)	5½ hr.	382×
19–5b	835 gm.	B	F	7 mo. (est.)	10 hr. 40 min.	660×
19–5c	1,270 gm.	?	F	?	21 hr.	255×

See illustrations on the opposite page

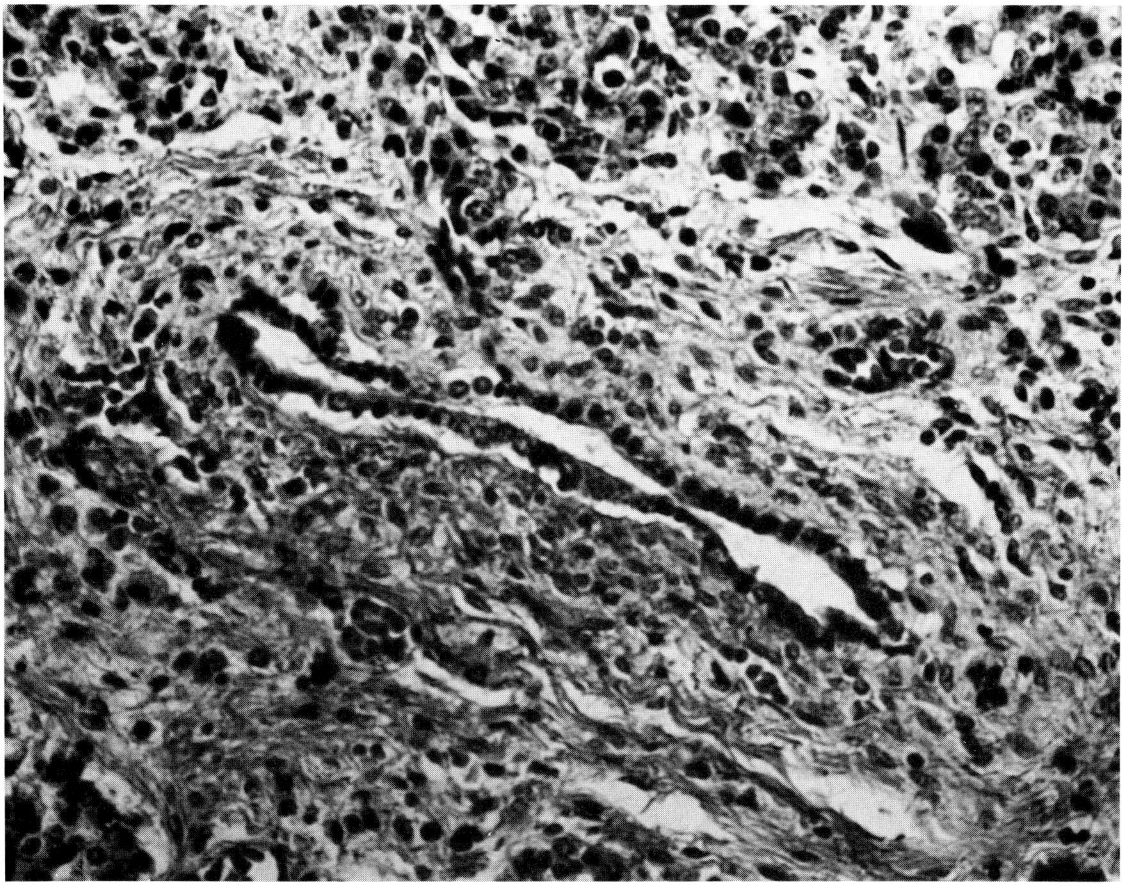

Figure 19-5a

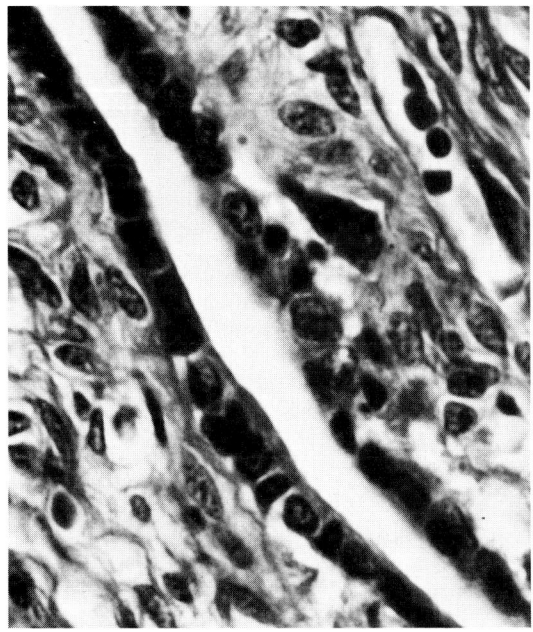

Figure 19-5b

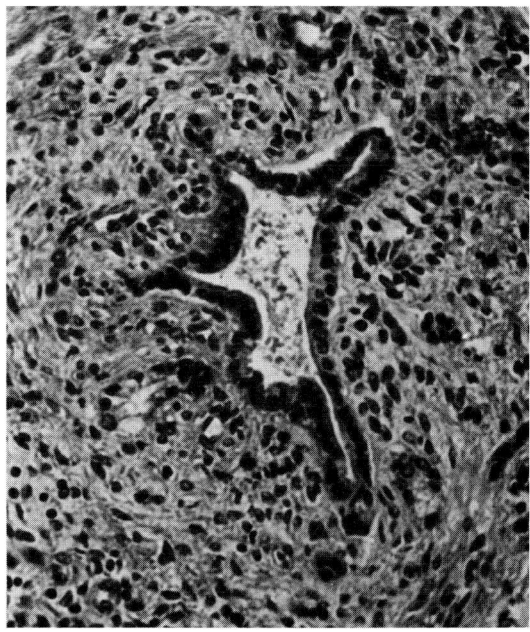

Figure 19-5c

See legend on the opposite page

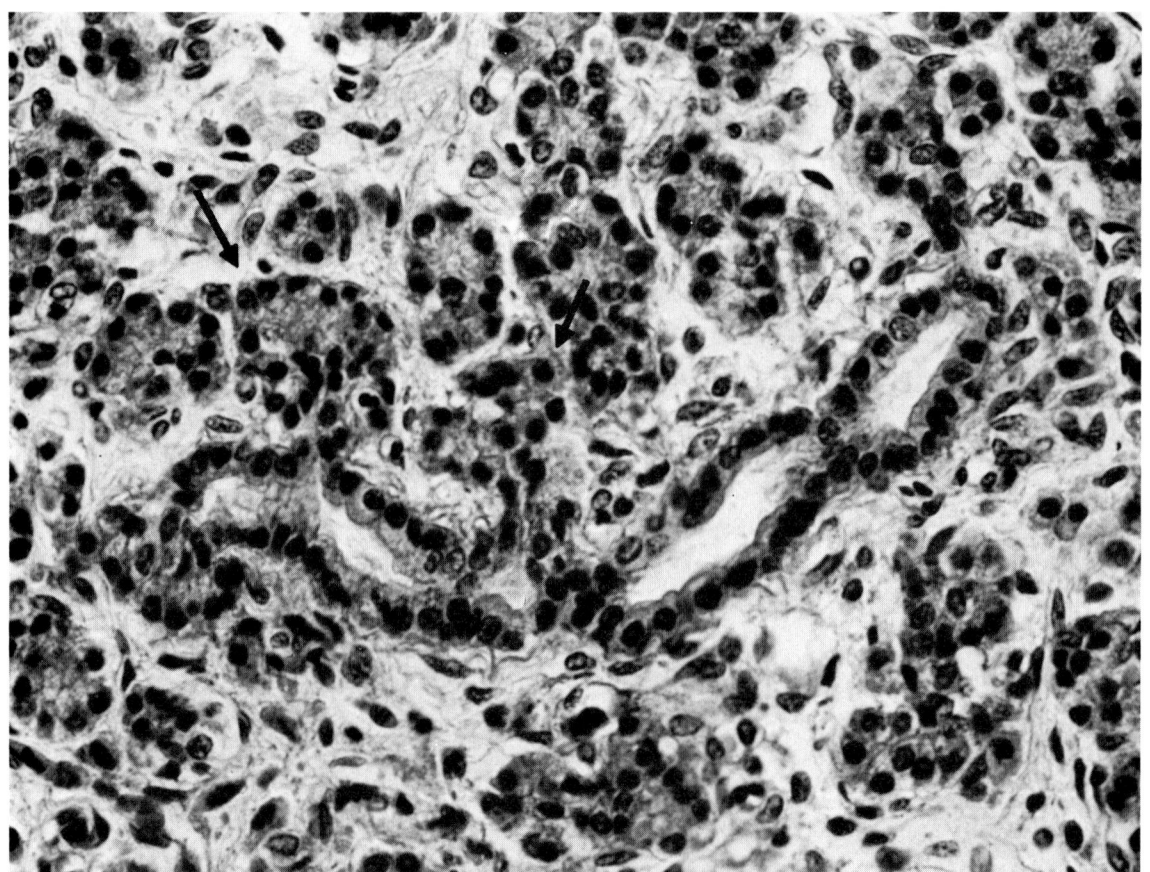

Figure 19–6

Figure 19–6. The exocrine part of the pancreas is, in fact, a lobulated branched acinar gland. In this illustration a narrow intralobular portion of a duct, that segment most peripherally located, is seen deep in the lobule. It is lined by a single layer of low cuboidal cells. As indicated by the arrows, two acini can be seen, on the left, as they open into this duct.

This section is from an 850 gram black female infant (estimated gestational age: 22 weeks) who lived for 10 minutes.

Hematoxylin and eosin stain. Mag. 450×.

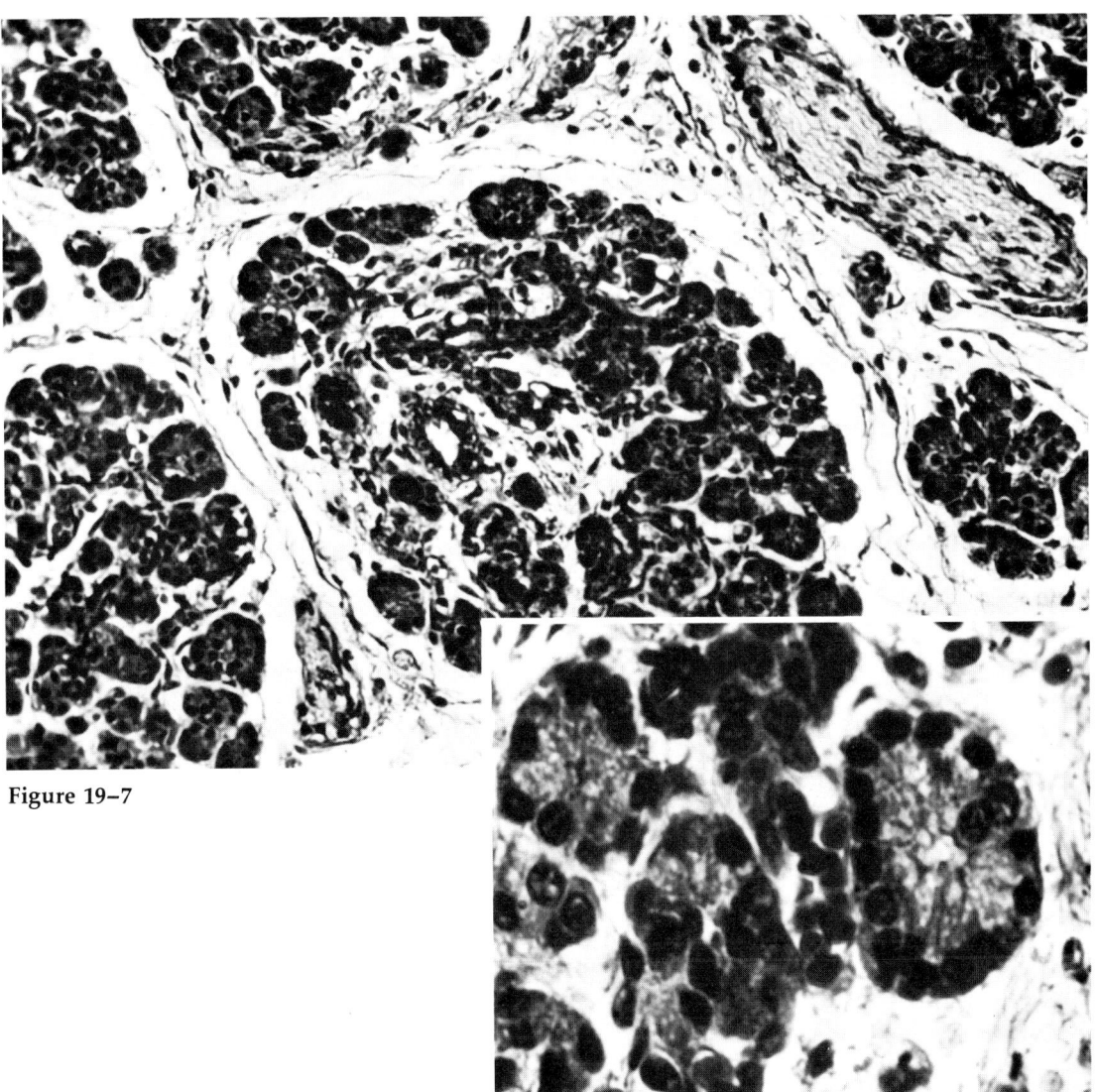

Figure 19–7

Figure 19–8

Figure 19–7. This photomicrograph shows a single pancreatic lobule from a prematurely born infant weighing 760 grams at thanatopsy. The baby, a black male, lived for 12 hours and 7 minutes. Characteristic of the immaturity of the organ is the abundant reticular supportive tissue within and around the lobule. Cross and longitudinal sections of the ductule appear in the midst of the acini.
Hematoxylin and eosin stain. Mag. 255×.

Figure 19–8. A single acinus, on the right, is seen in detail. This section is from a black male infant, weighing 1,055 grams at autopsy, who survived for 4 hours and 56 minutes. (Estimated gestational age: 29 weeks.)
Hematoxylin and eosin stain. Mag. 660×.

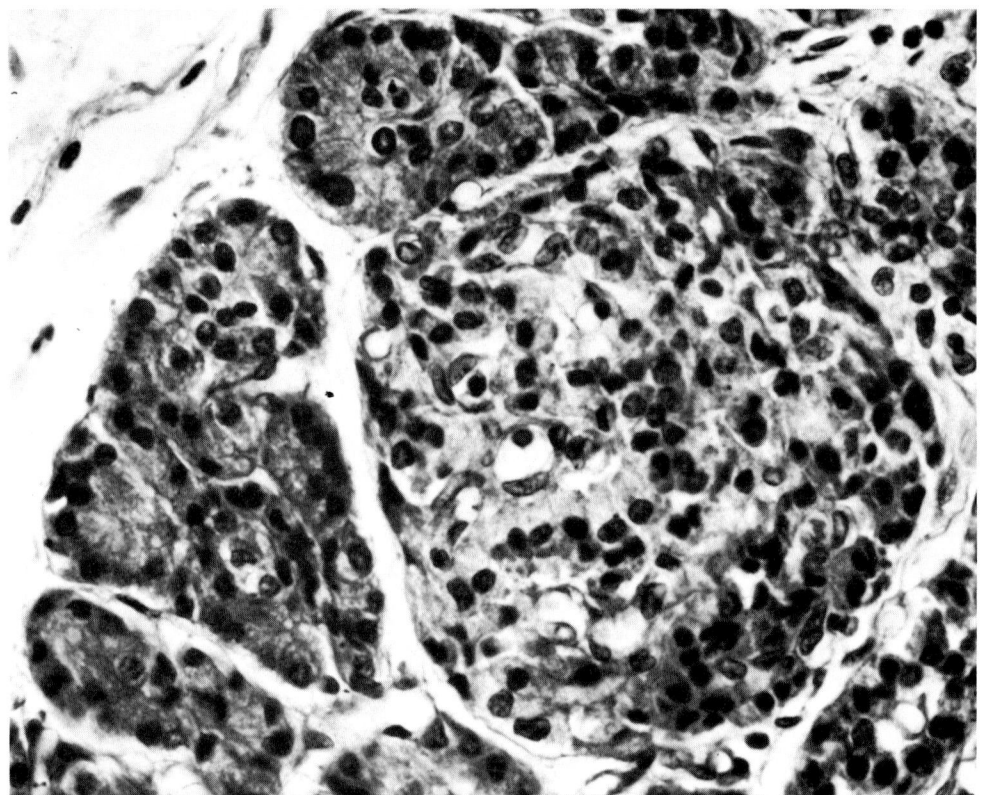

Figure 19-9

Figure 19-9. A pancreatic islet of a one day old white male born at term. Body weight at postmortem examination was 3,180 grams.

The islet is composed of a rounded clump of pale-staining cells, fairly sharply delineated, separated from the surrounding acinar cells by a delicate envelope of reticular tissue. Particularly in smaller prematurely born infants, the distinction between islet cells and acinar cells may be quite obscure.

In this routine histologic preparation, all of the islet cells appear to be similar. Special stains are necessary to distinguish one cell type from another.

Hematoxylin and eosin stain. Mag. 450×.

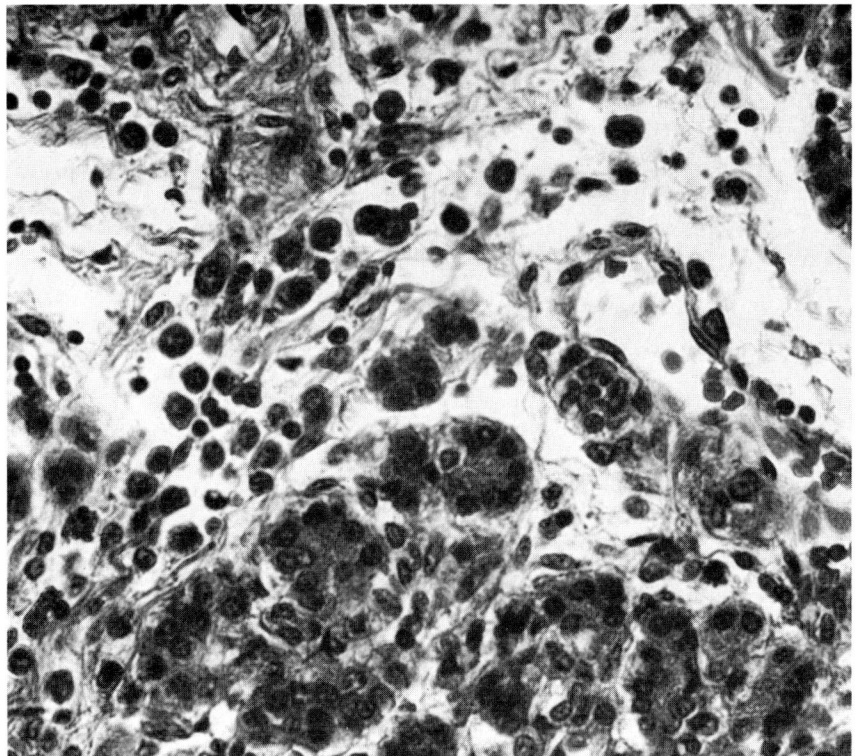

Figure 19–10

Figure 19–10. One of the characteristic features of the histologic appearance of the immature pancreas is the presence of clusters of hematopoietic cells within bands of interlobular connective tissue.

An arc of such cells is seen here swinging upward from left to right in the direction of the right upper corner of the photograph. (An adjacent lobule occupies the lower middle portion of the picture.) Blast forms can be identified within the group.

Section from a 615 gram white male infant born at 22 to 24 weeks of gestation, who lived for 5 hours and 42 minutes.

Hematoxylin and eosin stain. Mag. 440×.

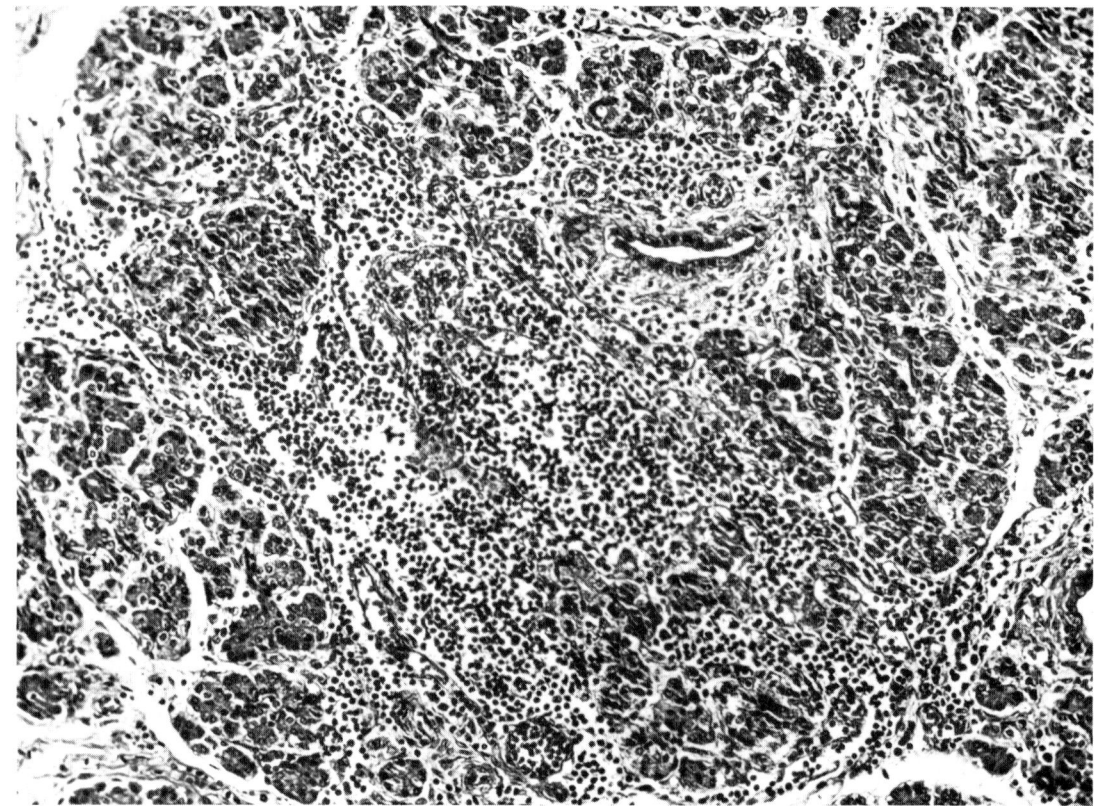

Figure 19–11

Figure 19–11. Another characteristic of the infant pancreas, particularly of the prematurely born, is the obvious presence of diffusely scattered, ill-defined areas of heavy lymphocytic infiltration such as is seen in this illustration. They tend to diminish in number and size with increasing maturation of the infant.

This is from a 1,720 gram black male infant who lived for 9 hours and 20 minutes. (Estimated gestational age: 32 weeks.)

Hematoxylin and eosin stain. Mag. 164×.

PANCREAS 283

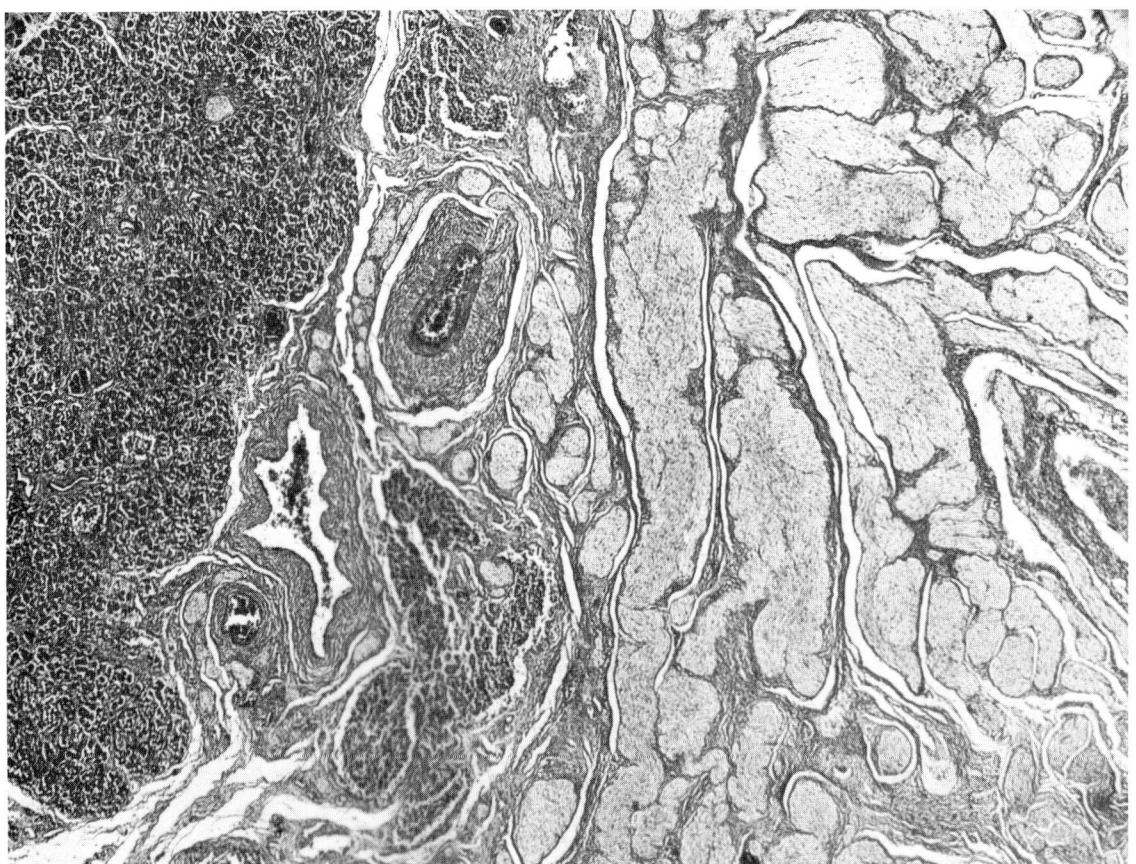
Figure 19-12

Figure 19-12. Sections of the infant pancreas often include, although not by intention, a portion of an adjacent autonomic nerve plexus, as illustrated here. The neural elements are at times surprisingly prominent.

This section was taken from a 500 gram black male infant (estimated gestational age: 20 weeks) who survived for 1 day and 2 hours.

Hematoxylin and eosin stain. Mag. 38×.

Part 7

RESPIRATORY SYSTEM

Chapter 20

THE UPPER RESPIRATORY TRACT

EMBRYOLOGY

Epiglottis

The earliest manifestation of the respiratory tree appears in the embryo of 3 mm. in about the third week of development. It is a groove oriented longitudinally in the floor of the gut just caudal to the pharyngeal pouches. The ventral pouch-like projection is directed caudally and becomes dilated somewhat at its distal end shortly after formation. It is referred to as the laryngotracheal ridge. There is a lateral furrow on each side, along the junction of the ridge and the esophagus dorsal to it, which becomes progressively deeper and splits off the laryngotracheal tube.

The proximal end of the laryngeal portion moves cranially until it lies between the fourth branchial pouches.

At the 4 mm. stage the laryngeal region opens proximally off the pharynx, and leads distally into a tubular trachea.

At the 5 mm. stage, a rounded prominence appears mid-ventrally from the bases of the third and fourth branchial arches, the first evidence of the evolving epiglottis. It soon changes its shape and becomes a transverse flap, concave on its laryngeal aspect. In the middle of fetal life a cartilage plate differentiates within it as its supporting framework.

Larynx

The larynx develops differently in its upper and lower halves. The part above the vocal cords evolves from the pharyngeal floor near the laryngeal orifice as a sort of vestibule, while the distal part takes shape from the cranial end of the trachea.

At the 5 mm. stage there is a mere slit, opening from the pharynx into the trachea, known as the primitive glottis. It is soon bounded on each side by a mound known as the arytenoid swelling, derived from the fourth and fifth arches. These two swellings grow and project upward like tongues. As they meet the primitive epiglottis, they arch against its caudal aspect. By the seventh week that union results in a change in the shape of the original vertical slit to a T-shaped laryngeal orifice. The entrance remains blind for some time because fusion of the epithelium obliterates the lumen; this union is dissolved by 10 weeks and the entrance becomes oval with a pair of lateral recesses, the laryngeal ventricles. Each ventricle is bounded cranially and caudally by a shelf; the caudal pair are the vocal folds.

Early in the seventh week, dense mesenchyme from the fourth and fifth arches condenses to form the first evidences of the laryngeal cartilages.

Trachea

The tracheal tube, which is bifurcated distally from the 4 mm. stage onward, elongates rapidly for a time; the point of bifurcation ultimately "descends" for a distance of eight body segments.

The epithelial lining is columnar in its early phases and changes finally to a ciliated pseudostratified type. Smooth muscle fibers and C-shaped incomplete cartilaginous rings differentiate from surrounding condensed mesenchyme at the end of the seventh week. The glands develop as ingrowths from the epithelium after the fourth month.[1]

Bronchi

Soon after its appearance, the "lung bud" bifurcates distally into two primary bronchi, the tubular system then assuming an inverted Y-shape. The right main bronchus extends more directly caudad than the left, a difference that is maintained throughout life. In the embryo of 7 mm. the right primary bronchus gives rise to two side buds while the left forms but one; the end of each main tube then constitutes the so-called stem bronchus, each destined to supply a future lobe.

ANATOMY

Epiglottis

The epiglottis of the newborn, especially the prematurely born infant, is not the thin leaf-like structure of the adult but is inclined to be relatively shorter and stouter with more rounded or blunt edges. It projects obliquely upward behind the tongue and the body of the hyoid bone, and in front of the entrance to the larynx. The free extremity is directed upward. The sides are attached to the arytenoid cartilages by the aryepiglottic folds of mucous membrane.[2]

Larynx

The cavity of the larynx extends from the laryngeal inlet, by which it communicates with the pharynx, to the level of the lower border of the cricoid cartilage, where it is continuous with the lumen of the trachea.[2]

The vestibule of the larynx is the part between the laryngeal inlet and the level of the vestibular folds; it is wide above and narrow below. Its anterior wall is much longer than its posterior wall and consists of the posterior surface of the epiglottis. Its lateral walls are formed by the medial surfaces of the aryepiglottic folds; its posterior wall consists of the mucous membrane connecting the arytenoid cartilages above the level of the vestibular folds or false vocal cords.

The middle part of the laryngeal cavity is the smallest. Its upper boundary is the false vocal cords, and its lower boundary is the true cords. On each side it opens through a slit between the vestibular and vocal cords (or false and true vocal cords) into a recess known as the laryngeal sinus or laryngeal ventricle. On each side there is an upward extension of the ventricle directed from the anterior part of the sinus and passing between the false vocal cords and the thyroid cartilage; it is conical and curved backward slightly (Fig. 20-6 and 20-7).

The lower part of the laryngeal cavity extends from the level of the true vocal cords down to the lower border of the cricoid cartilage. Its upper part is elliptical; the lower part becomes circular as it continues into the trachea.[2]

Trachea

The trachea is a cartilaginous and membranous tube extending from the lower border of the larynx down to its division into the two principal bronchi. It lies mainly in the midline, although its point of bifurcation is usually a little to the right of that.

It is not quite cylindrical, being flattened in the posterior or membranous part. In the first year of life its internal diameter does not exceed 3 mm.

Its wall is supported by a series of 16 to 20 incomplete cartilaginous rings, the membranous segment of each being located posteriorly. The cartilages are oriented horizontally one above the other, and are separated by narrow intervals.[2]

Bronchi

In the extrapulmonary bronchi the cartilages are shorter and narrower than those of the trachea, but have the same shape and arrangement.

HISTOLOGY

Epiglottis

The anterior surface of the epiglottis (Figs. 20-2 to 20-5), the upper half of its posterior surface, the aryepiglottic folds, and the vocal cords are all covered with stratified squamous epithelium. Ciliated epithelium clothes the lower part of the posterior surface of the epiglottis (Fig. 20-3) and continues downward to line the remainder of the larynx, trachea, and bronchi (Figs. 20-10, 20-14, and 20-17).

There are mucous glands in the mucosa of the epiglottis, particularly near the base, both anteriorly and posteriorly; they tend to lie in pits on the faces of the cartilage (Figs. 20–3 and 20–4). In addition, the cartilage is penetrated in places by vessels and nerves (Figs. 20–1, 20–2, and 20–5). The cartilage plate itself is of hyaline character and its surface is, as mentioned, pitted.

Larynx

The walls of the larynx are supported by hyaline and elastic cartilage associated with connective tissue, and striated muscles. Of the cartilages comprising the framework, the thyroid (Fig. 20–6) and cricoid (Fig. 20–11), both unpaired, and the lower parts of the arytenoids are hyaline cartilage as is that of the epiglottis. The remainder of the arytenoids, corniculate and cuneiform, are elastic.

Except for the vocal cords, which are covered with stratified squamous epithelium, the larynx is lined by epithelium of the respiratory type (Figs. 20–7 through 20–10). The glands of the larynx are of tubuloacinous, mixed mucous variety (Figs. 20–8 to 20–10). The alveoli secrete mucus and may have serous crescents.

The true vocal cords contain vocal ligaments. Each consists of a band of elastic tissue bordered laterally by the thyroarytenoid muscle and medially by a thin mucous membrane consisting of stratified squamous epithelium.

Trachea

The lining of the trachea is composed of pseudostratified ciliated columnar epithelium that rests on an unusually thick basement lamina. The lamina propria contains an abundance of elastic fibers and many glands like those of the larynx (Figs. 20–12 to 20–16). Most of these glands are external to a layer of elastic fibers beneath the lining epithelium. They open by short ducts onto the free surface of the lining epithelium. In the posterior portion of the trachea, the glands extend through the muscular layer. The lamina propria occasionally contains accumulations of lymphoid tissue.

The supporting framework of the trachea is a series of C-shaped hyaline cartilages, 11 to 16 in number, which encircle it on its ventral and lateral aspects. They are separated from one another by spaces bridged by fibroelastic tissue. Some of the cartilages branch obliquely around the trachea. The cartilages are surrounded externally by dense connective tissue, which may contain many elastic and reticular fibers.

The posterior wall of the trachea, adjacent to the esophagus, is devoid of cartilage. In that place is a thick layer of smooth muscle bundles. In the main, they run transversely. They are inserted into the elastic fiber bundles surrounding the cartilages and are joined to the mucosa by a layer of loose connective tissue.

Bronchi

The histologic structure of the major bronchi is practically identical with that of the trachea (Fig. 20–17). As long as they are extrapulmonary they possess cartilage rings, which are no longer present in the intrapulmonary bronchi. As a consequence of those rings, their shape is not cylindrical but flattened on one side.

The lining is pseudostratified ciliated columnar epithelium. The lamina propria consists of a small amount of reticular and collagenous connective tissue and many elastic fibers. It contains some lymphoid cells and is set off from the epithelium by a prominent basal lamina (Fig. 20–17). The glands are mucous and mucoserous.

The outermost layer of the bronchial wall consists of dense connective tissue containing many elastic fibers, and surrounds the cartilage rings.[3]

References

1. Arey, L. B. Developmental Anatomy, rev. 7th ed. Philadelphia, W. B. Saunders Co., 1974, pp. 263–266.
2. Warwick, R., and Williams, P. L.: Gray's Anatomy, 35th British ed. Philadelphia, W. B. Saunders Co., 1973, pp. 1175–1184.
3. Bloom, W., and Fawcett, D. W.: A Textbook of Histology. Philadelphia, W. B. Saunders Co., 1975, pp. 746–748.

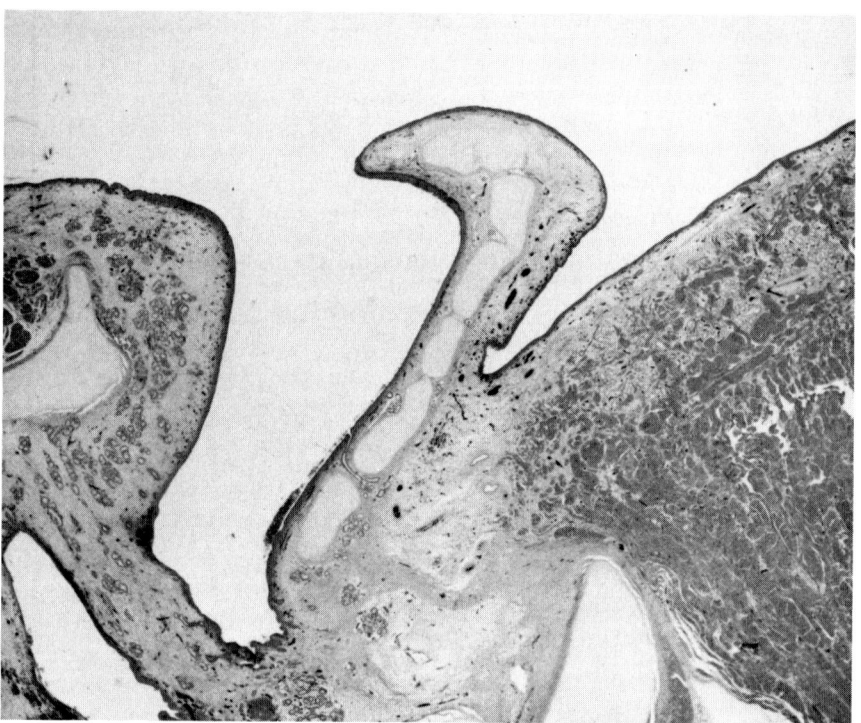

Figure 20–1

Figure 20–1. This is a survey view of a sagittal section taken to one side of the midline of the tongue (to the right side of the photograph), the epiglottis, the inlet to the larynx, and, on the lower left, a laryngeal ventricle. The characteristic woven pattern of the skeletal muscle of the tongue is clearly visible on the lower half of the right side. Glands of the larynx are apparent on the left.

This infant, an 860 gram white male, was 3 days of age at death. (Gestational age: 32 weeks.) Hematoxylin and eosin stain. Mag. 13×.

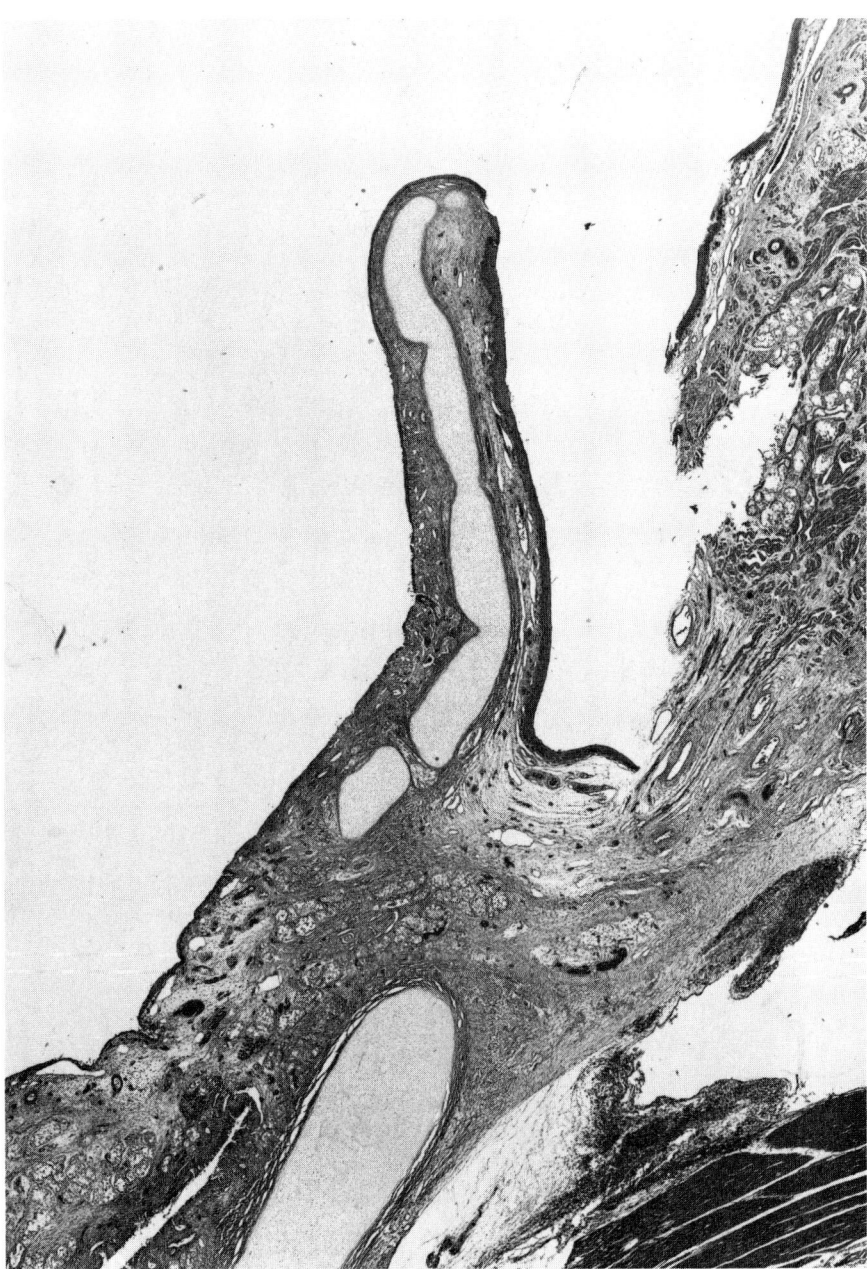

Figure 20–2

Figure 20–2. This is a sagittal section taken near the midline, including the base of the tongue (upper right), the epiglottis, and the inlet to the larynx. This photograph shows clearly the relationship of the cartilage of the epiglottis to the thyroid cartilage (lower left).

The infant is a newborn, not otherwise identifiable.

Hematoxylin and eosin stain. Mag. 18×.

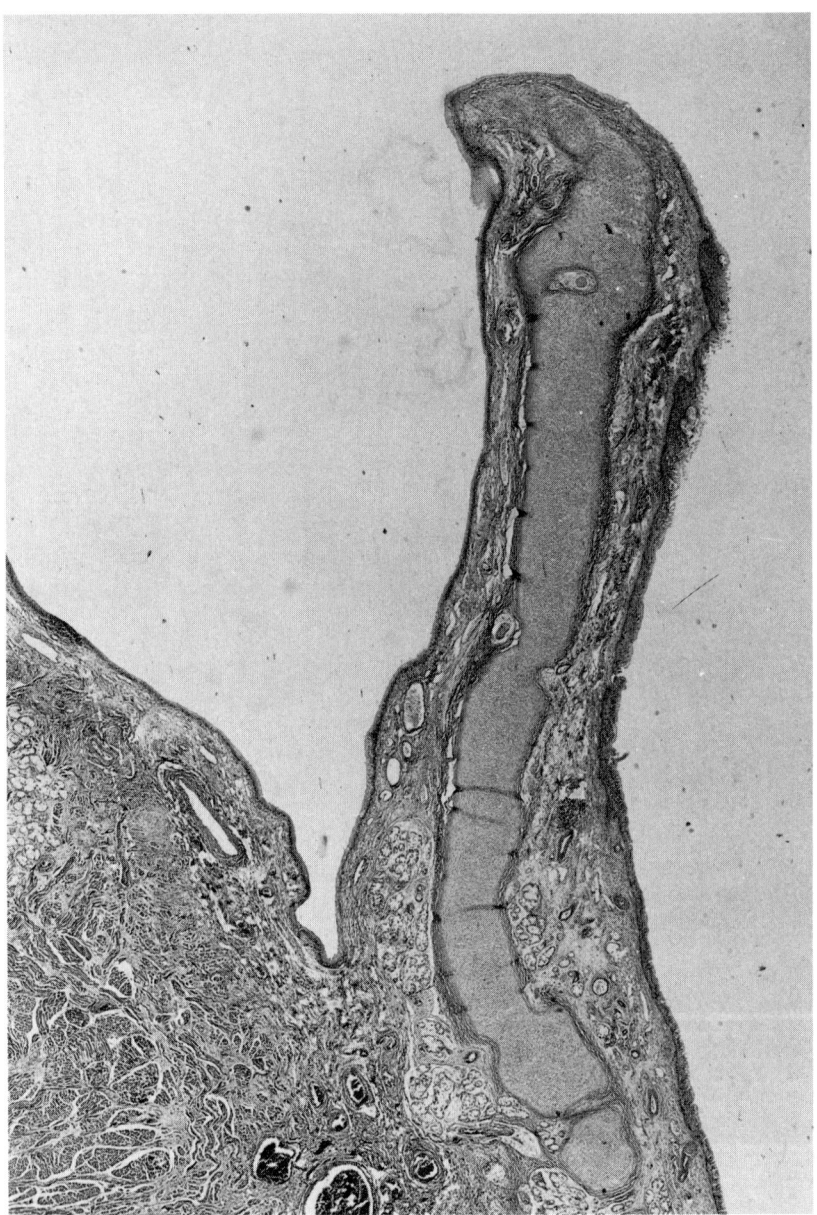

Figure 20-3

Figure 20-3. This is a longitudinal section through the epiglottis in the sagittal plane. The base of the tongue appears in the lower left corner. Glands are clearly visible anterior and posterior to the cartilage, near the inferior end of the cartilage plate of the epiglottis.

The covering epithelium is stratified squamous over the anterior aspect of the epiglottis and approximately the upper half of the posterior aspect; the inferior portion is clothed in epithelium of the respiratory type.

This infant was a one hour old white male whose body weight at autopsy was 2,420 grams. The gestational age was 38 to 40 weeks by history.

Hematoxylin and eosin stain. Mag. 45×.

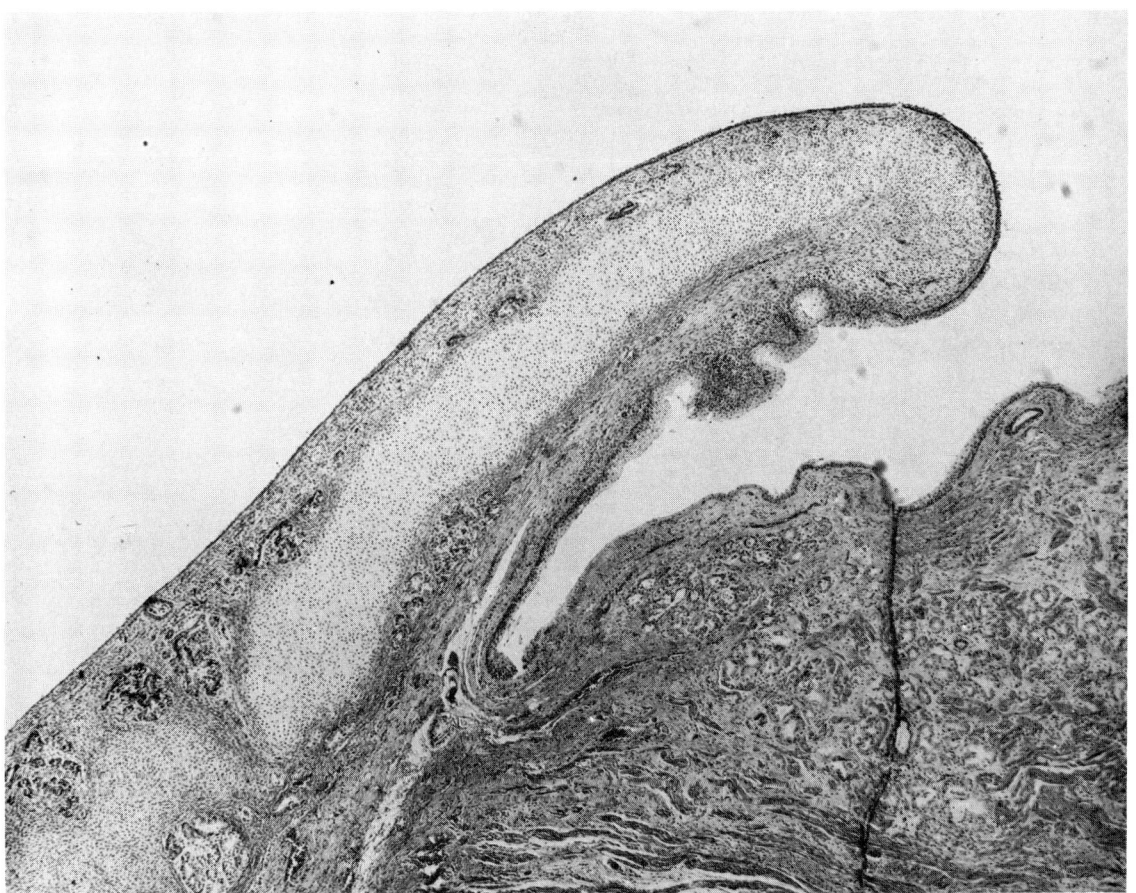

Figure 20–4

Figure 20–4. Another sagittal section of the epiglottis and base of the tongue. Stratified squamous epithelium over the anterior aspect of the epiglottis is clearly visible here. It tends to be pale staining.

The body weight of this six hour old black male was 735 grams. The gestational age was 24 weeks.

Hematoxylin and eosin stain. Mag. 45×.

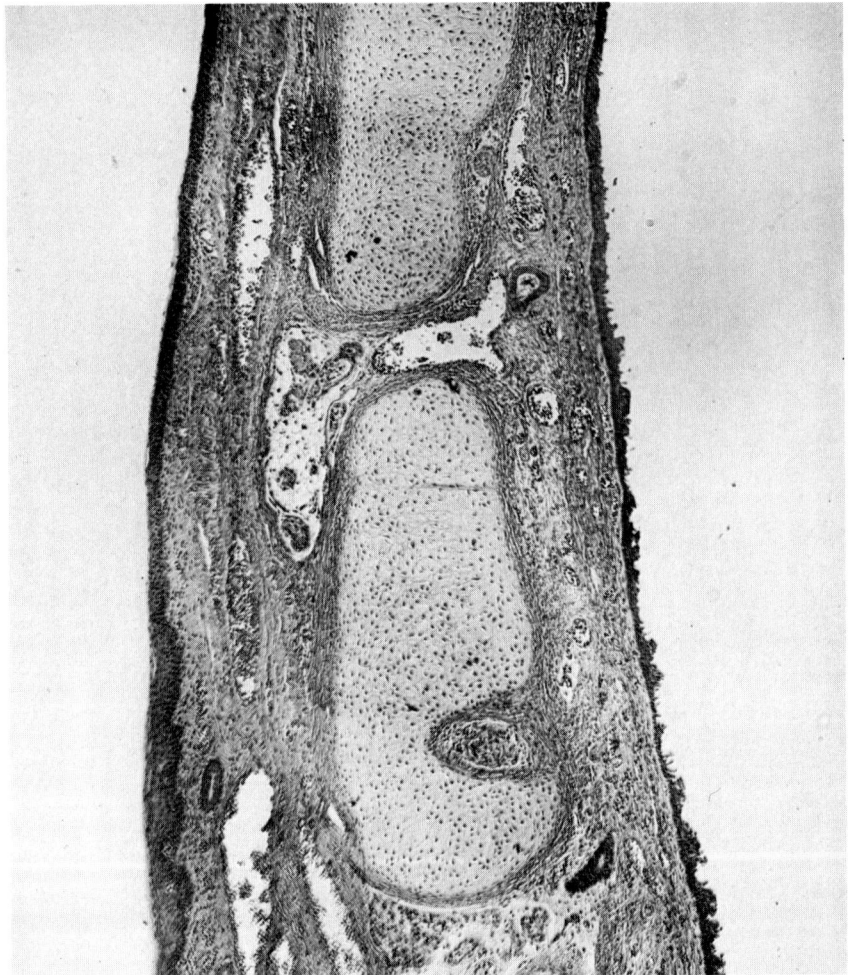

Figure 20–5

Figure 20–5. This photomicrograph depicts the epiglottis at high magnification. On the left is the anterior (or superior) aspect of the epiglottis, covered by stratified squamous epithelium. On the right, or posterior, is ciliated columnar epithelium. Elastic fibrocartilage forming the skeleton of the epiglottis is seen centrally.

This black male infant was born at term. His body weight at autopsy was 4,225 grams. Hematoxylin and eosin stain. Mag. 50×.

THE UPPER RESPIRATORY TRACT 297

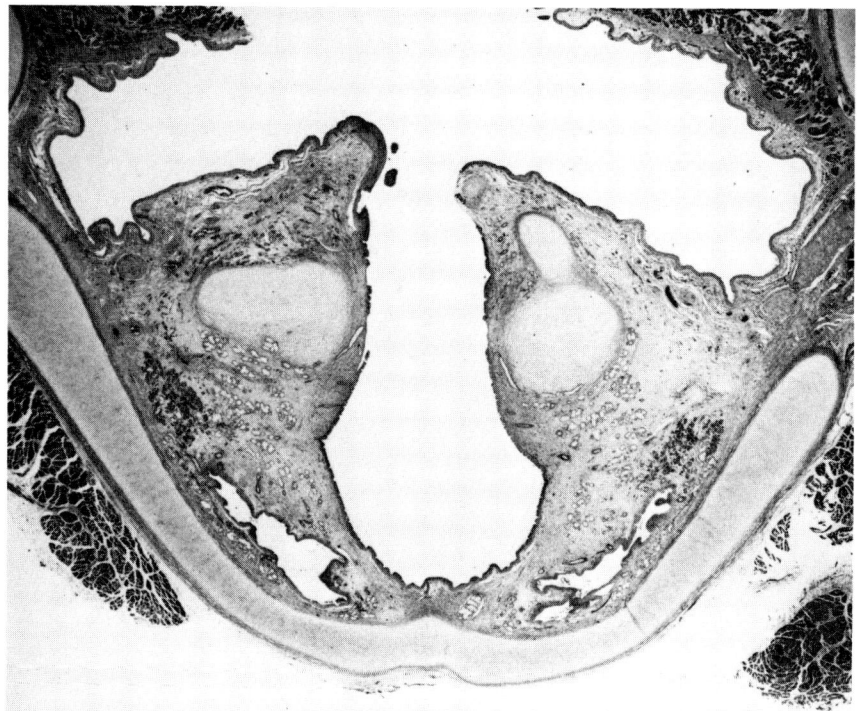

Figure 20–6

Figure 20–6. A horizontal section through the larynx and posterior pharynx. The U-shaped arc of cartilage inferiorly is thyroid cartilage. Portions of the extensions of the two laryngeal ventricles appear on the sides of the midline inferiorly.

This section was taken from a stillborn black female of 26 weeks gestation whose body weight at autopsy was 680 grams.

Hematoxylin and eosin stain. Mag. 12×.

298 THE UPPER RESPIRATORY TRACT

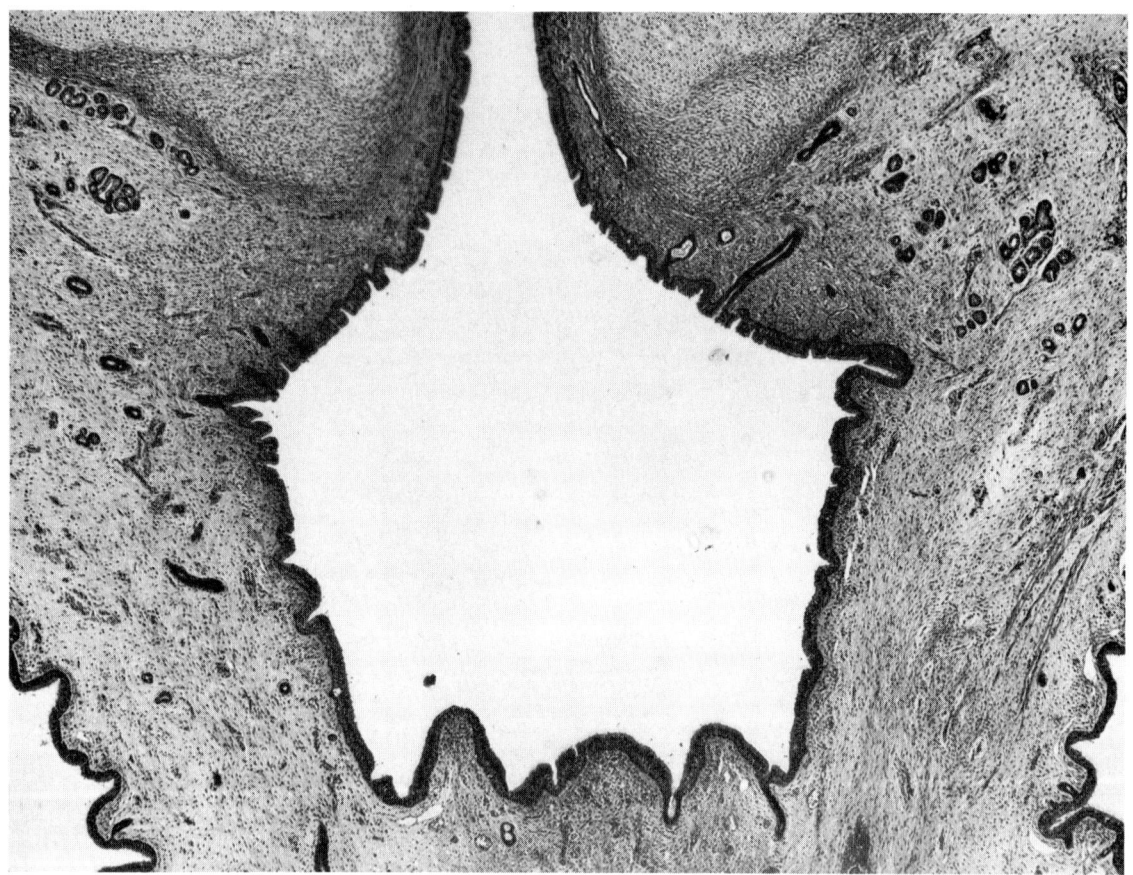

Figure 20-7

Figure 20-7. At higher magnification, this is another horizontal section of the larynx; portions of the extensions of the two laryngeal ventricles appear in the lower corners of the photograph. The lining of the larynx here is composed of ciliated columnar epithelium.

The infant from whom this section was taken weighed 370 grams and was stillborn. Hematoxylin and eosin stain. Mag. 45×.

THE UPPER RESPIRATORY TRACT 299

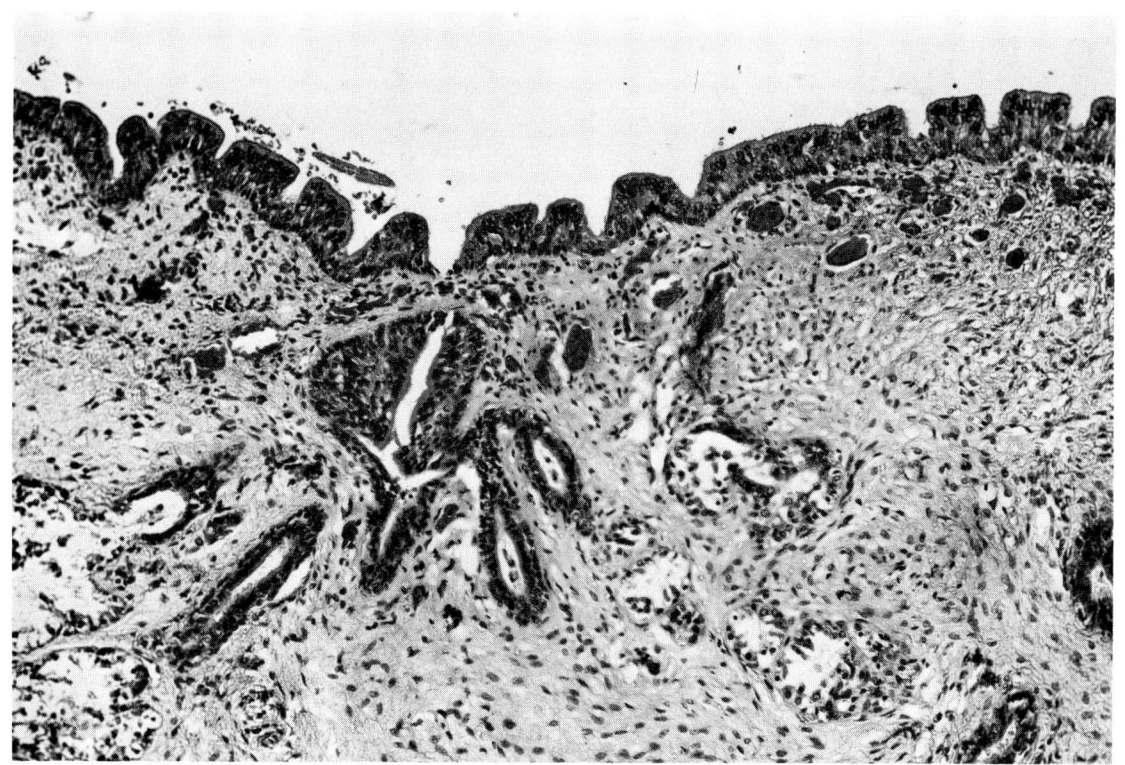

Figure 20-8

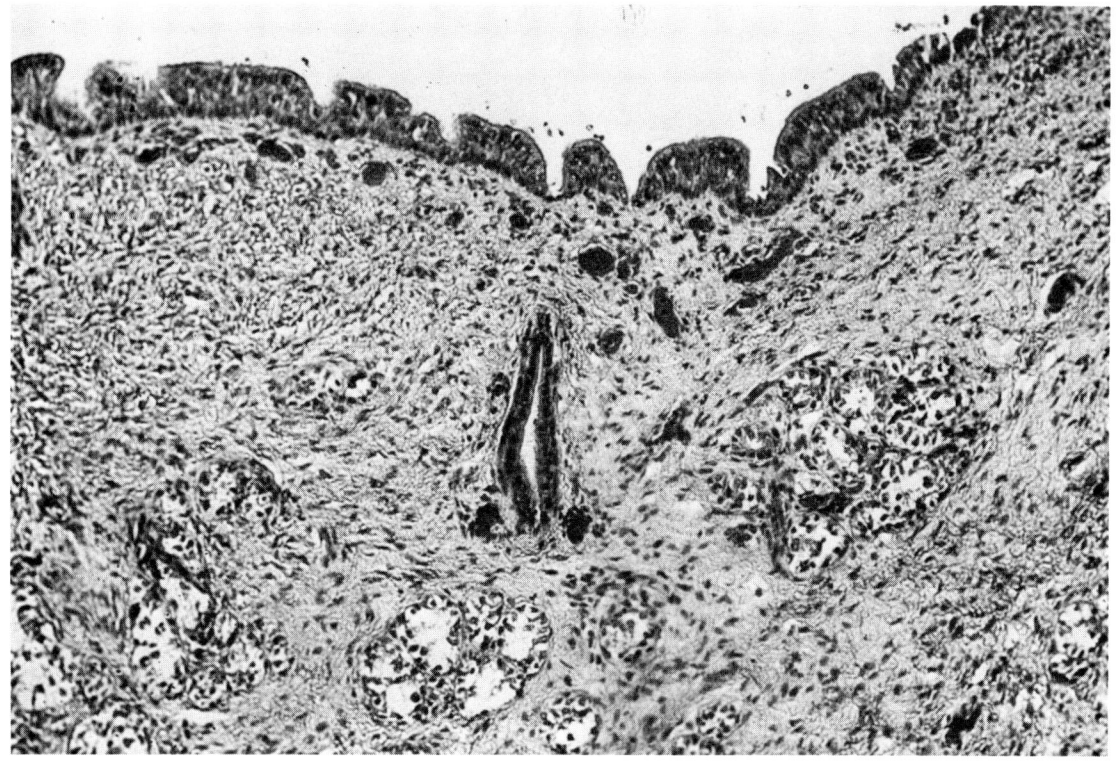

Figure 20-9

300 THE UPPER RESPIRATORY TRACT

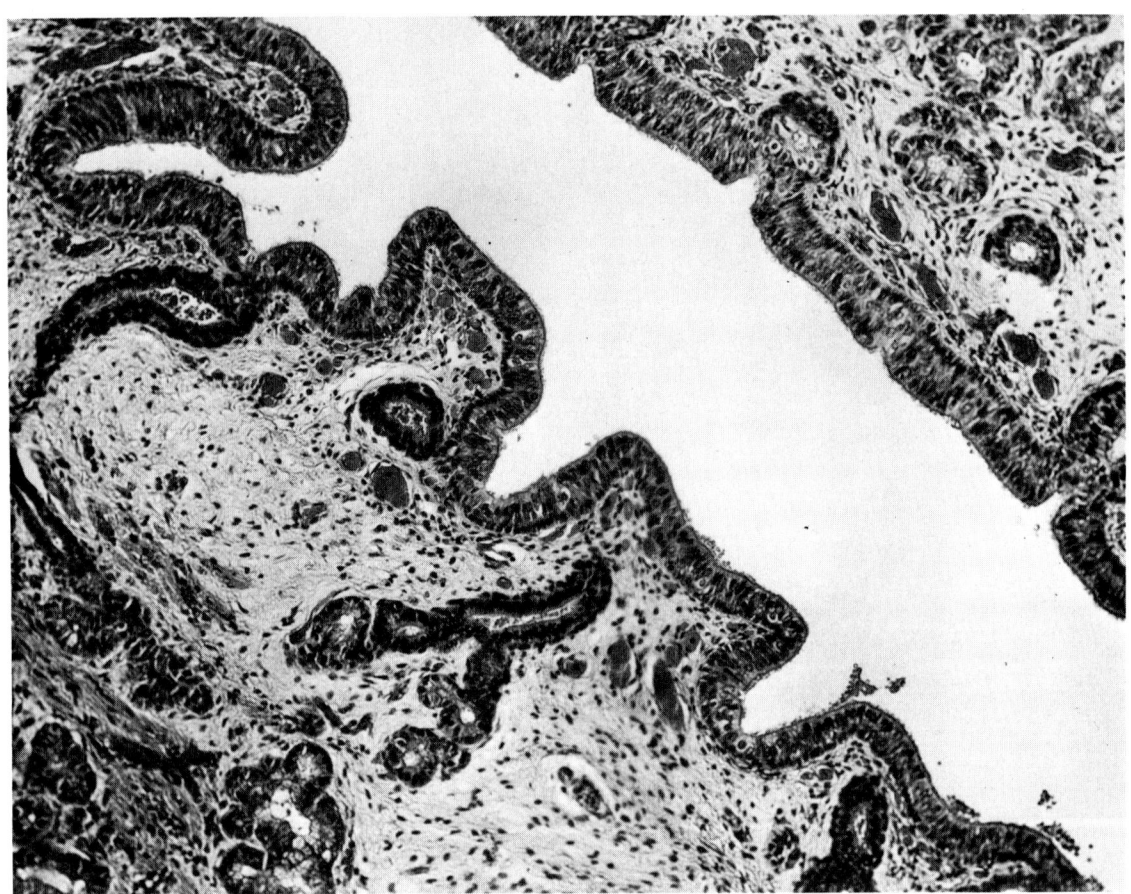

Figure 20–10

Figures 20–8, 20–9, and 20–10. Figs. 20–8 and 20–9 illustrate the lining of the major portion of the lumen of the larynx. The epithelium is ciliated columnar. The glands are tubuloacinous, mixed mucous variety. Ducts of those glands are visible in both of the photographs.

Fig. 20–10 shows the lining of the laryngeal ventricle and the relationship of glands and ducts to its lining.

Figs. 20–8 and 20–9 are from an 860 gram infant, a male, who survived for 10 hours. Fig. 20–10 is from a 1,280 gram infant who lived for 43 hours.

Hematoxylin and eosin stain. Mag. 142×.

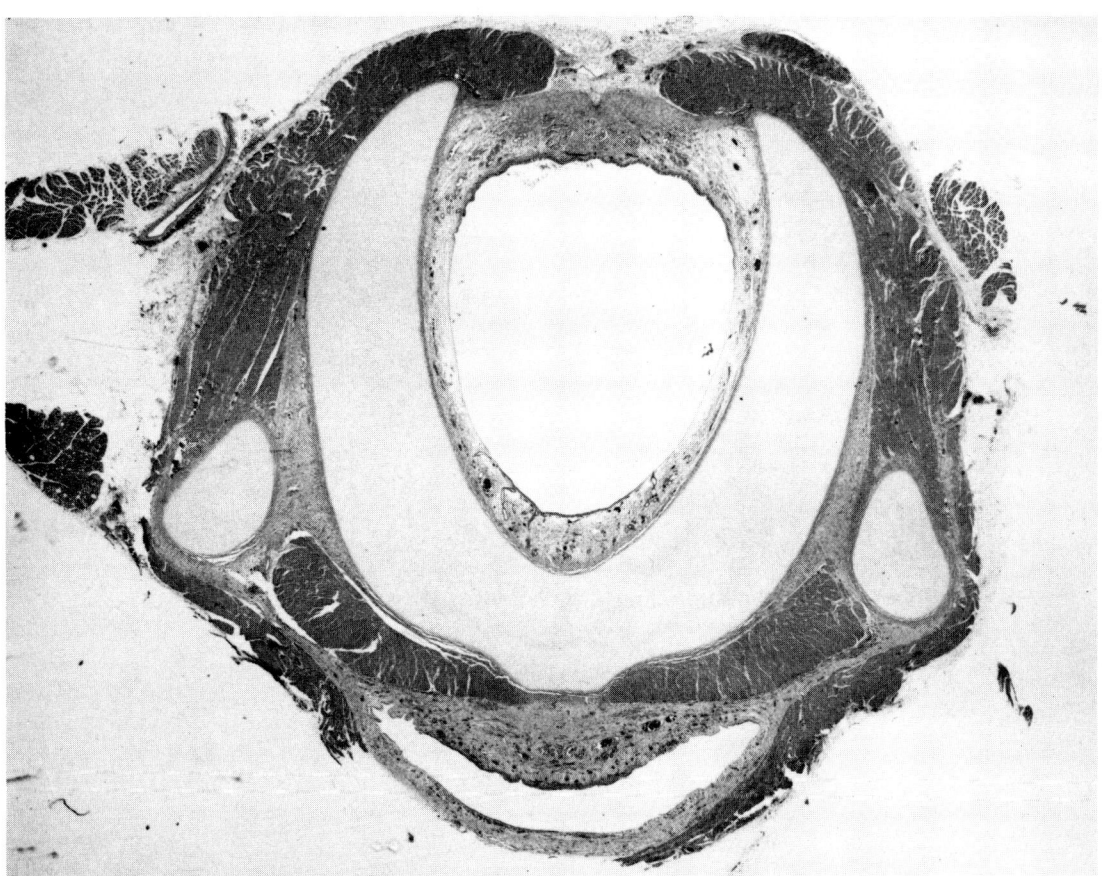

Figure 20–11

Figure 20–11. This is a horizontal section of the airway. The C-shaped cartilage is the cricoid. On each side of that, inferiorly, are the inferior horns of the thyroid cartilage. At the bottom edge, the C-shaped opening represents the pharynx. The major lumen centrally is that of the upper airway.

This infant was a 1500 gram black male born in the 30th week of gestation. He survived for one day.

Hematoxylin and eosin stain. Mag. 11.1×.

302 THE UPPER RESPIRATORY TRACT

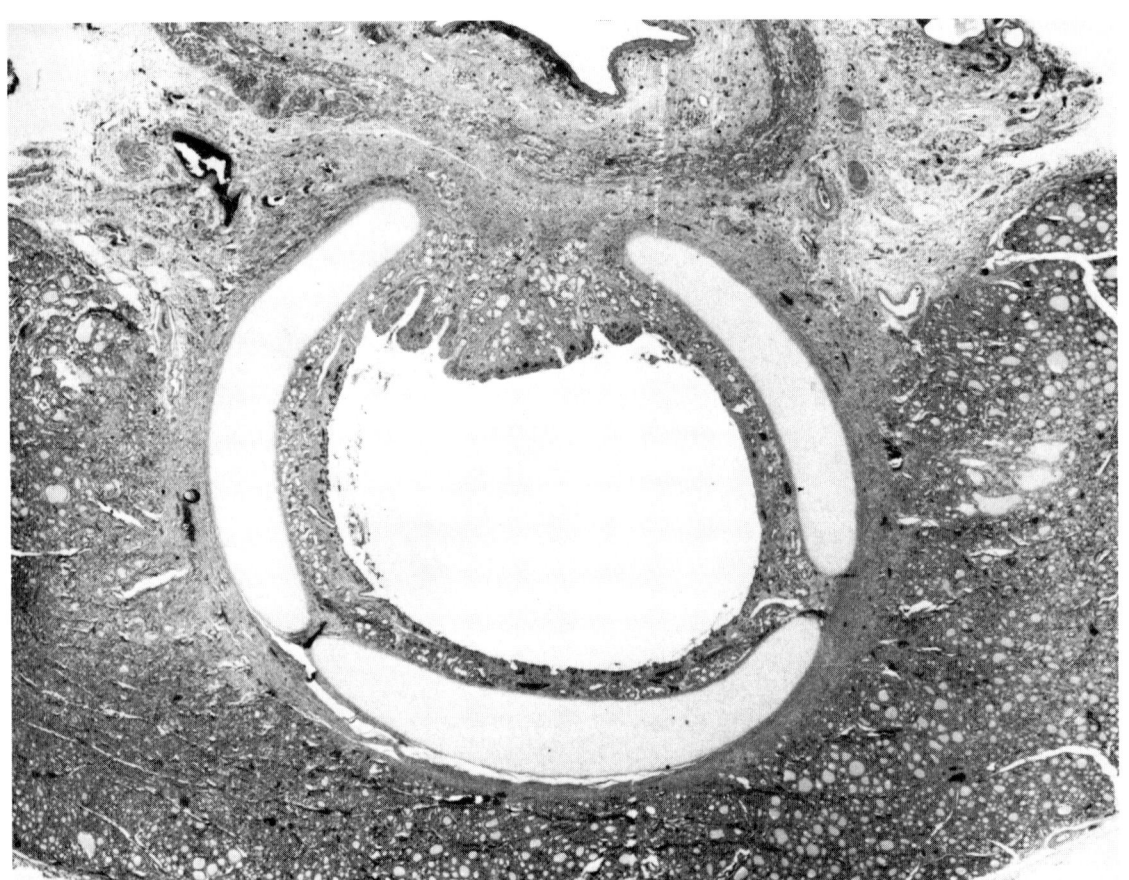

Figure 20–12

Figure 20-12. This is a cross section of the trachea of a prematurely born infant, taken at the level of the isthmus of the thyroid. A portion of a cross section of the esophagus appears posteriorly, and the two lateral lobes of the thyroid are seen at the sides.

This infant was born in the 30th week of gestation and weighed 1,500 grams at autopsy. Hematoxylin and eosin stain. Mag. 55×.

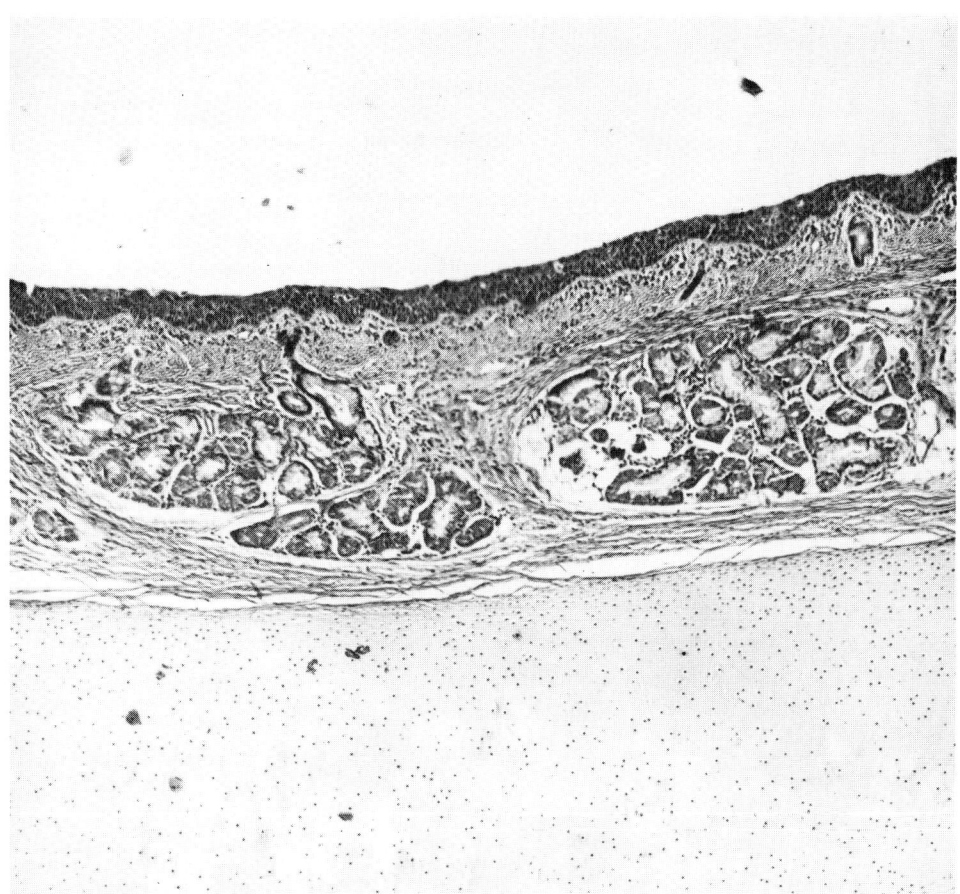

Figure 20-13

Figure 20-13. This is a cross section of the mucosal lining of the trachea. The epithelium is ciliated pseudostratified columnar, resting on an unusually thick basal lamina. The lamina propria contains many small glands similar to those in the larynx. The glands open by means of short ducts onto the free surface of the epithelium. In the lower third of the photograph is seen the supporting framework of the trachea, the C-shaped incomplete ring of hyaline cartilage.

The infant from whom this section was taken was not a neonate but was 9 months of age at death and weighed 8,275 grams.

Hematoxylin and eosin stain. Mag. 55×.

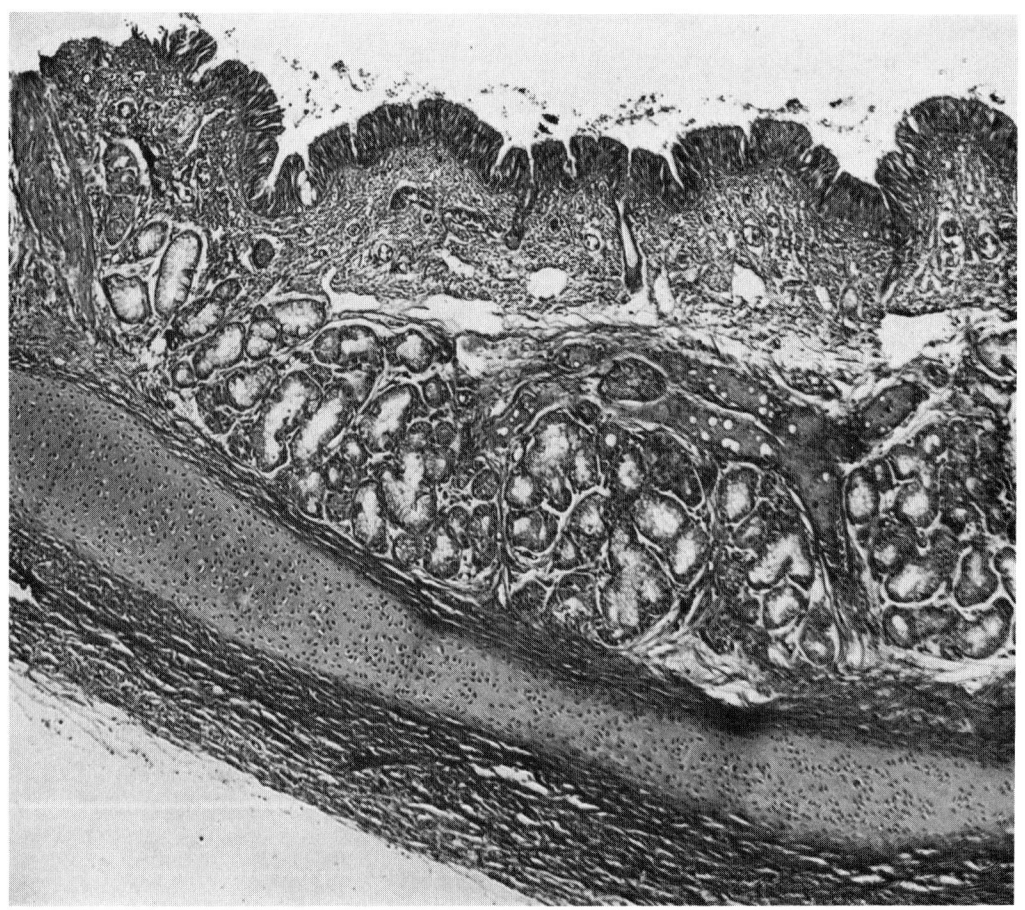

Figure 20-14

Figure 20-14. Depicted here is the entire thickness of the wall of the trachea of a newborn. Even the cilia of the tall pseudostratified columnar epithelium are visible, particularly just to the left of the center of the photograph.

Hematoxylin and eosin stain. Mag. 55×.

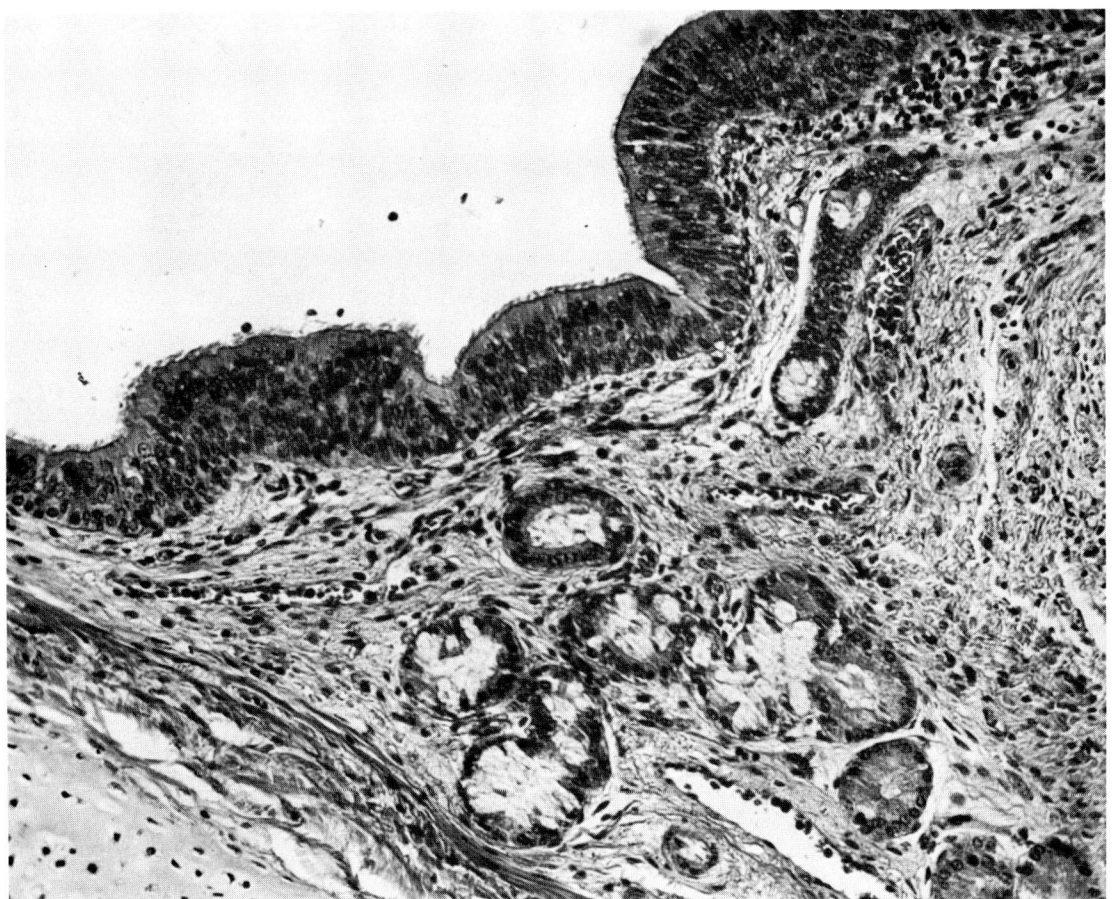

Figure 20-15

Figure 20-15. The mucosa of the trachea is illustrated here at considerably higher magnification. The mixed mucous glands and their ducts and the ciliated pseudostratified tall columnar epithelium are easily visible.

This infant lived for seven days. He was a black male who weighed 1,100 grams at the time of post-mortem examination.

Hematoxylin and eosin stain. Mag. 197×.

306 THE UPPER RESPIRATORY TRACT

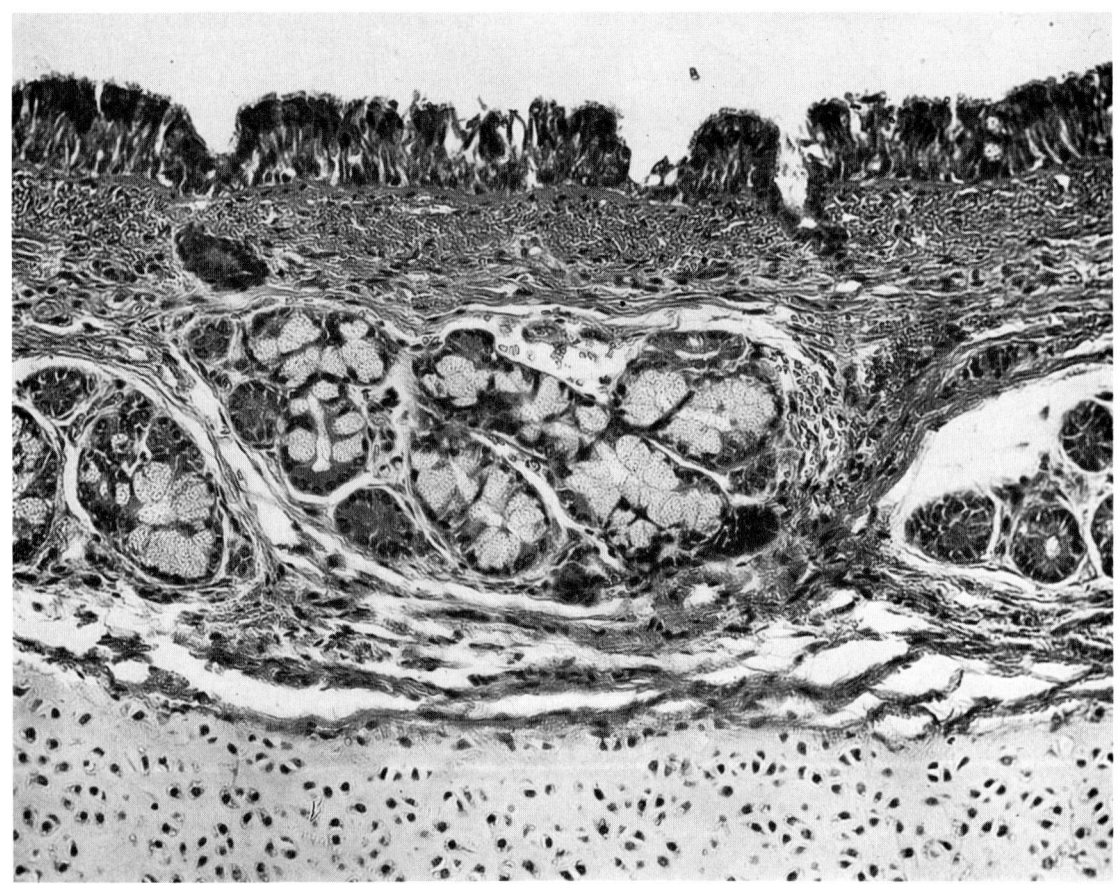

Figure 20–16

Figure 20–16. Shown here at the same high magnification is the mucosa of the trachea of an infant born at term, a 3,300 gram stillborn. Most of the glands are external to a superficial layer of the lamina propria that is rich in elastic fibers.
Hematoxylin and eosin stain. Mag. 197×.

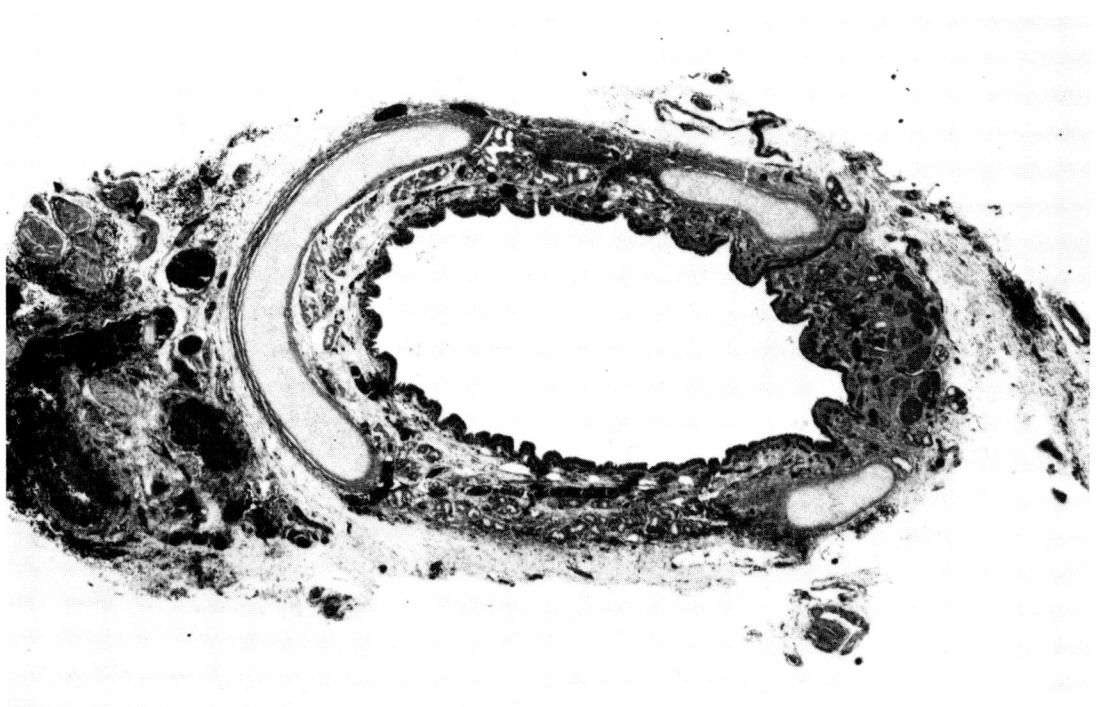

Figure 20–17

Figure 20–17. This is a cross section of a major bronchus from a newborn infant. Three different plaques of cartilage appear in the wall. Numerous glands can be seen in the mucosa.

This infant was a one day old black male, born at the 30th week of gestation. His body, at autopsy, weighed 1,500 grams.

Hematoxylin and eosin stain. Mag. 25×.

Chapter 21

THE LOWER RESPIRATORY TRACT

EMBRYOLOGY

The lung first appears in the fourth week of gestation, as a ventral diverticulum of the foregut, as previously mentioned. The endodermal lining of this early respiratory primordium develops within a median mass of mesenchyme located dorsal and cranial to the main peritoneal cavity. The original right and left bronchial buds grow out laterally from it into their respective pleural cavities, each carrying before it a dome-shaped investment of mesenchyme covered peripherally with mesothelium. The airways then branch within that bed of mesenchyme as it grows into the thoracic cavity on each side. The mesenchyme adapts itself to the shape of each bronchial tree; gradually the external lobation of the two lungs takes form, including the subdivision of lobes into bronchopulmonary segments. Internally each lobe becomes subdivided into lobules.[1]

The mesenchyme encasing the bronchial tree ultimately differentiates into muscle, connective tissue, cartilage plates of the walls of the bronchi, and the supporting tissue of the alveoli. Into this connective tissue grow blood vessels and nerve fibers.[1]

As far as the bronchi are concerned, their branching process is like the branching of a compound gland into a bush-like set of tubules. Their prenatal development may be thought of as occurring in three phases, occupying consecutive periods of time as follows:
1. Establishment of the larger conducting tubes, bronchi, and bronchioles (5 weeks to 16 weeks).
2. Laying down of the respiratory bronchioles (16 to 24 weeks).
3. Extension into a system of alveolar ducts and the differentiation of early alveoli (24 weeks to term). During this last period of time the lung loses its glandular appearance and becomes highly vascular.[1]

These three classic stages have been referred to as the:
1. Glandular (5 to 16 weeks)
2. Canalicular (16 to 24 weeks)
3. Alveolar (24 to 40 weeks).[2]

These latter terms serve best to describe the histologic appearance of the lung during each of these time periods.

From 16 to 23 generations of bronchial branches are formed during fetal life. In the fetus of six weeks, segmental bronchi are present. Between 10 and 14 weeks there is rapid branching of the airways, and by 16 weeks all pre-acinar airways are present. From 16 weeks to birth there is some further airway branching of channels, but only of prospective respiratory bronchioles and alveolar ducts. (Some further alveolar ducts develop after birth.)

During the canalicular period of development from 16 to 24 weeks, there is rapid growth of the mesenchymal tissue associated with the peripheral portions of the bronchial tree. Connective tissue cells and fibrils become prominent and an extensive system of capillaries develops. The capillaries are closely associated with air channels in a manner not unlike their relation to the respiratory membrane in the adult. (No alveoli are present at this stage.)[4]

In the alveolar stage of development, from 24 to 40 weeks, the lung loses its glandular character and becomes increasingly vascular. The bulbous expansions at the ends of the bronchial tree branch further, and alveoli arise as shallow evaginations from the channel walls. The connective tissue fibers become distributed around the alveolar openings. The epithelium becomes attenuated, and the capillaries establish a close relationship to the future respiratory surface.[4]

At birth there are 24 million alveoli. These multiply rapidly, and by eight years the adult number of 300 million has been attained.[3]

The arteries branch with the airways and develop at the same time, so that by 16 weeks of gestation all pre-acinar branching is complete. The veins develop at the same time but run independently in the lung. After birth there is rapid multiplication of arteries and veins peripherally.

During fetal life the high pulmonary resistance is associated with thick-walled pulmonary arteries. After birth there is a drop in resistance, and even after three days there is a drop in the thickness of the walls of small pulmonary arteries. By four months all pulmonary arteries are thin-walled.[3]

ANATOMY

The lungs of the fetus and the newborn are pale pink. Even when the infant has breathed for some period of time they are inclined to be of rubbery consistency; no air is visible or palpable within them and they may sink in watery fluid. (To a large extent this is due to their marked elasticity, so that when no negative pressure is brought to bear on them, the thick, elastic alveolar walls tend to force them into a collapsed state — or relatively collapsed state — as they were *in utero*.) The weight is dependent upon age, and the right lung is consistently heavier than the left.

The apex is rounded, lying in the plane of the thoracic inlet. The base is semilunar and concave; it rests upon the convex surface of the diaphragm. The concavity on the right is deeper than that on the left. The costal aspect is smooth and convex, and corresponds to the form of the cavity of the chest, which is deeper behind than in front. The mediastinal aspect exhibits a deep concavity which corresponds to the pericardium; it is larger and deeper on the left than on the right. Above and behind that concavity is a triangular depression known as the hilus, where the structures which form the root of the lung enter and leave the organ. The inferior border is thin and sharp where it separates the base from the costal surface, and it extends into the costodiaphragmatic recess. Medially, where it divides the base from the mediastinum, it is blunt and rounded.

The left lung is divided into a superior and inferior lobe by an oblique fissure. The superior lobe lies above and in front of the fissure, and the inferior below and behind it. The right lung is divided into three lobes, superior, middle, and inferior, by two fissures; one separates the inferior from the other two and corresponds to the oblique on the left. The second, a short horizontal fissure, separates the superior from the middle lobe.

The visceral pleura is a thin transparent layer composed of a single layer of mesothelium situated on its underlying lamina propria (Fig. 21–30), inseparably connected with the main mass of lung tissue which it invests.

The lung lobules are the important functional units of structure; each is a small polyhedral mass of lung tissue which receives a bronchiole together with terminal ramifications of vessels and nerves. The lobules are delineated on the surface of the lung by connective tissue septa (Fig. 21–31).

The intrapulmonary conducting passages branch repeatedly in dichotomous fashion. Each secondary bronchus supplies a lobe, each tertiary an individual bronchopulmonary segment. Within the lung, in the infant, the walls of the bronchi bear cartilage plaques which become smaller near the periphery, until finally they disappear in the walls of bronchioles.

Each terminal bronchiole gives rise to a number of respiratory bronchioles and each of these, in turn, opens into several alveolar ducts, thin-walled tubes which branch into expanded passages, the atria. These in turn lead into sacs. The walls of the ducts, atria, and sacs are studded with small pouches, the alveoli, separated from each other by thin septa composed of connective tissue elements and the capillary beds of the pulmonary blood supply.[5]

HISTOLOGY

Bronchi within the lungs are supported by a framework of cartilage plates; as a result, they and their branches are cylindrical and not flattened on one side as the extrapulmonary bronchi are. As one follows the air passages peripherally, the cartilage plates become smaller and irregularly distributed around the tube while the muscular layer completely surrounds the bronchus. The cartilage disappears from the wall as the bronchi become bronchioles.

The bronchus is lined by a mucous membrane like that of the trachea. The epithelium is ciliated columnar throughout the system in the infant (Figs. 21–1 through 21–10). The lamina propria consists of a small amount of reticular and collagenous connective tissue and many elastic fibers. Not infrequently it contains small clusters of lymphoid cells (Fig. 21–7). The mucosa, in histologic sections, shows a marked longitudinal folding, produced by contraction of the smooth muscle in the wall (Figs. 21–1 to 21–4 and 21–7).

Beneath the mucosa is a layer of smooth muscle fibers in bundles that are arranged around the tube, but which never form a closed ring as in blood vessels and the intestinal tract. Instead, the muscles form an interlacing feltwork, the meshes of which become larger in the smaller bronchioles (Figs. 21-1 to 21-4 and 21-7). Numerous elastic fibers are associated with the smooth muscle cells, and a dense network of small blood vessels accompanies the myoelastic layer.

The external layer of the bronchial wall, dense connective tissue with many elastic fibers, surrounds the plates of cartilage; it is continuous with the connective tissue of the surrounding pulmonary tissue and with that accompanying large vessels (Figs. 21-1, 21-4, and 21-7). Mucous and mucoserous glands may be seen as far out along the bronchial tree as the cartilage extends (Fig. 21-7). The glands are usually situated deep to the muscular layer, through which their ducts penetrate to open on the free surface.

Collections of lymphoid tissue appear commonly in the mucosa and in the fibrous tissue about the cartilage.

With the progressive decrease in the size of the bronchi and bronchioles toward the periphery, the layers of their walls become thinner. In some of them the various elements intermingle to form a single layer. The smooth muscle, however, is distinct up to the end of the respiratory bronchioles (Fig. 21-8), and a few strands continue even into the walls of the alveolar ducts.[4]

The *respiratory bronchioles* are short tubes lined in their first part with ciliated columnar epithelium (Figs. 21-6, 21-9, and 21-10). A short distance down the bronchioles, the ciliated columnar epithelium loses its cilia and becomes low cuboidal (Figs. 21-9 and 21-10). These bronchioles lack cartilage, and branch into radiating alveolar ducts (Fig. 21-10). They are surrounded by alveoli that have arisen from adjacent ducts.

The *alveolar ducts* are thin tubes with highly discontinuous walls (Fig. 21-9). They usually follow a long, tortuous course and give off several branches, which in turn may branch again. They are closely set with thin-walled outpouchings, the alveolar sacs, in the infant born at term. However, in immature infants such is not the case.

In the nineteenth week of gestation, as seen in Figure 21-11, there are no alveolar sacs but only alveolar ducts. This is in the midst of the so-called canalicular phase. Dense thick walls of connective tissue separate these epithelium-lined elements from one another. The microscopic appearance by 36 weeks of gestation is quite different, as attested by Figure 21-15; in Figure 21-16 one can see many *alveolar sacs,* as little hollows, arranged close to one another around the alveolar ducts.

In the fetus of 12 to 16 weeks (in the so-called glandular stage), the potential air spaces are lined by a single layer of prominent cuboidal cells with clear cytoplasm (Figs. 21-17 and 21-18). In the fetus of 18 weeks gestation, however, these cells begin to diminish in size and number (Fig. 21-19). By 20 weeks they are scarcely visible at all, nor are they seen thereafter (Figs. 21-20 to 21-22).

The interalveolar septa in the infant of 19 to 20 weeks are normally thick and cellular, almost as thick as the potential air spaces are wide (Figs. 21-19 and 21-20). After that they become almost, although not quite, as thin as the interalveolar septa of the adult. The epithelial cells lining the alveoli from the twentieth week on are very flat indeed (Figs. 21-21 and 21-24).

There is great variability in the size of the air spaces in sections of the lung of the infant, even one born at term, depending upon the state of distension or collapse of the organ at the time of death and of fixation of the section (Fig. 21–25).

Alveoli in the lung of an infant born near term have a configuration, under ordinary circumstances, which is very irregular and which Dr. Edith Potter has described as resembling that of a crumpled paper bag. Many times, however, attempts at resuscitation just prior to death lead to trapping of air in over-expanded alveolar ducts and alveoli, which lends to the section an unusual and completely artifactual spongy appearance (Fig. 21–28). The edges of these spaces are abnormally smooth in contour and sharply delineated; furthermore normal anatomical branching patterns are unduly clearly visible.

Aparently there is, under normal circumstances, a small tidal exchange moving fluid in and out of the lungs of the fetus in the latter part of gestation. This seems to carry keratinized squamous cells — which are ordinarily suspended in the amniotic fluid at that time — into the farthest reaches of the lung, where one can see them from time to time in histological sections (Fig. 21–29). The presence of a small number of these cells is considered to be within limits of normal.

Small pulmonary arteries, during fetal life, have relatively thick walls because of high pulmonary artery resistance. It is said by Doctors Hislop and Reid, however, that even three days after birth there is a measurable decrease in the thickness of the walls of these arteries. By four months, they say, all pulmonary arteries are thin-walled.[3]

The *visceral pleura* consists of a thin layer of collagenous tissue, containing some fibroblasts and several prominent layers of elastic fibers oriented at various angles to the outer surface[4] (Fig. 21–30). It is covered by a single layer of mesothelial cells. It is rich in blood capillaries and lymphatic vessels.

References

1. Arey, L. B. Developmental Anatomy, rev. 7th ed. Philadelphia, W. B. Saunders Co., 1974, pp. 266–271.
2. Loosli, C. G., and Potter, E. L. The prenatal development of the human lung. Anatomical Record, *109*:320–321, 1951.
3. Hislop, A., and Reid, L.: *In* Scientific Foundations of Paediatrics, ed. J. A. Davis and J. Dobbing, London, Heinemann, 1974.
4. Bloom, W., and Fawcett, D. W.: A Textbook of Histology. Philadelphia, W. B. Saunders Co., 1975, pp. 762–763.
5. Warwick, R., and Williams, P. L.: Gray's Anatomy, 35th British ed. Philadelphia, W. B. Saunders Co., 1973, pp. 1196–1201.

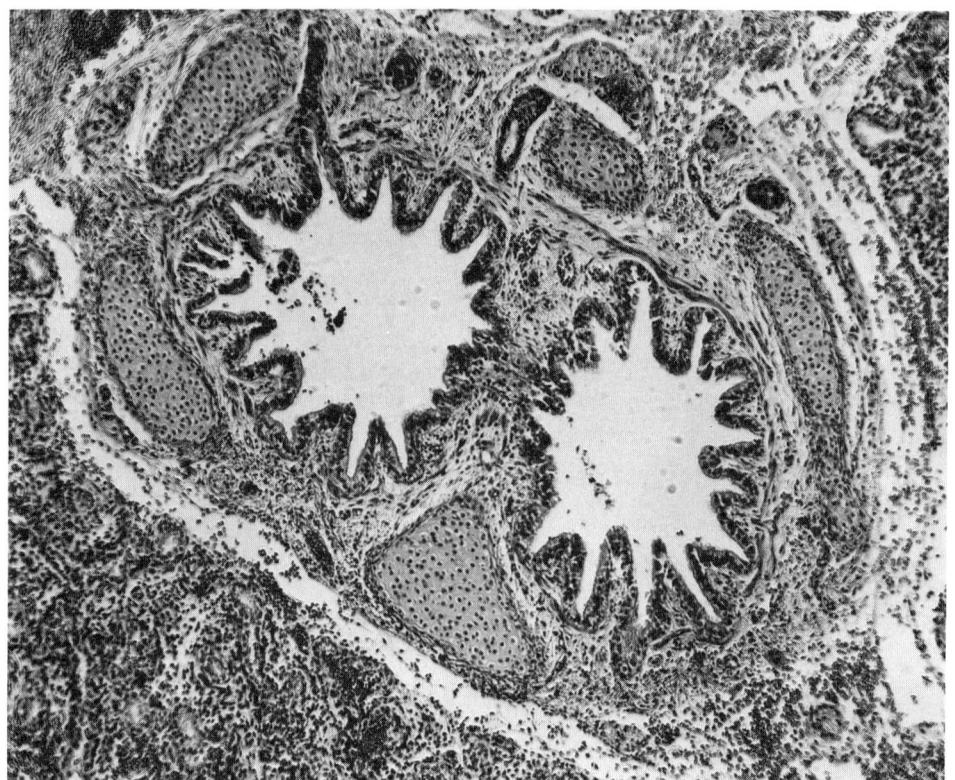

Figure 21–1

Figures 21–1 through 21–4. This set of four photomicrographs, taken at slightly different magnifications, illustrates some of the larger intrapulmonary bronchi in three infants of progressively greater gestational age, the first about 20 weeks, the second approximately 32 weeks, and the last two from the same infant of about 36 weeks.

Figure 21–1. These are cross sections of two large bronchi from an immature infant. They are sectioned just distal to the point of bifurcation.

This is a section from the autopsy of a black female infant born at 20 weeks of gestation, who survived for 37 minutes. Her body, at post-mortem examination, weighed 312.5 grams.

Hematoxylin and eosin stain. Mag. 100×.

THE LOWER RESPIRATORY TRACT 315

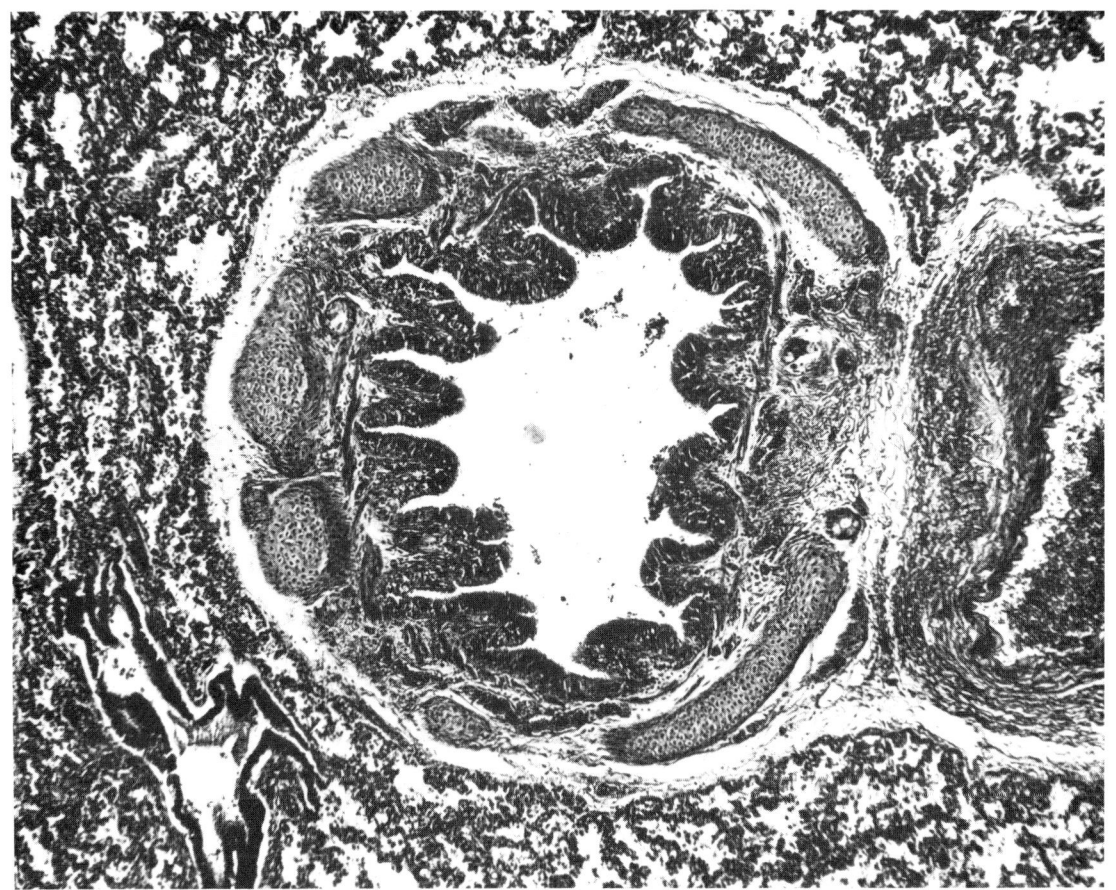

Figure 21-2

Figure 21-2. Seen here at relatively low magnification is a large bronchus from an infant born near term. Notice the rather intricate infolding of the mucosa, the prominent bundles of smooth muscle in the wall, and the many plaques of cartilage.

This section was taken from a 9 hour old black male who, at autopsy, weighed only 2,000 grams. (Estimated gestational age: 32 weeks.)

Hematoxylin and eosin stain. Mag. 81×.

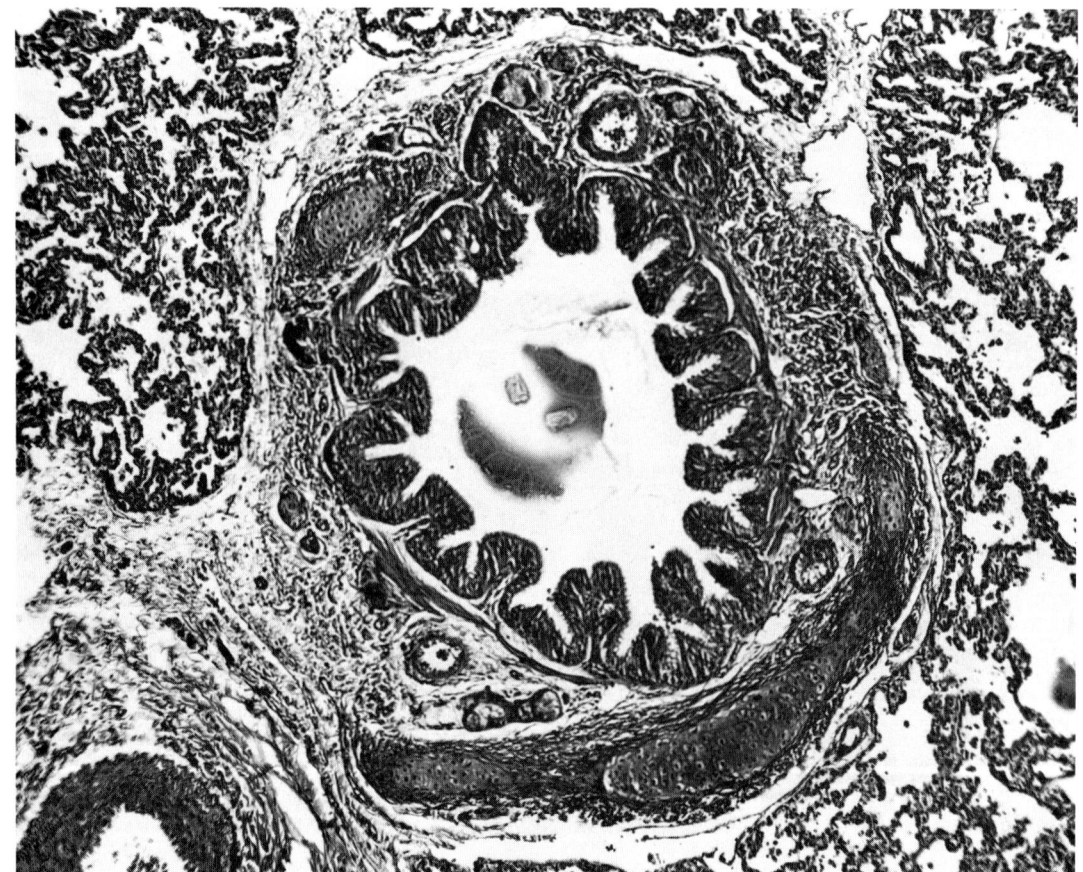

Figure 21–3

Figure 21-3. This is a cross section of a medium-sized bronchus from an infant born near term. The baby, a white female, lived for nine days. Her body weighed 2,420 grams at autopsy. Hematoxylin and eosin stain. Mag. 100×.

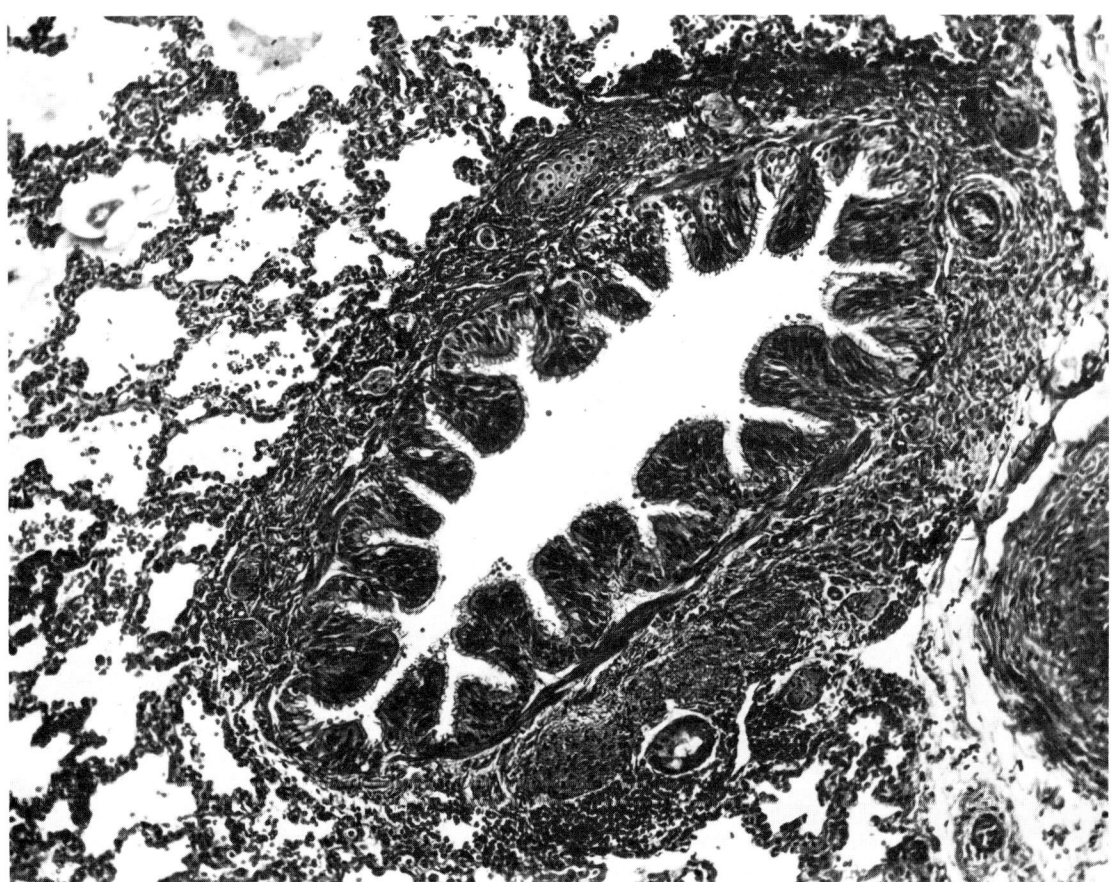

Figure 21-4

Figure 21-4. This is a tangential section of a bronchus of somewhat smaller caliber, depicted at higher magnification than the preceding.

Prominent cilia are apparent here, as are multiple bundles of smooth muscle in the wall. As it is a smaller bronchus, the cartilage plates are fewer and smaller also. Two glands are seen on the right side of the bronchus.

This section was taken from the same infant described in the legend for Fig. 21-3.

Hematoxylin and eosin stain. Mag. 142×.

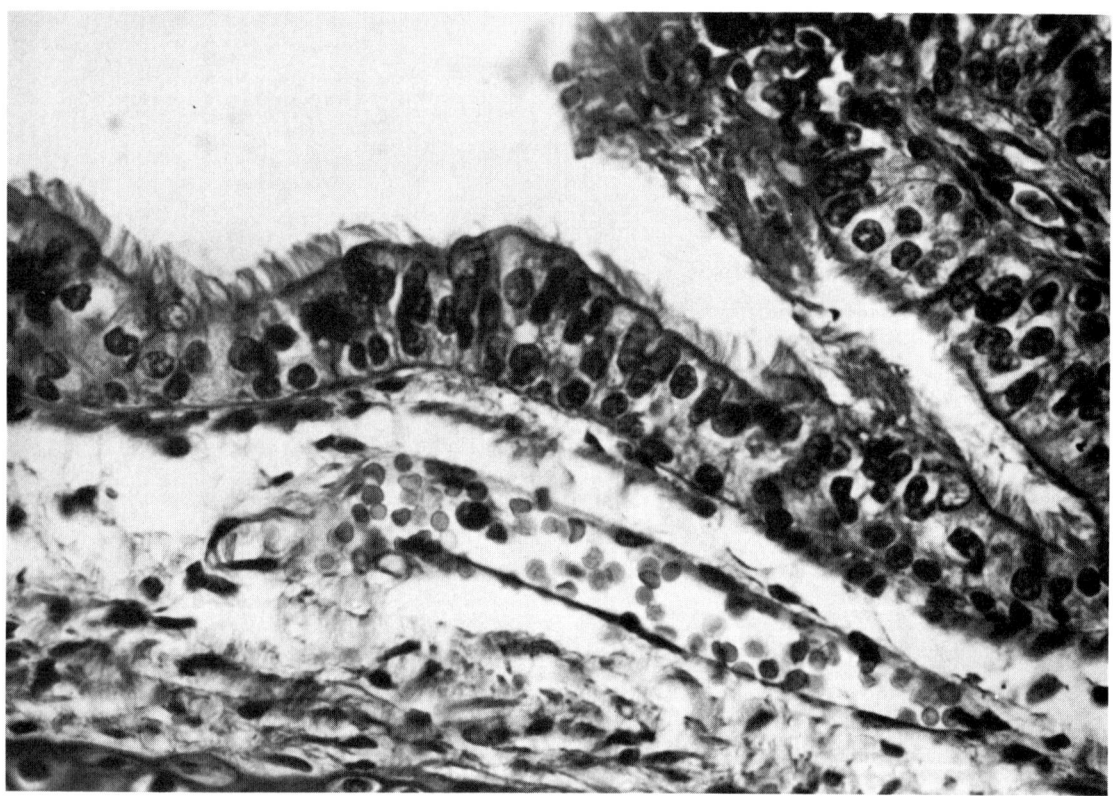

Figure 21–5

Figure 21–5. This is an illustration of the epithelial lining of a bronchus, in detail. The individual cells are tall columnar, with nuclei at various levels. The fine cilia are prominent here. A bit of cartilage appears in the lower left corner.

This patient was a 1 day old white male whose weight at autopsy was 2,180 grams. (Estimated gestational age: 32 weeks.)

Hematoxylin and eosin stain. Mag. 471×.

THE LOWER RESPIRATORY TRACT 319

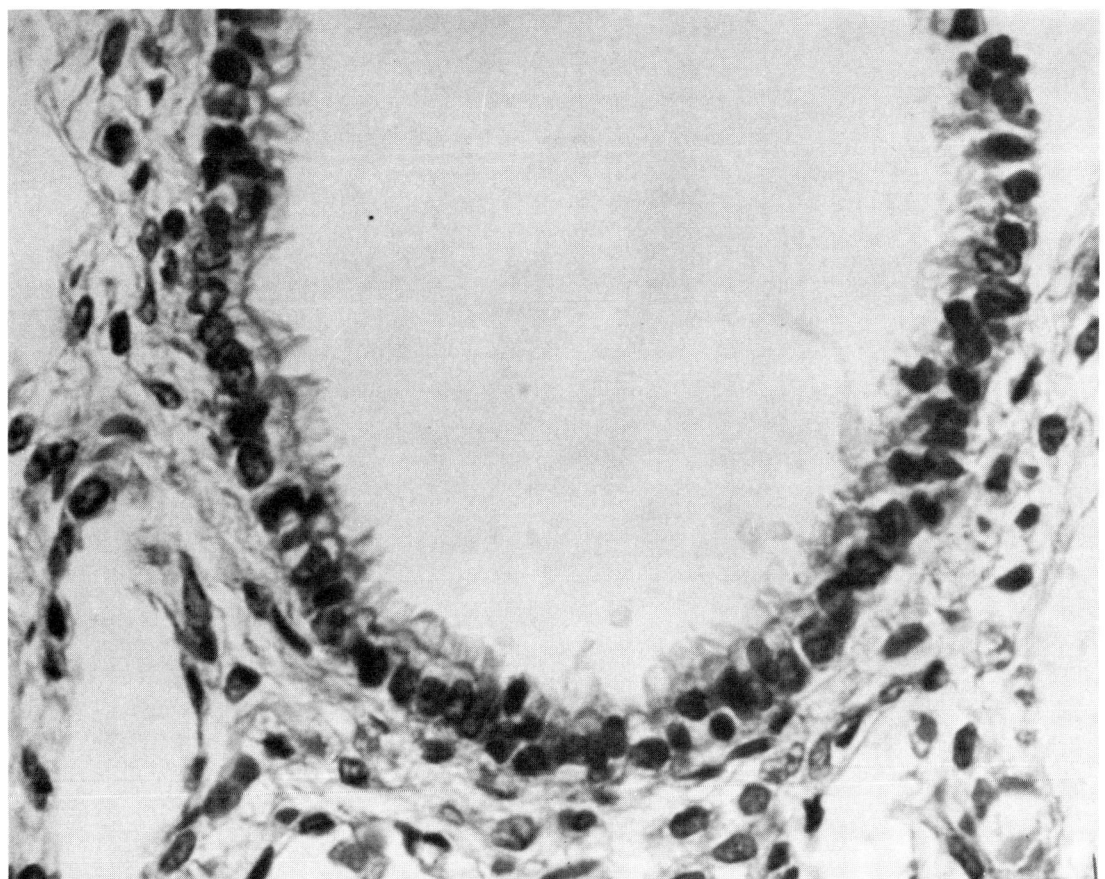

Figure 21-6

Figure 21-6. Seen here at very high magnification is the epithelial lining of a small bronchiole. Even though this is from an infant of comparable age and body weight, the epithelium at this extremity of the bronchial tree is considerably less tall than that seen in the bronchus in Fig. 21-5; the nuclei are not so staggered. The cilia, however, are just as prominent.

The subject was a 12 day old white male whose body, at necropsy, weighed 2,300 grams. (Estimated gestational age: 33 weeks.)

Hematoxylin and eosin stain. Mag. 660×.

320 THE LOWER RESPIRATORY TRACT

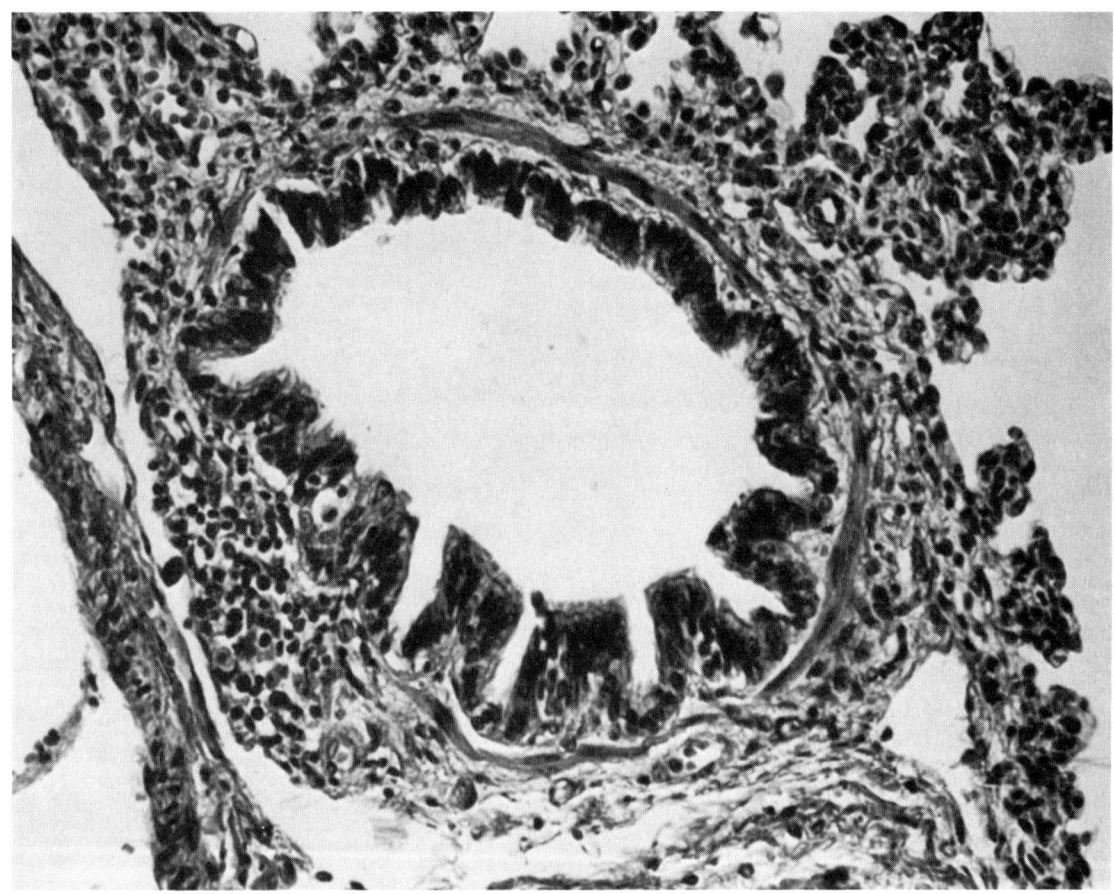

Figure 21-7

Figures 21-7 and 21-8. These two are direct cross sections of the bronchioles. one large and one small, from the lungs of term infants.

Note the considerable plication of the mucosal lining of the larger, Fig. 21-7, and the slender band of smooth muscle in the wall of each, more prominent in 21-7 than in 21-8.

Notice also the small artery, in cross section, adjacent to the bronchiole in Fig. 21-8.

Figure 21-7. From a 4 hr. old white male whose body weighed 2,850 grams at autopsy. Hematoxylin and eosin stain. Mag. 304×.

THE LOWER RESPIRATORY TRACT 321

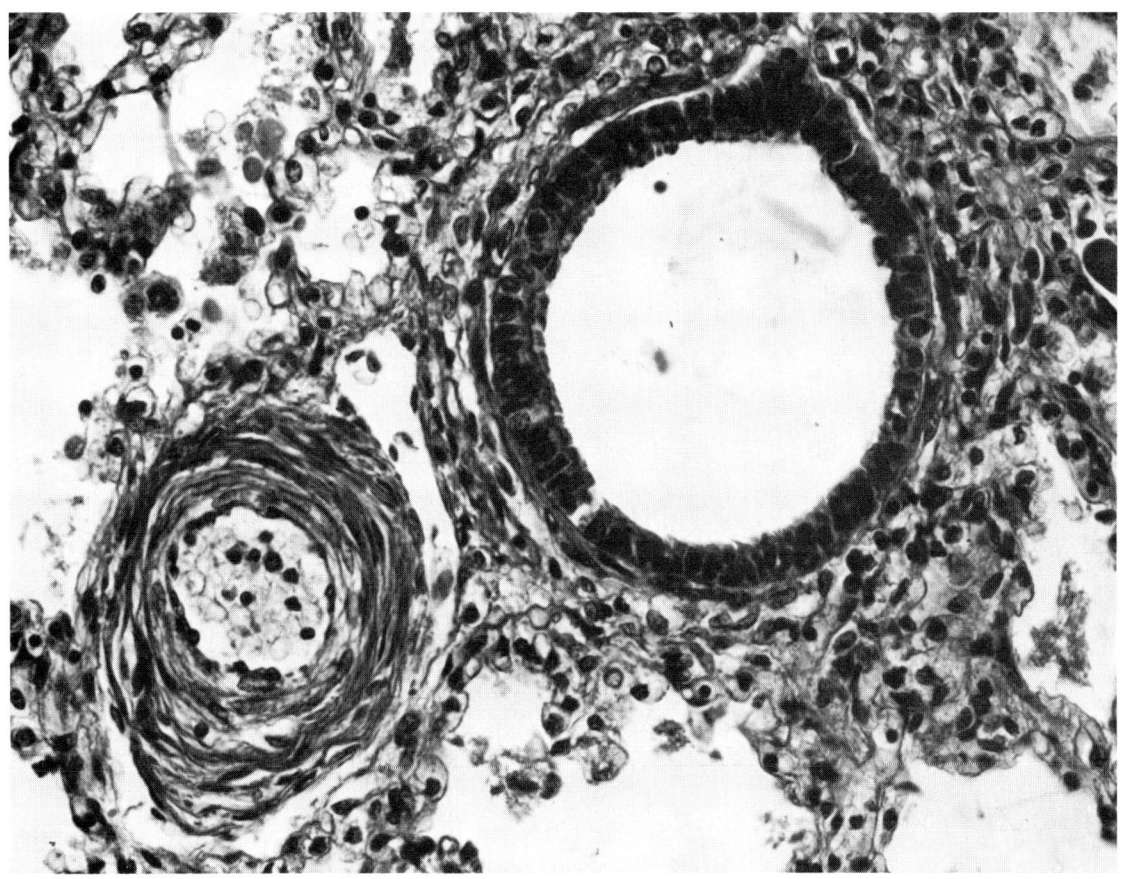

Figure 21-8

Figure 21-8. From a 3 week old white male, whose body weighed 3,850 grams at autopsy. (Estimated gestational age: 40 weeks.)
Hematoxylin and eosin stain. Mag. 370×.

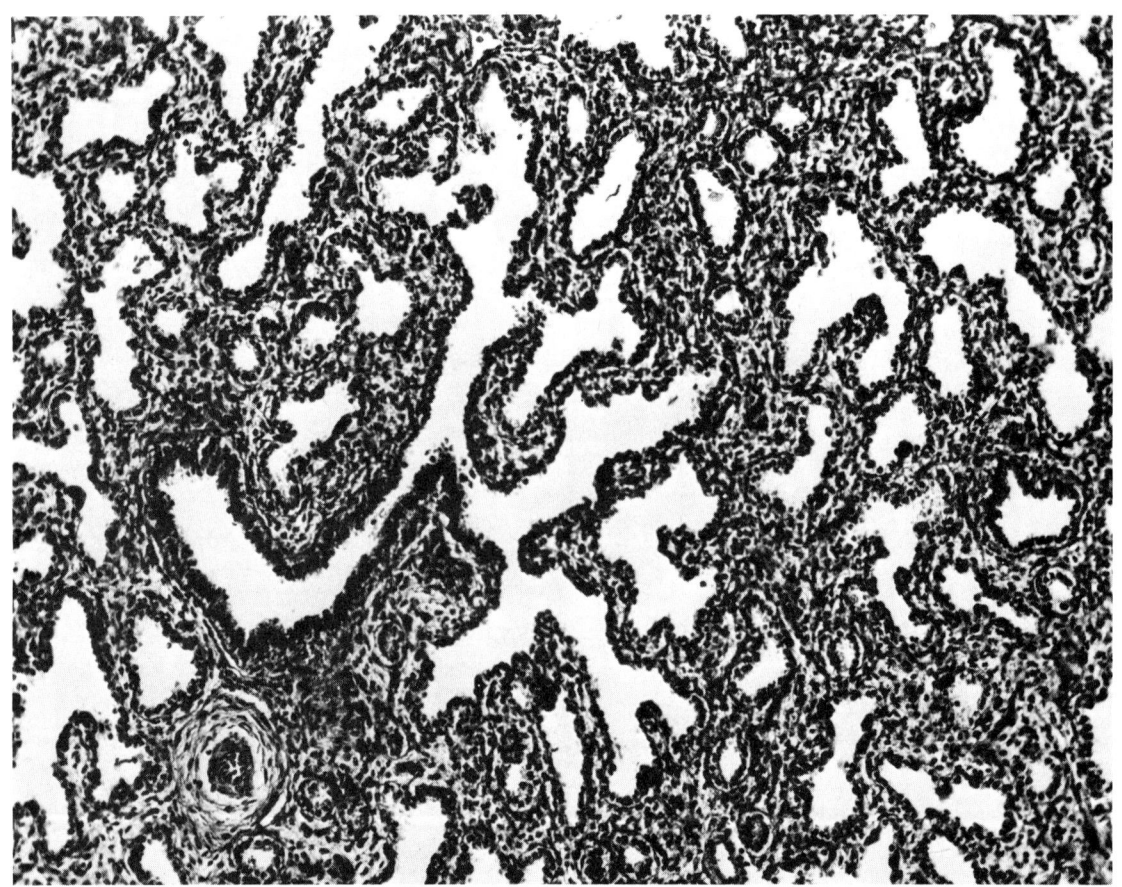

Figure 21-9

Figure 21-9. This photograph illustrates the termination of a respiratory bronchiole in multiple alveolar ducts and alveolar sacs in an immature male infant. The fetus was aborted at 16 to 18 weeks of gestation. Body weight at autopsy was 430 grams.

Hematoxylin and eosin stain. Mag. 153×.

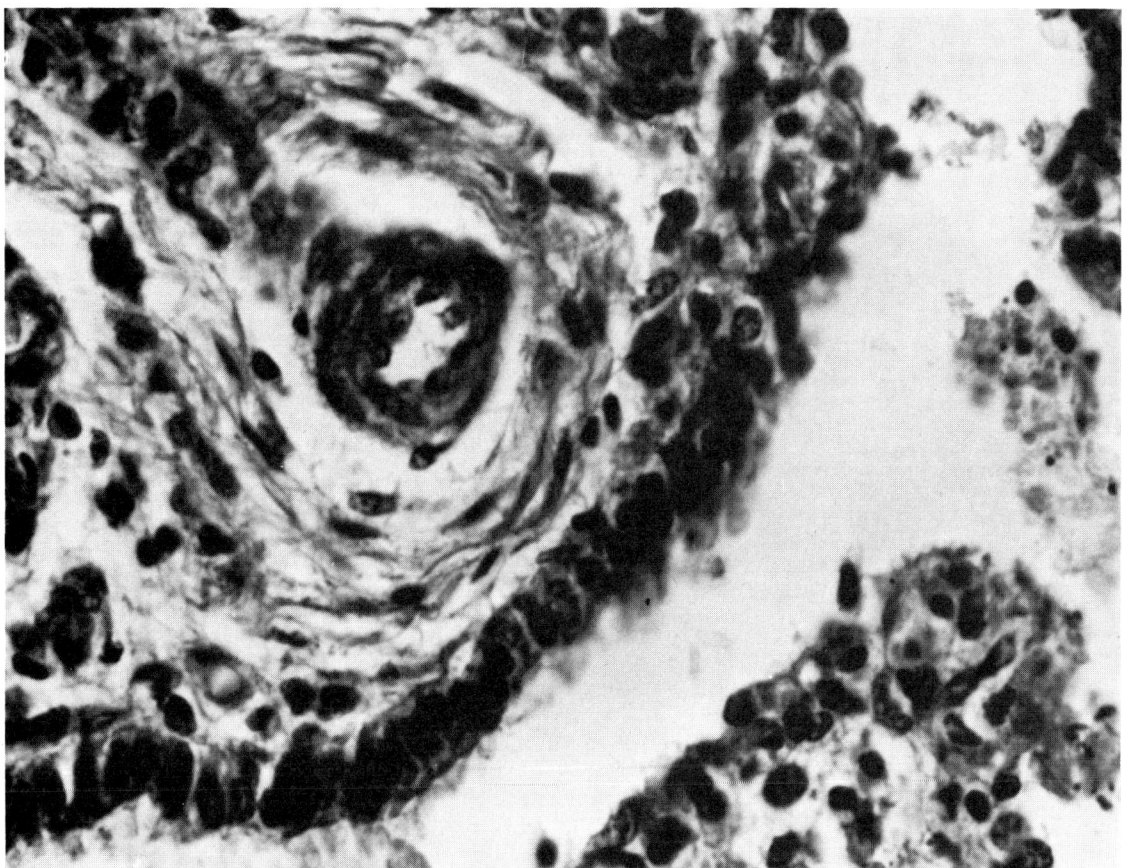

Figure 21–10

Figure 21–10. Seen here at higher magnification is the termination of a respiratory bronchiole in what are probably two alveolar ducts. An arteriole, cut in cross section, appears just above the terminal bronchiole.

The patient was a black male infant, the product of a 30 week gestation, who died at four hours of age. His body weight at autopsy was 1,070 grams.

Hematoxylin and eosin stain. Mag. 660×.

Figures 21–11 through 21–16. This series of six photomicrographs, all taken at the same low magnification, illustrates the evolution of the histologic pattern of the lung during the latter half of gestation and early postnatal life.

Note the gradual diminution in relative amount of interstitial or supporting tissue with increasing development.

Potential air spaces in the 230 gram stillborn are relatively small, widely separated from one another, and all lined by prominent epithelial cells. These lining cells are still visible in Fig. 21–12 but not in succeeding photographs.

In Figs. 21–15 and 21–16, alveoli are present and all air spaces have the shapes of crumpled paper bags.

Hematoxylin and eosin stain. Mag. 76×.

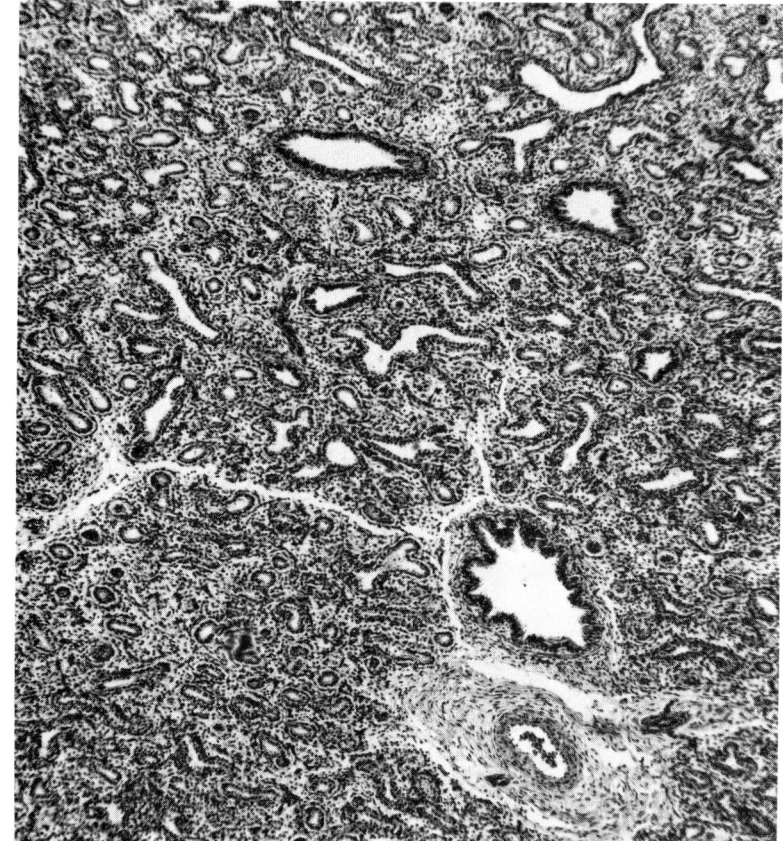

Figure 21-11. 230 grams White male. Approx. 19 wks. gest. Stillborn.

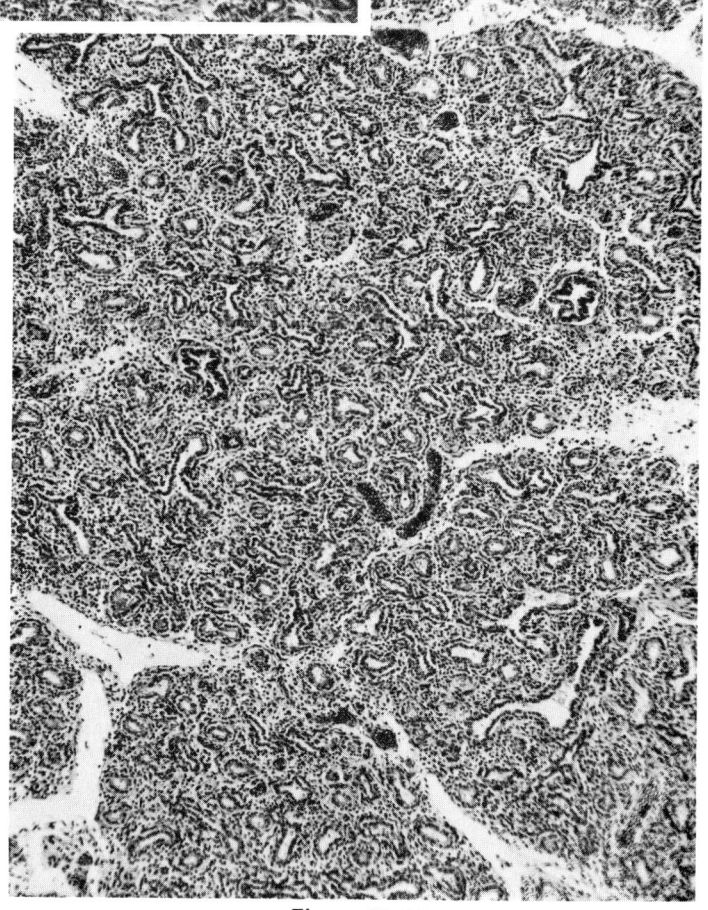

Figure 21-12. 312.5 grams Black female. 20 wks. gest. Age: 37 min.

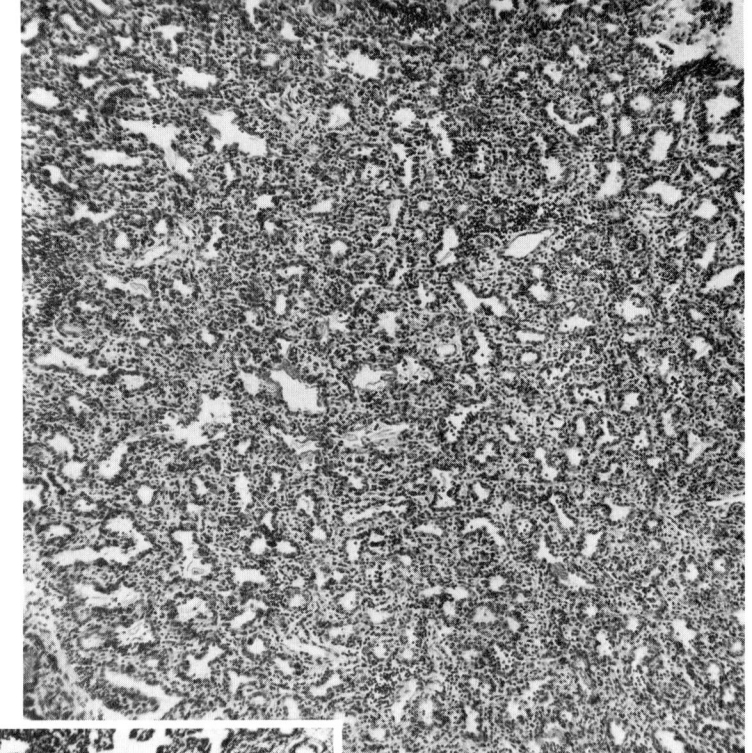

Figure 21–14. 610 grams Black female. Age: 6 hrs. 18 min.

Figure 21–14

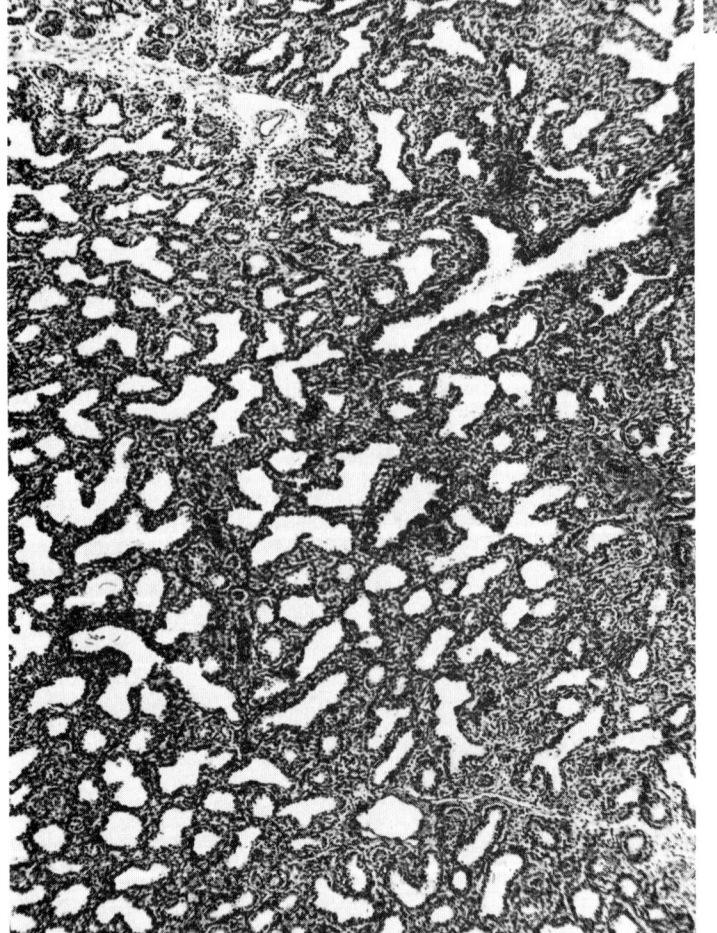

Figure 21–13. 430 grams Male. 16–18 wks. gest. Stillborn.

Figure 21–13

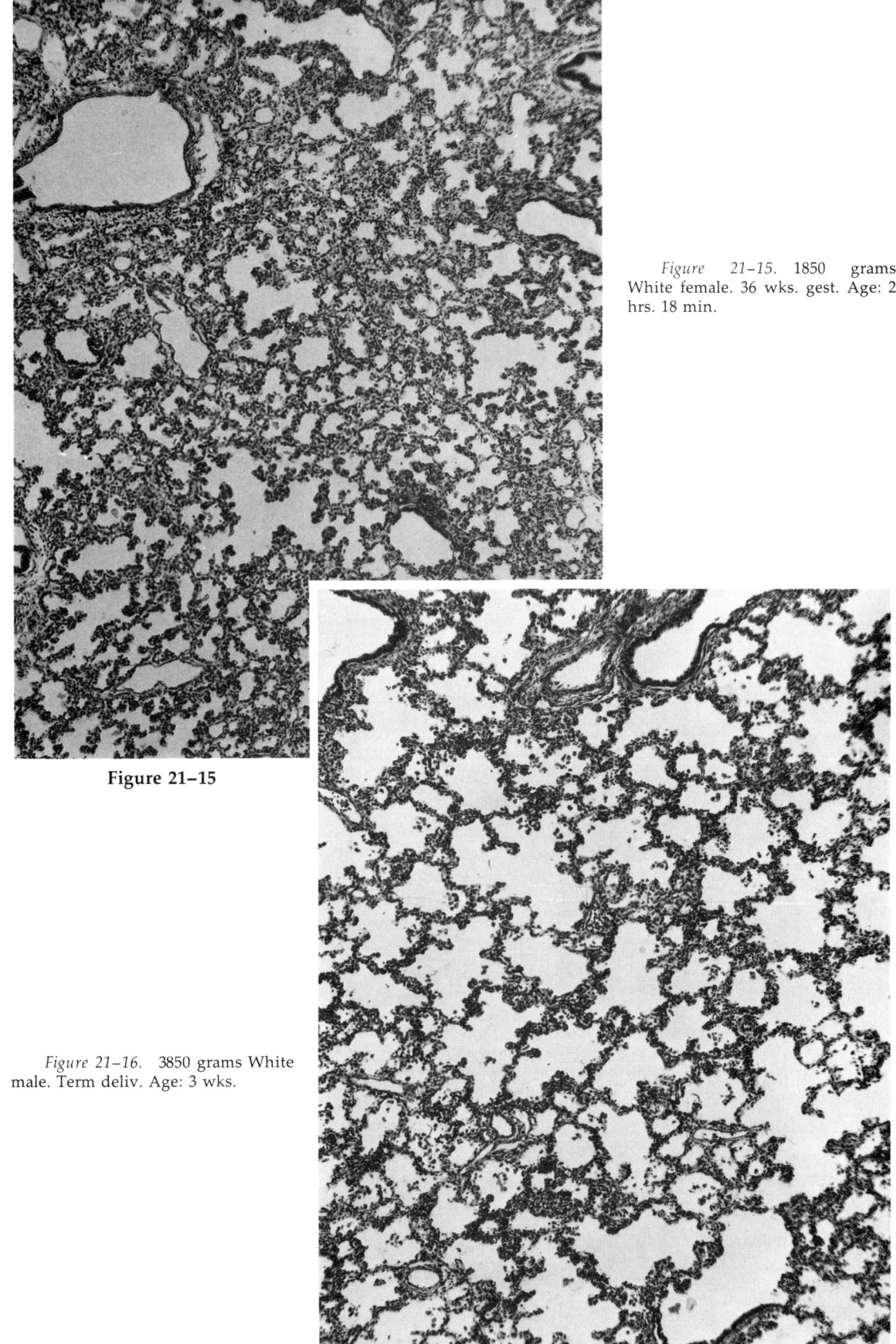

Figure 21–15. 1850 grams White female. 36 wks. gest. Age: 2 hrs. 18 min.

Figure 21–15

Figure 21–16. 3850 grams White male. Term deliv. Age: 3 wks.

Figure 21–16

328 THE LOWER RESPIRATORY TRACT

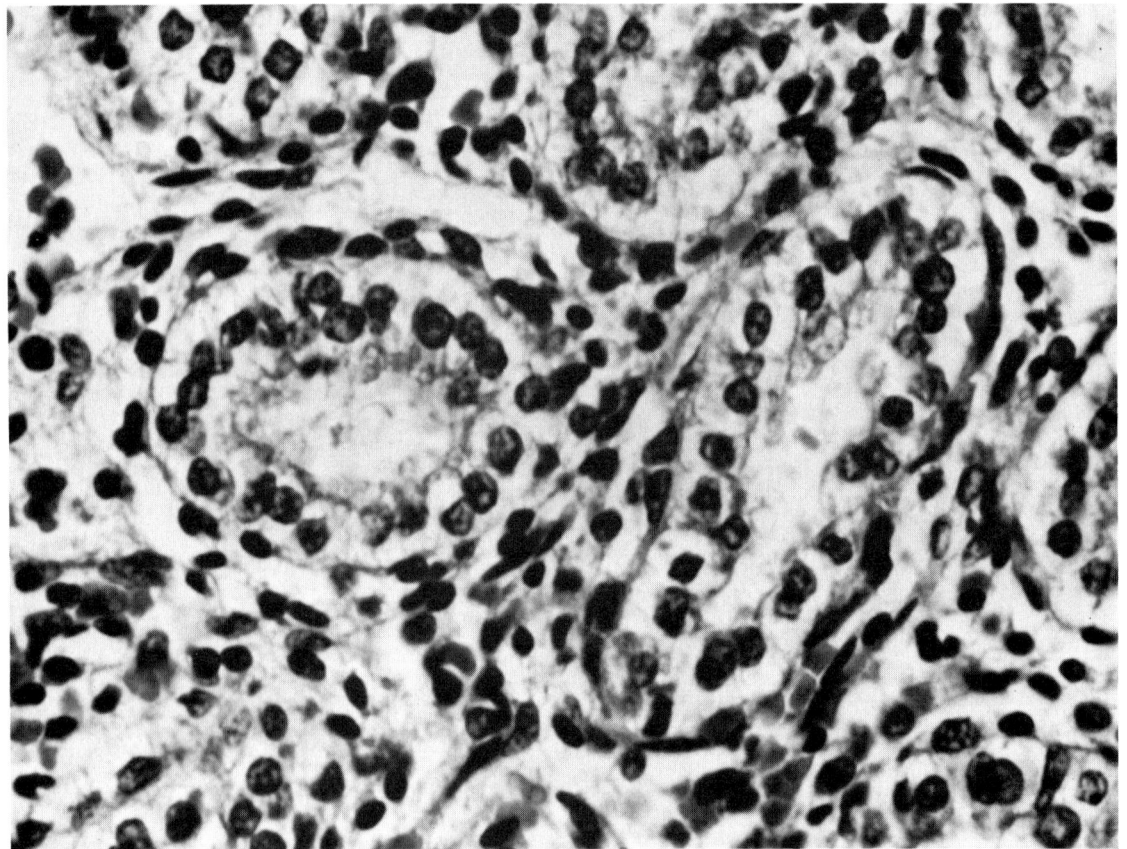

Figure 21–17

Figures 21–17 through 21–22. The following set of six photomicrographs illustrates in detail the changing character of the lining cells of the potential air spaces and alveoli and the evolution of the nature of their walls.

Initially, in the fetus of 16 to 20 weeks, lining cells of potential air spaces are prominent, cuboidal, and in some instances almost columnar (Fig. 21–17). In the stillborn infant pictured in Fig. 21–22, on the other hand, they are quite flat as in the adult lung.

Walls of air spaces in the 16th to 20th weeks of gestation are very thick and cellular, whereas in the term infant the walls of the alveoli appear to consist of little more than a meshwork of capillaries.

Hematoxylin and eosin stain. Mag. 660×.

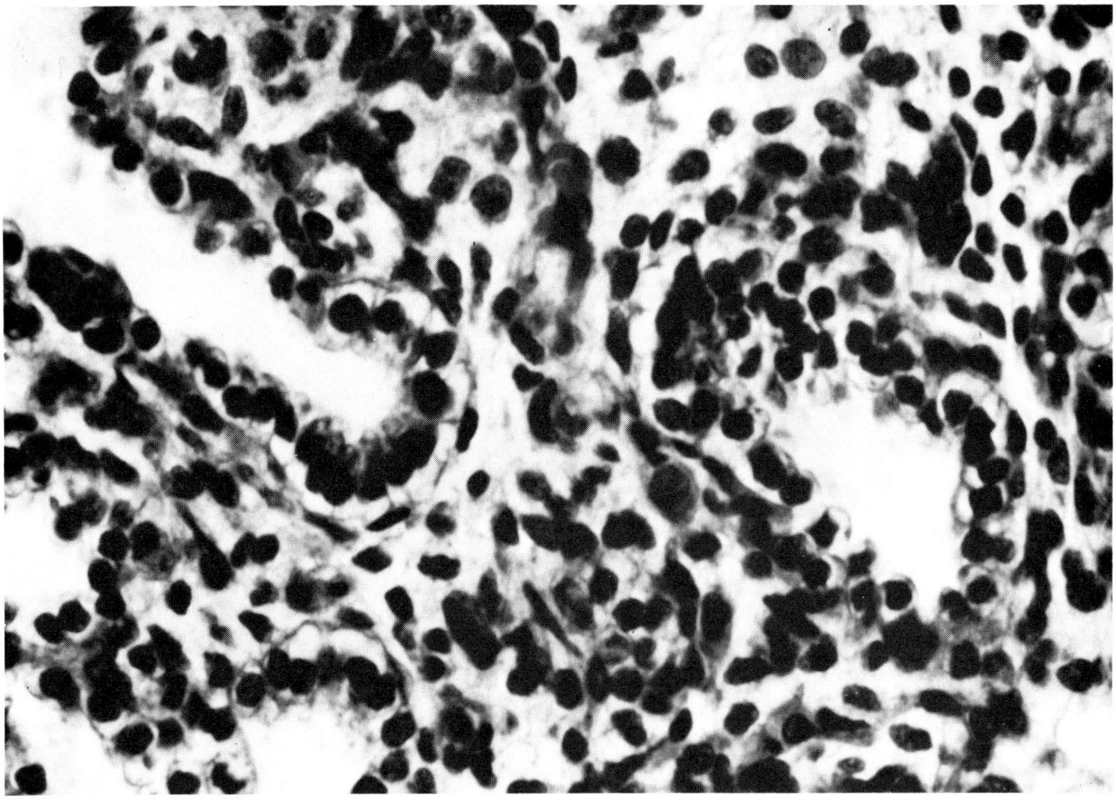

Figure 21–18

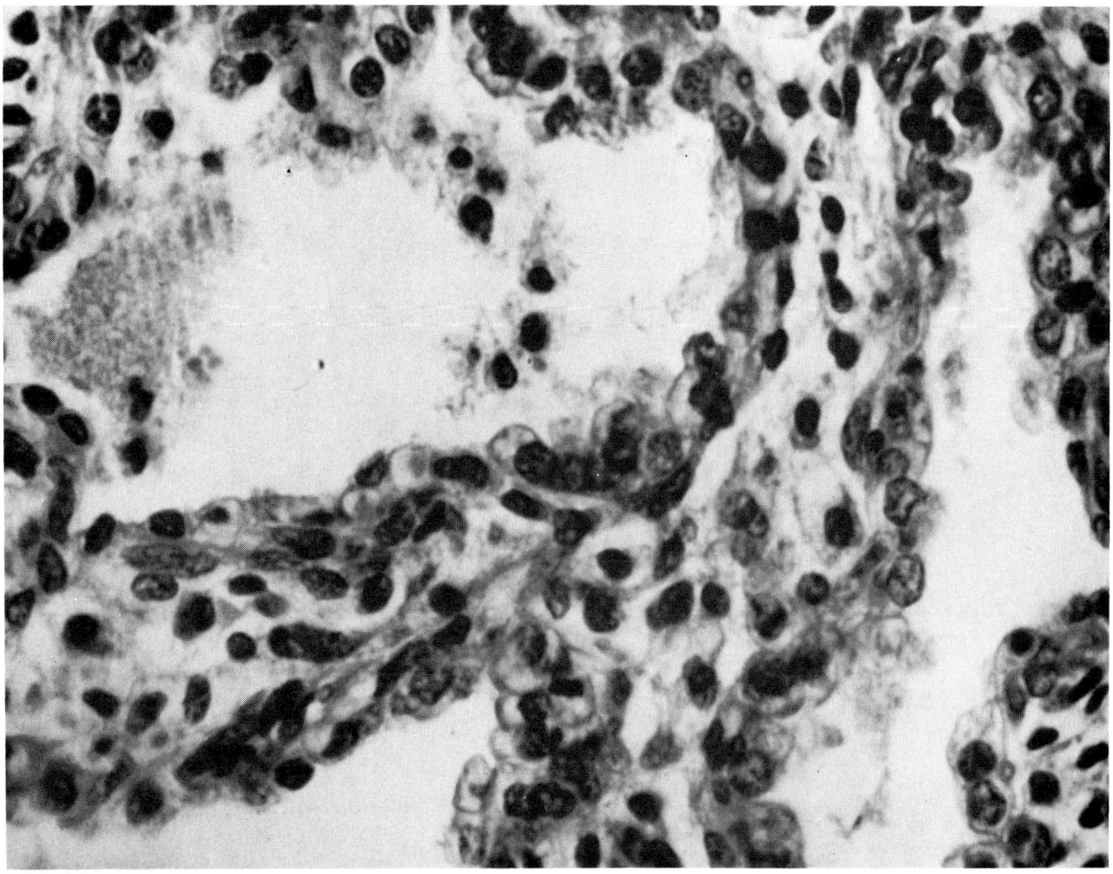

Figure 21–19

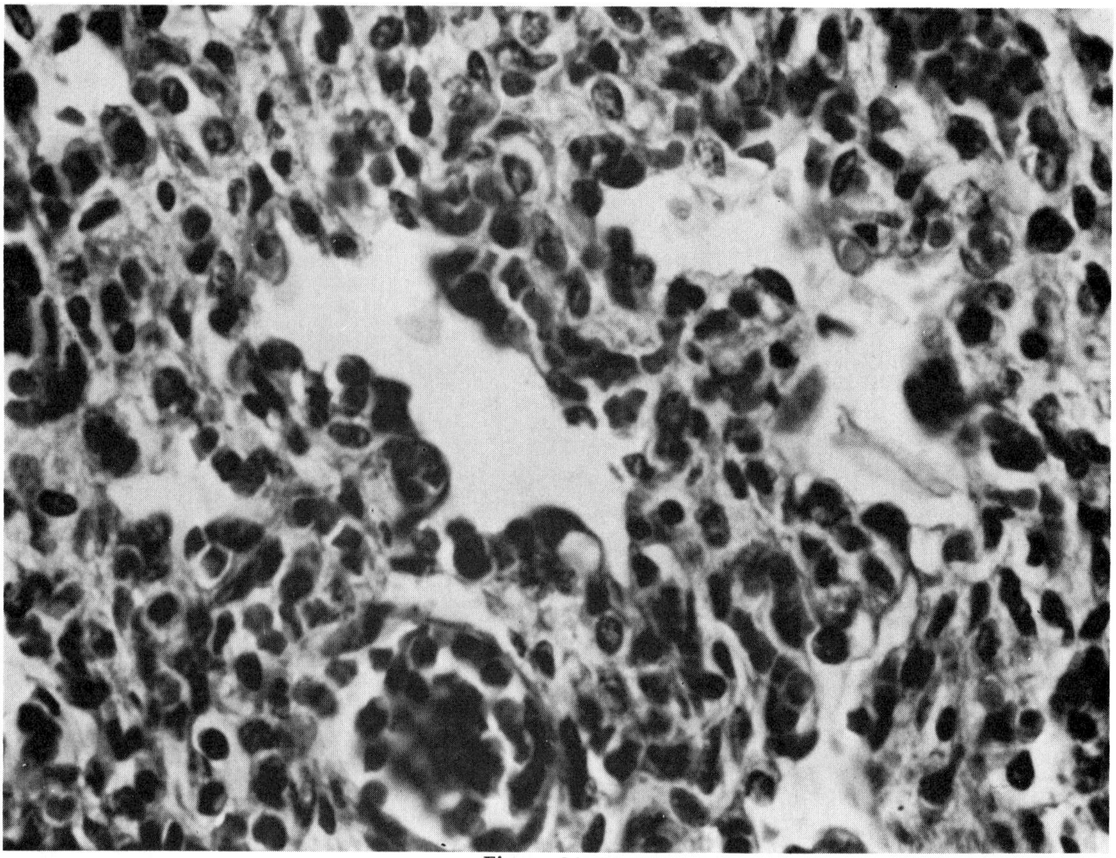

Figure 21-20

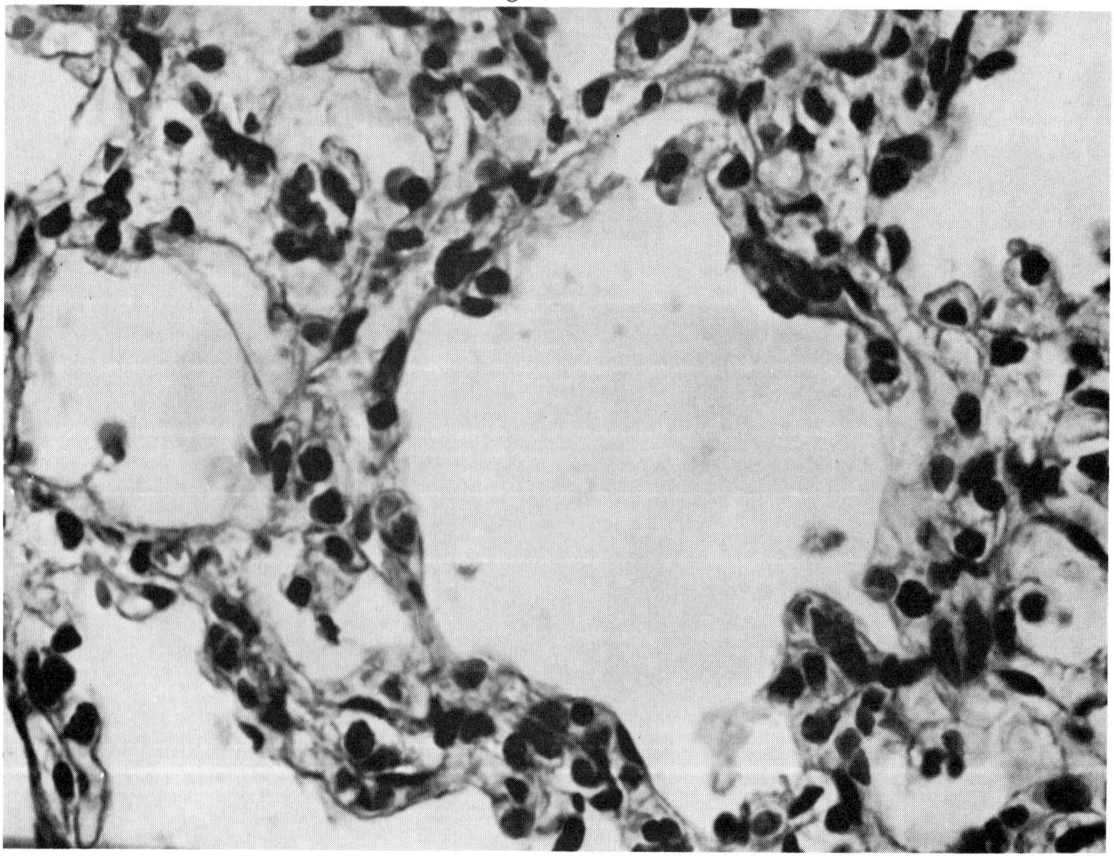

Figure 21-21

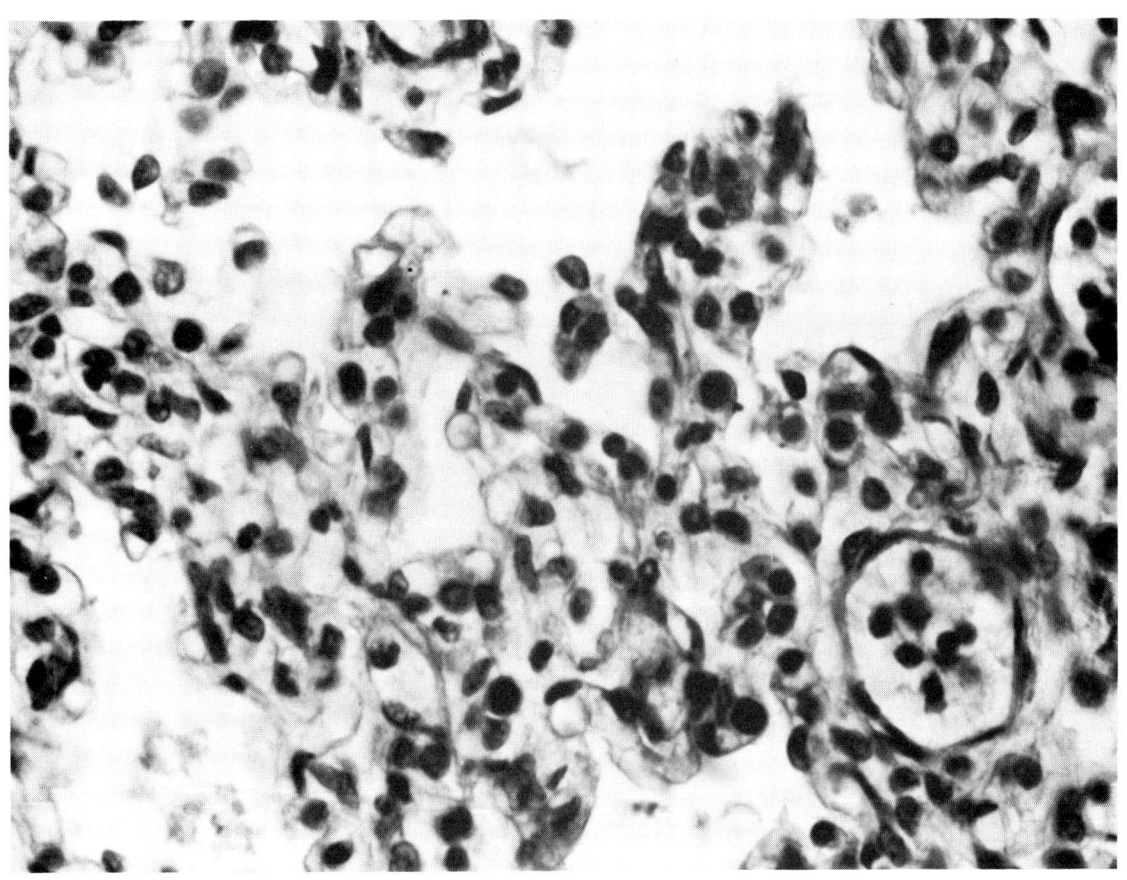

Figure 21–22

Fig.	Weight	Race	Sex	Gestation	Age
21–17	312.5 gm.	B	F	20 wk.	37 min.
21–18	430 gm.	?	M	16–18 wk.	Stillborn
21–19	510 gm.	B	F	?	1½ hr.
21–20	925 gm.	B	F	?	Stillborn
21–21	1,780 gm.	B	M	32 wk. (est.)	27 hr.
21–22	3,020 gm.	B	F	?	Stillborn

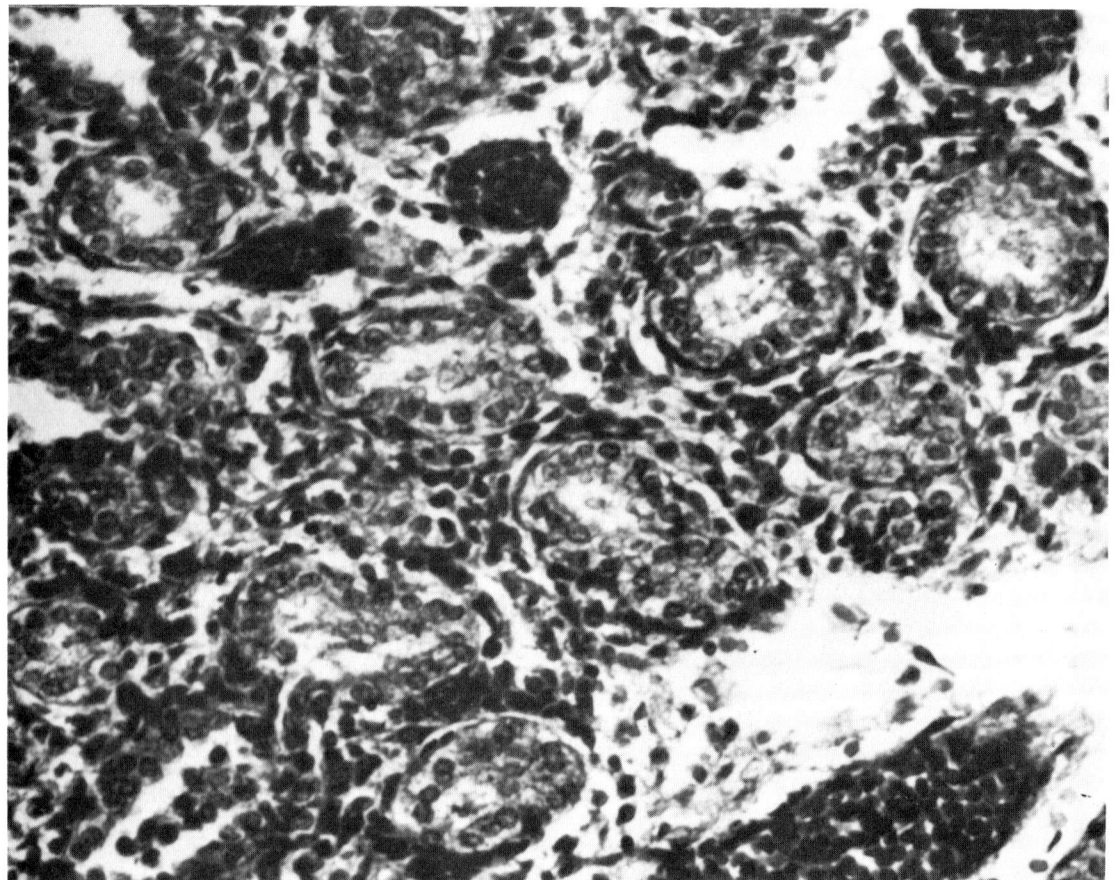

Figure 21–23

Figures 21–23 and 21–24. These two figures illustrate the histologic appearance of the alveoli of infants at the extremes of the span of life dealt with in this atlas. Fig. 21–23 depicts the air spaces or potential air spaces of a fetus at approximately 20 weeks of gestation, whereas Fig. 21–24 shows the alveoli of a 3 week old infant born at term.

Figure 21–23. The potential air spaces here are small and lined by a continuous single layer of prominent cuboidal (almost tall columnar in places) epithelium. They are separated from one another by cellular interstitium.

This patient was a male infant, stillborn at 20 weeks of gestation, whose body at post-mortem examination weighed 270 grams.

Hematoxylin and eosin stain. Mag. 382×.

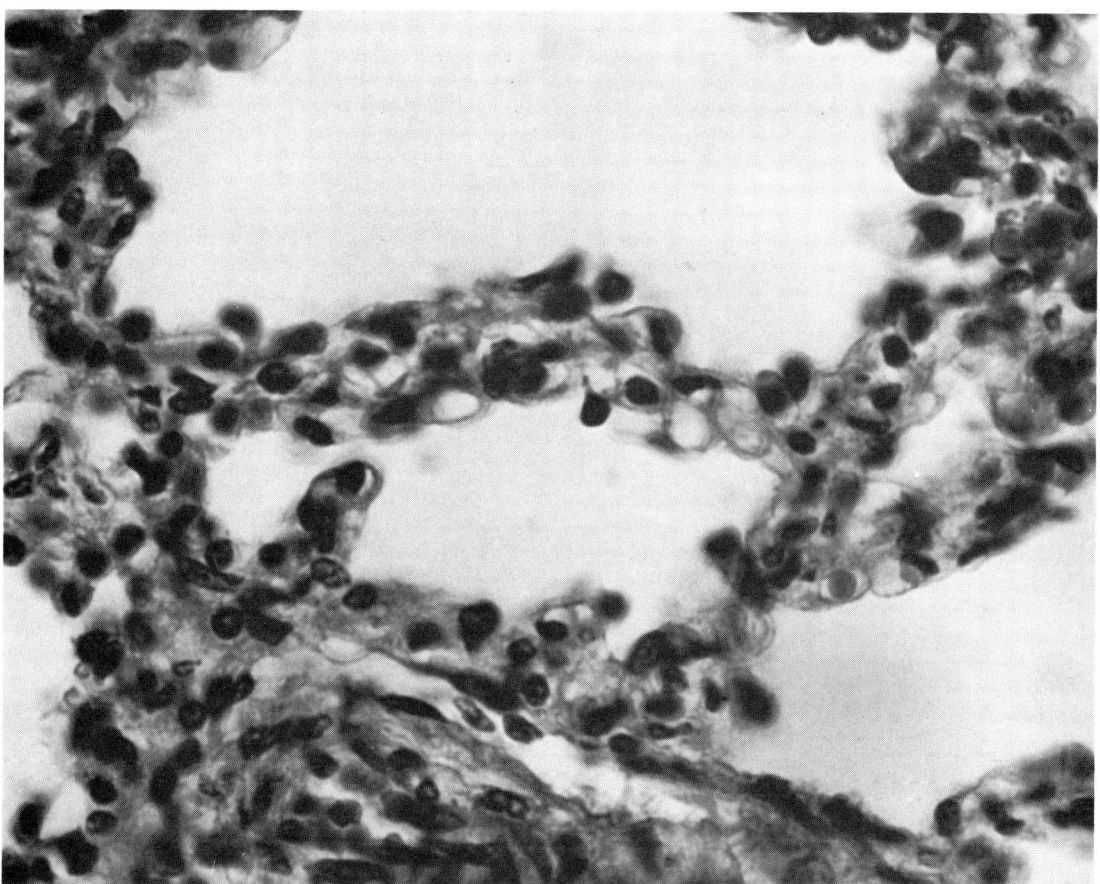

Figure 21-24

Figure 21-24. The alveolar walls in this figure are delicate and composed of little more than a plexus of capillaries, the lumens of some of which are clearly visible here.

The patient, a white male infant born at term, survived for 3 weeks. At autopsy he weighed 3,850 grams.

Hematoxylin and eosin stain. Mag. 660×.

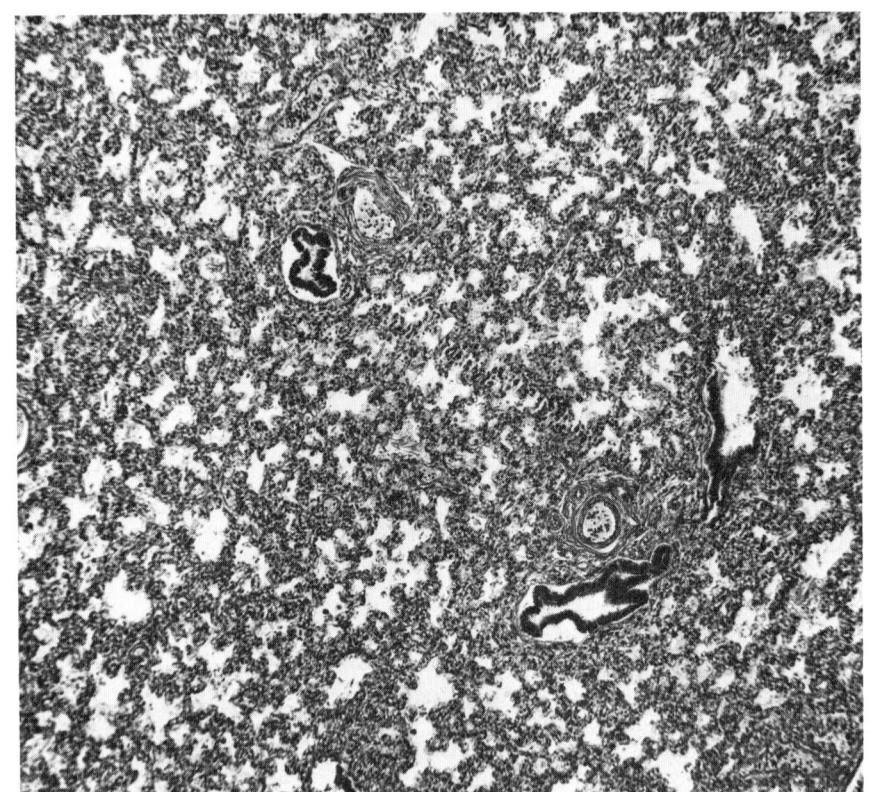

Figure 21-25a

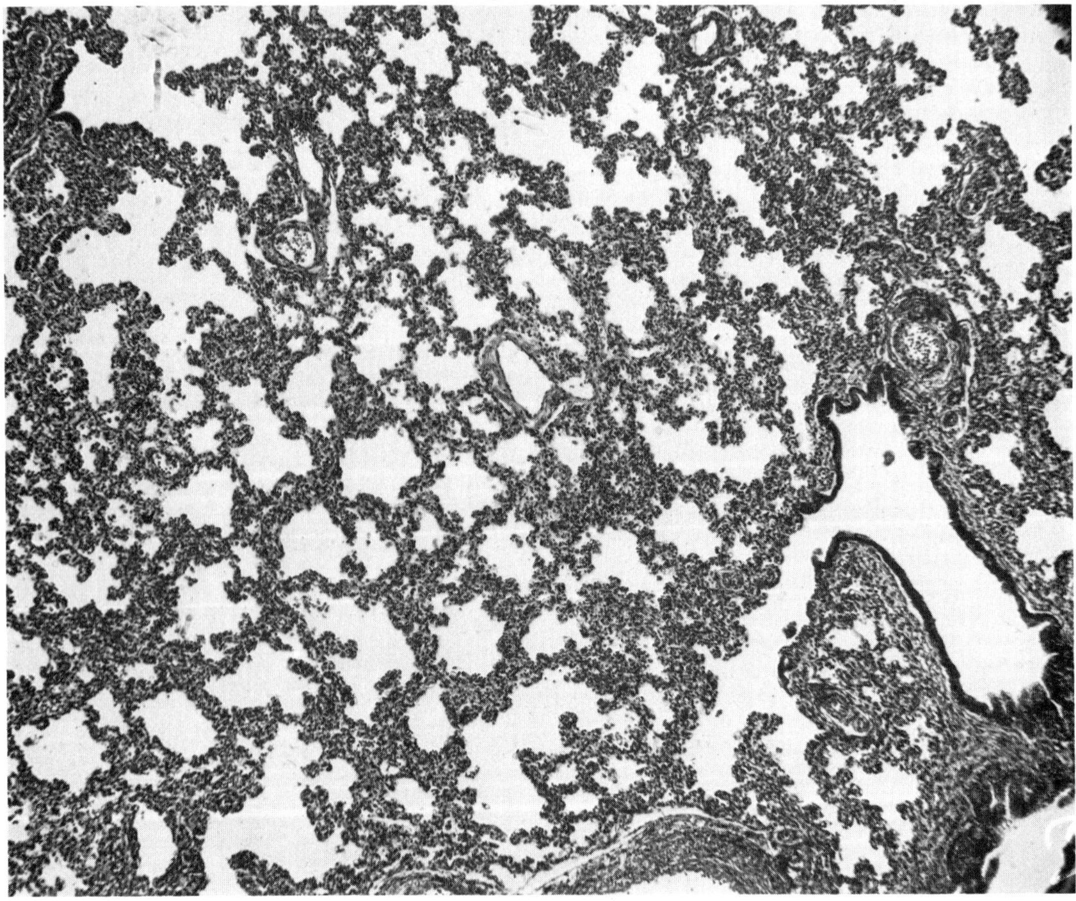

Figure 21-25b

334

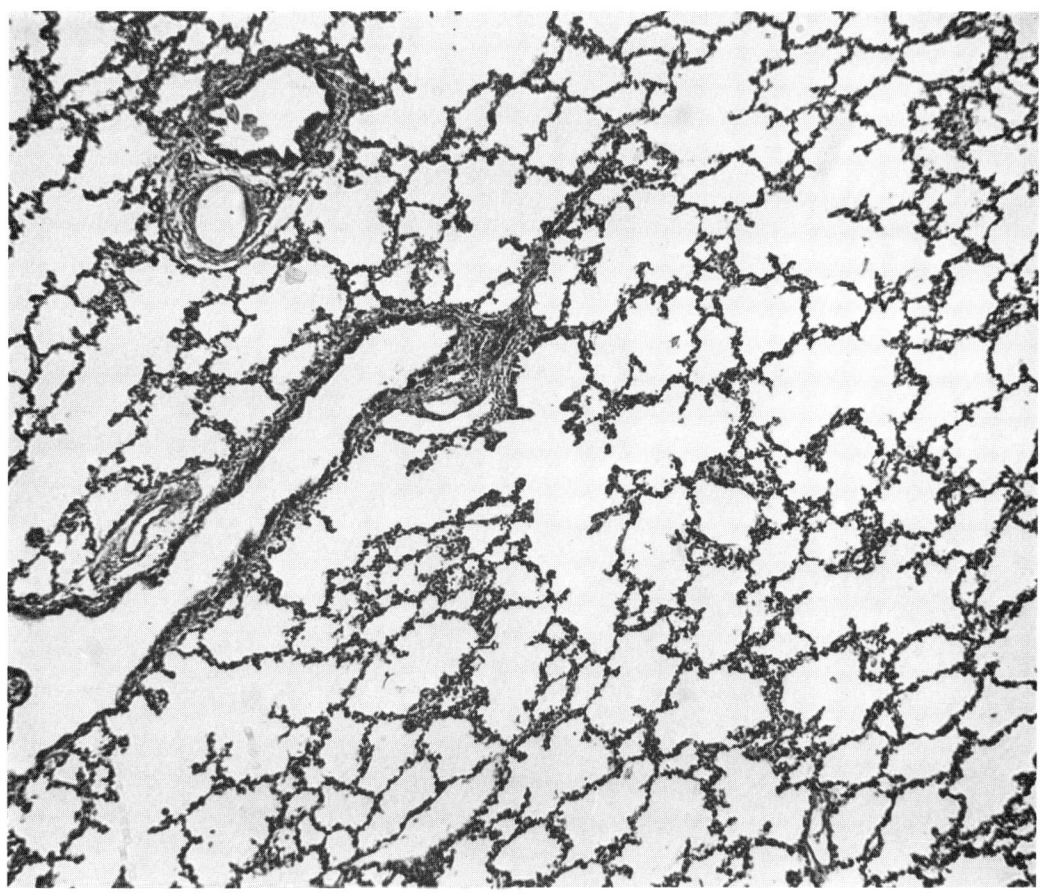

Figure 21–25c

Figure 21–25. All three of these photographs were taken at the same low or survey magnification, and illustrate the range of normal histology among the lungs of infants born at term. All are derived from sections taken at autopsy; the differences in state of expansion are artifactual. The impression derived is that alveolar walls vary considerably in thickness, whereas, in fact, that appearance is predominantly a reflection of their elasticity (or contractility) in the face of a variety of states of aeration or collapse.

Hematoxylin and eosin stain. Mag. 76×.

Fig.	Weight	Race	Sex	Gestation	Age
21–25a	2,850 gm.	W	M	?	4 hr.
21–25b	3,850 gm.	W	M	40 wk.	3 wk.
21–25c	2,850 gm.	B	F	40 wk.	1 hr. 20 min.

Figures 21–26, 21–27, and 21–28. This set of three photomicrographs depicts the shape of the alveolar ducts, alveolar sacs, and alveoli as they appear at autopsy when the infant has died with normal respiratory activity, as opposed to their appearance following artificial respiration, accomplished during the agonal period by a variety of means.

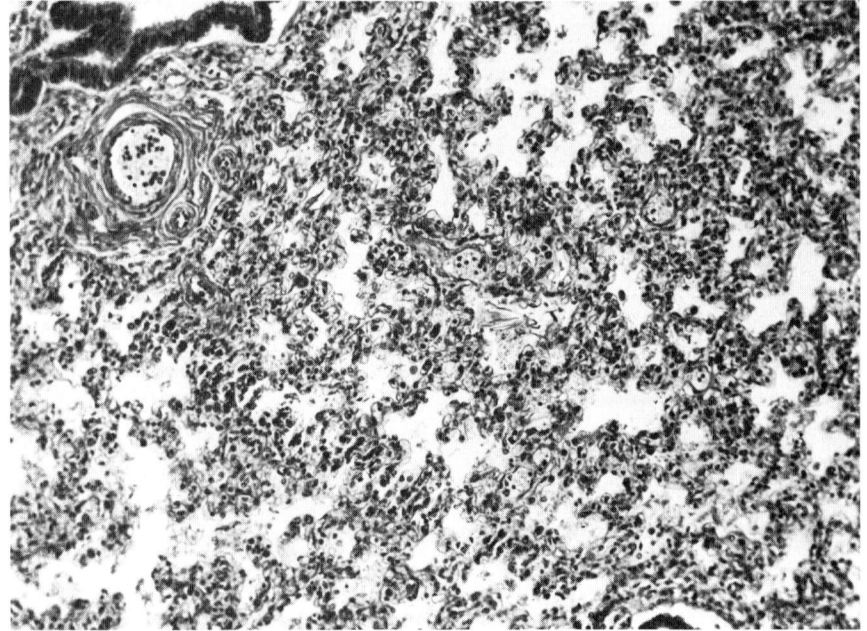

Figure 21–26

Figure 21–26. This photomicrograph shows alveoli of a near-term infant. As Dr. Edith Potter has described them, they have the shape of crumpled paper bags.

This section is from a 4 hour old white male infant who weighed 2,850 grams at autopsy. Hematoxylin and eosin stain. Mag. 142×.

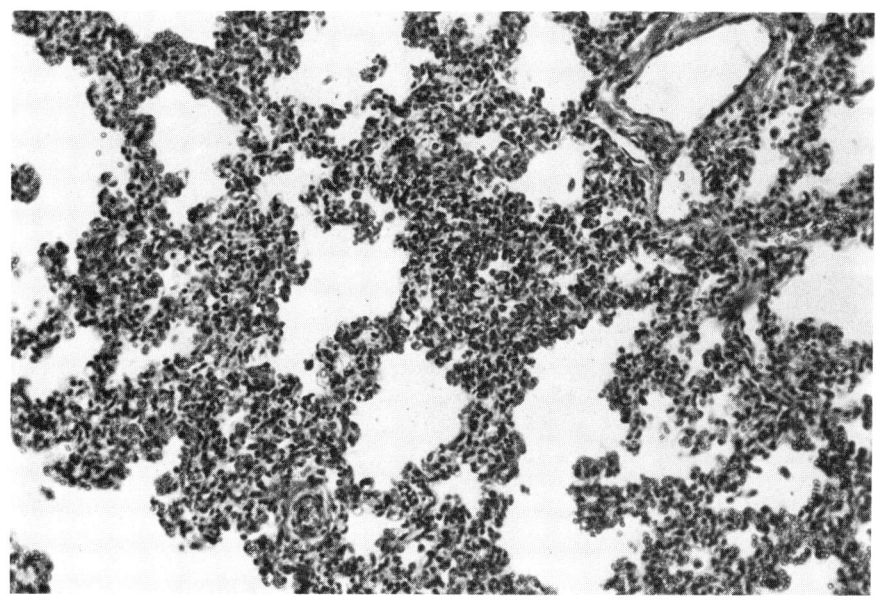

Figure 21-27

Figure 21-27. Here, at higher magnification, is essentially the same sort of pattern. Alveolar walls are irregularly infolded.

This is from a 3 week old white male infant, born at 40 weeks of gestation, who weighed 3,850 grams at autopsy.

Hematoxylin and eosin stain. Mag. 142×.

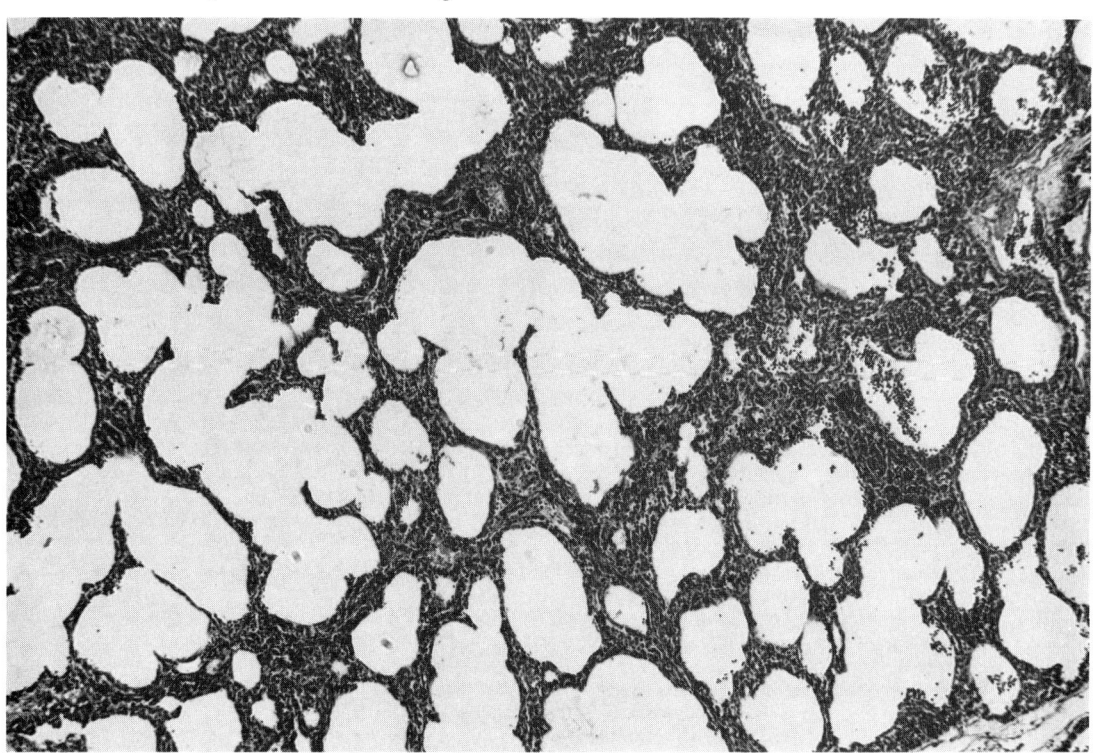

Figure 21-28

Figure 21-28. Seen here at half the magnification of Fig. 21-27 is the lung of an infant, born prematurely, to whom artificial respiration was administered just before death. The shape of the alveoli and alveolar ducts is totally abnormal; with tree-like branching, they are blown up like balloons. Each air space has perfectly regular, sharp, evenly rounded edges. This is typical of the history of air administered under pressure just prior to death.

This patient was a white male born at 7 months of gestation, whose body weight at autopsy was 1,115 grams. He lived for 11 days.

Hematoxylin and eosin stain. Mag. 76×.

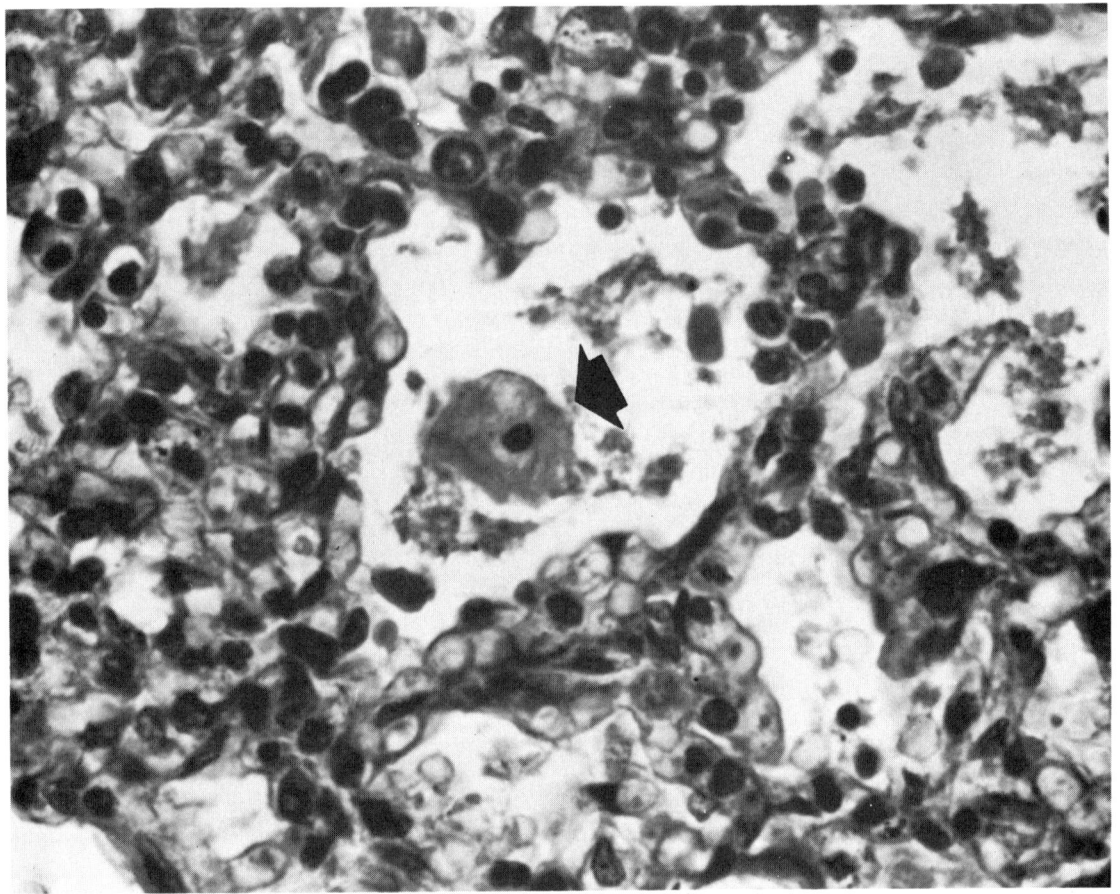

Figure 21–29a

Figure 21–29. Apparently normal infants, at birth, exhibit a few widely scattered, adult-type keratinized stratified squamous epithelial cells within alveolar lumina. These cells are initially suspended in the amniotic fluid, having been sloughed off of the surface of the infant's skin. When the cells are seen laid out flat (which is rare), as in Fig. 21–29a, they appear large and pavement-like, with bright pink-staining relatively homogeneous cytoplasm.

More often, however, they are sectioned on edge and are thus darkly stained, slender, sharply demarcated linear structures as in Fig. 21–29b.

When infants are born following episodes of intrauterine hypoxia, especially if protracted, their lungs show much more marked aspiration of squamae than is seen here, a situation which is, of course, pathologic.

Figure 21–29a is from a 4 hour old white male infant, who weighed 2,850 grams at autopsy.

Fig. 21–29b is from a 9 day old white female, born at 40 weeks of gestation, whose body at postmortem examination weighed 2,420 grams.

Hematoxylin and eosin stain. Mag. 660×.

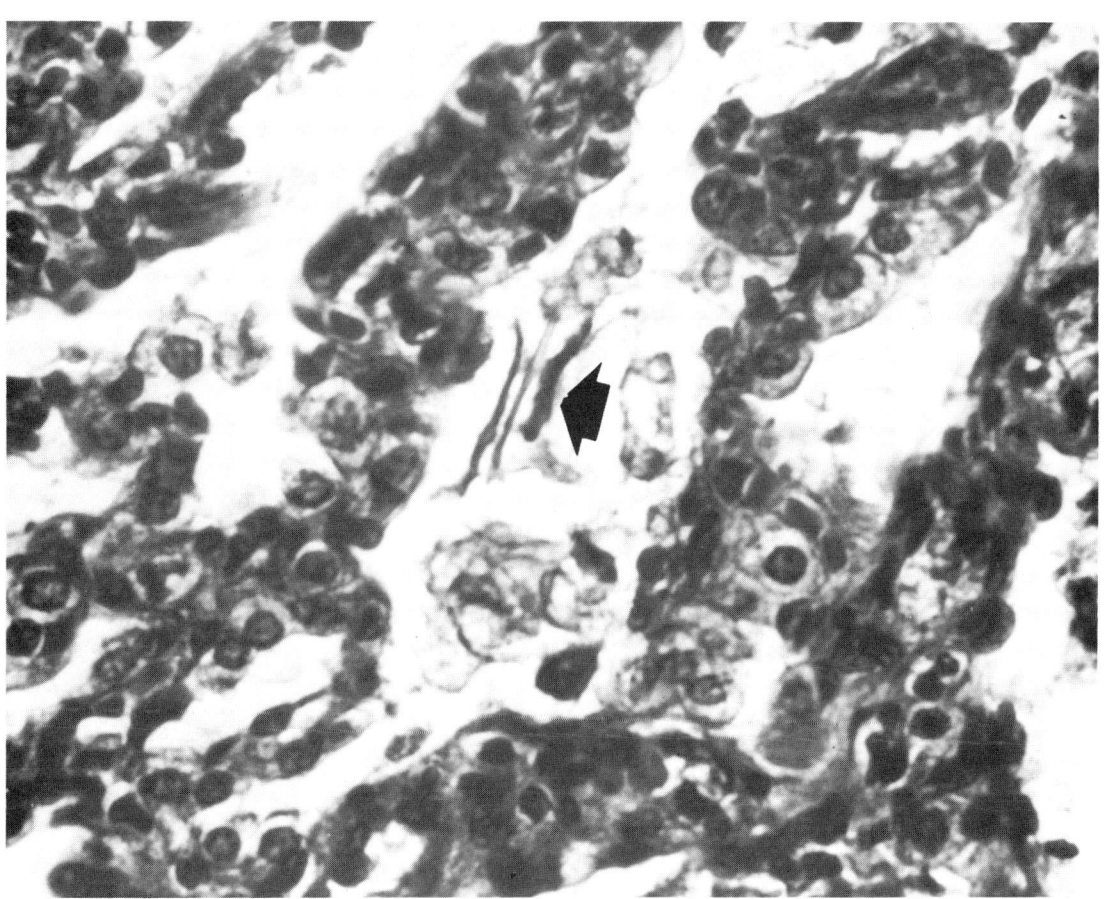

Figure 21-29b

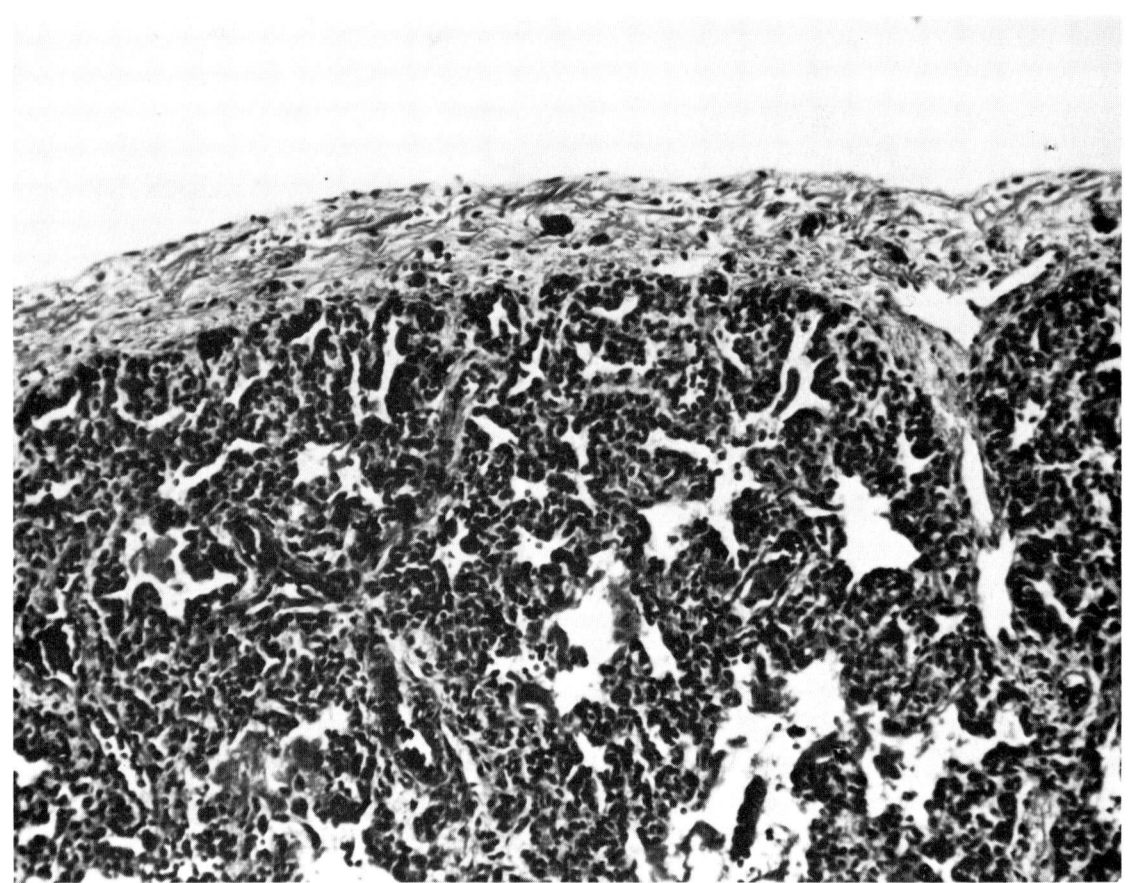

Figure 21-30

Figure 21-30. The visceral pleura is depicted in this illustration. It consists of multiple layers of collagenous connective tissue covered on the surface by a single layer of squamoid mesothelial cells, best observed in the left upper corner of the photograph.

The visceral pleura bears many small blood vessels and lymphatics, one of which appears on the right.

This section is from a 2,760 gram white female infant who died at the age of 34 hours. Hematoxylin and eosin stain. Mag. 382×.

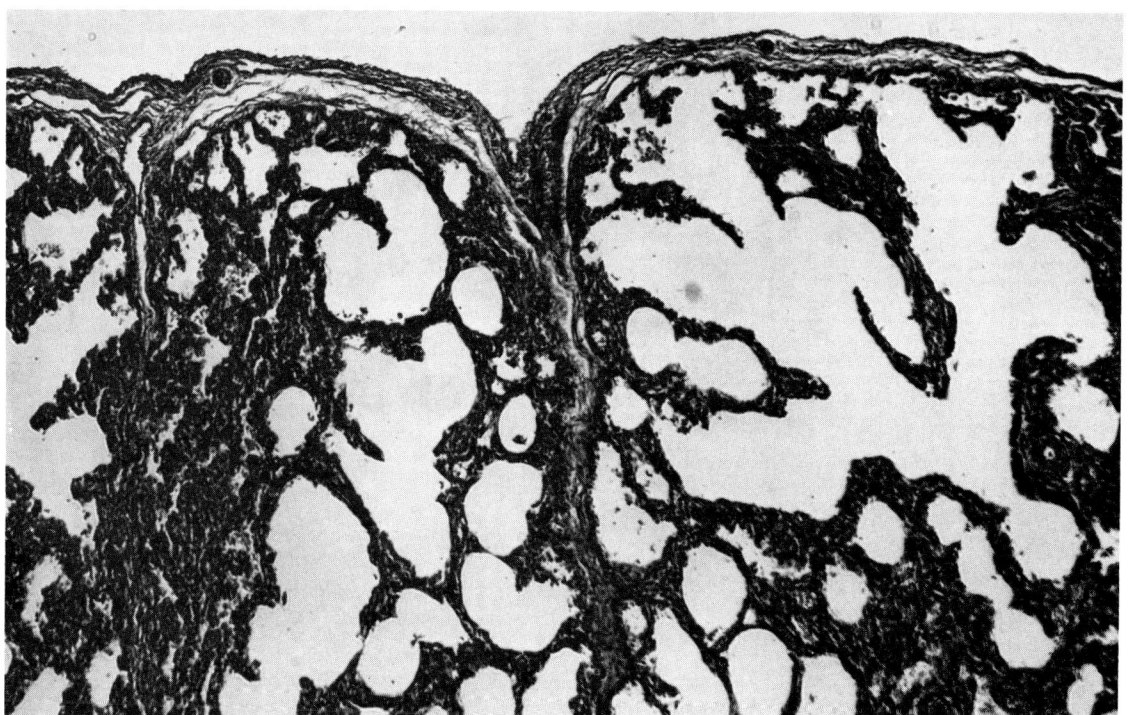

Figure 21–31

Figure 21–31. This photomicrograph illustrates the junction of an interlobular septum with the visceral pleura.

The distinctive pattern for the distribution of air in this section is the result of forceful artificial aeration, probably administered terminally, which "blows out" or overexpands alveolar ducts and alveoli.

This section is from a five day old black male whose body weight at autopsy was 2,075 grams. Hematoxylin and eosin stain. Mag. 60×.

Part 8
URINARY SYSTEM

Chapter 22

KIDNEY

EMBRYOLOGY

There is probably no organ in the human that better illustrates the recapitulation of phylogeny than the kidney. In the embryo it evolves by way of three sequential phases — in position and in time — from the pronephros, or "head kidney," caudally, through the mesonephros, or "middle kidney," to the metanephros or ultimate kidney. The vestigial, functionless "head kidney" appears at the junction of the future neck and upper thorax; it develops and degenerates by the time the embryo has attained a length of only 5 mm. From one month to two months of gestation the "middle kidney" predominates; it disappears at approximately the end of the fourth month. The development and function of the definitive or permanent kidney overlap those of the mesonephros; the metanephric primordium appears in the embryo of 5 mm. (at the stage of complete disappearance of the pronephros). Differentiation of new tubules within the metanephros is complete at about the eighth month of gestation.

The pronephros consists of several matched pairs of primitive tubules, which arise as dorsolateral sprouts from a longitudinally oriented nephrogenic cord located dorsally and a bit lateral to the midline on each side. Although the cord hollows out to become an excretory duct, the tubules never join it.

After the tubules disappear, the excretory duct persists, finally reaching caudally to the cloaca and perforating that structure.

The *metanephros*, unlike the pronephros, is at least temporarily an excreting organ; this obtains for the human until about the tenth week. Like the pronephros, it is made up of a series of tubules which at their distal extremities open into the same longitudinally oriented common excretory duct; from this point forward in time it is known as the mesonephric or Wolffian duct. These tubules differ, however, from those of the pronephros in that each bears an internal glomerulus that indents its proximal blind end and that filters excreta out of the blood and into the tubule. As the developing tubules enlarge and elongate they create, in aggregate, an elongate ventrolateral bulge into the coelom on each side of the dorsal midline, the mesonephric ridge. The glomeruli form a medial column in the gland; the common excretory duct is laterally situated, and the tubules are between the two. Branches from the aorta supply the glomeruli.

After the end of the first month of gestation, the more cranial mesonephric tubules degenerate and disappear in sequence as new tubules appear at the caudal end of the ridge; thus, the upper five-sixths is lost by the end of the second month.

As is true of the mesonephros, the more caudally placed metanephros consists of an aggregate of tubules that drain into a common excretory duct on each side. The more complex system of drainage ducts, however, comprising the ureter, pelvis, calyces, papillary ducts, and straight collecting tubules, develops as a bud growing out of the common excretory mesonephric duct. Each secretory unit or nephron arises, as do the pronephric and mesonephric tubules, from the nephrogenic cord; each consists of Bowman's capsules, the convuluted tubules, and the loop of Henle. The proximal secretory and distal collecting tubules unite secondarily.[1]

The ureteric duct arises dorsally as a hollow bud or diverticulum from the mesonephric duct in the embryo of about four weeks. It pushes cranially into the most caudal part of the metanephrogenic mass. That mass soon embraces the dilated pelvic upper end of the ureteric duct. The ureteric pelvis flattens and bifurcates, and then sends out secondary and tertiary branches into the metanephrogenic mass. Branching is repeated radially until, at five months, some twelve generations of collecting tubules have been developed; the branching proceeds but little thereafter. At completion of the process there are about nine minor calyces, into each of which up to 25 papillary ducts enter; these have been referred to as the "trunks of the tubular trees" (Figs. 22–1 and 22–2). Ultimately, each of the nine or so papillae serves as a common outlet for several pyramids.

Early on, the simple metanephric cap is composed of a deep section comprising the nephrons and an external loose layer destined to become the interstitial connective tissue and the capsule.

As the primitive ureteric pelvis branches, the metanephric cap responds by dividing into a corresponding number of masses, one lump embracing the end of each pelvic subdivision. As new orders of collecting tubules arise, each cap enlarges and subdivides.

Finally, the renal cortex is composed of two kinds of structures, the medullary rays, or upward extensions of the collecting tubules (Fig. 22–10), and the labyrinth of secretory tubules derived from the metanephros (Fig. 22–8).

ANATOMY

The kidneys of the human, which arise quite caudally as the bilateral metanephros, come to lie much more cranially as the embryo develops. Much of this apparent migration is attributed to straightening of the body curvature combined with marked growth of the lumbosacral region. By eight weeks of gestation the growing kidneys have met the caudally migrating adrenal glands.

As the kidneys rise out of the pelvis, they also rotate 90 degrees, so that the original dorsal border is finally the lateral border and the hilus faces medially rather than ventrally.

As the cortex differentiates, that portion which caps each pyramid becomes divided from neighboring caps by a deep groove. Later, as the pyramids divide, there is an increase in the number of caps or lobes. This division of lobes creates the pattern, so familiar in the fetal and neonatal kidney, known as *fetal lobulation*. The number of individual lobes may reach a maximum of 20 in the newborn. Within each lobe there are lobules, each of which contains all of the tubules belonging to one particular medullary ray (Fig. 22–8).

The fetal kidney is capable of secretion early in the third fetal month.[1]

HISTOLOGY

From the sixteenth week of gestation, the kidney is clearly divided into cortical and medullary portions, which are clearly delimited (Figs. 22–1 to 22–8). Early on, the cortex is relatively thin (Fig. 22–1) and there are few recognizable glomeruli between the capsule and the base of the pyramid. In time, the number of glomeruli in any such cortical lobule increases as new glomeruli are added in the nephrogenic zone just beneath the capsule (Figs. 22–2 to 22–8). As they increase in number, so do the cortical tubules; the depth of the cortex also increases.

At every stage in this process it is apparent that the largest and most well developed glomeruli are located nearest the pyramid; conversely, the most immature are nearest the nephrogenic zone (Figs. 22–11 to 22–14).

Throughout this period there is very little visible supporting connective tissue in the cortex, and only slightly more than that in the medulla and medullary rays (Fig. 22–10).

In the fetus of 22 weeks gestation, the nephrogenic zone appears as a subcapsular, very cellular, compact layer of darkly stained and rather S-shaped structures (Fig. 22–15). At 27 weeks (Fig. 22–16) it is still quite prominent. At 37 weeks, however (Fig. 22–17), it is no longer present.

Those glomeruli which are deep in the cortex and adjacent to the bases of pyramids are not fully matured in the fetus of 22 weeks (Fig. 22–15). The most peripherally placed nuclei are intensely stained and have an almost cuboidal appearance. This impression is retained in the fetus of 27 weeks (Fig. 22–16) but has almost completely vanished by 37 weeks (Fig. 22–17).

The character of the convoluted tubules and the loops of Henle changes little from 24 to 36 weeks of gestation (Figs. 22–20 and 22–21).

In the normal newborn infant, and even in the premature, scattered individual glomeruli will be partly or completely sclerotic. This apparently has no particular functional clinical significance, and its cause is unknown. One such glomerulus appears in Figure 22–22.

The juxtaglomerular apparatus is not easily identified in routine sections of the neonatal kidney. It is depicted here, however, in a section from the kidney of a six year old boy (Fig. 22–23).

The *urinary pole* of Bowman's capsule in a newborn appears in Figure 22–24. Here the cavity or Bowman's space is continuous with the lumen of the next segment of the nephron, the proximal tubule.

In Figures 22–25 and 22–26 are seen the prominent, pale-staining epithelial cells lining the collecting tubules. In each pair the upper illustration represents the tubule at its inception, high in the pyramid, close to the junction of cortex and medulla; the lower illustration is of the most distal segment, near the very apex of the pyramid. The epithelial cells are cuboidal and very distinctly outlined. They have darkly staining round nuclei and clear cytoplasm.

In Figures 22–27 and 22–28, the large straight tubules or papillary ducts of Bellini are illustrated as they open on the area cribrosa at the apex of the papilla. The epithelium lining these intrarenal excretory ducts is quite different from that of the various other parts of the nephron (see Figs. 22–25 and 22–26).

In Figure 22–29, the epithelial clothing of the tip of the pyramid is shown in detail. The individual cells are rather tall and the nuclei are staggered.

In Figure 22–30, the epithelium covering the pyramid appears above the calyceal space and that lining the remainder of the calyx, which at least here appears to be somewhat thicker. The breadth of the calyx is seen, at somewhat lower magnification, in Figure 22–31; this is from a term infant.

The wall of the ureter is very thin in the newborn, and particularly so in the immature baby. Note the isolated and rather sparse smooth muscle bundles deep in the wall in Figure 22–32. The inner surface is lined with a mucous membrane of transitional epithelium; there is no apparent submucosa.[2]

References

1. Arey, L. B.: Developmental Anatomy. A Textbook and Laboratory Manual of Embryology. Philadelphia, W. B. Saunders Co., 1974, pp. 295–307.
2. Bloom, W., and Fawcett, D. W.: A Textbook of Histology, 10th ed. Philadelphia, W. B. Saunders Co., 1975, pp. 766–799.

Figures 22-1 through 22-8. This set of eight matched photomicrographs depicts the gradual change in the morphology of the cortex of the kidney during the latter half of gestation, beginning with that of a fetus of 16 weeks (Fig. 22-1) and ending with that of an infant born at term (Fig. 22-8).

Note the steady increase in depth of the cortex and the increasing numbers of generations of glomeruli.

Hematoxylin and eosin stain. Mag. 45×.

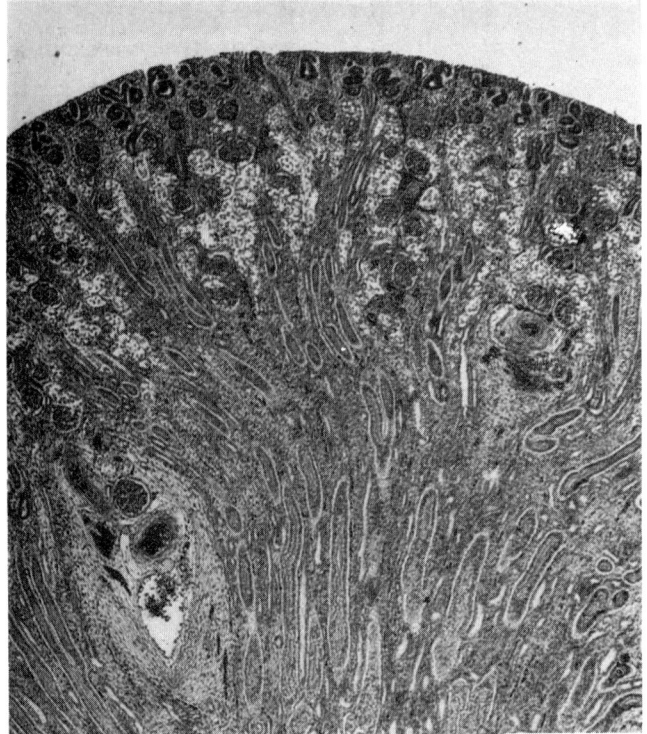

Figure 22-1. Cortex and pyramid of the kidney of a 250 gram fetus, the product of a 16 week gestation, who lived for one hour.

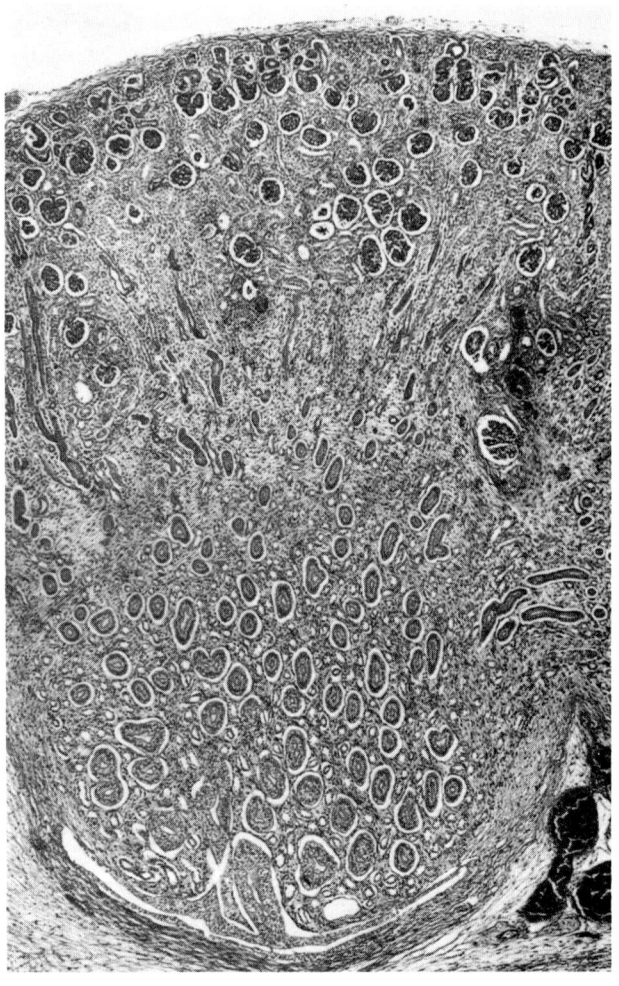

Figure 22-2. Cortex and pyramid of a 320 gram fetus, the product of a 16 week gestation, who was stillborn.

Figure 22–3. Cortex and pyramid of a 450 gram fetus, born at 23–25 weeks of gestation, who lived for 48 hours.

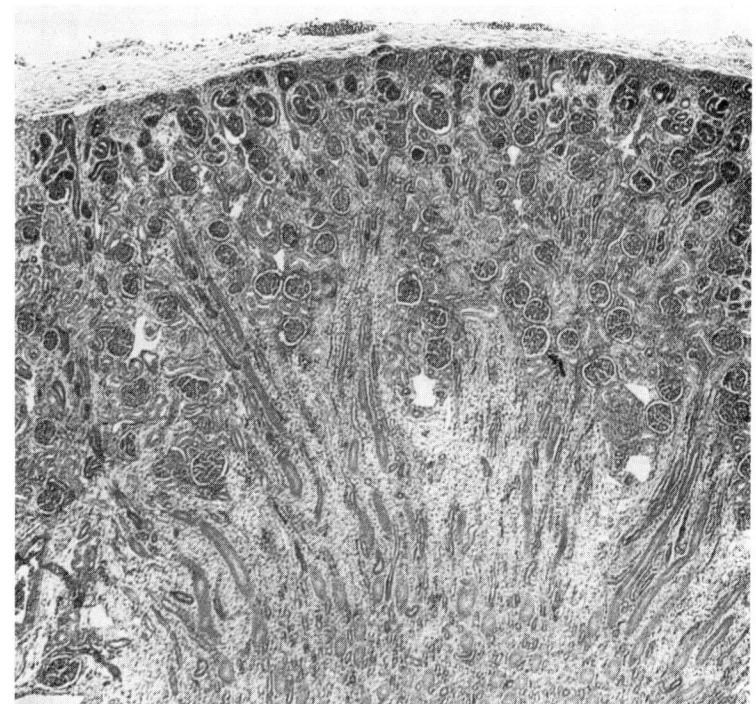

Figure 22–3

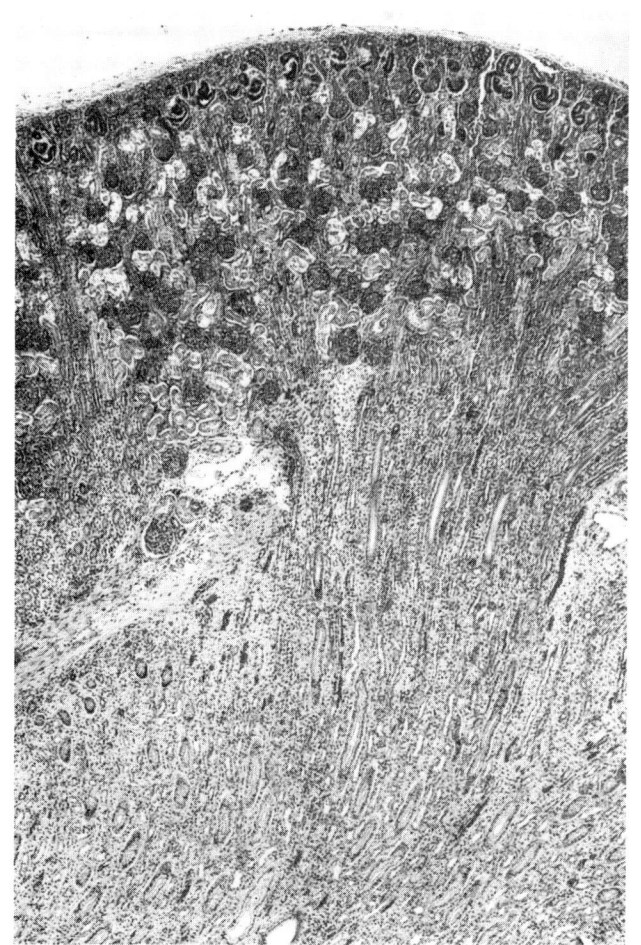

Figure 22–4

Figure 22–4. Cortex and pyramid of a 520 gram fetus, born after 24 weeks of gestation, who survived for 4½ hours.

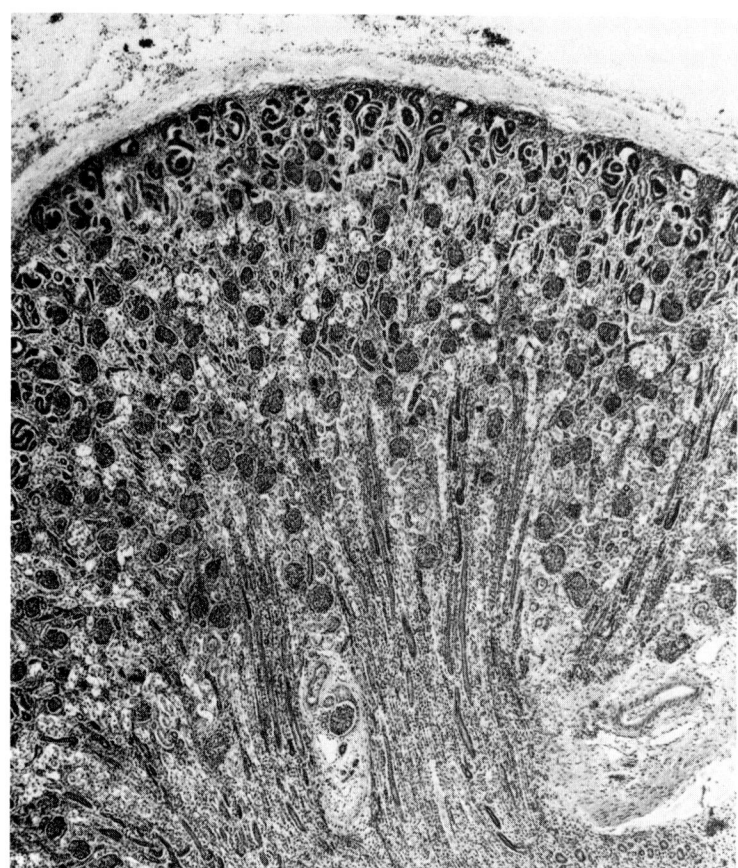

Figure 22–5

Figure 22–5. Cortex of the kidney of a male infant born at 27 weeks of gestation, who lived for 45 hours.

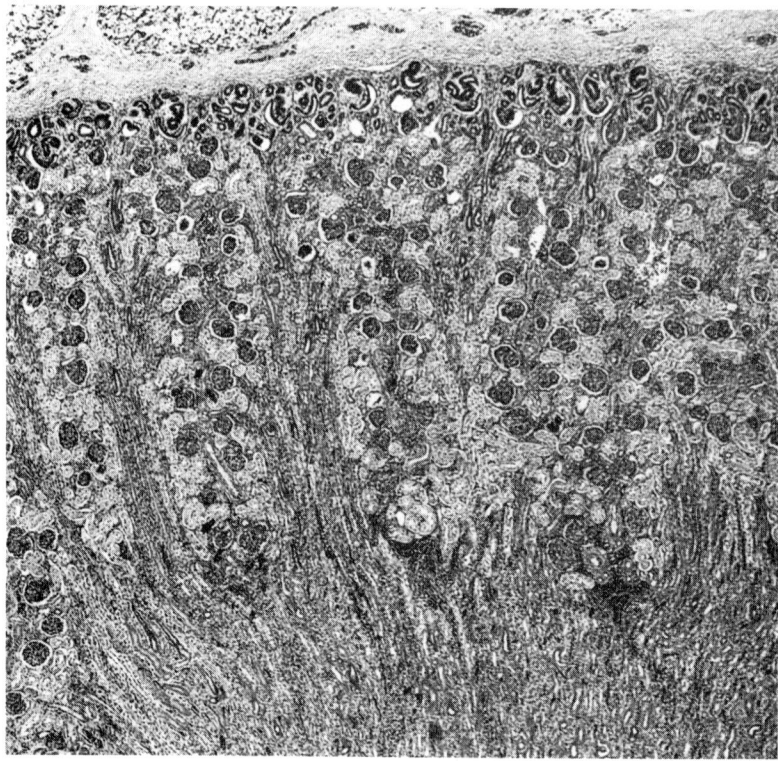

Figure 22–6. Cortex and a bit of the base of a pyramid of the kidney of a 1,300 gram infant, the product of a 28 week gestation, who survived for 48 hours.

Figure 22–6

KIDNEY

Figure 22-7. The cortex and some of the base of a pyramid of a 2,500 gram infant born at 37 weeks of gestation, who lived for 30 days.

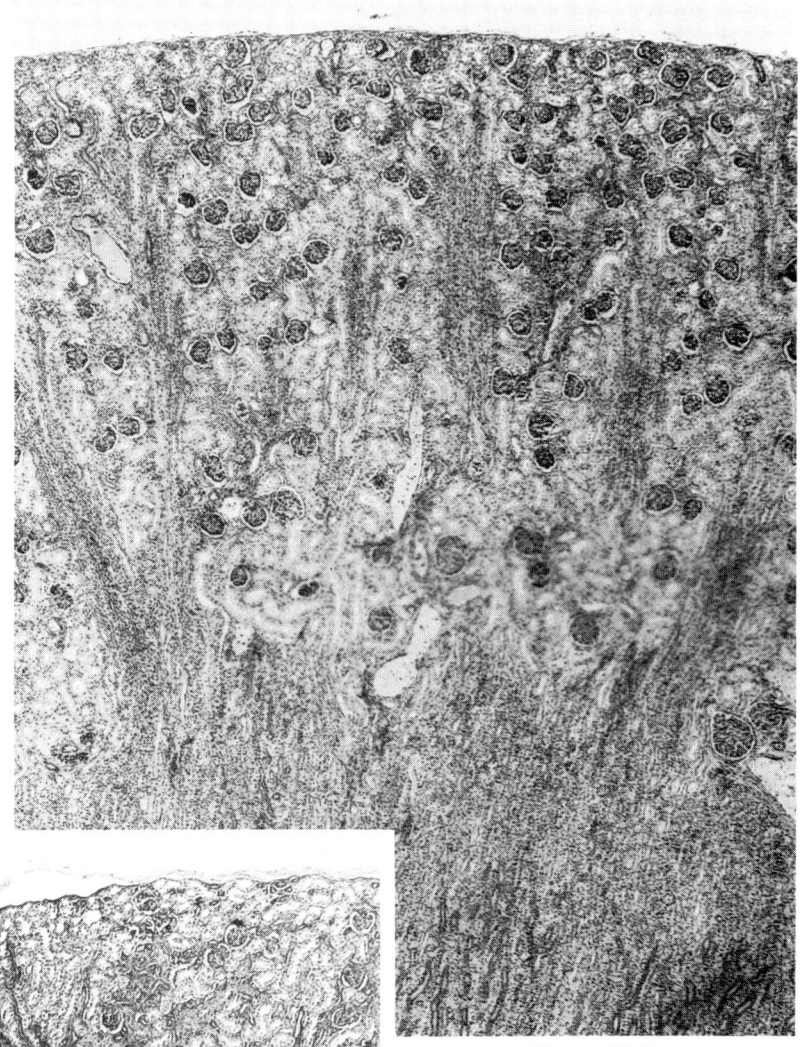

Figure 22-7

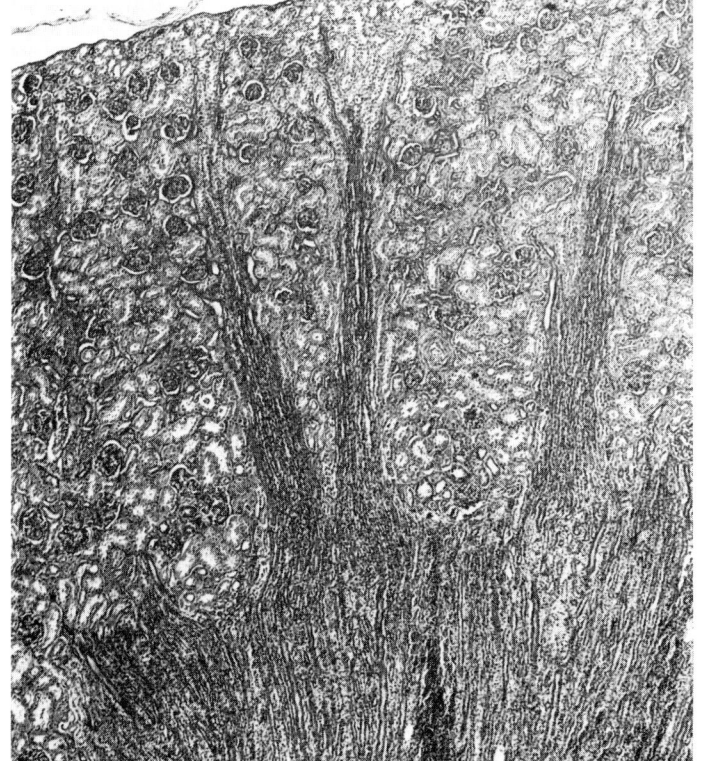

Figure 22-8. Cortex and base of a pyramid of the kidney of an infant born at term, who lived for 11 hours. His body at autopsy weighed 3,197 grams.

Figure 22-8

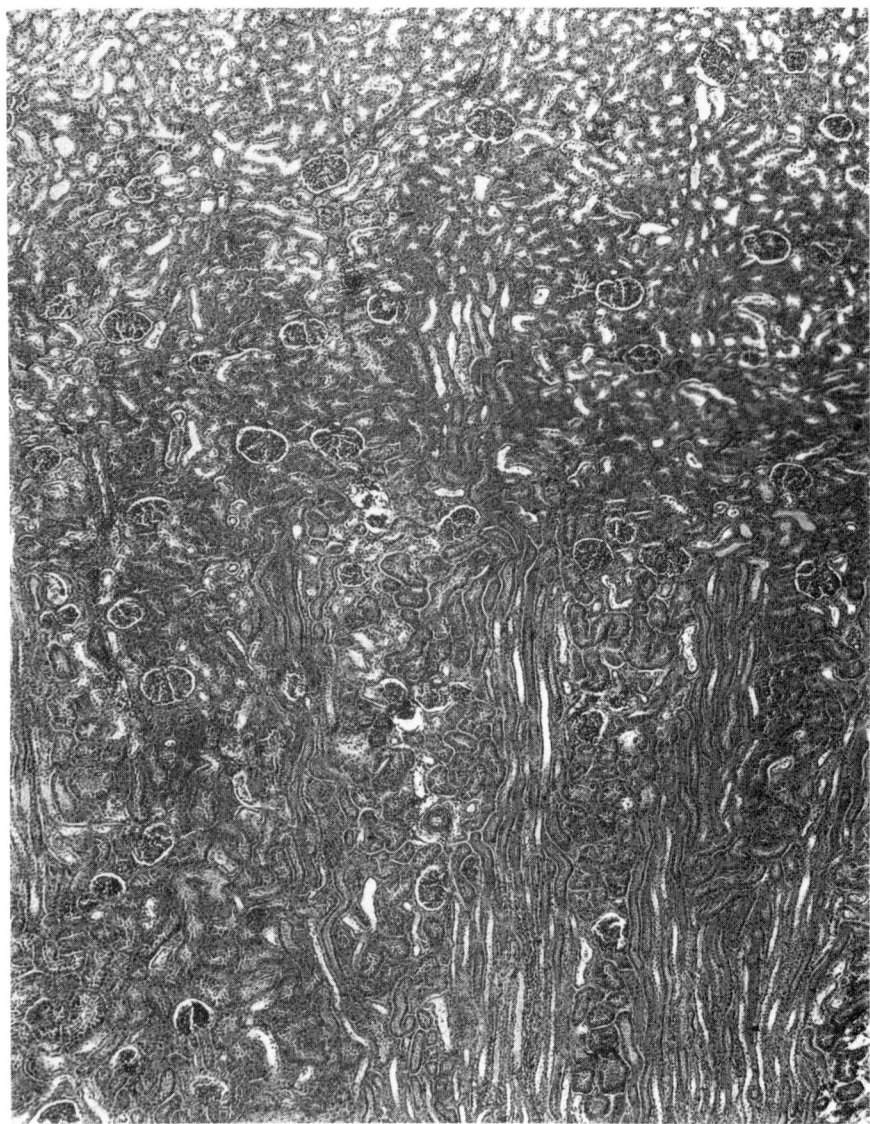

Figure 22-9

Figure 22-9. By contrast with Fig. 22-1 through 22-8, we see here, at the same magnification, the cortex of the kidney of a 19 month old infant. Note the complete disappearance of the zone of glomerulogenesis, and also the maturity of the most superficial glomeruli.

Hematoxylin and eosin stain. Mag. 45×.

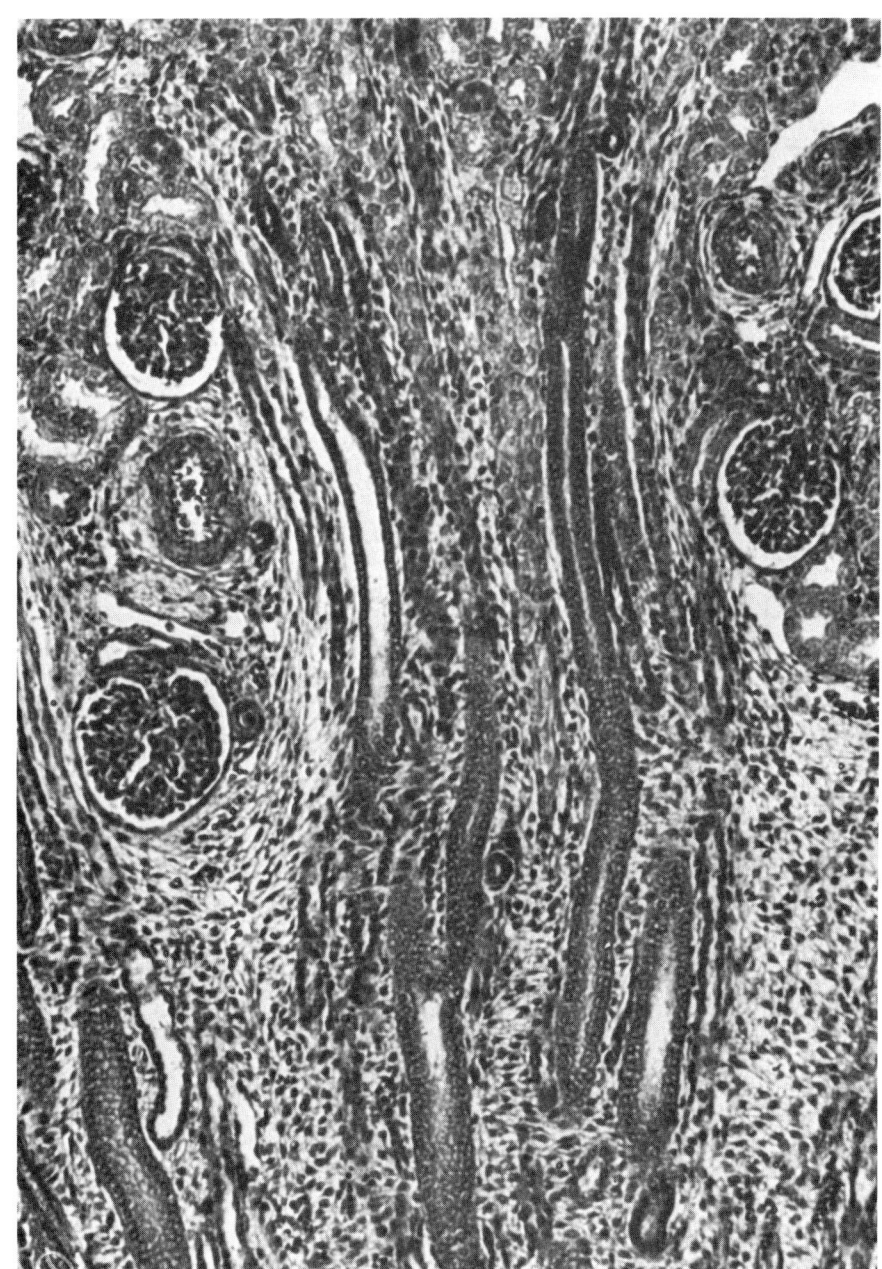

Figure 22–10

Figure 22–10. Medullary ray in an immature kidney. This patient was a 520 gram female infant, born at 24 weeks of gestation. She lived 4½ hours.
Hematoxylin and eosin stain. Mag. 200×.

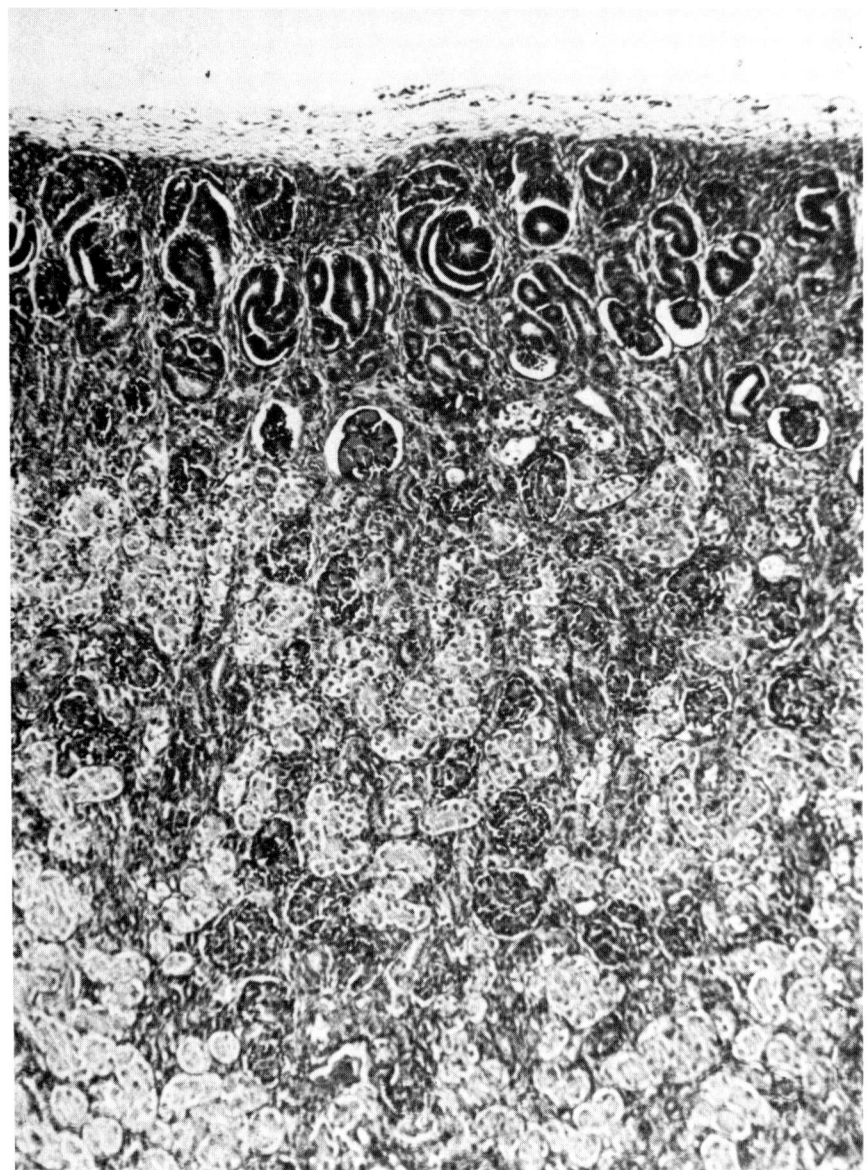

Figure 22–11

Figures 22–11 to 22–14. This series of four photomicrographs depicts the changing morphology of the cortex of the kidney, particularly that portion which lies immediately beneath the capsule, as the infant develops, from mid-gestation through the first month of extrauterine life.

Figure 22–11. The patient was a 525 gram female, the product of a 22 week gestation. Hematoxylin and eosin stain. Mag. 132×.

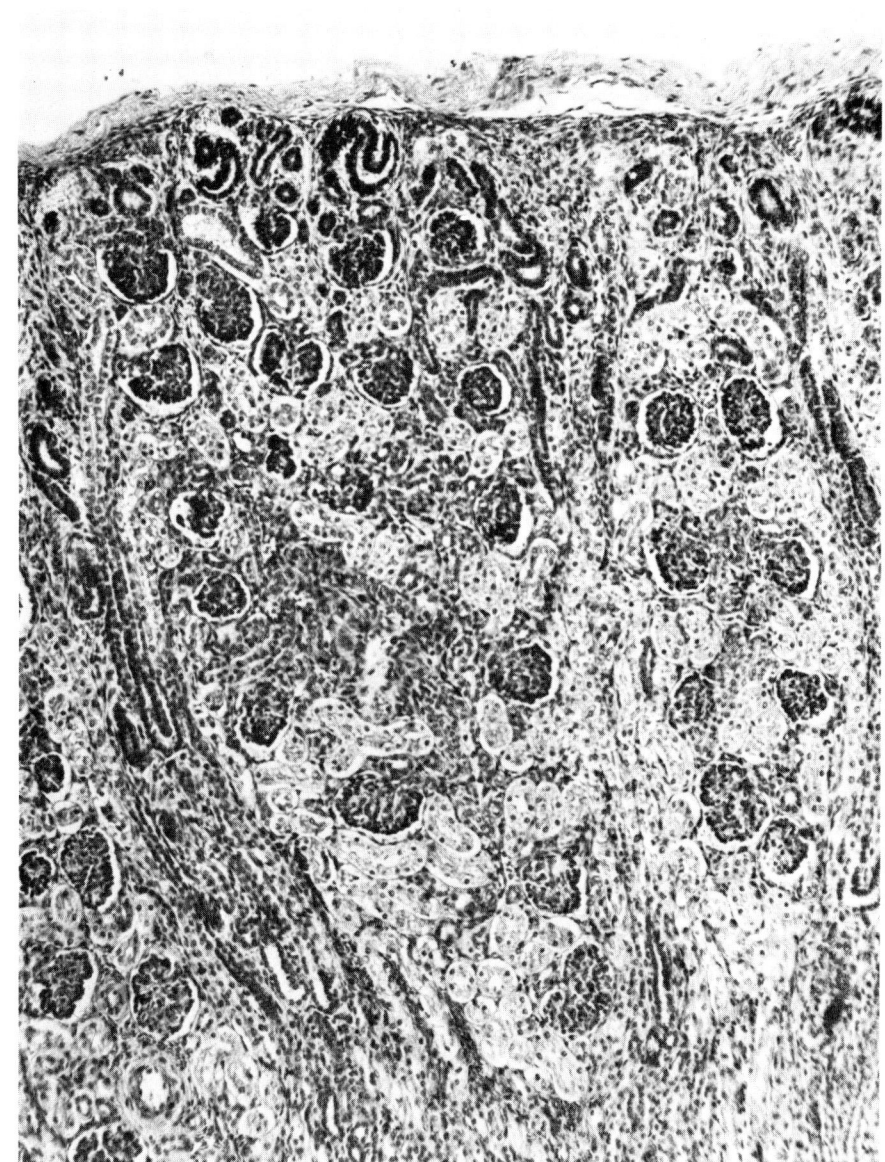

Figure 22-12

Figure 22-12. Note the considerable reduction in prominence of the nephrogenic zone as the kidney matures.

The subject was a 1,300 gram infant, born following 28 weeks of gestation; the infant survived for 48 hours.

Hematoxylin and eosin stain. Mag. 132×.

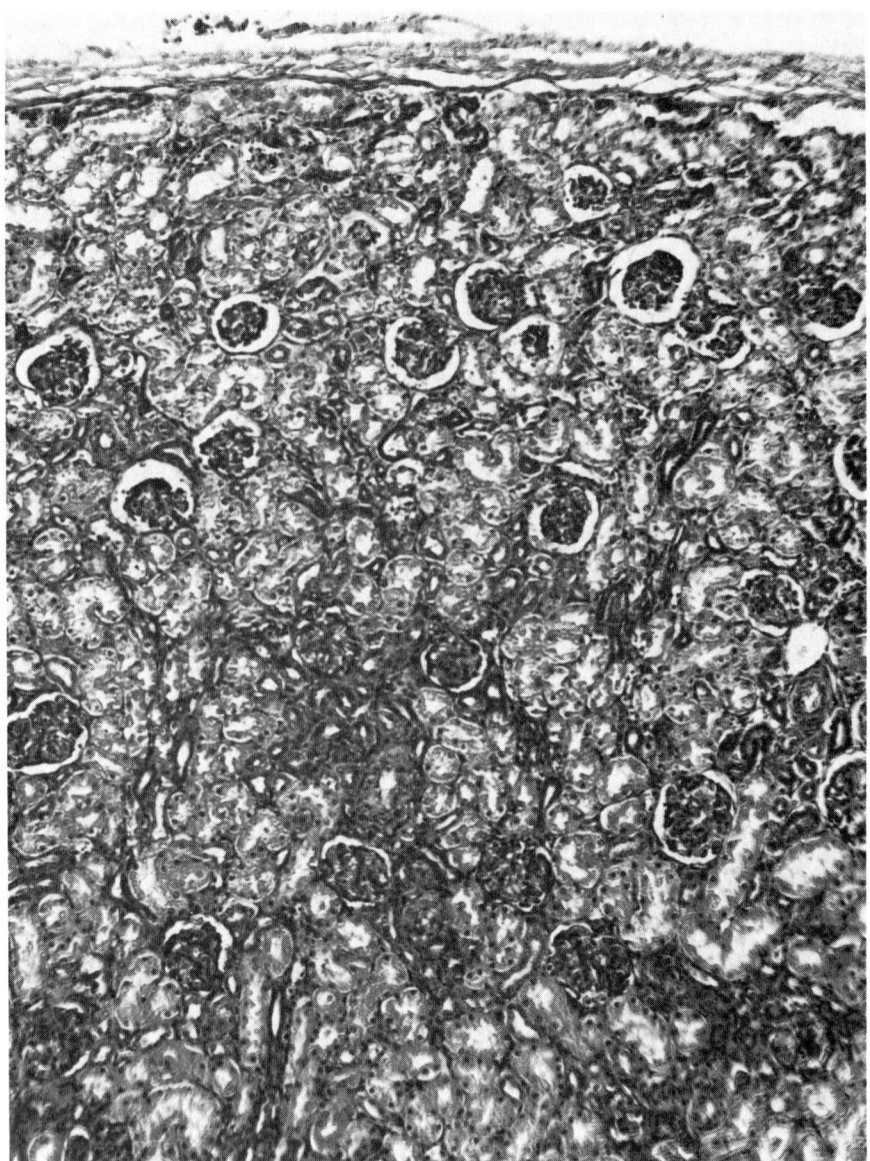

Figure 22–13

Figure 22–13. One expects the nephrogenic zone to have disappeared completely as the infant reaches term.

This infant was born at 37 weeks of gestation. Body weight at autopsy was 2,500 grams. The patient lived for 30 days.

Hematoxylin and eosin stain. Mag. 132×.

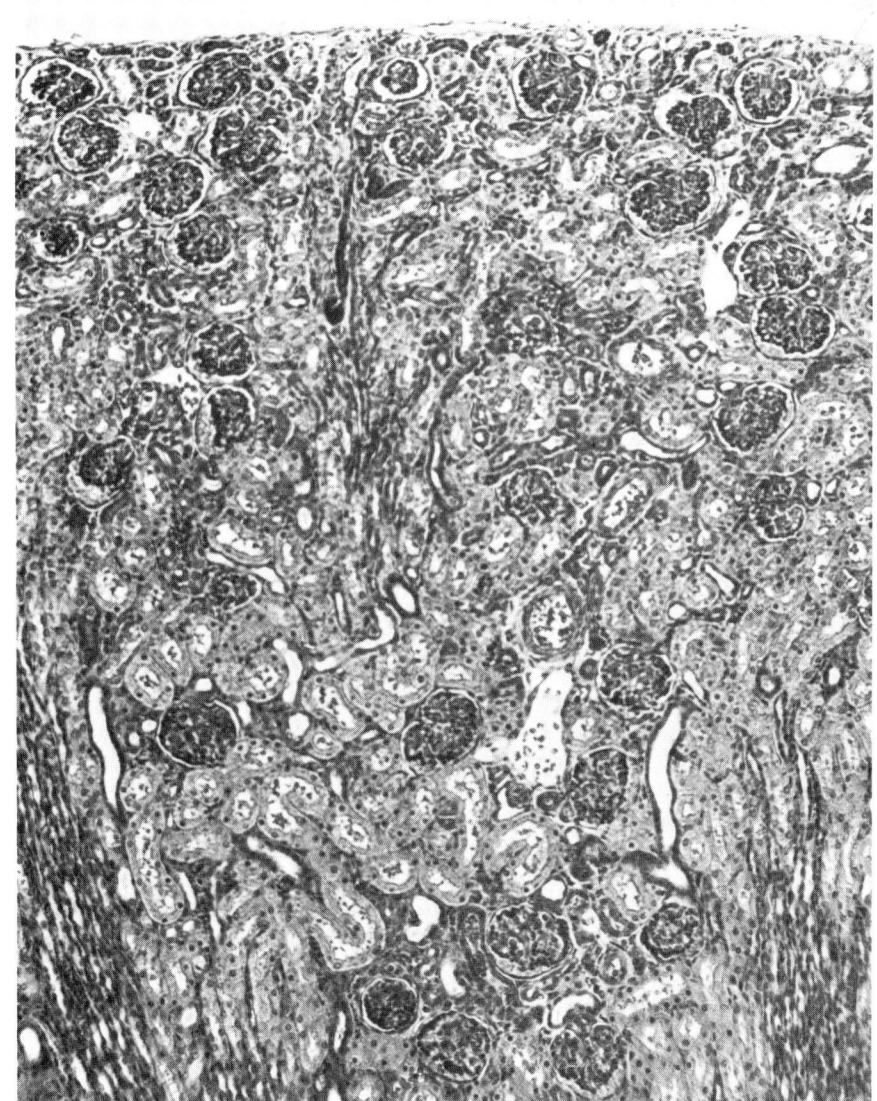

Figure 22–14

Figure 22–14. This patient, a 4,050 gram male infant, was born after 36 weeks of gestation and lived for two days.
Hematoxylin and eosin stain. Mag. 132×.

Figures 22-15 to 22-19. The paired illustrations in these figures depict, in some detail, the changing morphology of the nephrogenic zone from mid-gestation to the middle of the second year of infancy.

In each pair, the upper section represents the nephrogenic zone, and the lower section shows that portion of the cortex which is adjacent to the medulla.

Hematoxylin and eosin stain. Mag. 382×.

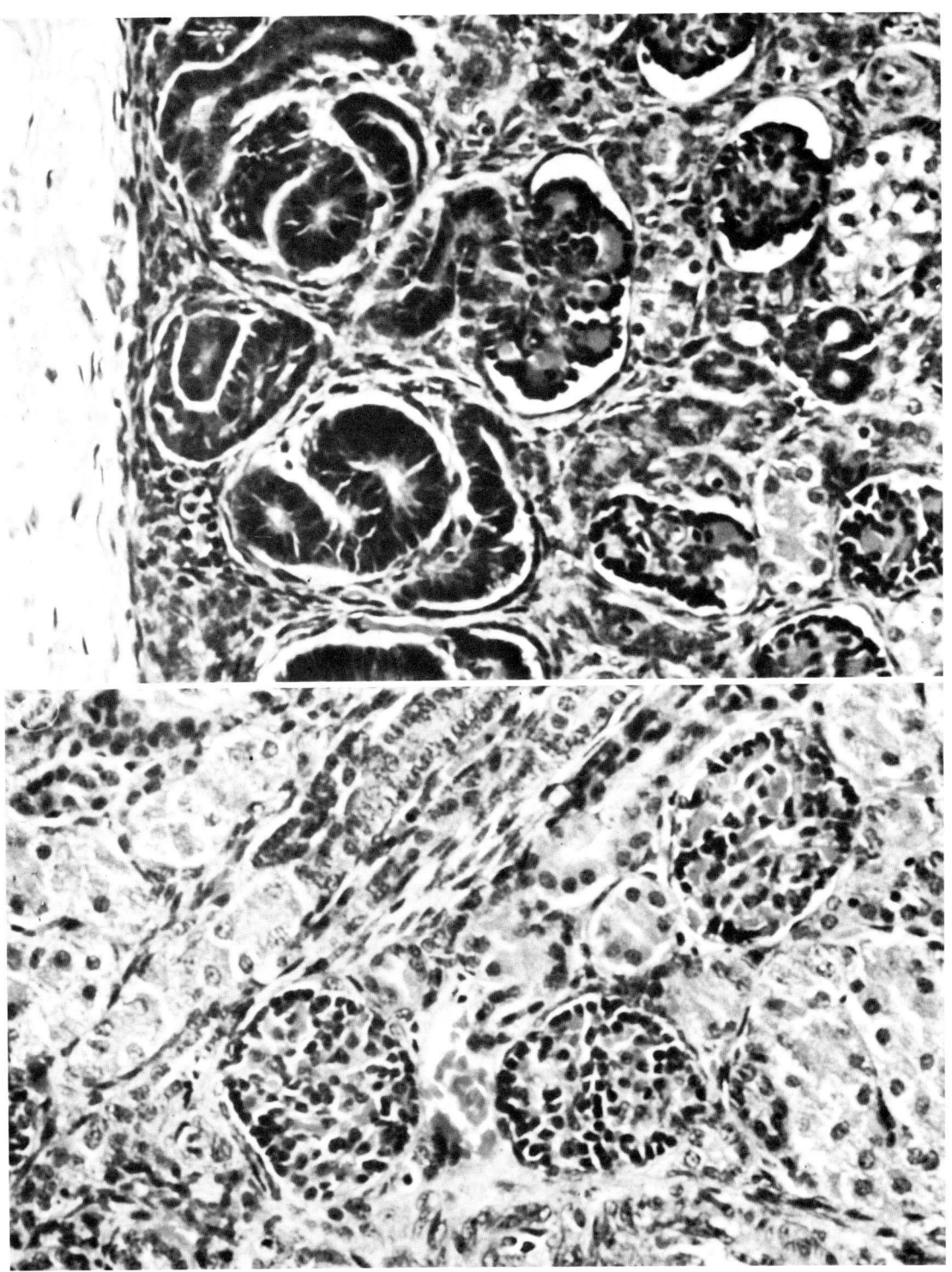

Figure 22–15. This patient was a 525 gram female infant, liveborn at 22 weeks of gestation.

362 KIDNEY

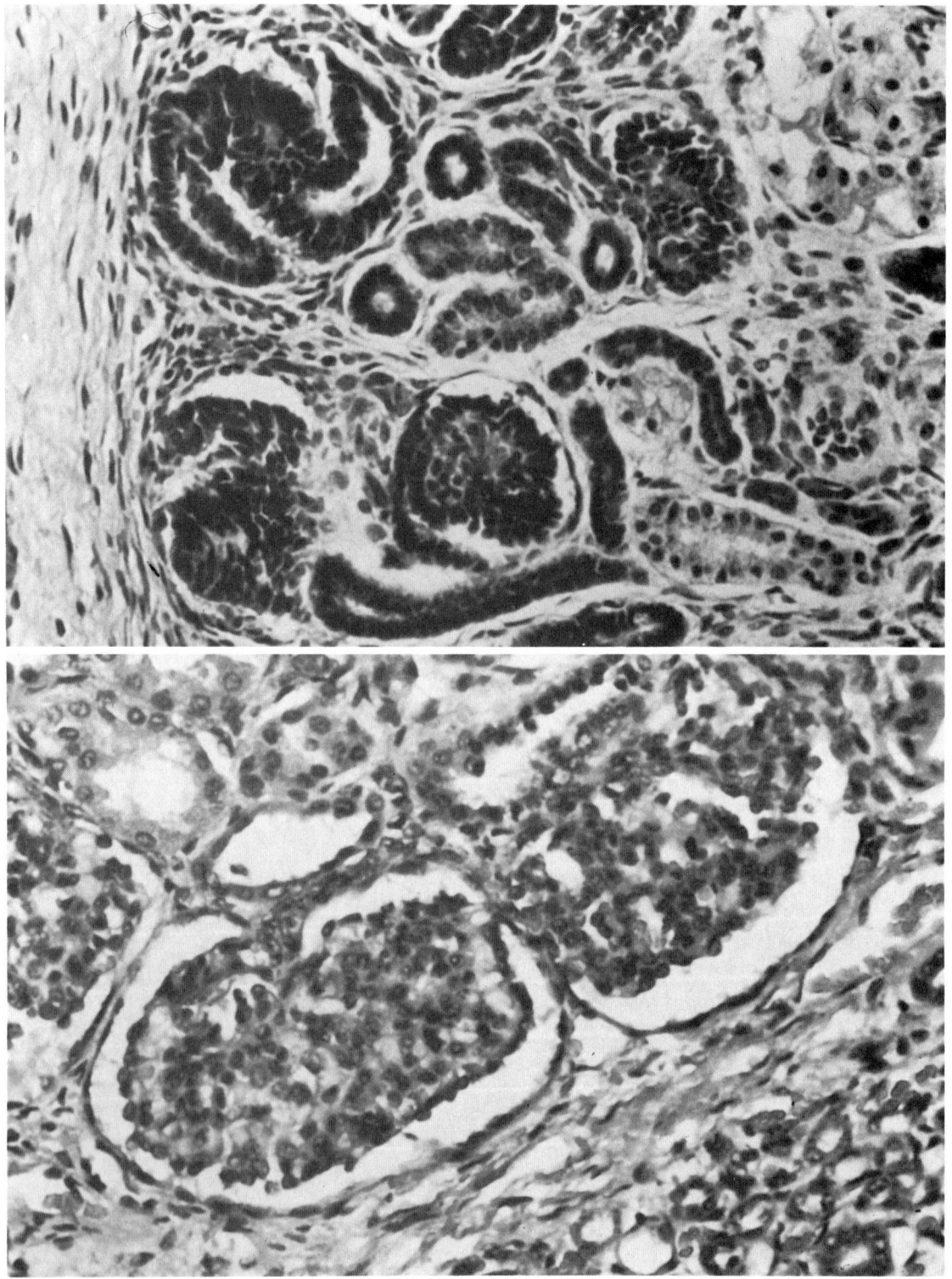

Figure 22–16

Figure 22–16. The patient was a male infant whose body weight at autopsy was 1,133 grams. The baby was born at 27 weeks of gestation and survived for 45 hours.

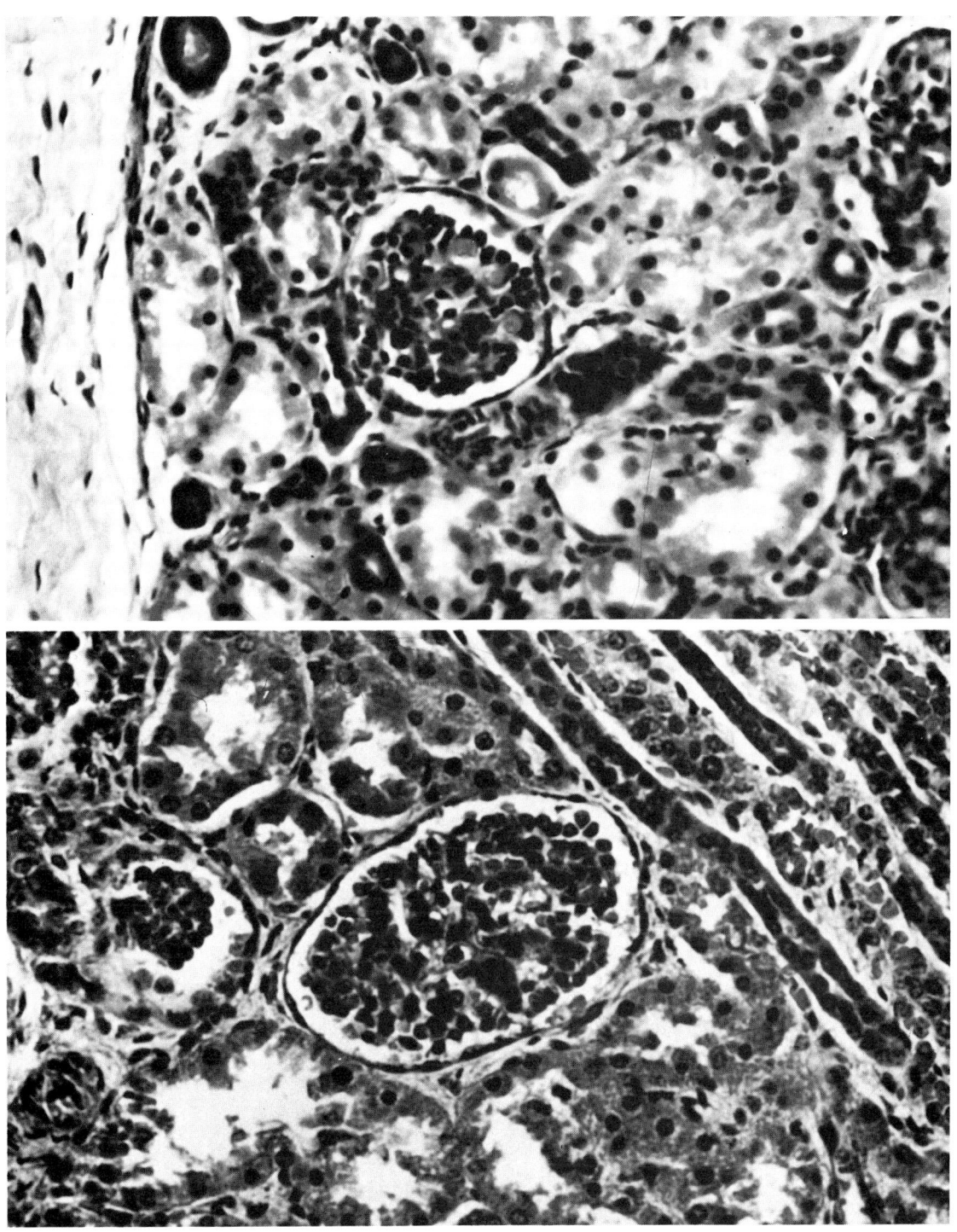

Figure 22–17

Figure 22–17. This patient was a 2,500 gram infant, born at 37 weeks of gestation, who lived for 30 days.

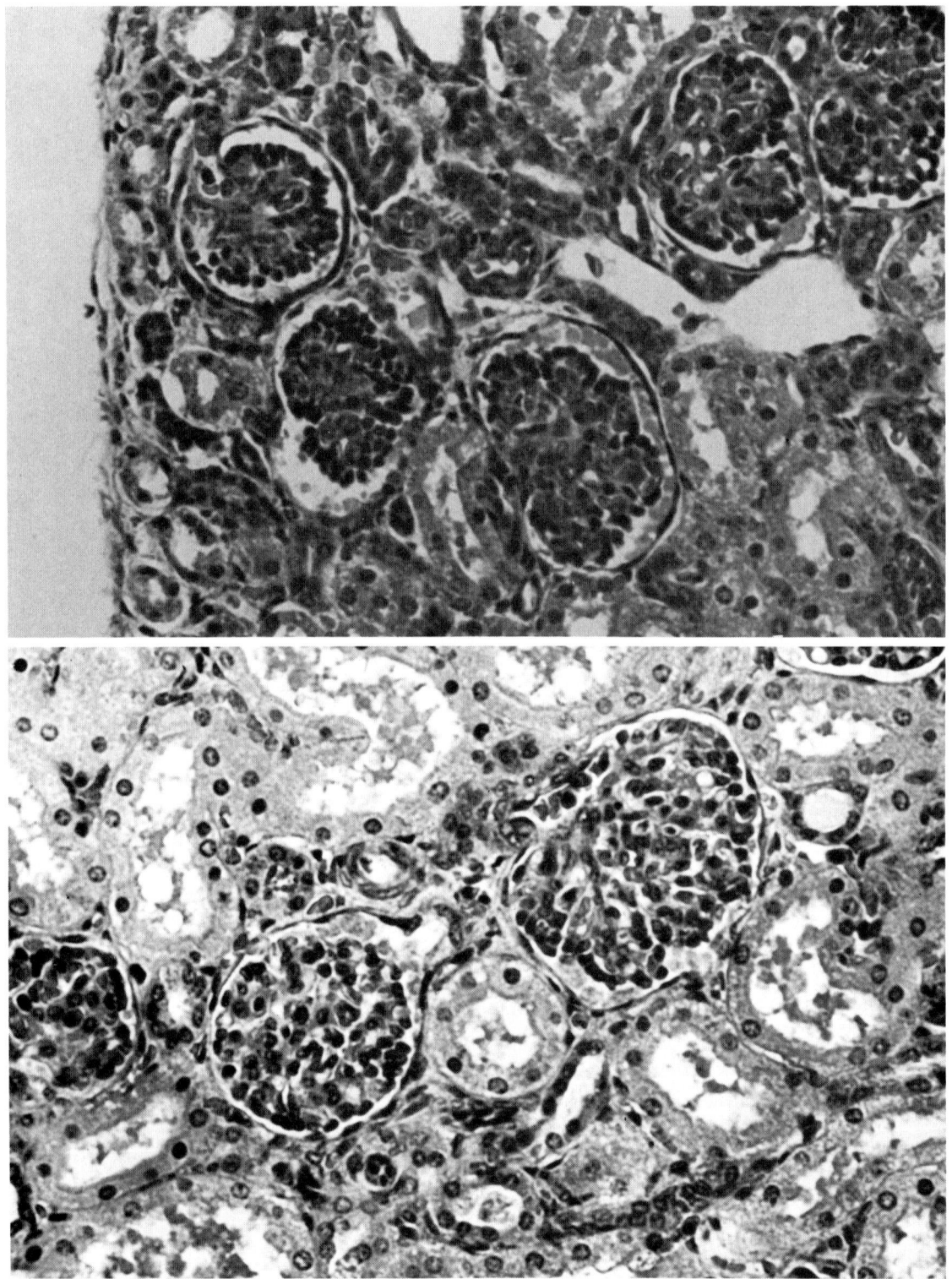

Figure 22-18

Figure 22-18. This infant, a male, was born at 36 weeks of gestation. At autopsy the body weighed 4,050 grams.

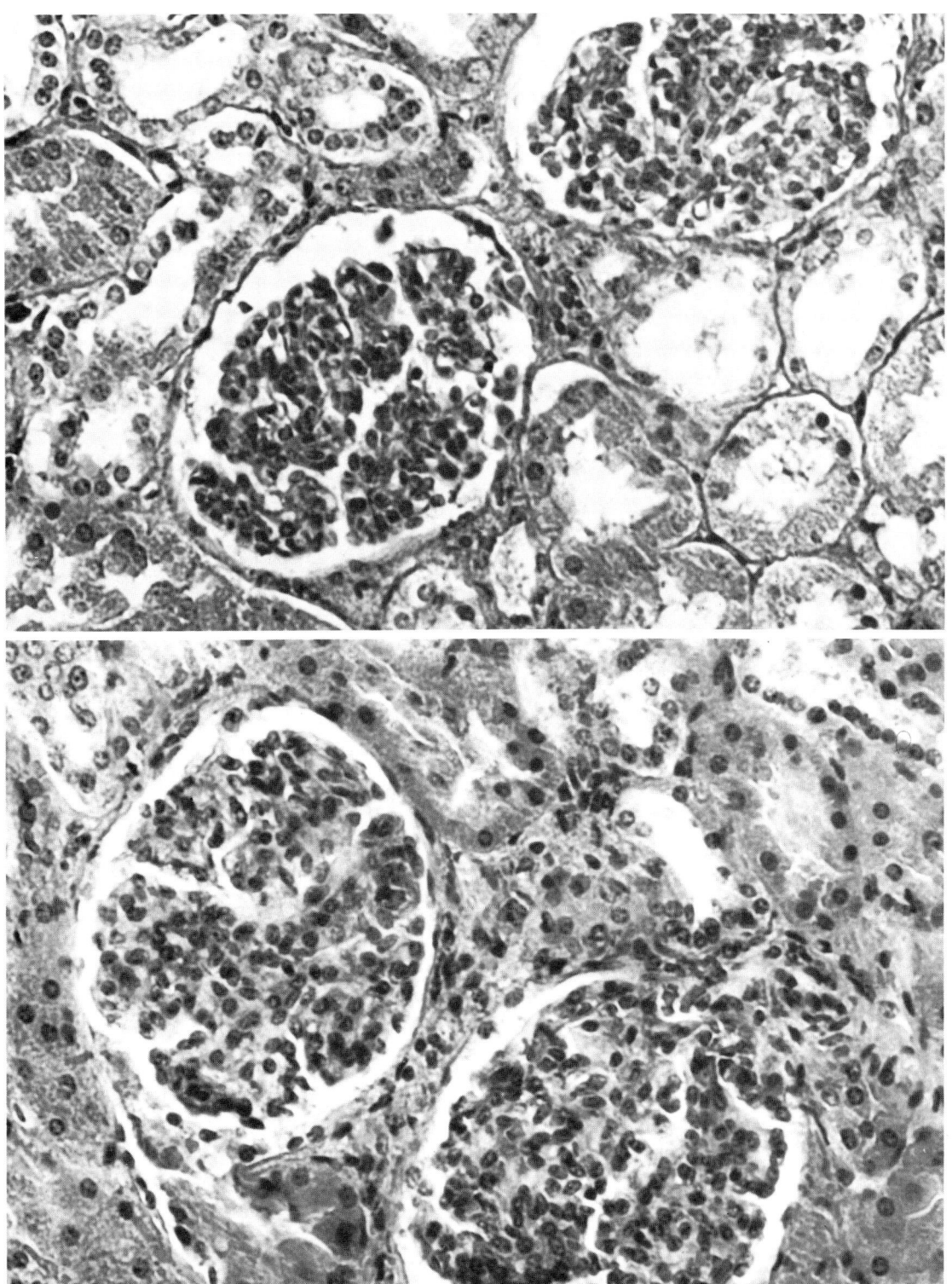

Figure 22-19

Figure 22-19. This infant, the product of 35 weeks gestation, lived for 19 months.

366 KIDNEY

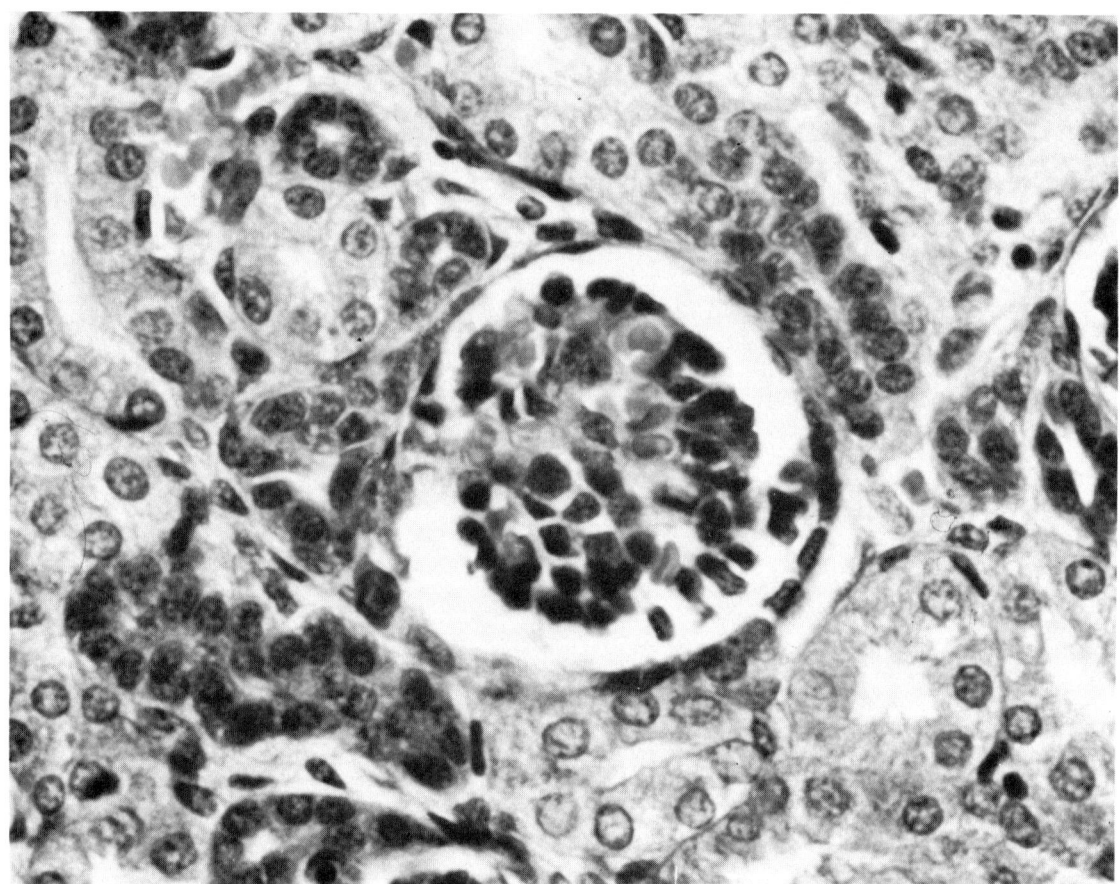

Figure 22–20

Figures 22–20 and 22–21. These two photomicrographs, taken at high magnification, illustrate both the glomeruli and cortical tubules and the contrast between them at mid-gestation and at term.

Figure 22–20. This infant was a female whose body, at autopsy, weighed 520 grams. Gestation was of 24 weeks duration.
Hematoxylin and eosin stain. Mag. 660×.

KIDNEY 367

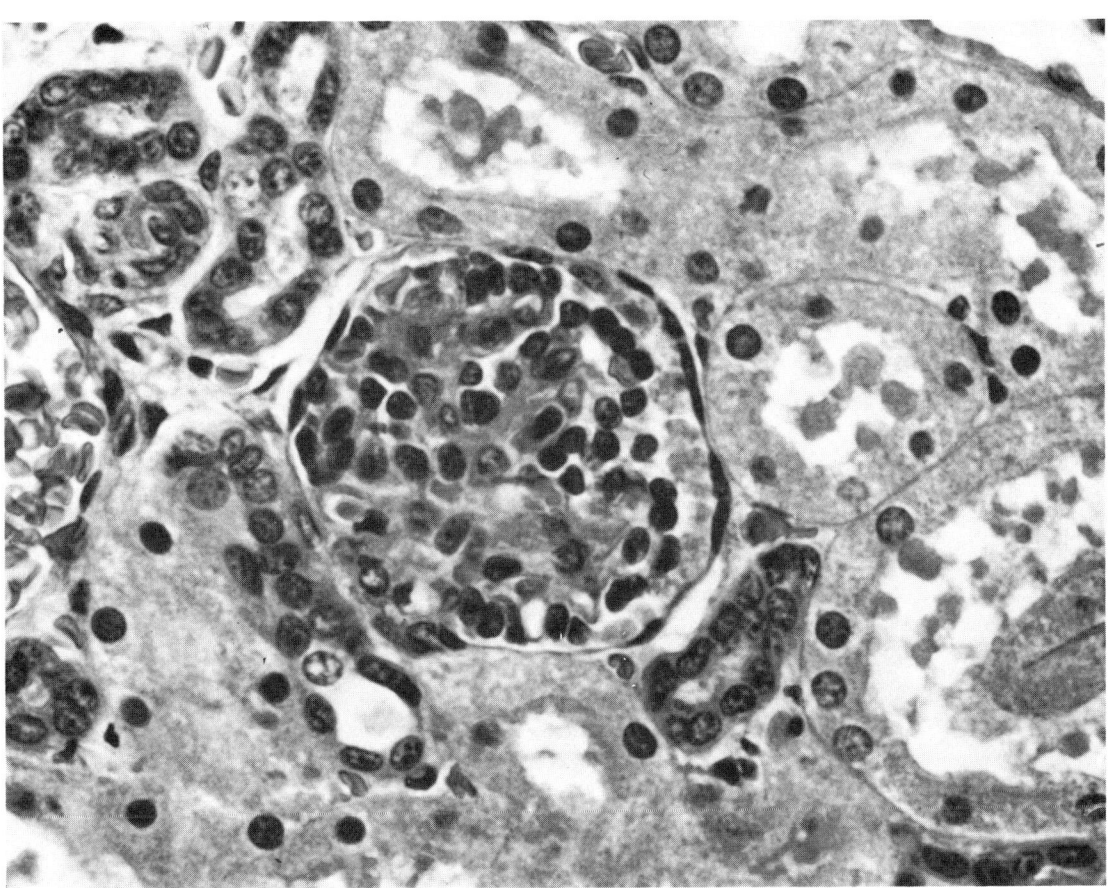

Figure 22-21

Figure 22-21. This male infant was born after 36 weeks of gestation and survived for two days. At post-mortem examination, the body weighed 4,050 grams.
Hematoxylin and eosin stain. Mag. 597×.

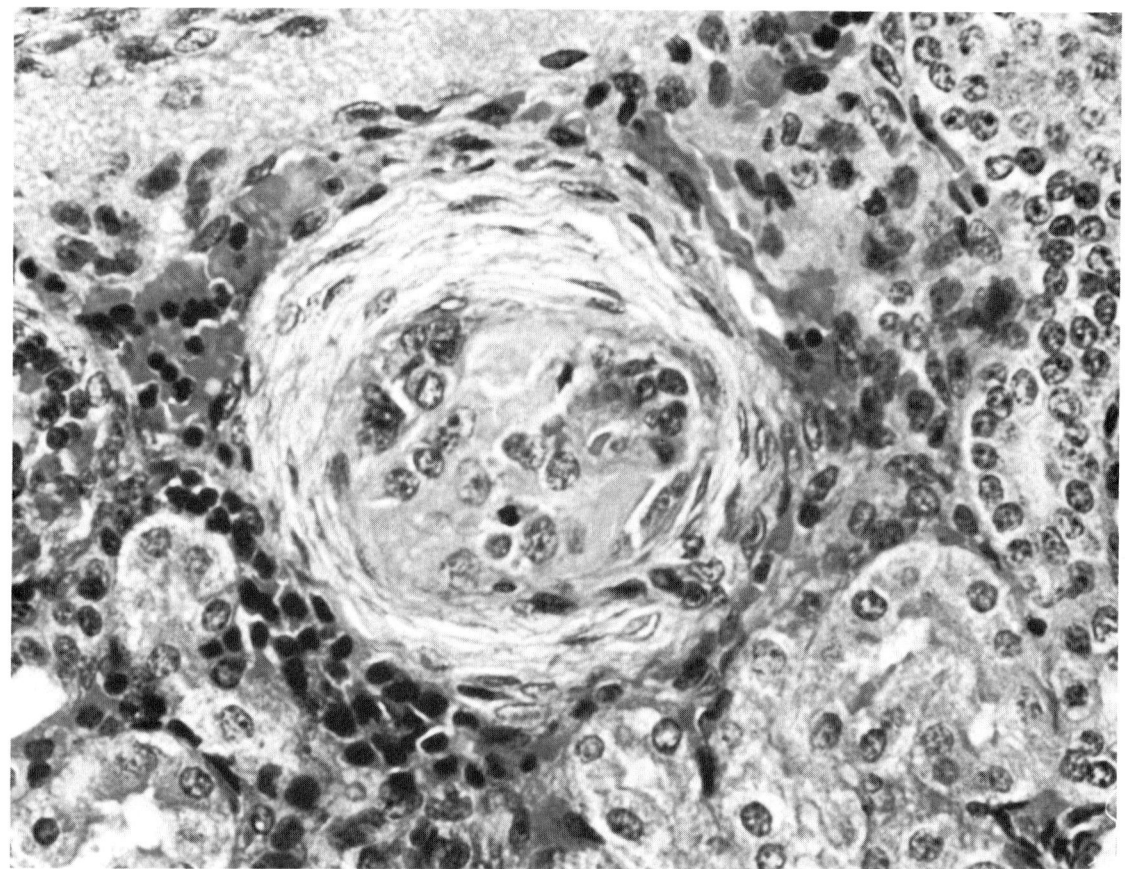

Figure 22–22

Figure 22–22. This photomicrograph illustrates a single glomerulus that has undergone so-called fetal glomerulosclerosis. Sclerotic glomeruli such as this are common in the neonatal kidney. Some have said that from 10 to 17 per cent of glomeruli may be so altered in a normal infant kidney.

This baby was a female of 30 weeks gestation. The infant lived for 26 hours. Her body weight at autopsy was 1,504 grams.

Hematoxylin and eosin stain. Mag. 492×.

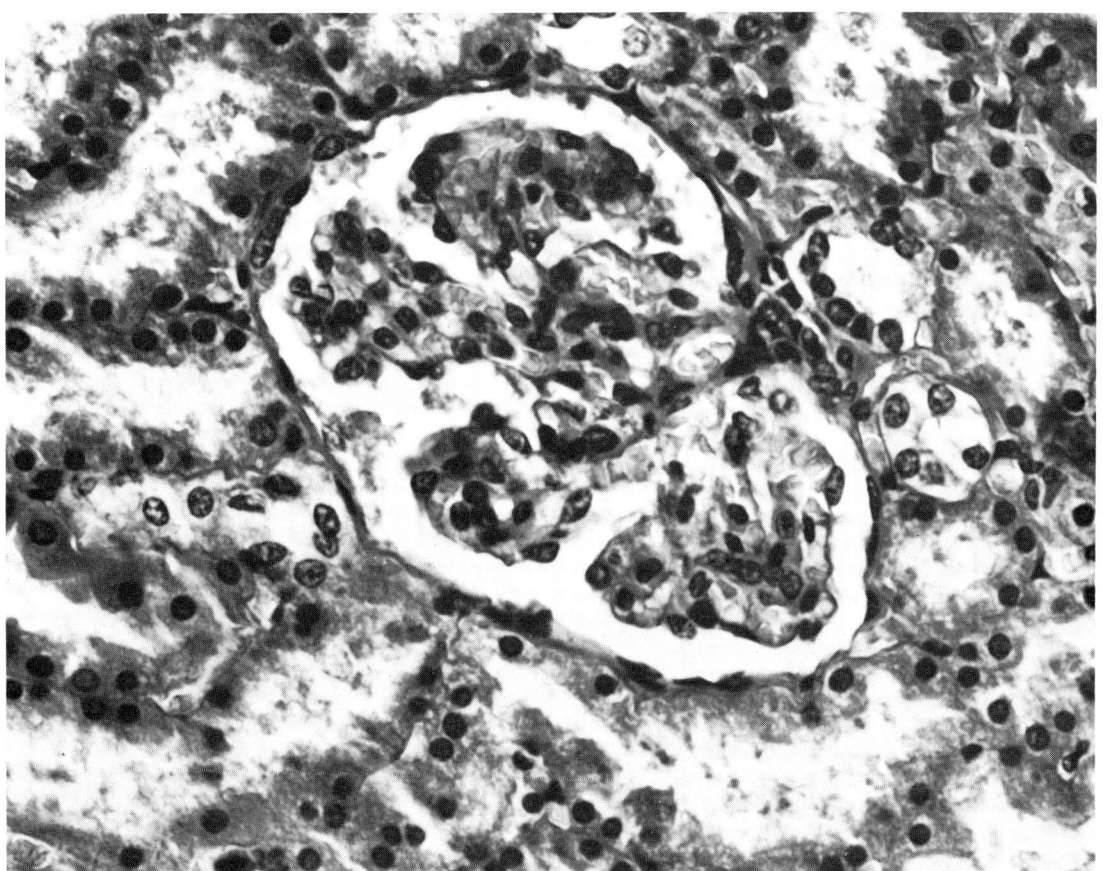

Figure 22–23

Figure 22–23. Although this is not a section from the kidney of an infant, but rather from that of a young child, it does illustrate the juxtaglomerular apparatus quite clearly. The juxtaglomerular cells appear in a triangular cluster just above and to the right of the visible glomerular arteriole. The macula densa, a segment of six prominent cuboidal cells in this photograph, appears again, just above and to the right of the aggregated juxtaglomerular cells, lining the adjacent portion of that particular tubule.

The patient was a six year old white male.
Hematoxylin and eosin stain. Mag. 492×.

370 KIDNEY

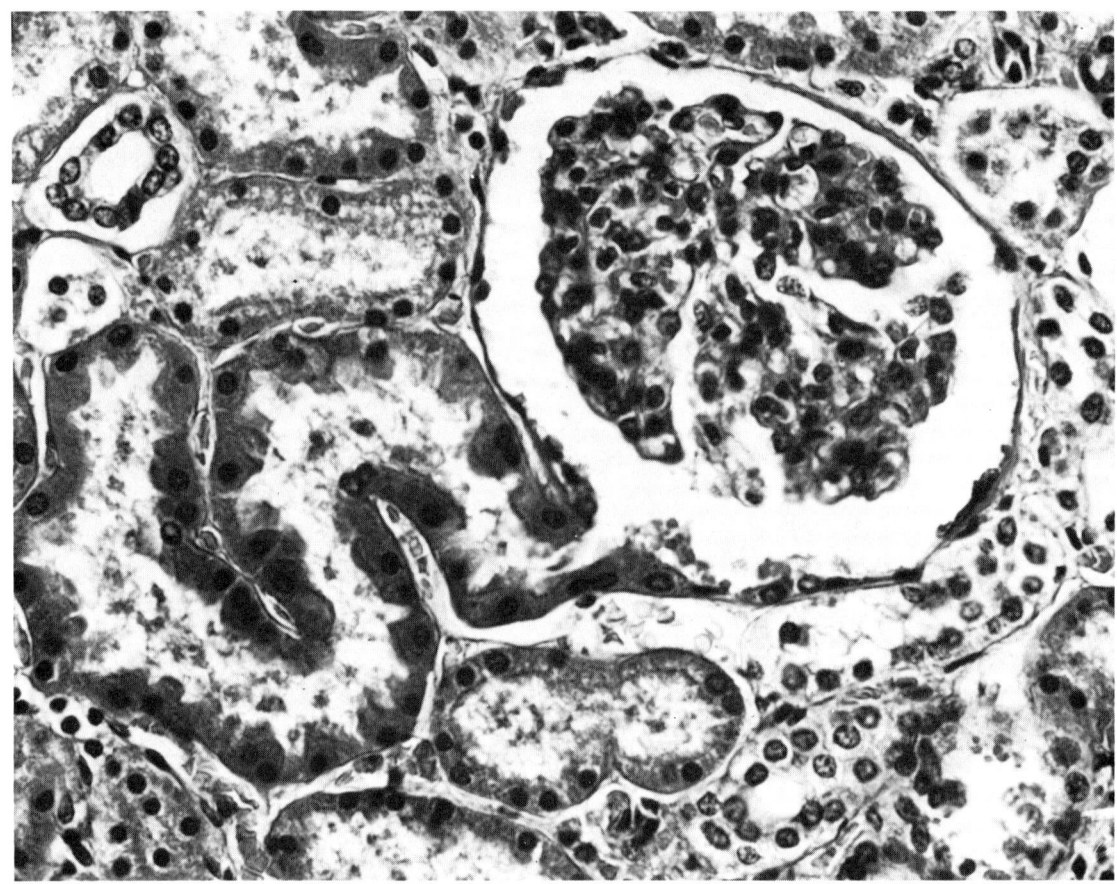

Figure 22–24

Figure 22–24. This photograph was taken from a section of the kidney of a six year old boy, but nevertheless seems to be appropriate in this series—simply because it illustrates so very well the origin of the tubule, from Bowman's space in this particular nephron.
Hematoxylin and eosin stain. Mag. 492×.

Figures 22–25 and 22–26. These two pairs of photomicrographs illustrate, at rather high magnification, the character of the cells that line the collecting tubules in the newborn infant. In each instance, the upper illustration depicts the tubule high in the pyramid, near the corticomedullary junction; the lower illustration is taken near the tip of the pyramid.

See illustrations on the following pages.

Figure 22–25. A 2,360 gram female born at 38 weeks, who lived 59 hours.

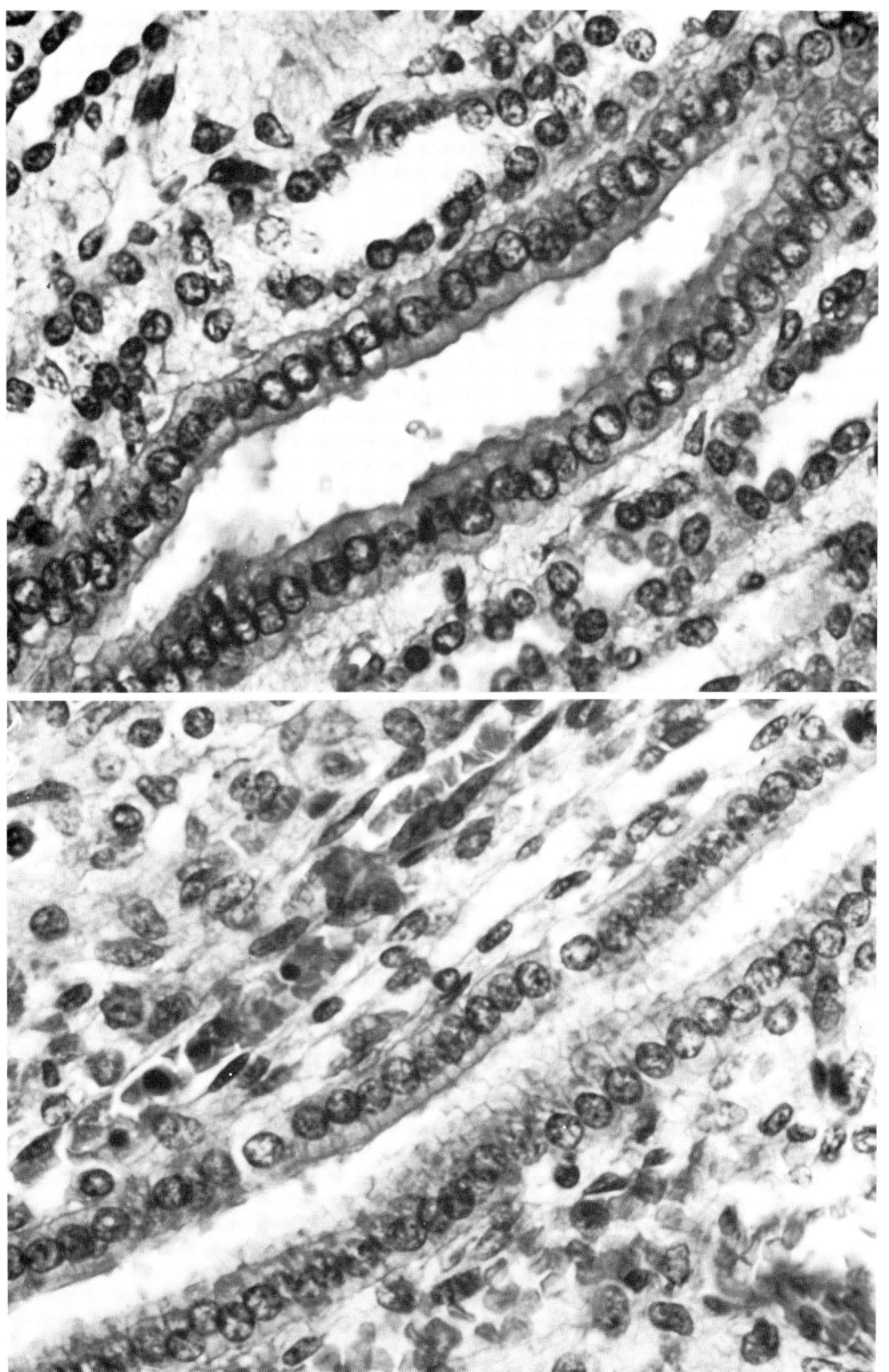

Figure 22–25

Figure 22–26. A 2,920 gram infant, born at term, who lived 2½ months. Hematoxylin and eosin stain. Mag. 660×.

See illustration on the opposite page.

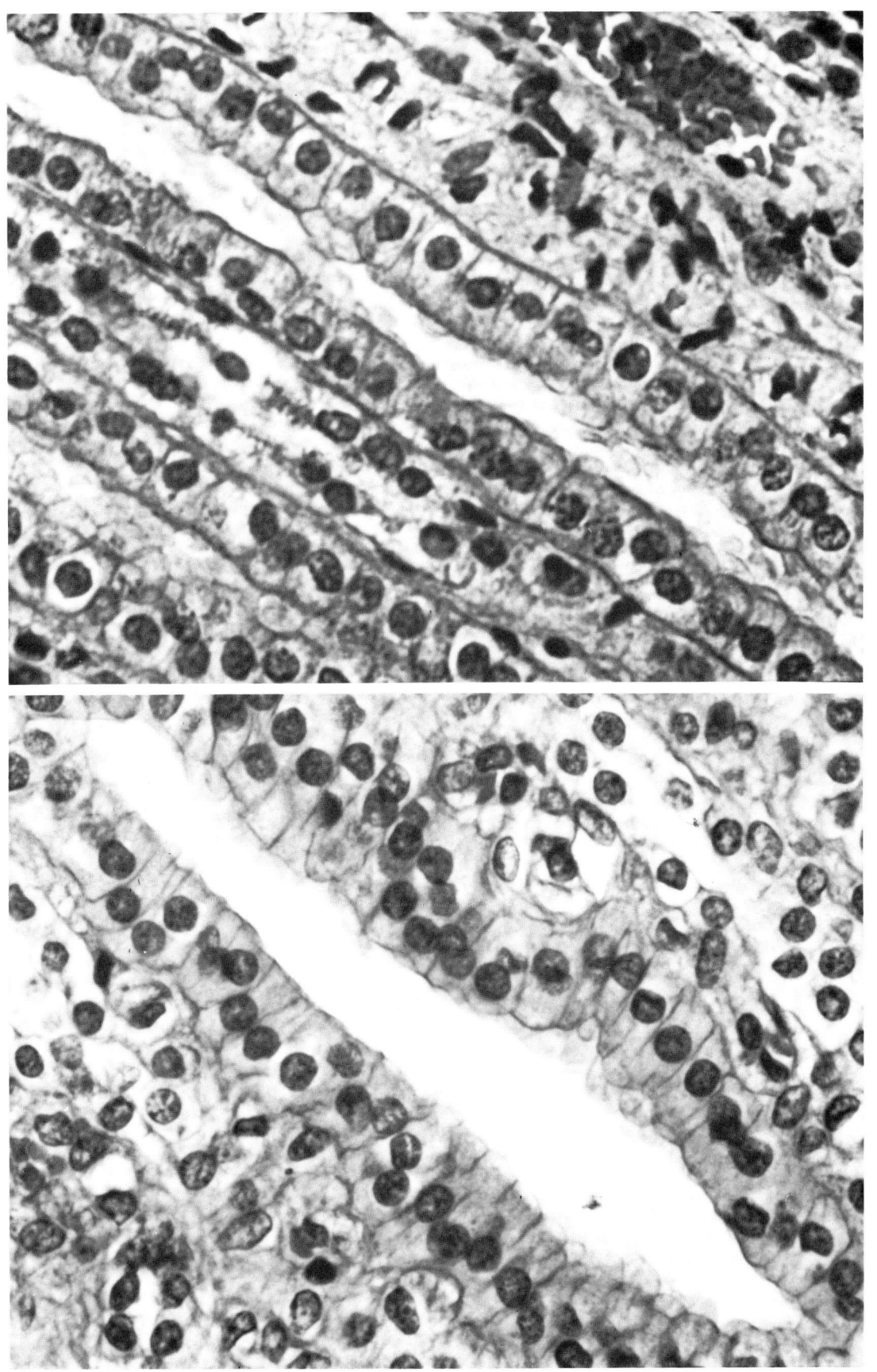

Figure 22–26

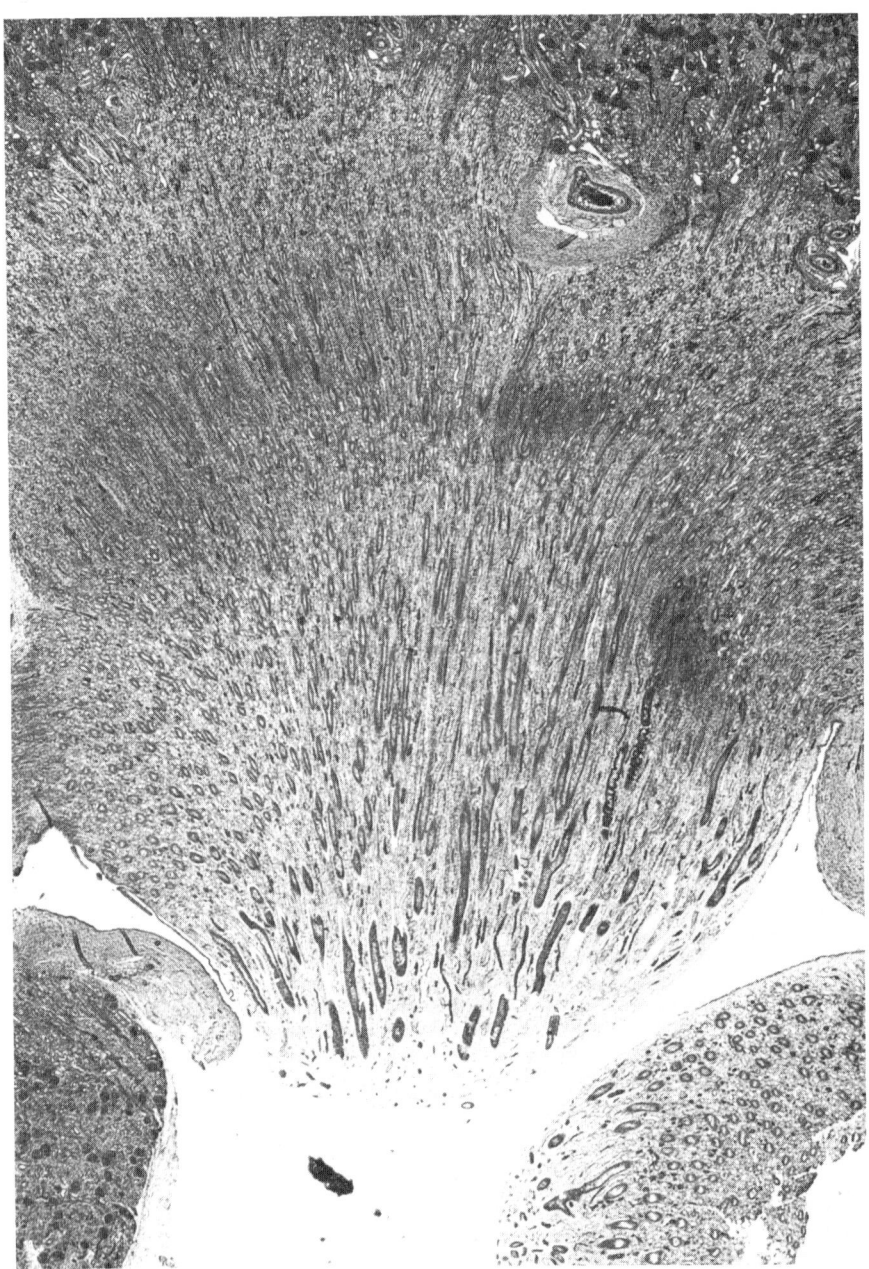

Figure 22-27

Figure 22-27. This is a photograph of the entire pyramid from a prematurely born infant. This male baby was born at 35 weeks of gestation and survived for 26 hours. His body weight at post-mortem examination was 1,505 grams.

Hematoxylin and eosin stain. Mag. 20.8×.

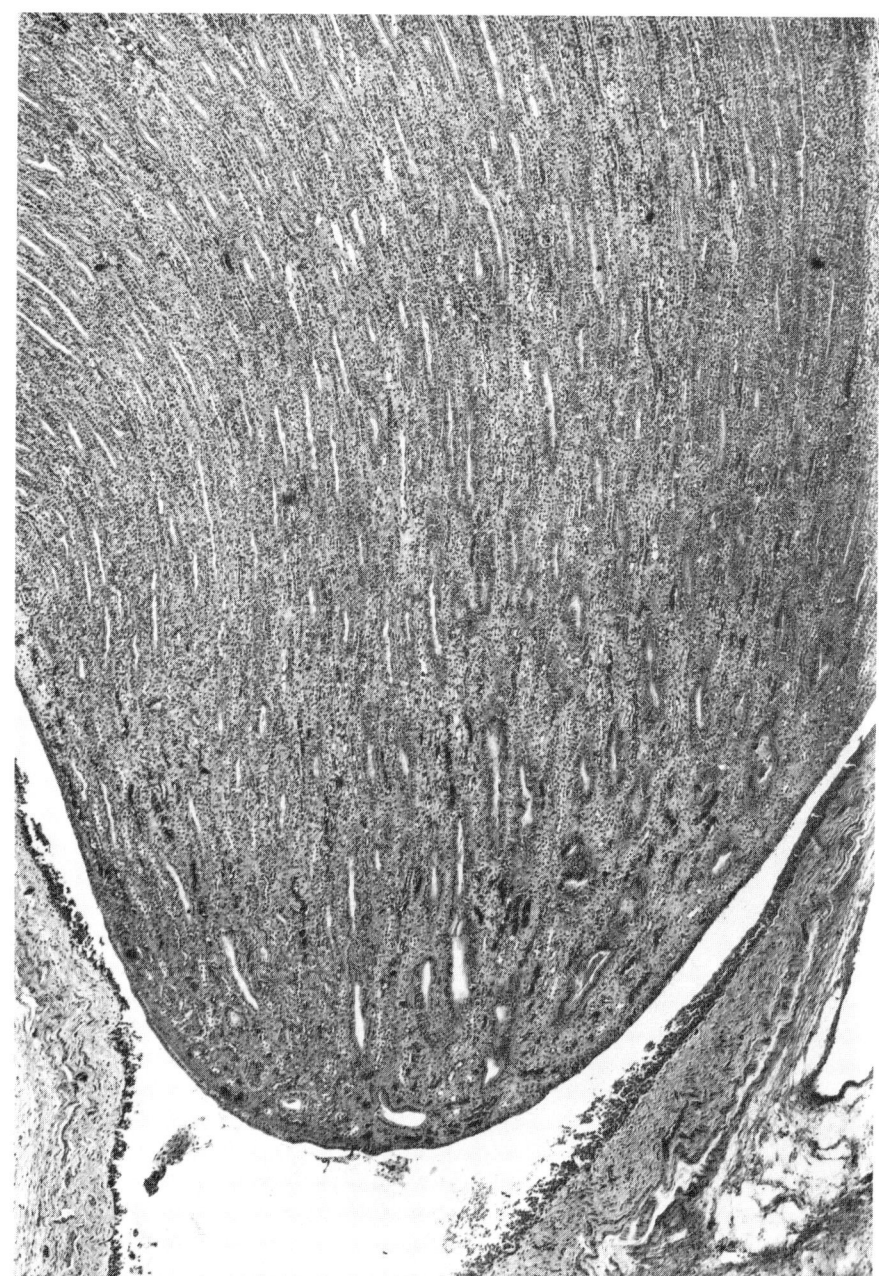

Figure 22–28

Figure 22–28. This illustration, taken at slightly higher magnification than Fig. 22–27, shows only the distal portion of the pyramid of a more mature infant.

This baby was born after 40 weeks of gestation and lived for 2½ months. His body, at autopsy, weighed 2,920 grams.

Hematoxylin and eosin stain. Mag. 45×.

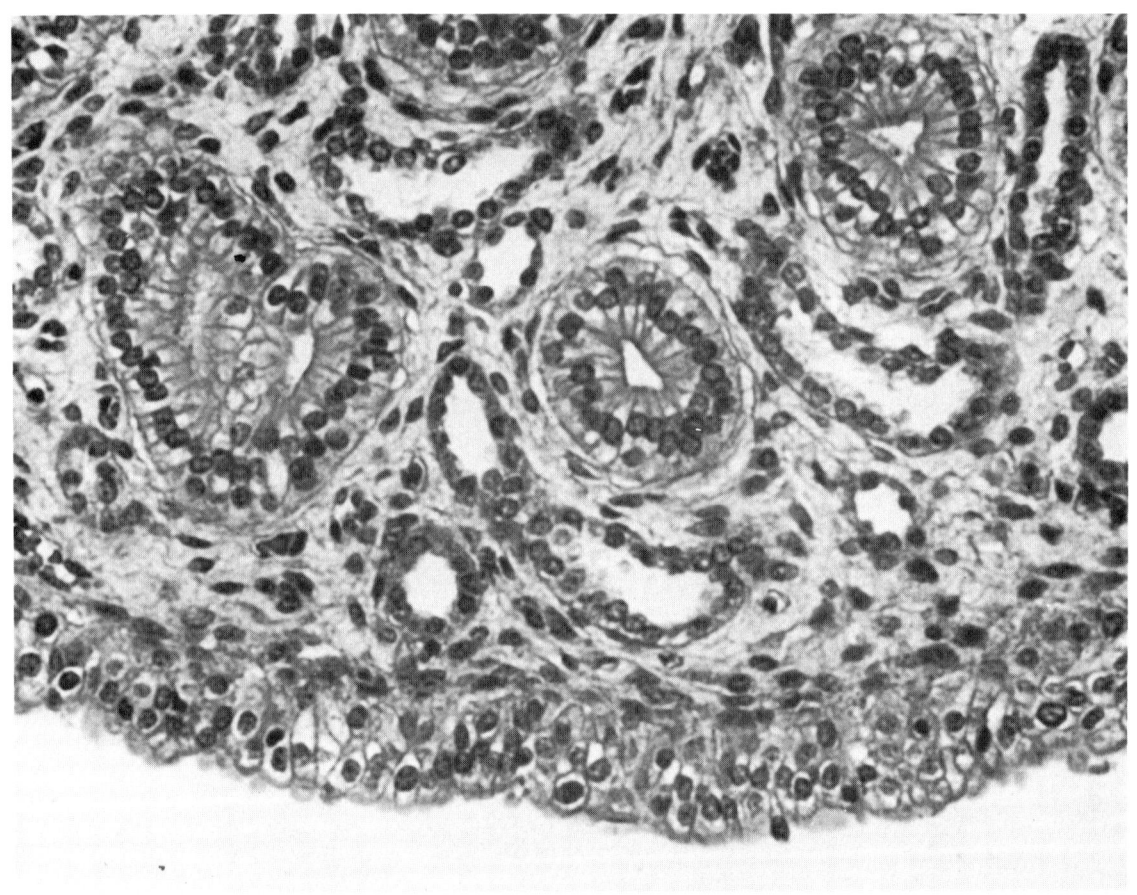

Figure 22–29

Figure 22–29. This photograph shows in some detail the kind of epithelium normally clothing the tip of the pyramid in a very small and immature infant.

This patient, a 370 gram female, was stillborn at 18 weeks of gestation.

Hematoxylin and eosin stain. Mag. 382×.

KIDNEY 379

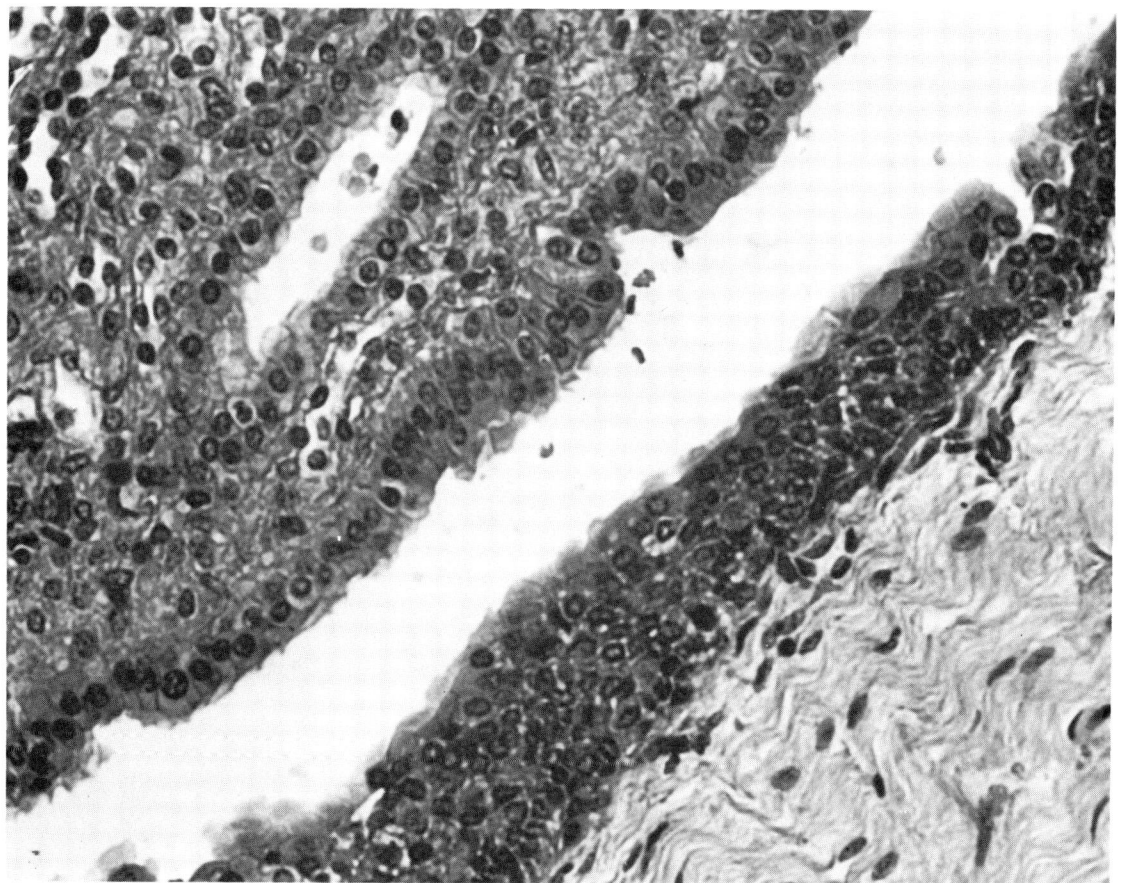

Figure 22-30

Figure 22-30. By contrast with Fig. 22-29, this illustration shows the cells which line the pelvis and clothe the tip of the pyramid in an older and more mature infant.

This baby, born at term, lived for 2½ months. His body weight at autopsy was 2,920 grams. Hematoxylin and eosin stain. Mag. 382×.

380 KIDNEY

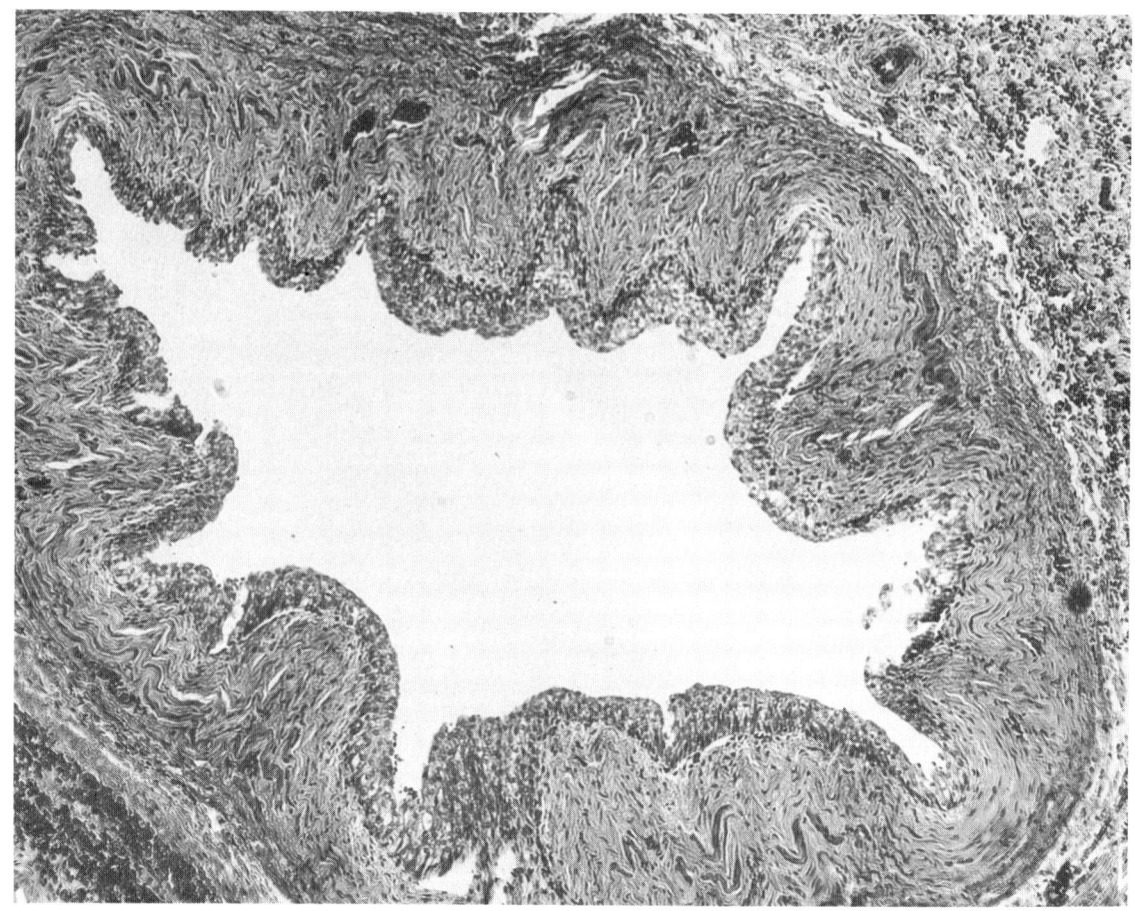

Figure 22–31

Figure 22–31. The calyx, represented here, is the first portion of the excretory passages conducting the urine from the kidney to the outside. This photograph shows the nature of its wall and lining cells in an infant born at 40 weeks gestation.

This male infant lived for 12½ hours, and his weight at necropsy was 3,530 grams.

Hematoxylin and eosin stain. Mag. 108×.

KIDNEY 381

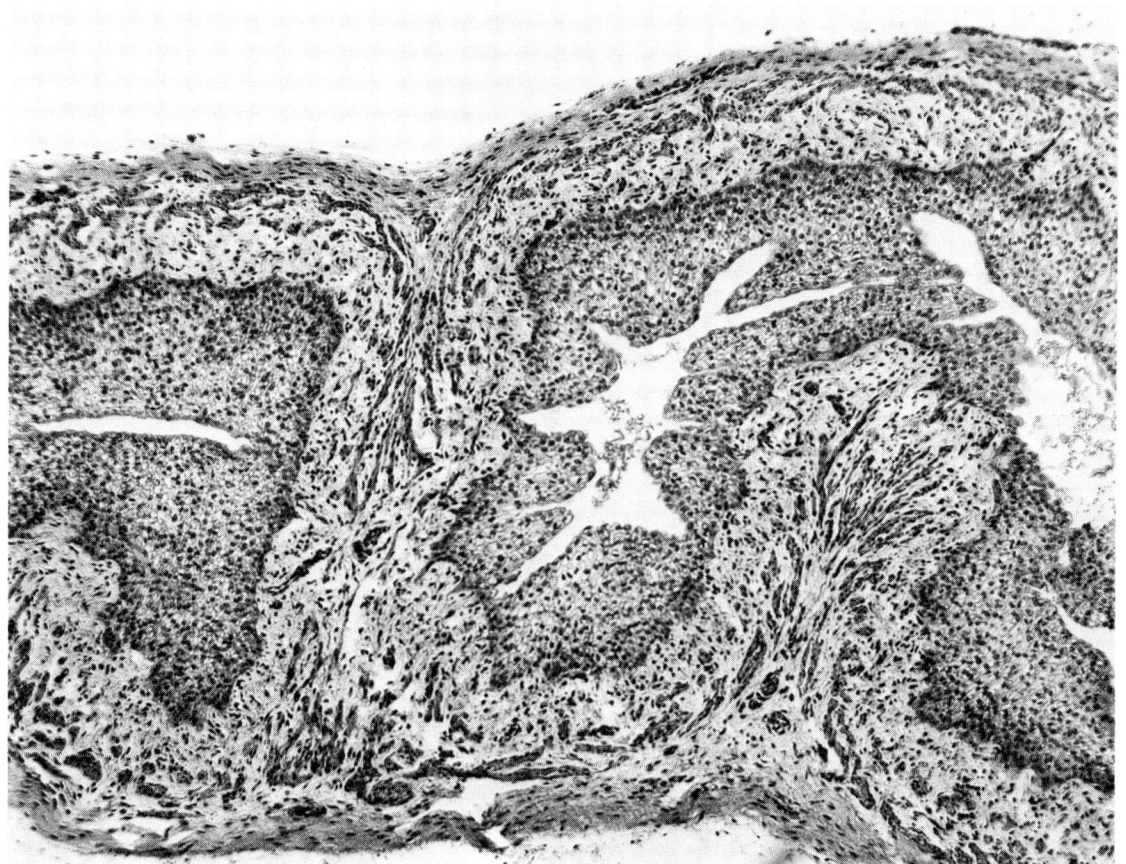

Figure 22-32

Figure 22-32. Depicted here are several sections of a ureter, another and lower portion of the system of excretory passages.

This patient, by contrast with that of Fig. 22-31, was a very small and immature infant, stillborn at 18 weeks of gestation, who weighed 370 grams at autopsy.

Hematoxylin and eosin stain. Mag. 108×.

Chapter 23

URINARY BLADDER AND URETHRA

EMBRYOLOGY

The urinary bladder is derived from the cranial or vesicourethral part of the primitive urogenital sinus, which is continuous with the allantois. The lining epithelium develops from the endoderm of the vesicourethral canal. The laminae propria, muscularis, and serosa develop from the adjacent splanchnic mesenchyme.[1]

As the bladder is taking shape, the allantois above it involutes to form a thick tube, the *urachus*. After birth, the urachus becomes a fibrous cord, the median umbilical ligament, extending from the apex of the bladder to the umbilicus.

As the bladder enlarges, the caudal portions of the mesonephric ducts are incorporated into its dorsal wall, initially contributing to the formation of the mucosa of the trigone; but this epithelium is soon replaced by the epithelium of the urogenital sinus.[2] As the mesonephric ducts are absorbed, the ureters come to open separately into the urinary bladder.

The epithelium of the prostatic portion of the *urethra*, proximal to the orifices of the ejaculatory ducts, is also derived from the endoderm of the vesicourethral canal of the urogenital sinus, and its lamina propria similarly forms from adjacent splanchnic mesenchyme. The epithelium of the remainder of the prostatic urethra and that of the membranous urethra are derived from the endoderm of the pelvic portion of the urogenital sinus. The epithelium of the penile urethra, except for the glandular portion, forms from cells derived from the phallic portion of the urogenital sinus. That of the glandular portion develops by canalization of an ectodermal cord of cells which extends into the glans from its tip.

The epithelial lining of the entire length of the female urethra is derived from exactly the same origins as the proximal portion of the prostatic segment of the urethra in the male.

ANATOMY

Urinary Bladder. The urinary bladder of the neonate is an almond-shaped structure extending well up out of the pelvis and blending imperceptibly at its apex with the still very obvious cord-like remnant of the urachus, which serves to anchor it to the umbilicus. Bladder and urachus are clearly flanked by the two umbilical arteries, one on each side, which are usually still patent though thick-walled.

The serosa of the bladder is shiny and white. Its muscular wall is thick in the collapsed state, and tough. On section its color is almost white. The mucosa is shiny, white, and (again in the collapsed state) very wrinkled. The trigone is usually readily visualized.

The apex of the bladder internally is quite acute, much more so than it ever is in the adult.

Urethra. The epithelial lining of the prostatic portions of the male urethra resembles that of the urinary bladder. That of the penile portion varies alternately from stratified columnar to stratified squamous. The glandular segment is lined exclusively by squamous cells. The lamina propria is made up of loose areolar tissue rich in elastic fibers.

Most of the lining epithelium of the female urethra is stratified squamous, although there may be interspersed segments of stratified columnar or pseudostratified epithelium. It is transitional near the bladder (Fig. 23-5).

Numerous minute urethral glands and pit-like urethral lacunae open into the female urethra. One group on each side possesses a tiny common duct, known as the paraurethral duct, which opens at the side of the external urethral orifice (Fig. 23-5). (These are the equivalent of the prostatic glands of the male.)

HISTOLOGY

Urinary Bladder. The wall of the urinary bladder consists of four coats, all of which are visible in Figure 23-2. The epithelial lining is of transitional type (Fig. 23-3). Its thickness varies with the degree of dilatation of the bladder. The lamina propria consists of loosely woven fibrous connective tissue in which there are moderate numbers of vessels.

The thick muscular coat consists of three imperfectly separated strata, the external, middle, and internal. The smooth muscle fibers of the external stratum are generally directed longitudinally (Fig. 23-2) in the median plane and obliquely in the more lateral portions. The middle stratum is composed of fibers which, for the most part, run circularly and form the most prominent part of the thickness of the muscular coat (Fig. 23-2). The internal stratum consists of a very thin layer of muscle fibers, most of which are directed longitudinally (Fig. 23-2). The serosa is relatively thin and composed of loose areolar connective tissue containing large vessels and nerves.

Ureter. The epithelial lining, like those of the renal pelvis and urinary bladder, is transitional and varies in thickness depending upon the degree of distention of the ureter. The lamina propria consists of collagenous connective tissue with some elastic fibers. There are no connective tissue papillae.

The muscular coat consists of two layers of smooth muscle, an inner longitudinal and an outer circular.

As the ureter is retroperitoneal, it is invested in an adventitia consisting of fibrous tissue containing vessels and nerves.

Urachus. In late fetal life and early infancy, the urachus is often quite stout. Sections taken near the fundus of the bladder show its wall to be composed of many intertwined bundles of smooth muscle (Fig. 23–4a). In the very center there may be a tiny nest of epithelial cells, usually solid, rather resembling stratified squamous epithelium (Fig. 23–4b).

Toward the umbilicus, the smooth muscle bundles diminish in number and size, and the central nidus of epithelium is less likely to be encountered.

References

1. Moore, K. L.: The Developing Human. Clinically Oriented Embryology. Philadelphia, W. B. Saunders Co., 1973, pp. 204–206, 213, and 224.
2. Gyllensten, L.: Contributions to embryology of the urinary bladder. Development of definitive relations between openings of the Wolffian ducts and ureters. Acta Anat., 7:305, 1949.

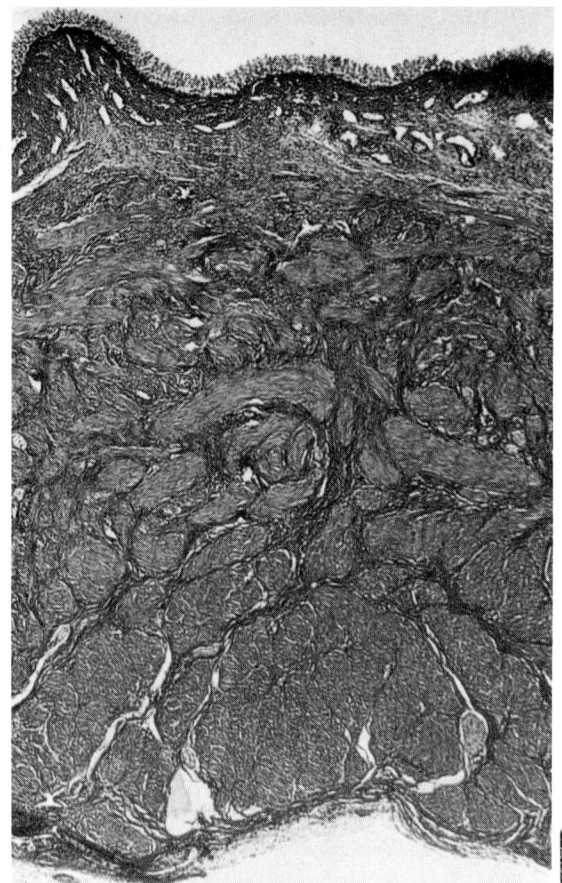

Figure 23-1a

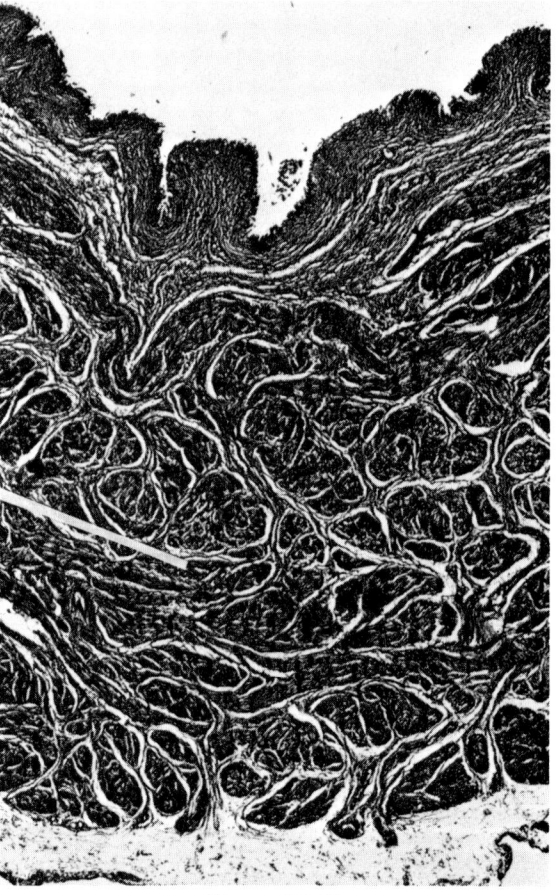

Figure 23-1b

Figure 23–1. The thickness of the wall of the urinary bladder and the number of layers that it comprises vary with the degree of dilatation. These are sections from four infants of different body weights, increasing from 23–1a to 23–1d. All are stained with hematoxylin and eosin.

Figure 23–1a. Section from the bladder of a 1,300 gram female infant who died at the age of 6 hours. Mag. 41×.

Figure 23–1b. Section from the bladder of a 12-day old male weighing 2,400 grams at death. Mag. 26.5×.

Figure 23–1d. Section from the bladder of a term infant who survived for 6 days. Body weight: 3,090 grams. Mag. 26.5×.

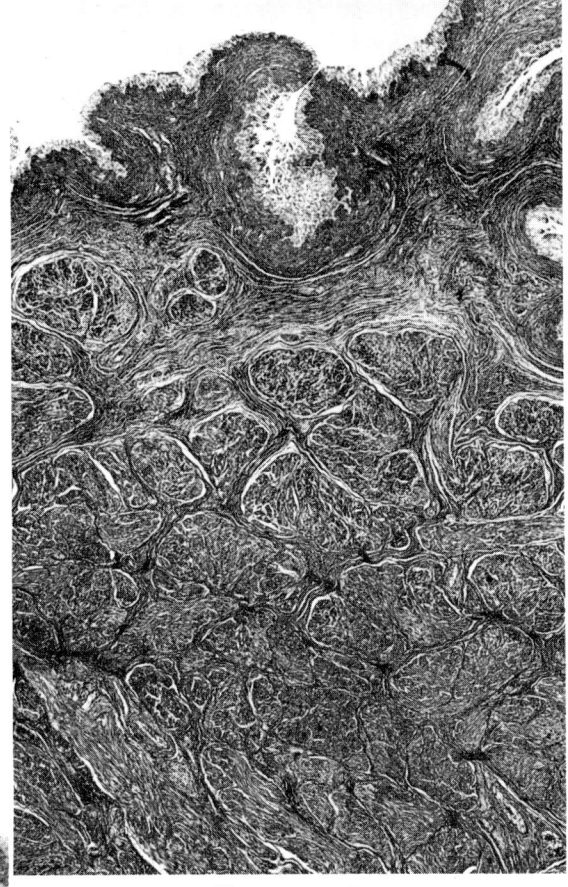

Figure 23–1d

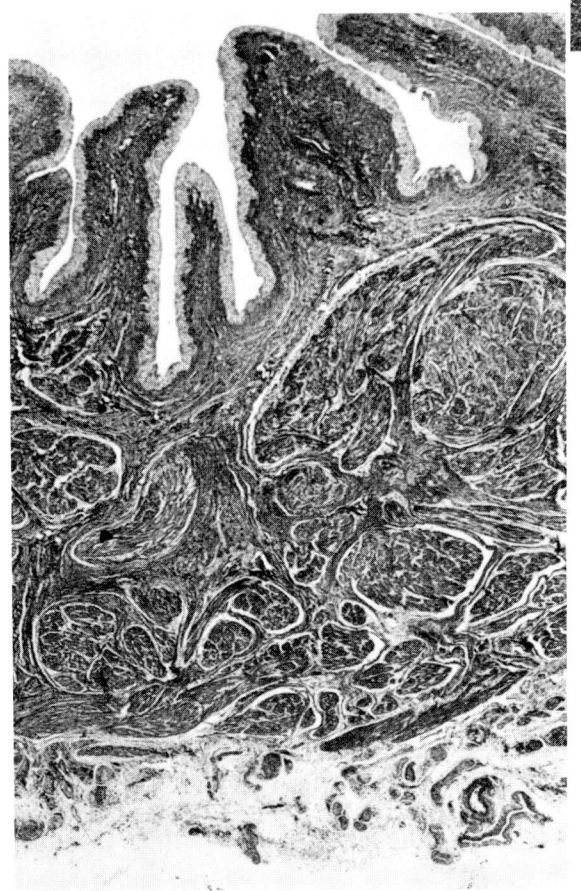

Figure 23–1c. Section of the urinary bladder of a 34-hour old white female who weighed 2,760 grams at death. Mag. 20.8×.

Note that although these four infants differ markedly in body weight, there is little difference among them in the histologic appearance of the wall of the bladder.

Figure 23–1c

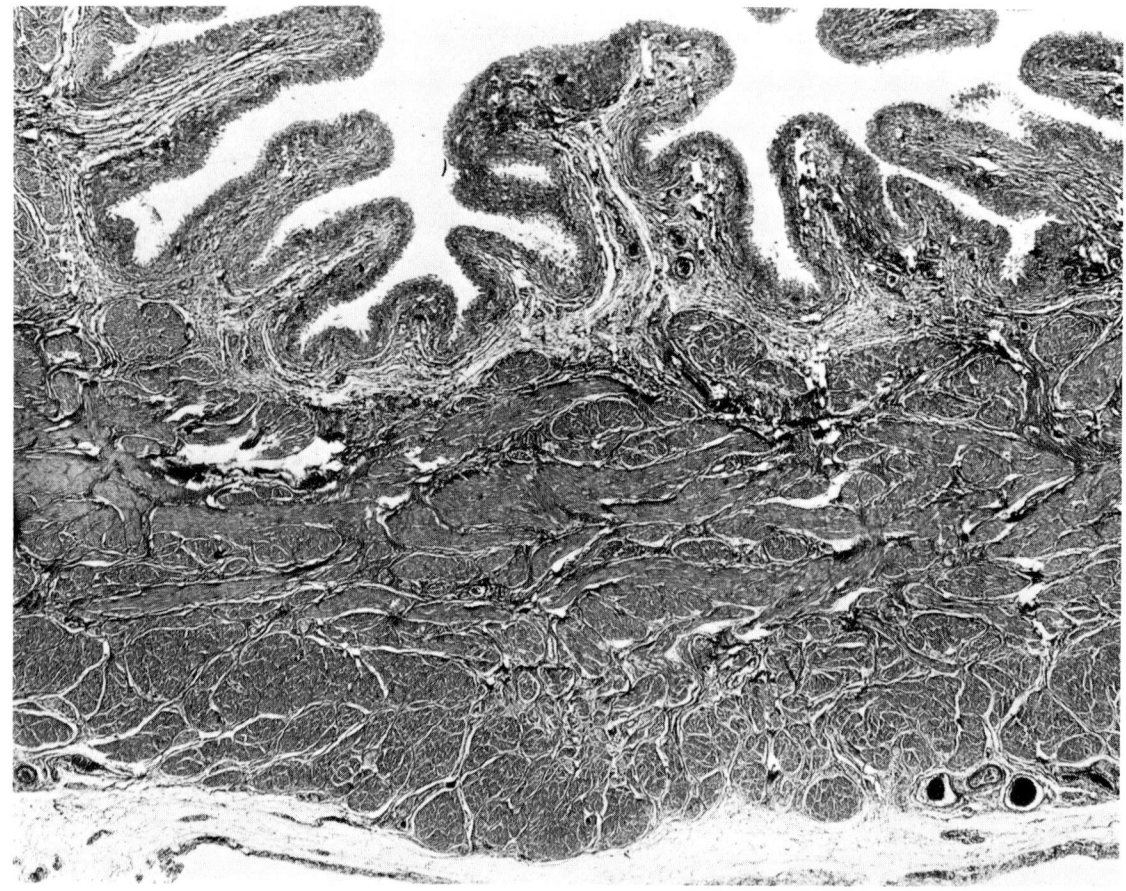

Figure 23–2

Figure 23–2. This is a survey view of the wall of the urinary bladder from a 3½ day old black male weighing 1,530 grams at autopsy. This illustrates the component parts of the wall. The mucosal lining consists of well differentiated transitional epithelium. The lamina propria is composed of loosely woven connective tissue bearing vessels. The muscular coat is made up of interlacing bundles of smooth muscle fibers. The pale staining serosa consists of loosely arranged fibrous connective tissue containing blood vessels and nerves.

Hematoxylin and eosin stain. Mag. 20.8×.

URINARY BLADDER AND URETHRA 389

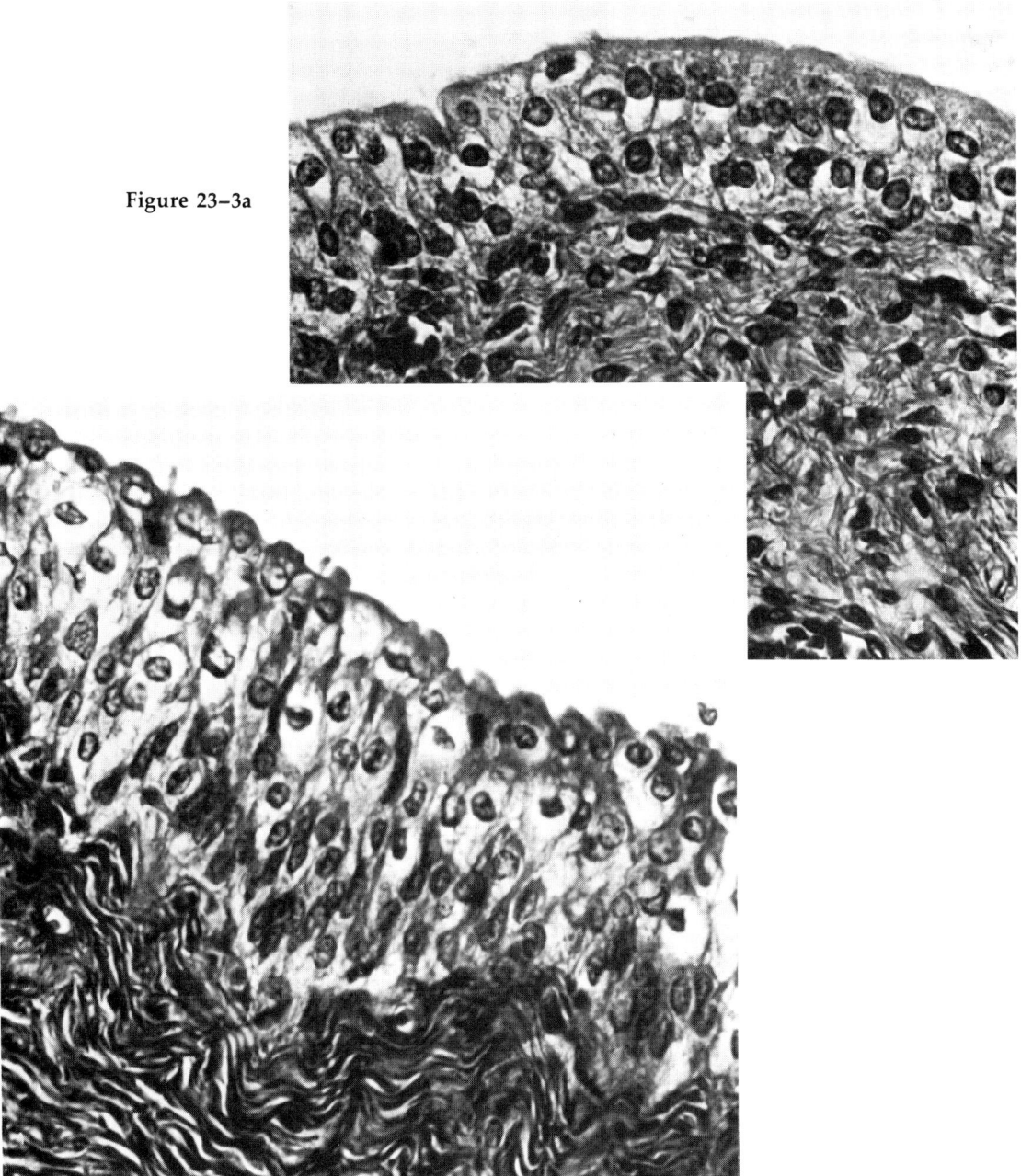

Figure 23–3a

Figure 23–3b

Figure 23–3. These two photographs illustrate, in detail, the microscopic appearance of the transitional epithelium lining the urinary bladder of the premature infant and the infant born at term.

Figure 23–3a. Section from a black male, weighing 1,010 grams, who lived 9 hours and 47 minutes. Mag. 450×.

Figure 23–3b. Section from a 6 day old white female who weighed 3,090 grams at autopsy. Mag. 450×.

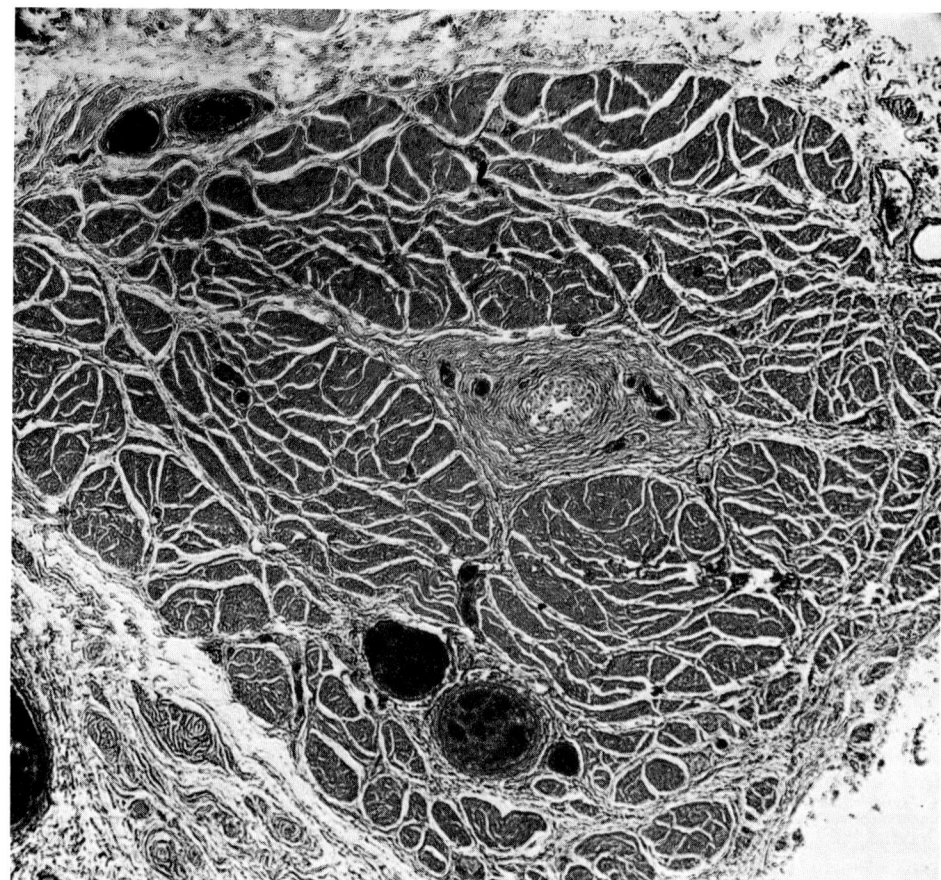

Figure 23–4a

Figure 23–4a. A cross section of the fundus of the urinary bladder of a 3,000 gram infant born after a 39 week gestation. The infant, a female, lived for 1½ hours.

At this level, a portion of the urachus is still visible and patent. The lining is of a transitional character.

Hematoxylin and eosin stain. Mag. 50×.

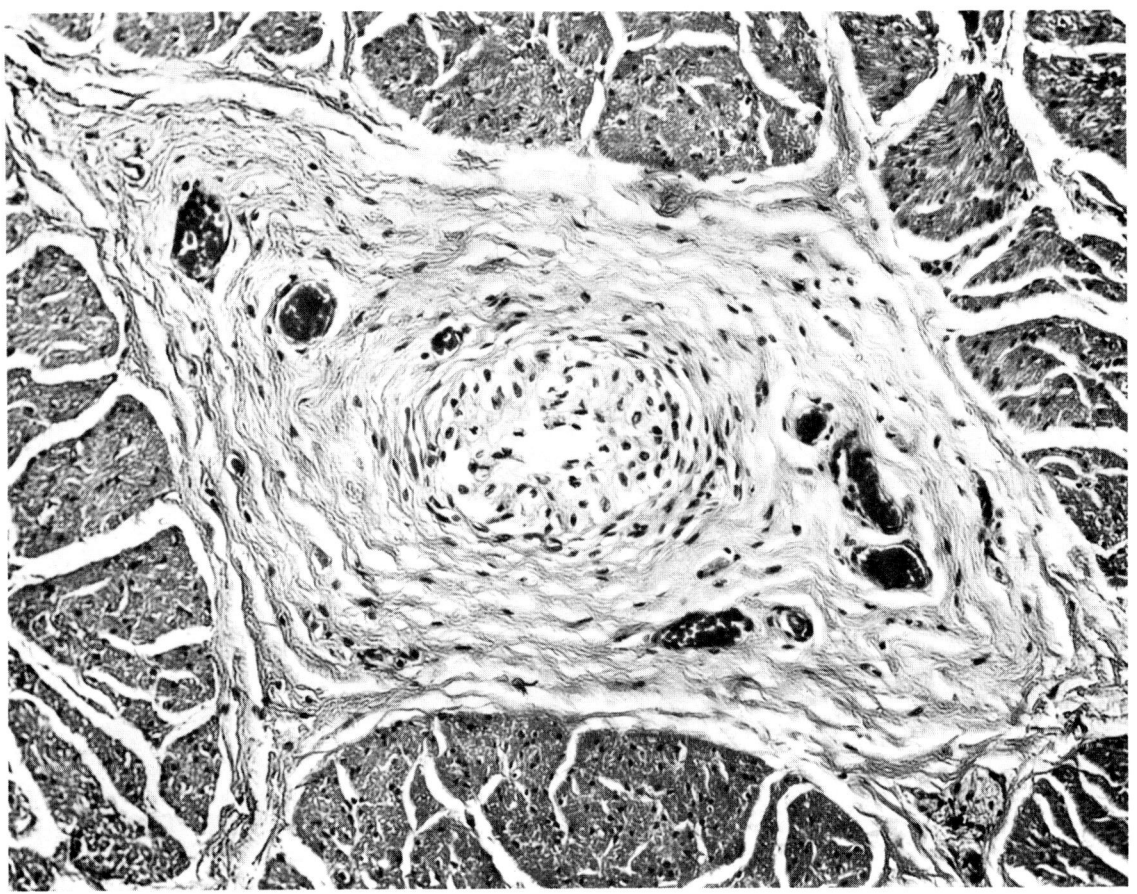

Figure 23–4b

Figure 23–4b. Higher magnification of the urachal remnants depicted in Fig. 23–4a. Hematoxylin and eosin stain. Mag. 197×.

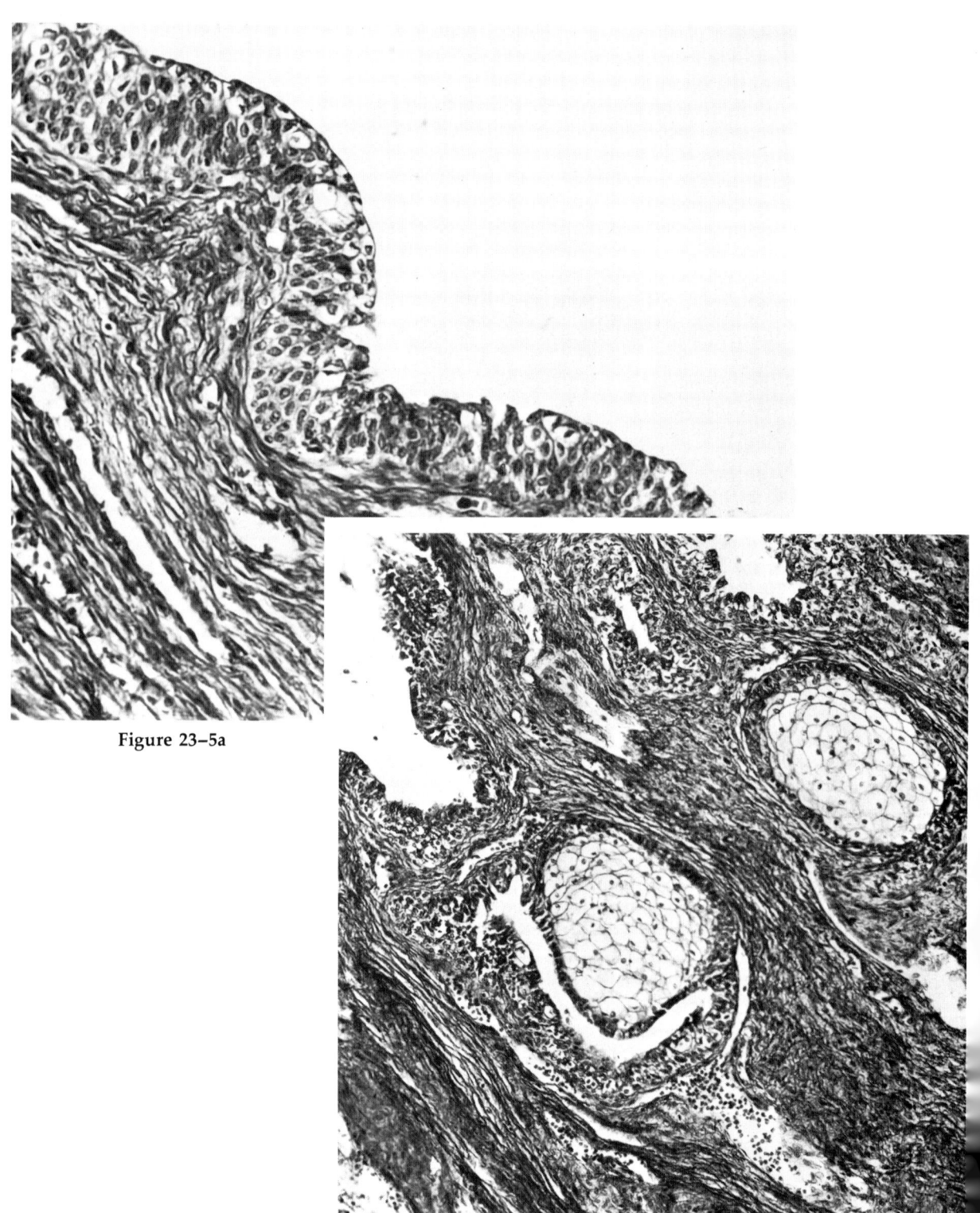

Figure 23–5a.

Figure 23–5b.

Figure 23–5a. The epithelial lining of the urethra of a female infant weighing 4,251 grams, who died at 16 hours and 40 minutes of age. Mag. 243×.

Figure 23–5b. Periurethral glands of the same infant. Note the islands of epithelium of rather squamous character interspersed. Mag. 142×.

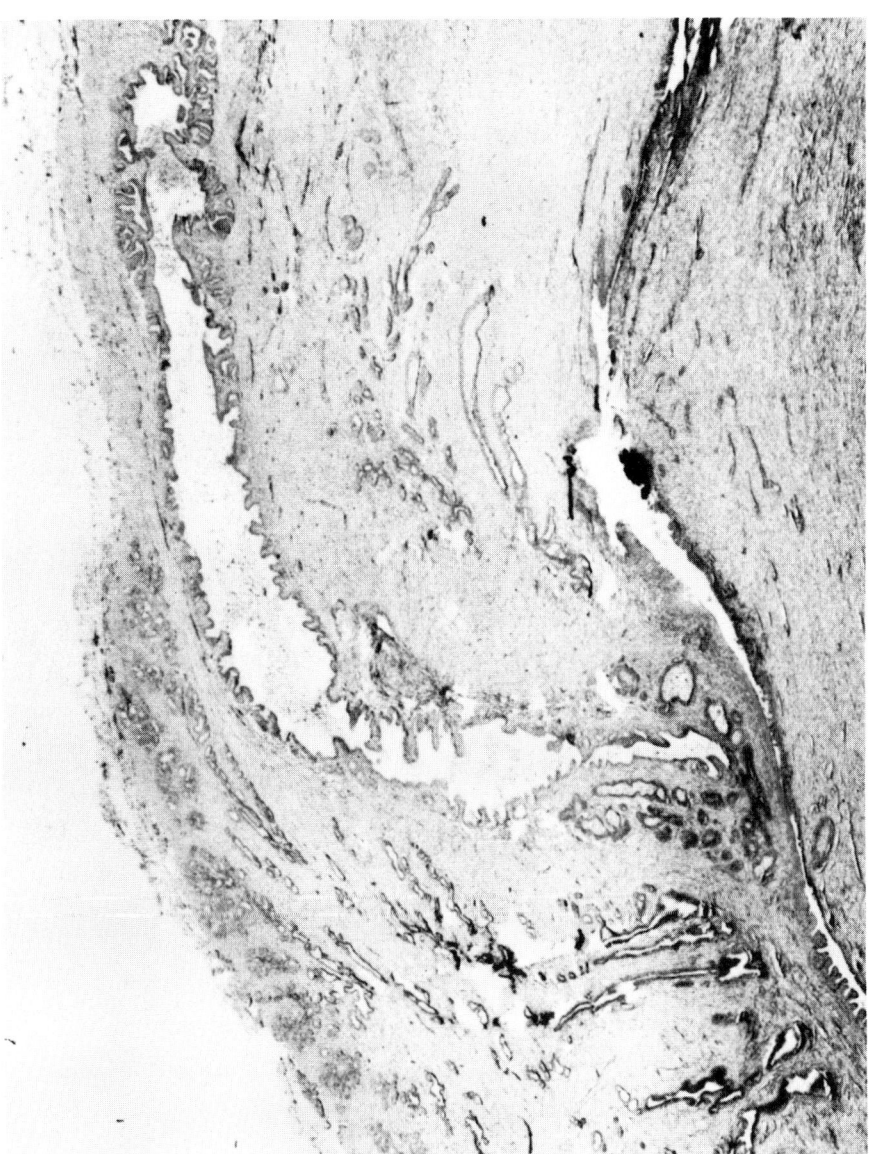

Figure 23-6

Figure 23-6. A section in the sagittal plane to demonstrate the entrance of the seminal vesicle into the urethra.

This infant, a white male, lived for four days. He had been born at term and his body weight at autopsy was 3,915 grams.

Hematoxylin and eosin stain. Mag. 28.8×.

Part 9

MALE REPRODUCTIVE SYSTEM

Chapter 24

TESTIS

EMBRYOLOGY

Testis. There is no morphologic indication of sex in the fetus until the seventh week of gestation, when the gonads begin to acquire distinctive sexual characteristics.[1] In embryos with an XY sex chromosome complex, the medulla of the early indifferent gonad differentiates into the testis, while the cortex regresses. Under the influence of the Y chromosome, with its strong testis-determining effect on the medulla, the primary sex cords that project into the gonad from the surface cortex (from which they originate) differentiate into the seminiferous cords. The hilar ends of these cords anastomose to form the rete testis. These seminiferous or testicular cords soon lose their peripheral connections with the covering germinal epithelium, as the latter structure is elevated and flattened by an underlying thick, fibrous capsule, the tunica albuginea, a characteristic and diagnostic feature of testicular development.

Gradually, the enlarging testis separates from the regressing mesonephros and becomes suspended by its own mesentery, the mesorchium. The seminiferous cords develop into the seminiferous tubules, the tubuli recti, and the rete testis.

The walls of the emerging seminiferous tubules (which, at this stage of development, have no lumens) are composed of two kinds of cells; the supporting or sustentacular cells of Sertoli, the most numerous, are derived from the germinal epithelium, while the spermatogonia are derived from the primordial germ cells.

During later development, the surface germinal epithelium flattens to form the mesothelium on the outer surface of the testis. The rete testis becomes continuous with 15 to 20 adjacent mesonephric tubules, which become the efferent ductules. The latter are connected with the mesonephric duct which forms the ductus epididymis.[1]

Genital Ducts. Two pairs of genital ducts develop in both sexes; these are the mesonephric (Wolffian) ducts and the paramesonephric (Müllerian) ducts.

The fetal testis produces at least two hormones: one stimulates development of the mesonephric ducts into the male genital tract, and the other suppresses the development of the paramesonephric ducts.[1] When the mesonephros degenerates, some of its tubules near the testis persist and are transformed into the efferent ductules or ductuli efferentes. These open into the mesonephric duct, which becomes the ductus epididymis in this region.[1]

Beyond the epididymis, the mesonephric duct acquires a thick investment of smooth muscle and becomes the ductus deferens or vas deferens.

A lateral outgrowth from the caudal end of each mesonephric duct gives rise to a seminal vesicle or, as it is currently referred to, the seminal gland. The part of the mesonephric duct between the seminal gland and the urethra becomes the ejaculatory duct.

Appendix Testis and Appendix Epididymis. Various authors attribute the embryologic origin of the appendix testis and appendix epididymis to either the mesonephric system or the paramesonephric system. There does not seem to be unanimity of opinion on this point.

ANATOMY

Testis. The testis of the newborn infant is usually ovoid and pale pink. It may be contained within the scrotal sac, or it may be in the canal. In premature infants, not uncommonly, the testis is located within the peritoneal cavity, usually rather close to the internal opening of the canal.

The neonatal testis ordinarily measures about 7 mm. in greatest diameter. Its exterior is smooth. It is suspended by the structures forming the spermatic cord.

The tunica albuginea is the fibrous covering of the testis.[2]

Genital Ducts. The epididymis is an aggregate of tortuous loops of a canal forming the first part of the efferent passage from the testis. Its head is directly connected with the cranial pole of the testis by the efferent ductules of the gland. Its tail is linked with the caudal pole by areolar tissue and a reflection of the tunica vaginalis.

The tunica vaginalis is the lowermost extremity of the processus vaginalis of the peritoneum, which, in the fetus, precedes the descent of the testis from the abdomen into the scrotum. Its visceral layer clothes all but the posterior border of the testis. The parietal layer is more extensive; its inner surface is smooth.

Appendix Testis and Appendix Epididymis. In the infant each appears as a tiny, almost white, ear-like appendage a few millimeters in greatest diameter, attached at or near the superior pole of either the testis or the epididymis.

HISTOLOGY

Testis. In Figure 24–1 we see, at very low magnification, a survey view of the testis of a term infant. The germinal epithelium is barely visible as a fine dark line on the very surface of the tunica albuginea at the top of the photograph. Individual lobules, radiating away from the hilus, are separated from one another by rather broad bands of connective tissue bearing prominent vessels.

Within each lobule the solid cellular convoluted tubules are somewhat crowded.

In Figure 24-2, a section of the testis taken from an infant born in about the fifth month of gestation, the tunica albuginea is scarcely visible at the anatomical border superiorly. Cells within the much convoluted tubules appear shrunken, but this is an artifact.

In Figure 24-3, the germinal epithelium is clearly visible on the surface of the organ as a single layer of typical mesothelial cells. The fibrous quality and relative density of the tunica albuiginea are apparent here, as is the solid cellular nature of the seminiferous tubules in the infant born at term.

Seminiferous Tubules. Figure 24-4 illustrates clearly the kinds of cells that populate the testicular tubule during this phase of life. The relatively few large, round cells with almost clear or pale-staining cytoplasm, nestled against the thin basement membrane, are the spermatogonia. On the other hand, the great majority of cells within these tubules are Sertoli or supporting cells; their small, round, darkly stained nuclei are dispersed fairly evenly from one wall of the tubule to the other. One notes in Figures 24-5 and 24-6, taken from a term infant at birth and a child three weeks of age respectively, that the character and relative distribution of cells within the tubules are not really different from those observed in the tubules of the prematurely born infant (in approximately the eighth month of gestation) depicted in Figure 24-4.

Interstitial Cells of Leydig. The developing seminiferous tubules are separated from one another by mesenchyme that gives rise to the interstitial cells of Leydig. These are rather plump cells with darkly stained cytoplasm, occurring in crowded clusters between tubules. They appear in large numbers in at least three areas in Figure 24-2, a section taken from an infant in approximately the fifth month of gestation. Their numbers diminish steadily during the latter part of intrauterine life, and they disappear during the first year of extrauterine life, not to be seen again until puberty. They are clearly visible in Figure 24-4a, where their cytoplasm appears to be relatively smooth and gray; when the section is stained with hematoxylin and eosin, the cytoplasm is bright pink. The nucleus may be either centrally located or eccentric. In Figures 24-5 and 24-6 one can appreciate the finely vacuolated quality of their cytoplasm, which is characteristic of these cells.

Genital Ducts. In Figure 24-7 is seen the epididymis of a prematurely born infant in the fifth month of gestation. Individual ductules are relatively few, and they have stout walls. In Figure 24-8 (taken at the same magnification) is seen a section from a considerably more mature infant. The tubules are much more numerous; they have thinner walls and wider lumina.

Figure 24-9 illustrates the range of epithelial cell types in the lining of these ductules in the premature infant at about seven months of gestation. In Figure 24-10, at the same magnification, are seen these same types of cells as observed in sections from two infants near term. Individual cells, on the average, appear to be larger.

Figure 24-11a depicts the histologic morphology of the ductus deferens in the vicinity of the testis in a term infant. Figure 24-11b, at much lower magnification, illustrates its appearance near the seminal gland in a premature infant; the wall is thinner and the lumen larger.

Figures 24-12 and 24-13 show the seminal glands of two infants who weighed 2,150 grams and 4,005 grams, respectively. The convoluted appearance of the lining of each is easily discernible. The epithelium is of pseudostratified cuboidal to columnar type.

Appendix Testis and Appendix Epididymis. The appendices are very similar if not identical in histologic appearance. They tend to be polypoid, with a fairly stout body and slender stalk (Fig. 24–14). The stroma is composed of cellular and moderately vascular fibrous connective tissue, and the covering consists of epithelial cells having a cuboidal to columnar character. Not infrequently, the covering epithelium is somewhat folded into the core; at times one will encounter a cyst-like space or spaces within the center of the appendix, completely lined by these same epithelial cells.

References

1. Moore, K. L.: The Developing Human. Clinically Oriented Embryology. Philadelphia, W. B. Saunders Co., 1973, pp. 207–211.
2. Warwick, R., and Williams, P. L.: Gray's Anatomy. 35th British ed. Philadelphia, W. B. Saunders Co., 1973, pp. 1336–1337.

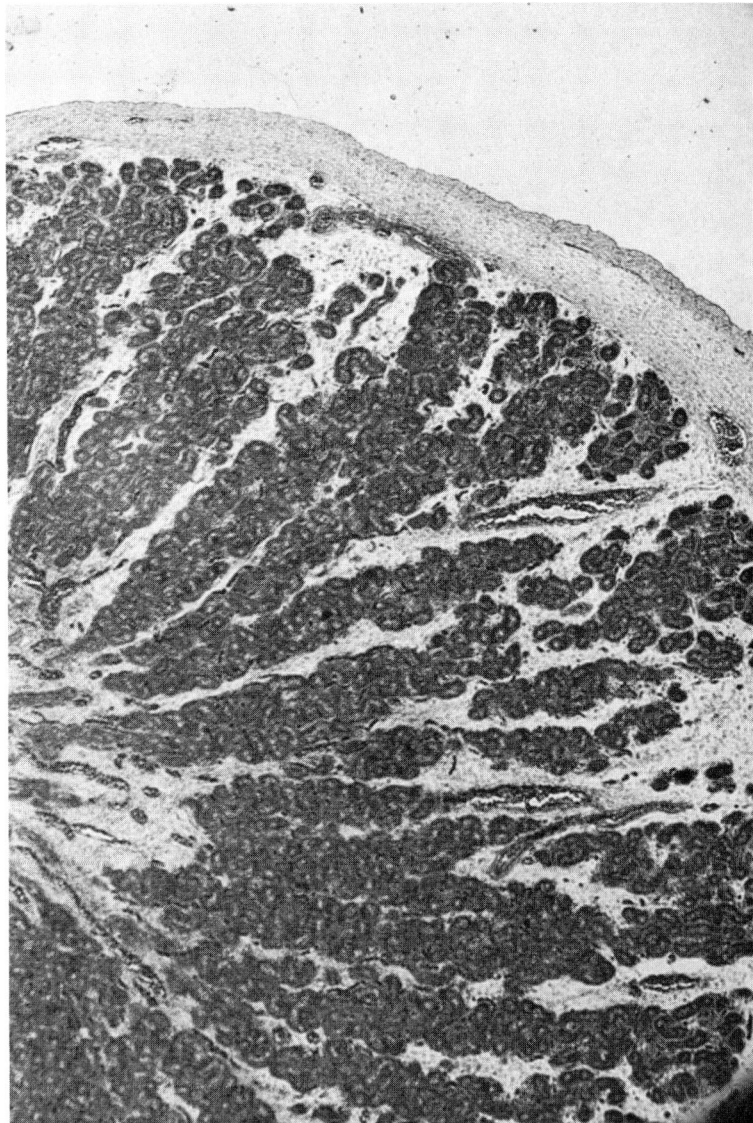

Figure 24–1

Figure 24–1. Survey view of the testis of an infant weighing 2,850 grams, who lived for 25½ hours. The tunica albuginea is visible along the upper margin of the image, and the rete testis in the lower left. Individual lobules of the testis are clearly visible, divided from one another by fibrous septa which radiate out into the organ from its hilus.

Hematoxylin and eosin stain. Mag. 24.5×.

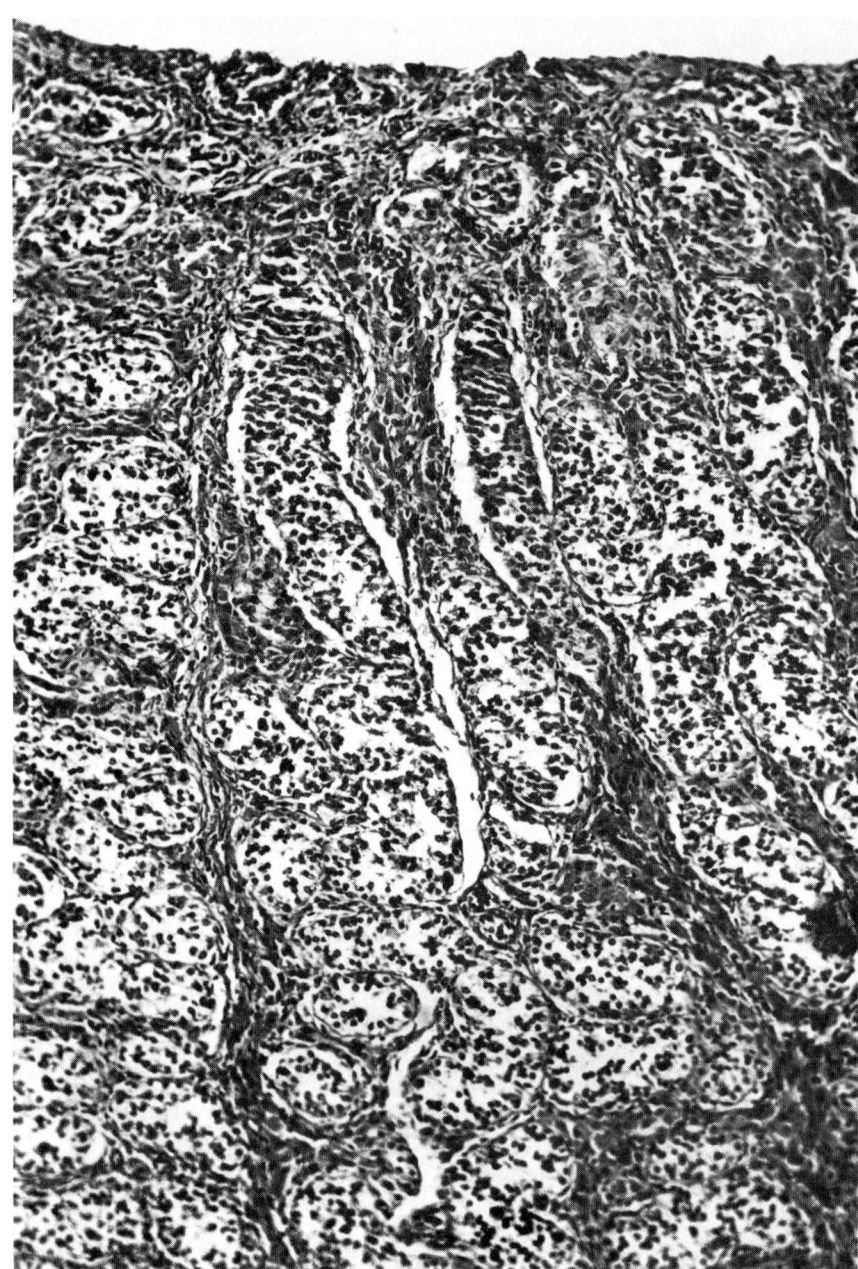

Figure 24–2

Figure 24–2. At somewhat higher magnification we see here the radiating arrangement of the seminiferous tubules as they appear peripherally, immediately beneath the tunica albuginea, in an infant weighing 476.5 grams who survived for 30 minutes.
Hematoxylin and eosin stain. Mag. 142×.

TESTIS 403

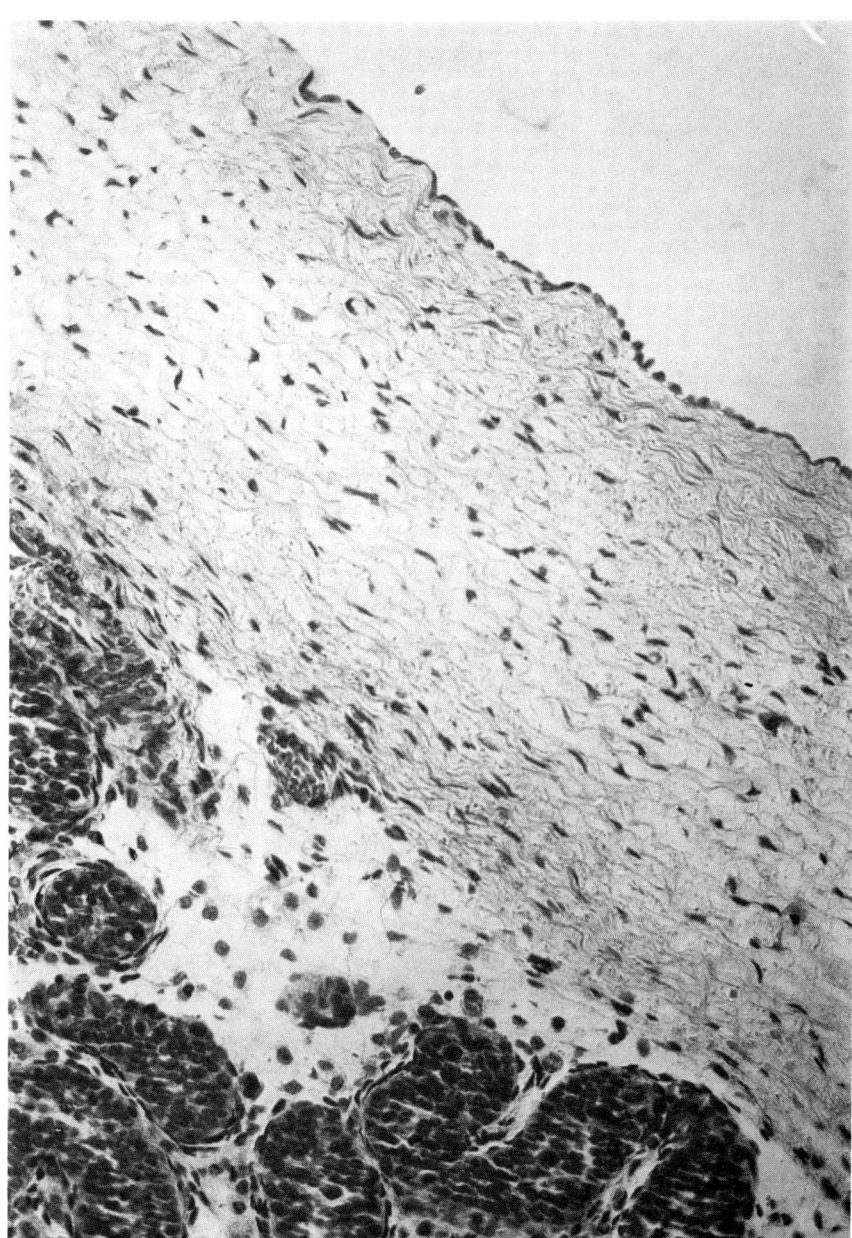

Figure 24–3

Figure 24–3. The tunica albuginea and germinal epithelium at higher magnification. This infant is the one referred to in the legend of Fig. 24–1.
Hematoxylin and eosin stain. Mag. 250×.

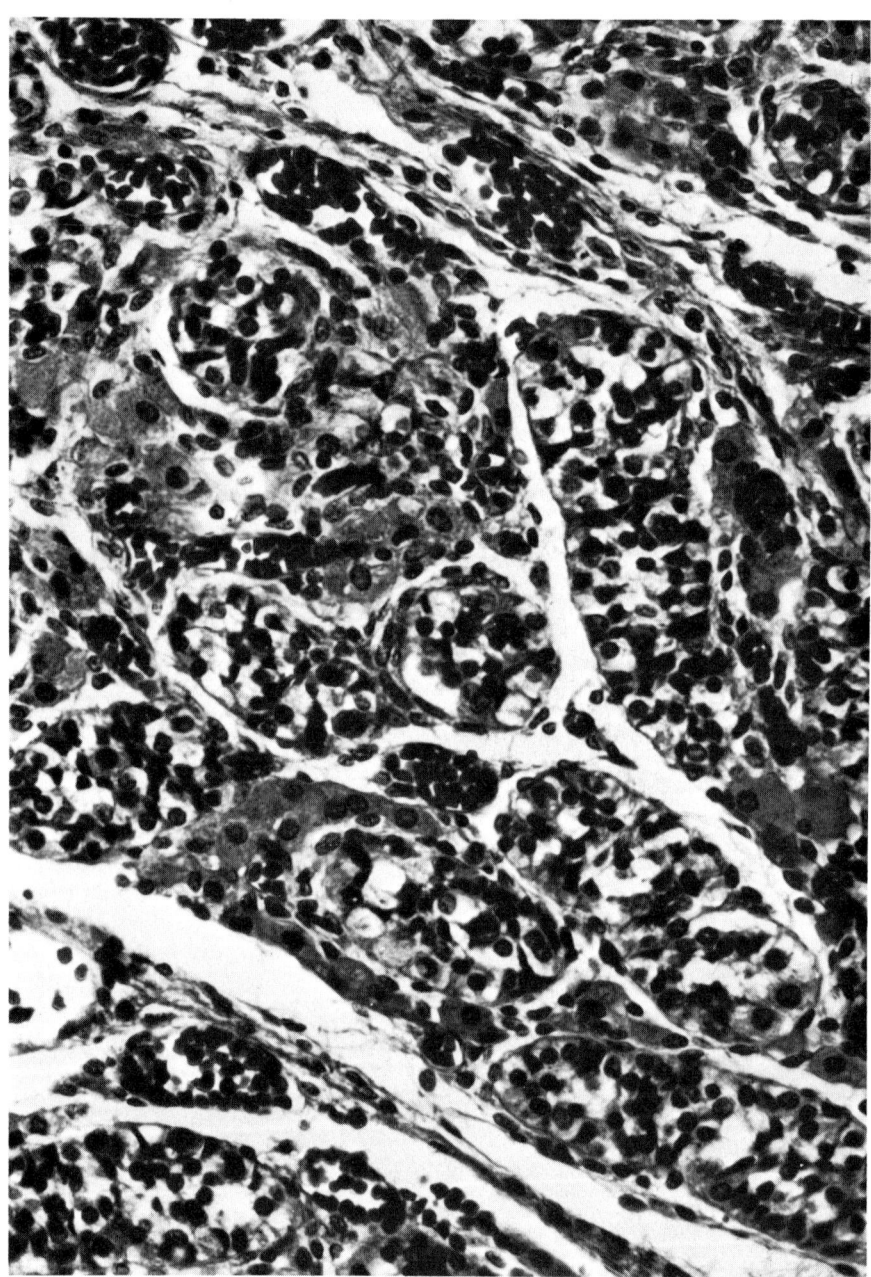

Figure 24–4

Figure 24–4. The seminiferous tubules of a liveborn infant weighing 1,720 grams, who lived for 9 hours and 20 minutes. Note the apparent absence of any lumen, the delicate basement membrane, and the large clear cells situated peripherally in each tubule. Crowds of Leydig cells with darkly stained cytoplasm are visible in nests between tubules.
Hematoxylin and eosin stain. Mag. 350×.

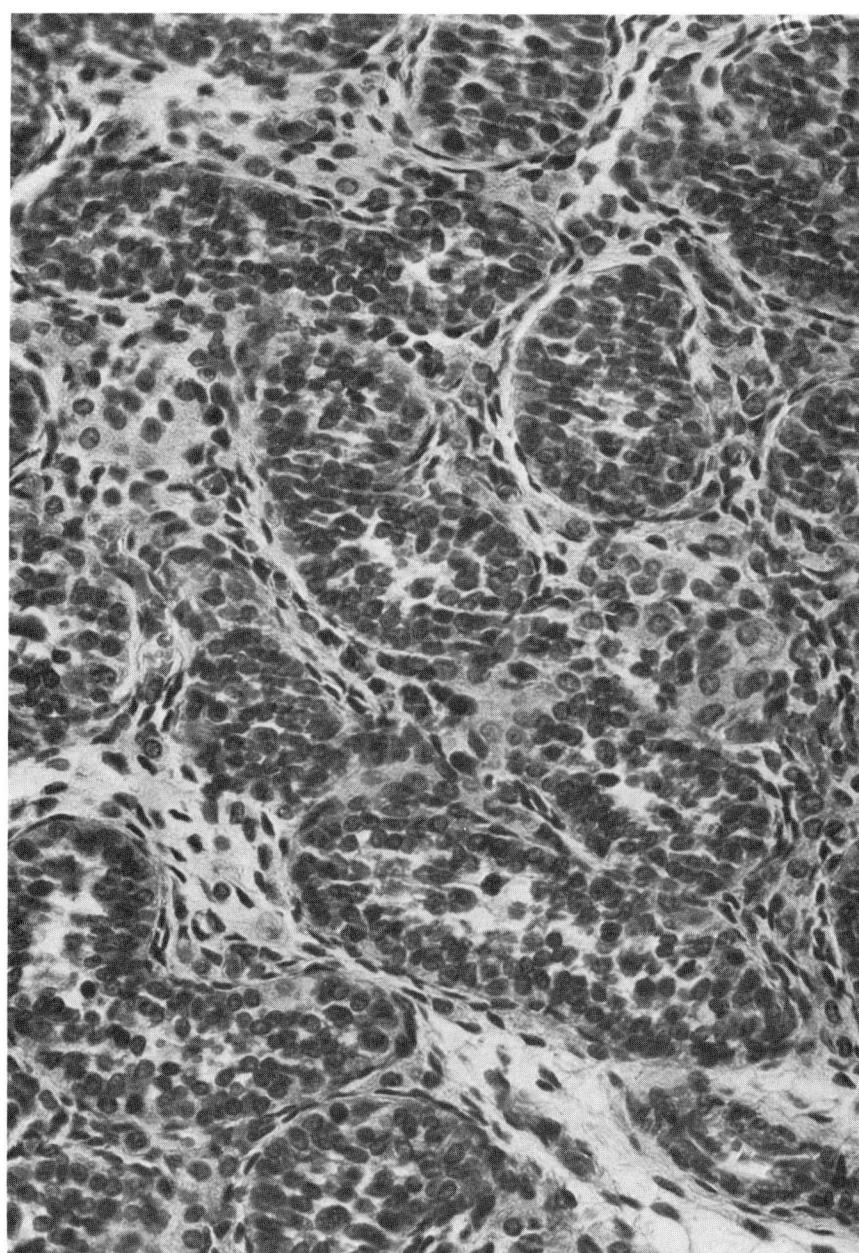

Figure 24–5

Figure 24–5. The seminiferous tubules of the infant referred to in the legends of Figs. 24–1 and 24–3. Even though this is a term infant, the tubules are quite like those of the premature depicted in Fig. 24–4.
Hematoxylin and eosin stain. Mag. 350×.

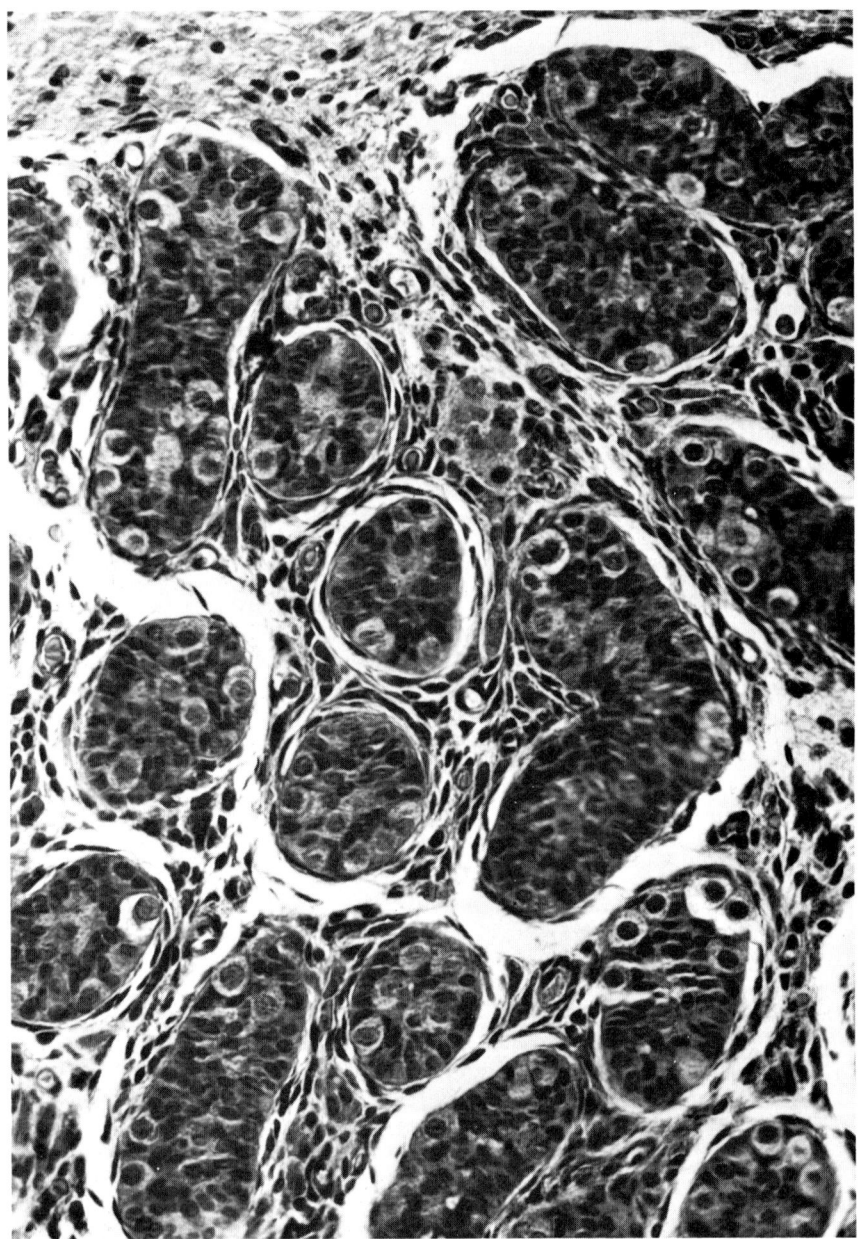

Figure 24–6

Figure 24–6. This section was taken from a surgical specimen from a 3 week old infant who weighed 3,362 grams. He had been born at 8½ months of gestation.

The histologic features are still quite like those of the prematurely born infant depicted in Fig. 24–4. The basement membrane is delicate. Spermatogonia are arranged peripherally in each tubule, close to the basement membrane. Leydig cells, however, do appear to be less numerous.

Hematoxylin and eosin stain. Mag. 350×.

TESTIS 407

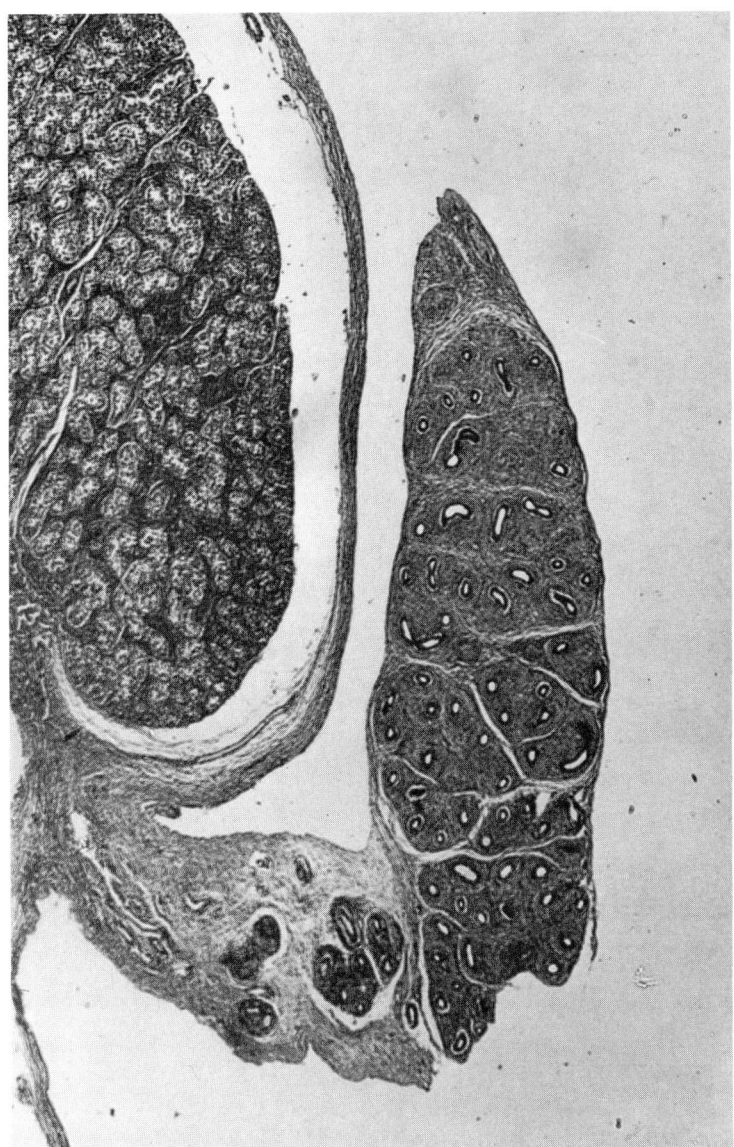

Figure 24–7

Figure 24–7. The epididymis of a 476.5 gram infant who lived for 30 minutes. The coiled ductules are arranged in lobules.
Hematoxylin and eosin stain. Mag. 37×.

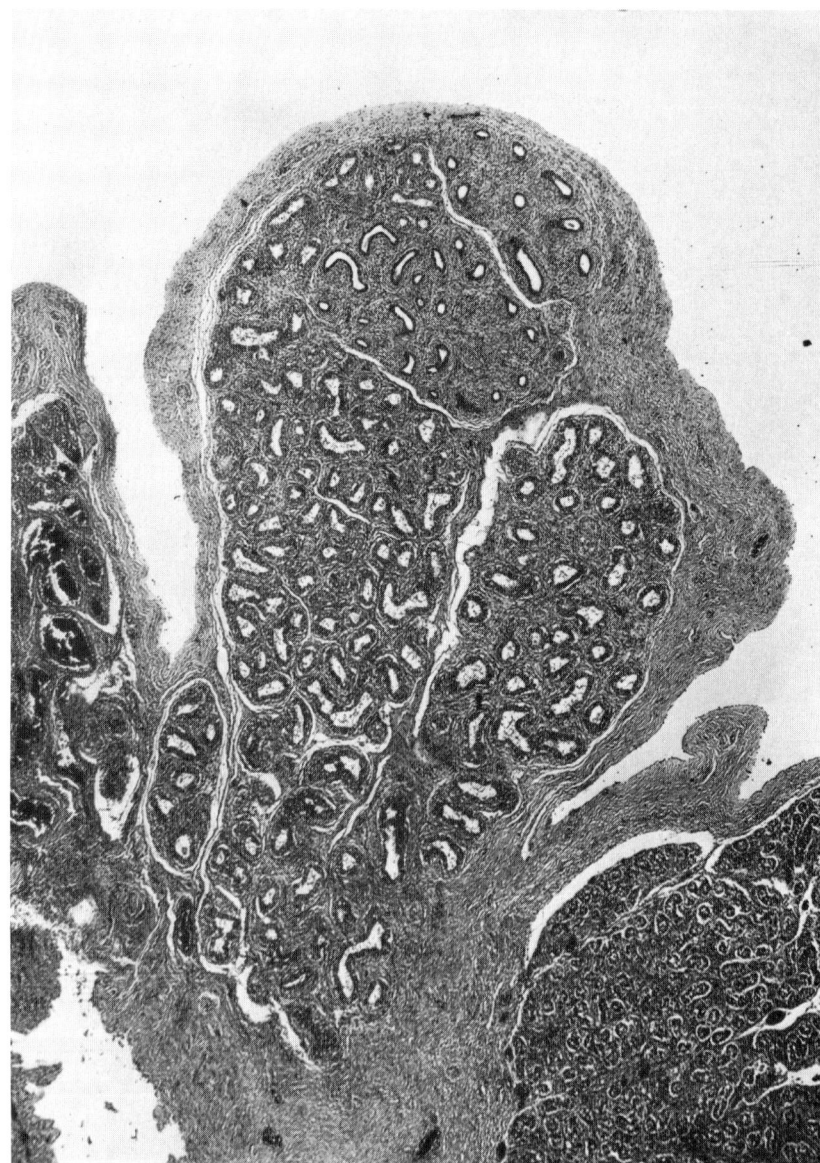

Figure 24–8

Figure 24–8. This is the epididymis of an infant having roughly twice the body weight of that described in the legend for Fig. 24–7, 1050 grams. Note that the lobular arrangement is still apparent. Hematoxylin and eosin stain. Mag. 37×.

TESTIS 409

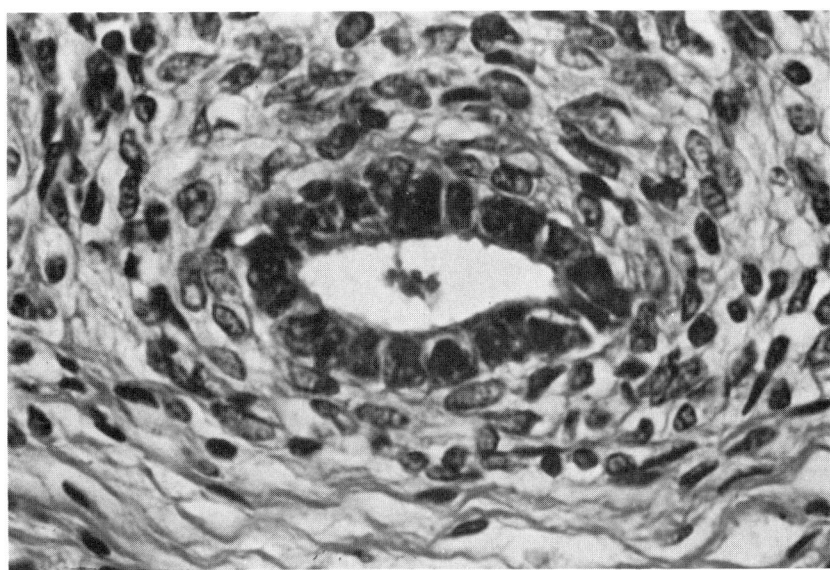

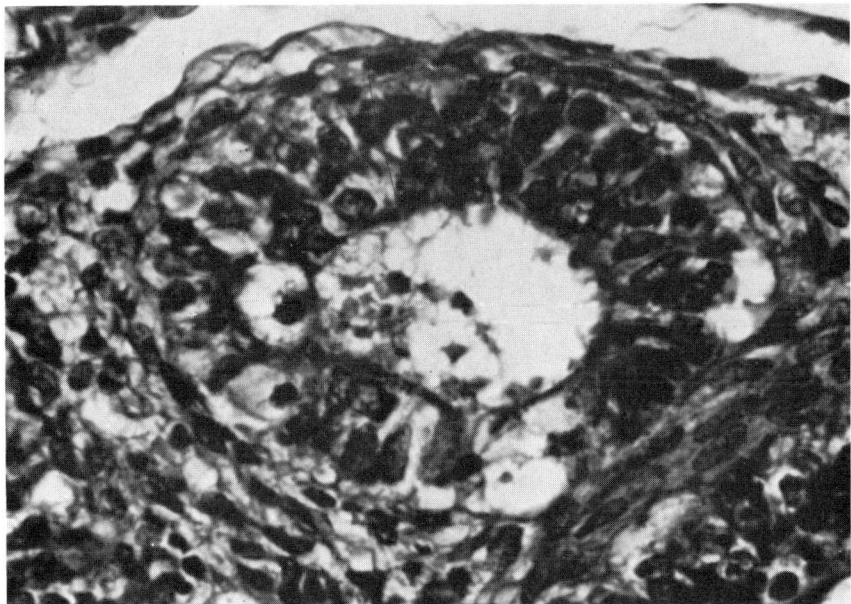

Figure 24-9

Figure 24-9. The epithelial lining of the ductules of the epididymis in the infant during the perinatal period ranges from cuboidal to columnar. These sections are both from an infant weighing 1,050 grams, who lived for 25 hours.
Hematoxylin and eosin stain. Mag. 597×.

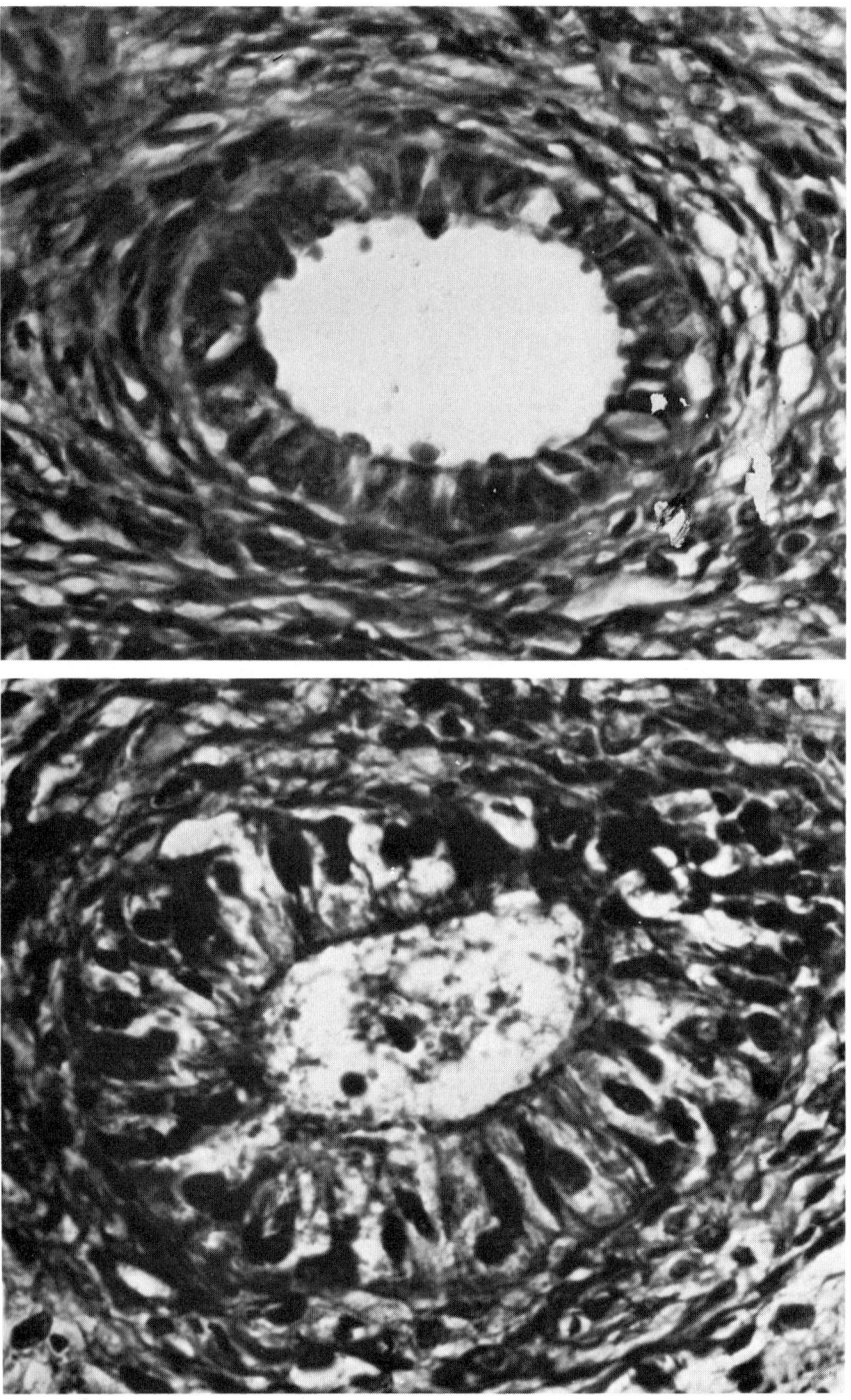

Figure 24–10

Figure 24–10. All components of the ductules appear magnified in these sections from two infants, both with body weight about 2,200 grams. The lumina of the ductules are larger than those in Fig. 24–9, and the lining cells are also larger.
Hematoxylin and eosin stain. Mag. 597×.

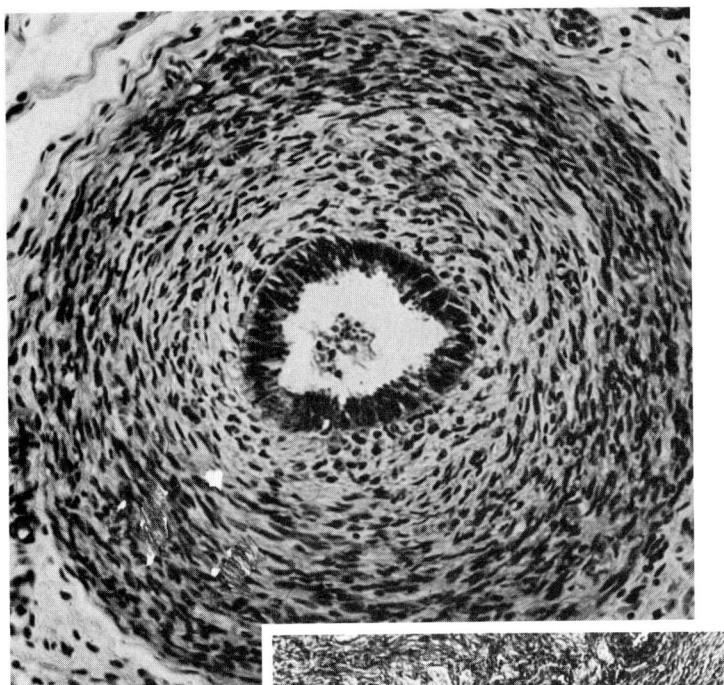

Figure 24–11a

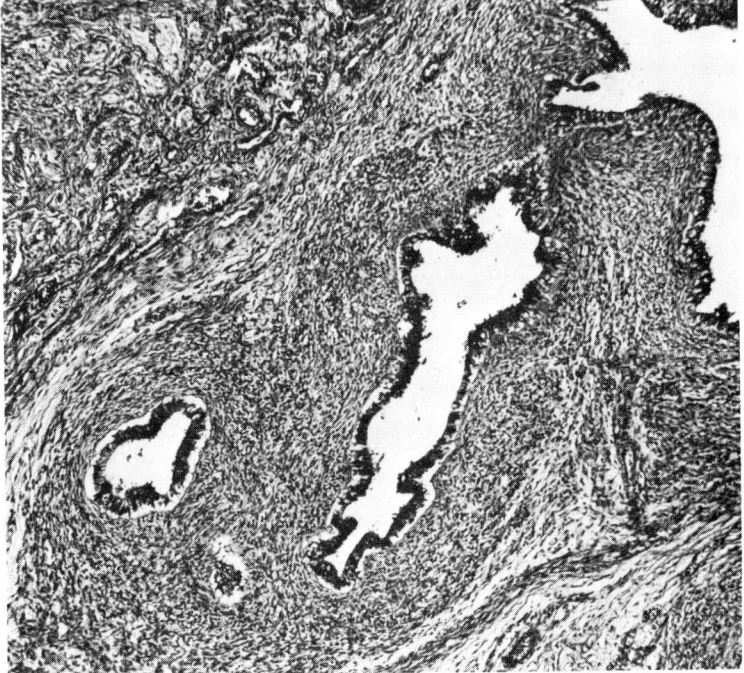

Figure 24–11b

Figure 24–11a. This section illustrates the ductus deferens in proximity to the testis. This is from a term infant weighing 2,501 grams, who lived for 17 hours.
Hematoxylin and eosin stain. Mag. 208×.

Figure 24–11b. This is the ductus near its ampulla and the seminal vesicle. This section is from an infant weighing 760 grams, who survived 12 hours and 8 minutes.
Hematoxylin and eosin stain. Mag. 92.5×.

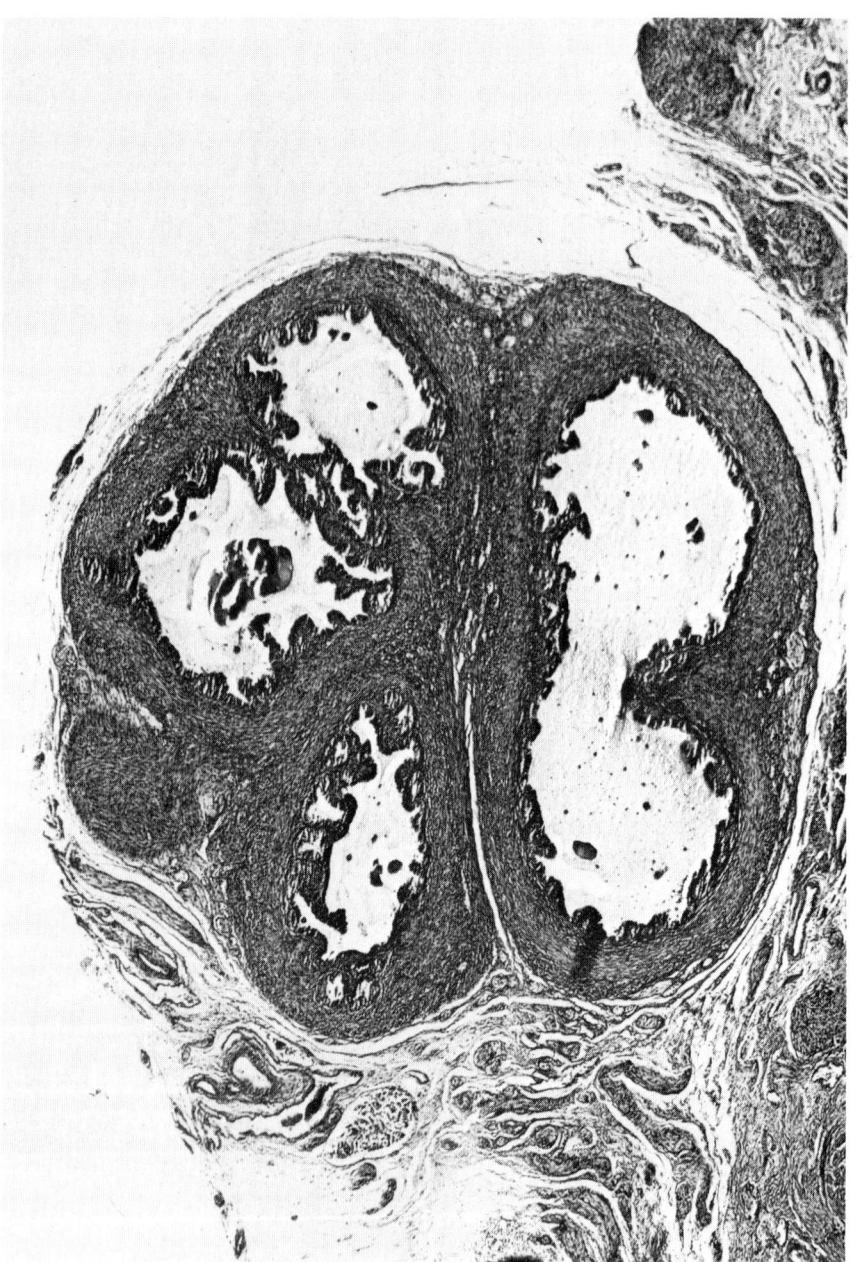

Figure 24–12

Figure 24–12. Cross section of the seminal gland of an infant who lived 11 days and whose body weight at death was 2,150 grams.
Hematoxylin and eosin stain. Mag. 45×.

TESTIS 413

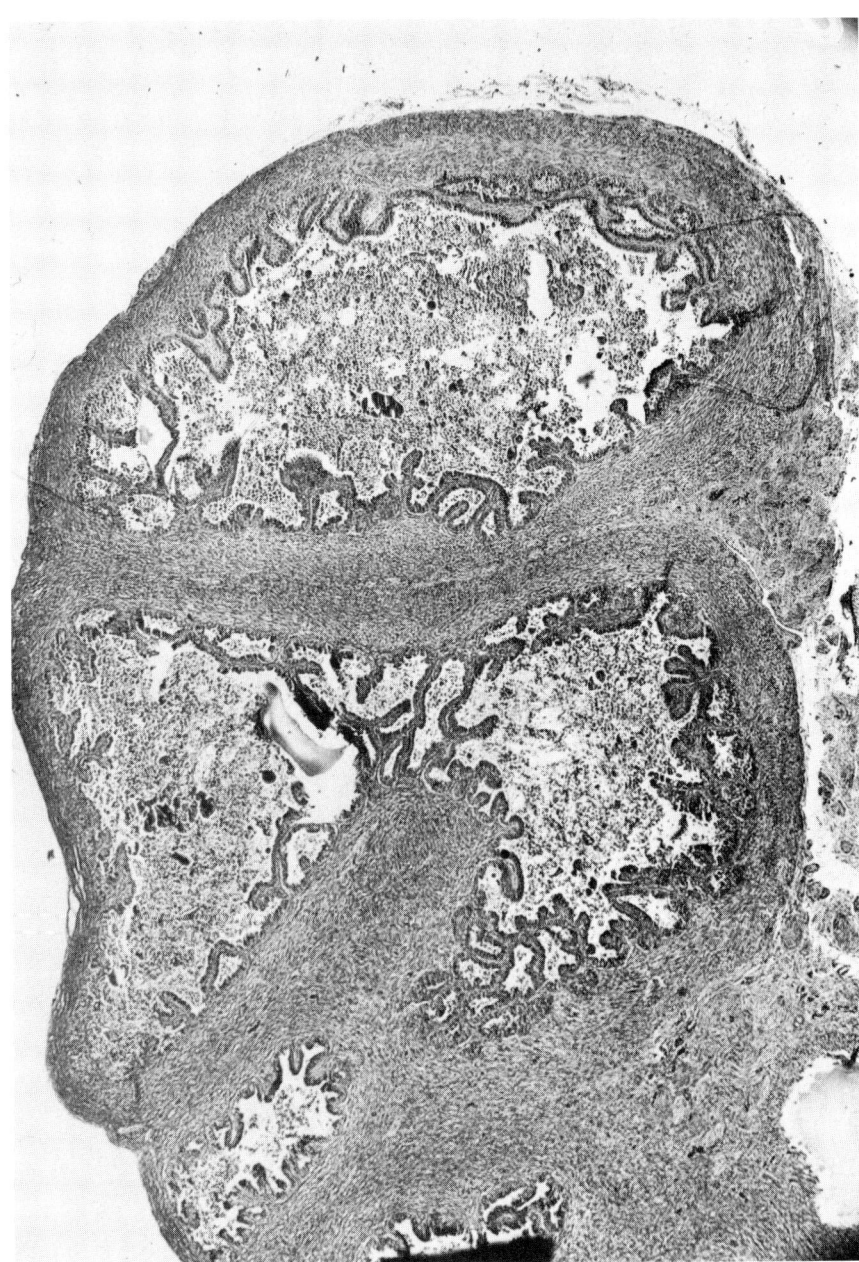

Figure 24–13

Figure 24–13. Cross section of the seminal gland of an infant who died at the age of one month and whose body weight at death was 4,005 grams.
Hematoxylin and eosin stain. Mag. 38×.

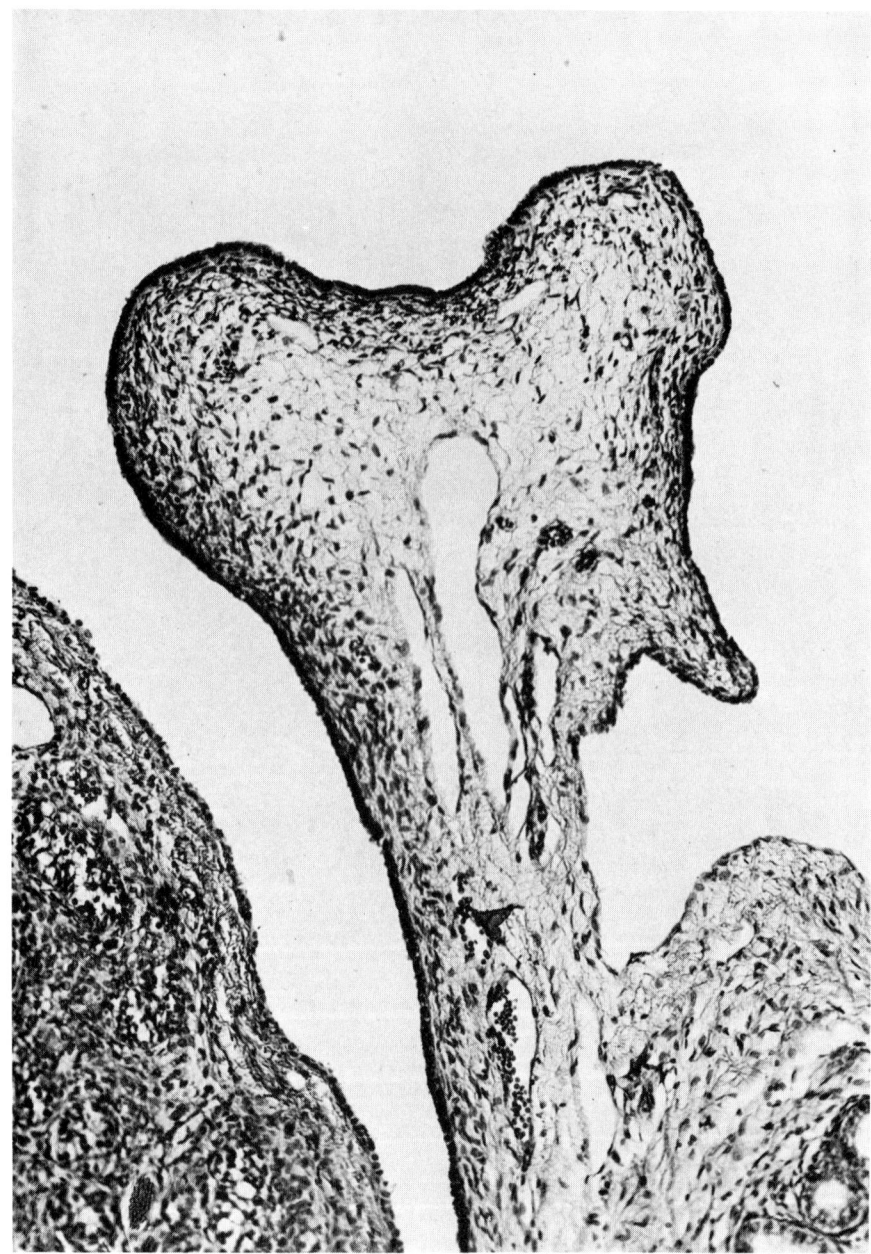

Figure 24-14

Figure 24-14. The appendix epididymis from an infant weighing 835 grams, who lived for 5 hours and 25 minutes.
Hematoxylin and eosin stain. Mag. 208×.

Chapter 25

PROSTATE

EMBRYOLOGY

Multiple endodermal outgrowths from the prostatic portion of the urethra grow into surrounding mesenchyme and constitute the emerging prostate. The glandular epithelium of prostatic ducts and glands is derived from these endodermal cells, and the associated mesenchyme differentiates into the dense fibrous and smooth muscular stroma.[1]

The fused caudal ends of the paramesonephric (Müller's) ducts in the male give rise to the prostatic utricle, the blind pouch which, in infants, is often surprisingly prominent, at times even cystically dilated (Fig. 25–4 to 25–6).

ANATOMY

The prostate encircles the urethra immediately distal to the neck of the bladder (Figs. 25–1 and 25–2). Although it comprises from 30 to 50 tubuloalveolar glands arranged in lobes, only a limited number are visible in any one cross section. The glands themselves, at this stage of development of the organ, are not nearly so conspicuous as they appear in sections taken from an adult.

HISTOLOGY

Throughout late fetal and neonatal life the stroma, which is the predominant element, is clearly made up of two distinct types of tissue, mature collagenous connective tissue and interweaving bundles of smooth muscle (Fig. 25–3).

As mentioned above, the prostatic utricle of the newborn is not uncommonly dilated to cystic proportions. It is lined by stratified squamous epithelium (Fig. 27–6) and may contain sloughed-off surface cells of that type (Fig. 27–4).

The groove on each side of the prostatic crest is known as the prostatic sinus, and into it the numerous major ducts of the prostatic glands open by minute apertures (Fig. 25–2). The lining of these major ducts is predominantly a sort of transitional epithelium, but frequently it includes sizeable segments of stratified squamous character (Figs. 25–7 and 25–8).

On each side of and slightly distal to the opening of the prostatic utricle are the paired ostia of the ejaculatory ducts (Fig. 25–9).

The large ducts of the glands within the body of the prostate, again, are lined by a kind of transitional epithelium with stratification of nuclei (Fig. 25–10 and 25–11). The tubuloalveolar glands themselves are very small and simple compared with those of the adult. The lumina are slender; their lining consists of simple cuboidal to very low columnar cells (Fig. 25–12). Prostatic concretions (corpora amylacea) are not seen in the prostate of the fetus or newborn.

Reference

1. Moore, K. L.: The Developing Human. Clinically Oriented Embryology. Philadelphia, W. B. Saunders Co., 1973, p. 214.

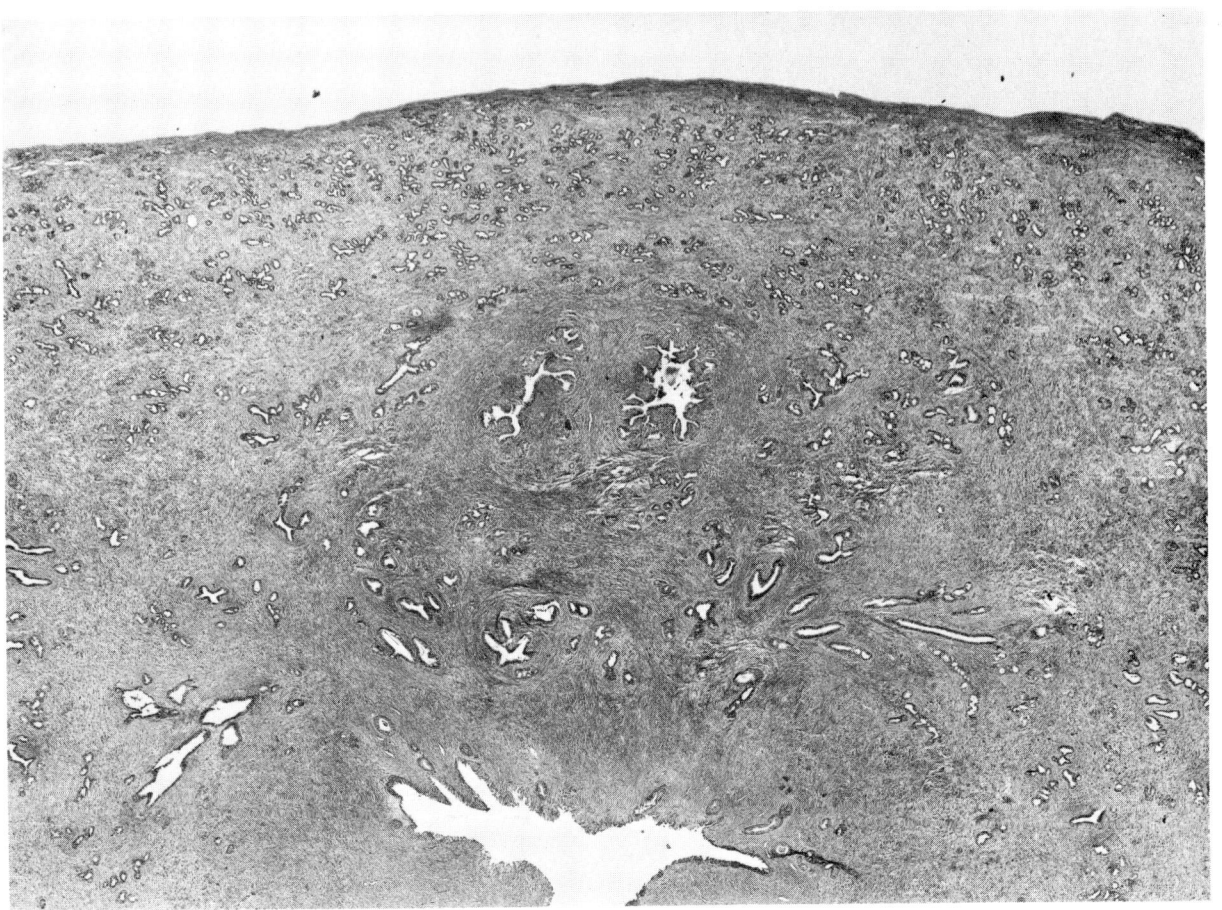

Figure 25–1

Figure 25–1. This photomicrograph, taken at very low magnification, represents an almost horizontal section through the prostate of an infant weighing 4,005 grams, who died at the age of one month. At the bottom of the photograph, in the center, a few of the major ducts are seen emptying into the prostatic portion of the urethra. Along the upper margin, tiny round tubuloalveolar glands appear. Near the center of the section there are two rather stellate isolated tubular structures, larger than all the rest, which are the ejaculatory ducts.

Hematoxylin and eosin stain. Mag. 17.3×.

418 PROSTATE

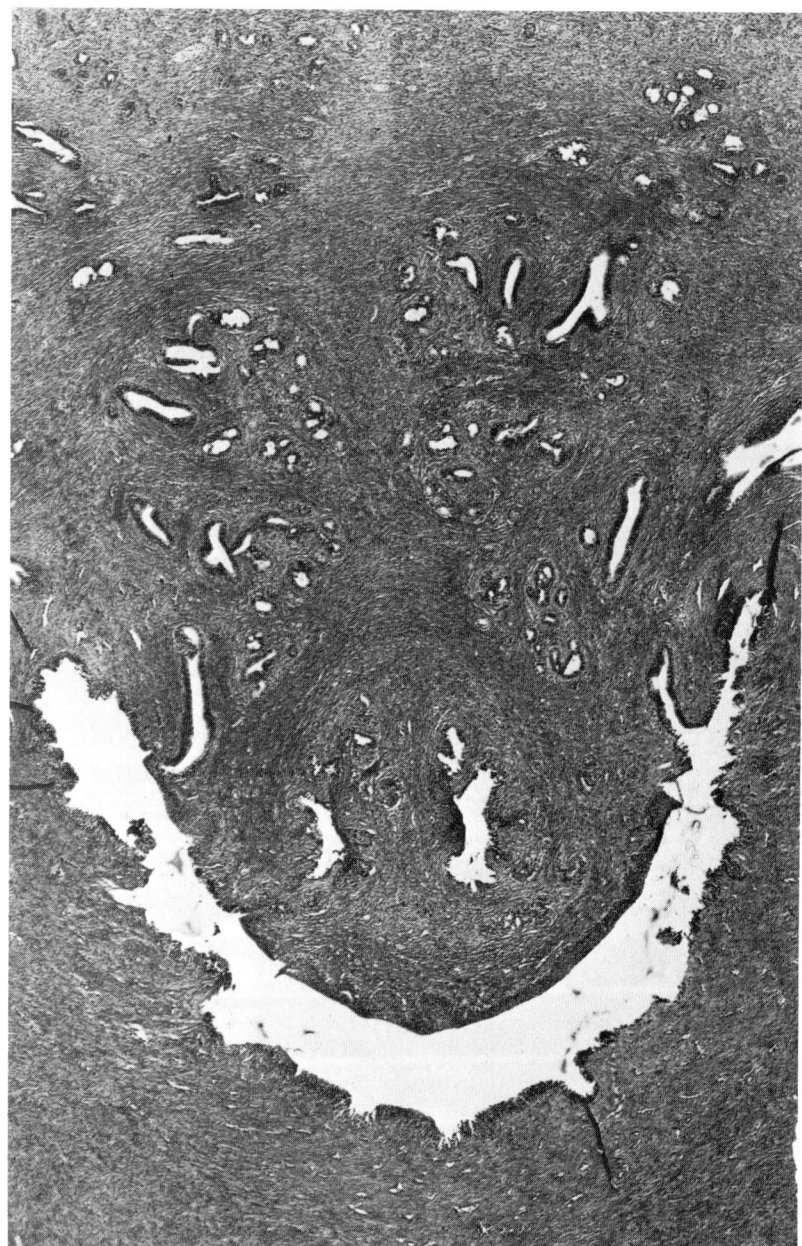

Figure 25–2

Figure 25–2. This is another section of the prostate from the infant described in the legend for Fig. 25–1. The urethral crest (verumontanum) projects downward into the prostatic urethra, which at this level assumes a crescentic shape. Into the two prostatic sinuses, on the sides of the urethral crest, prostatic ducts empty.

Hematoxylin and eosin stain. Mag. 31×.

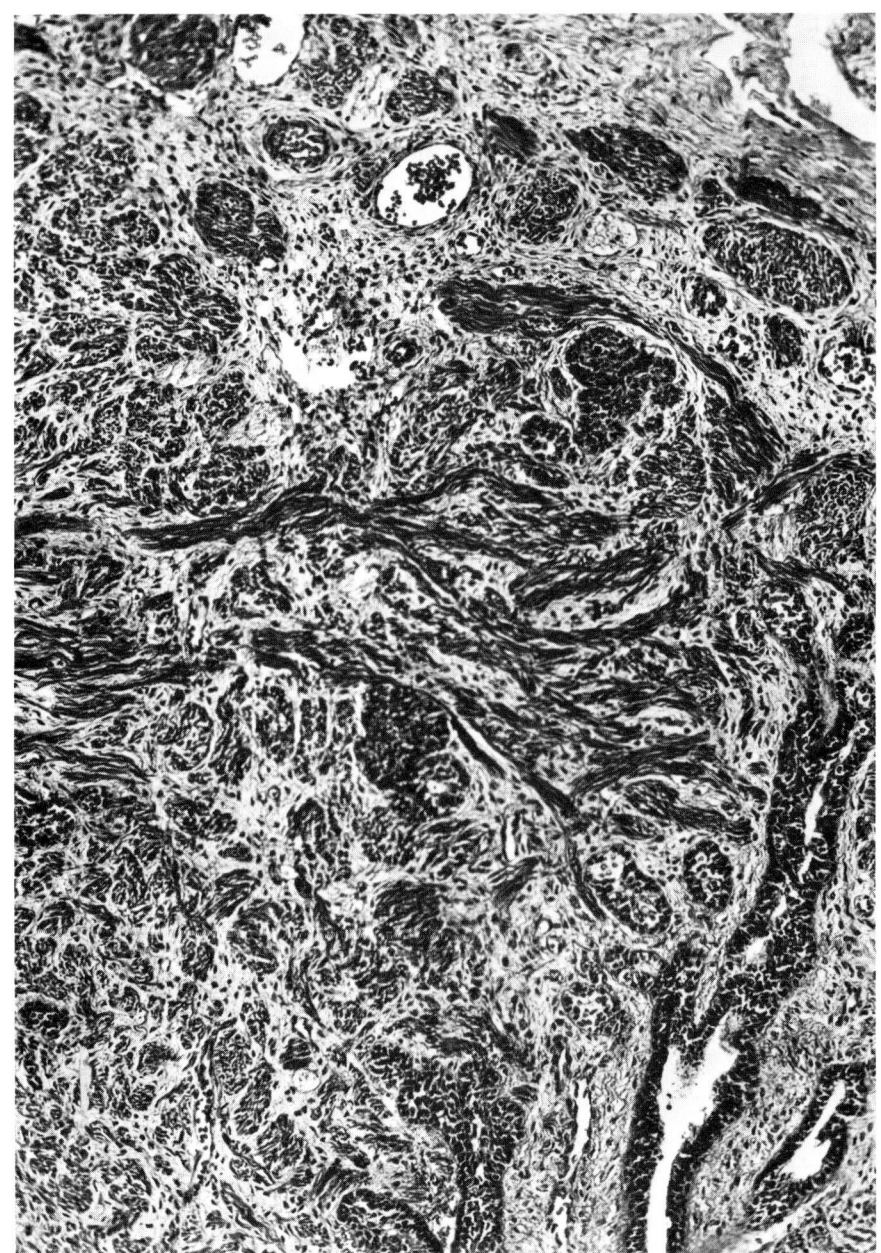

Figure 25–3

Figure 25–3. Photomicrograph of the fibromuscular stroma of the prostate of an infant who weighed 1,720 grams and who lived 9 hours and 20 minutes. The interweaving smooth muscle bundles are darkly stained.
Hematoxylin and eosin stain. Mag. 142×.

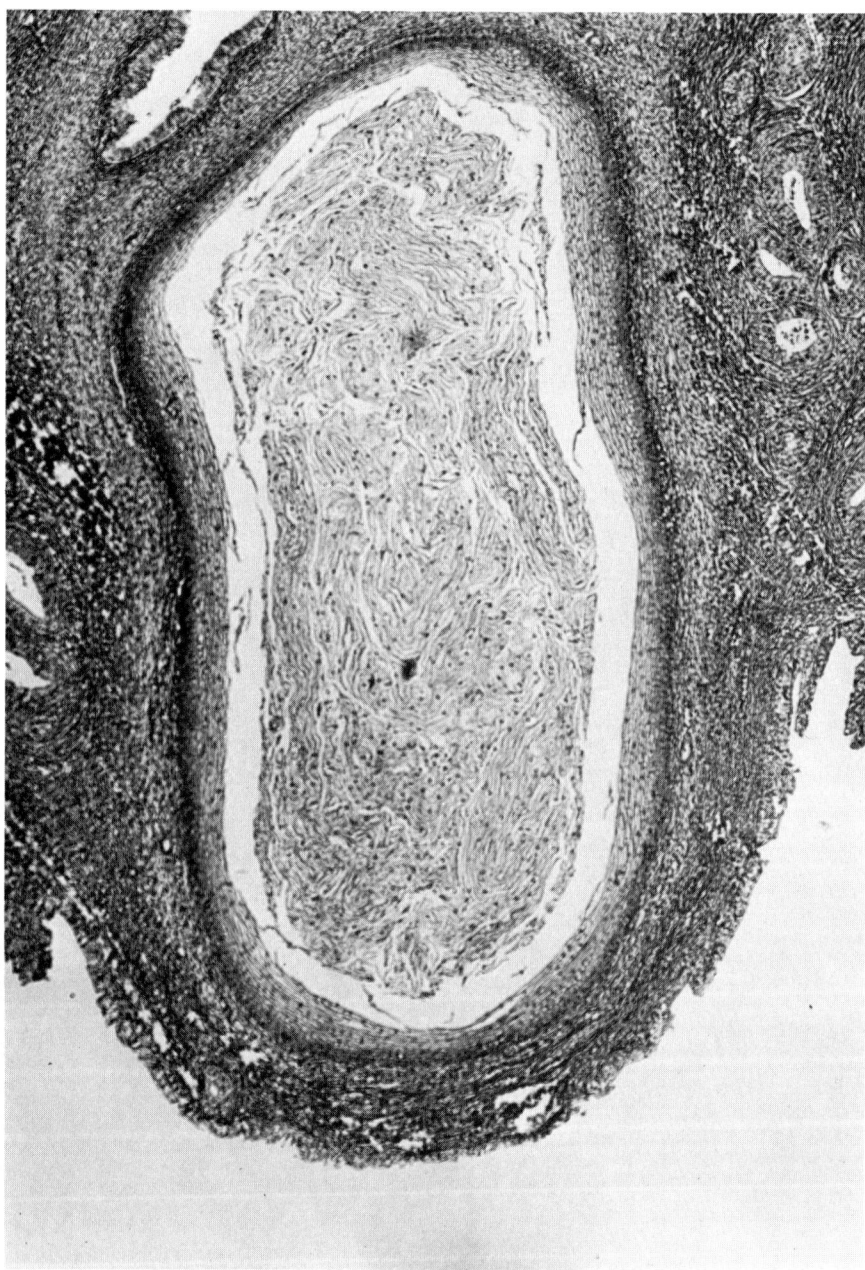

Figure 25–4

Figure 25–4. Horizontal section of the urethral crest from an infant of 615 grams who died at 5 hours and 42 minutes of age. The large, almost cystically dilated structure in the center of the photograph is the prostatic utricle. It is completely lined by stratified squamous epithelium here, and the lumen is filled with cast-off epithelial cells.

Hematoxylin and eosin stain. Mag. 88.5×.

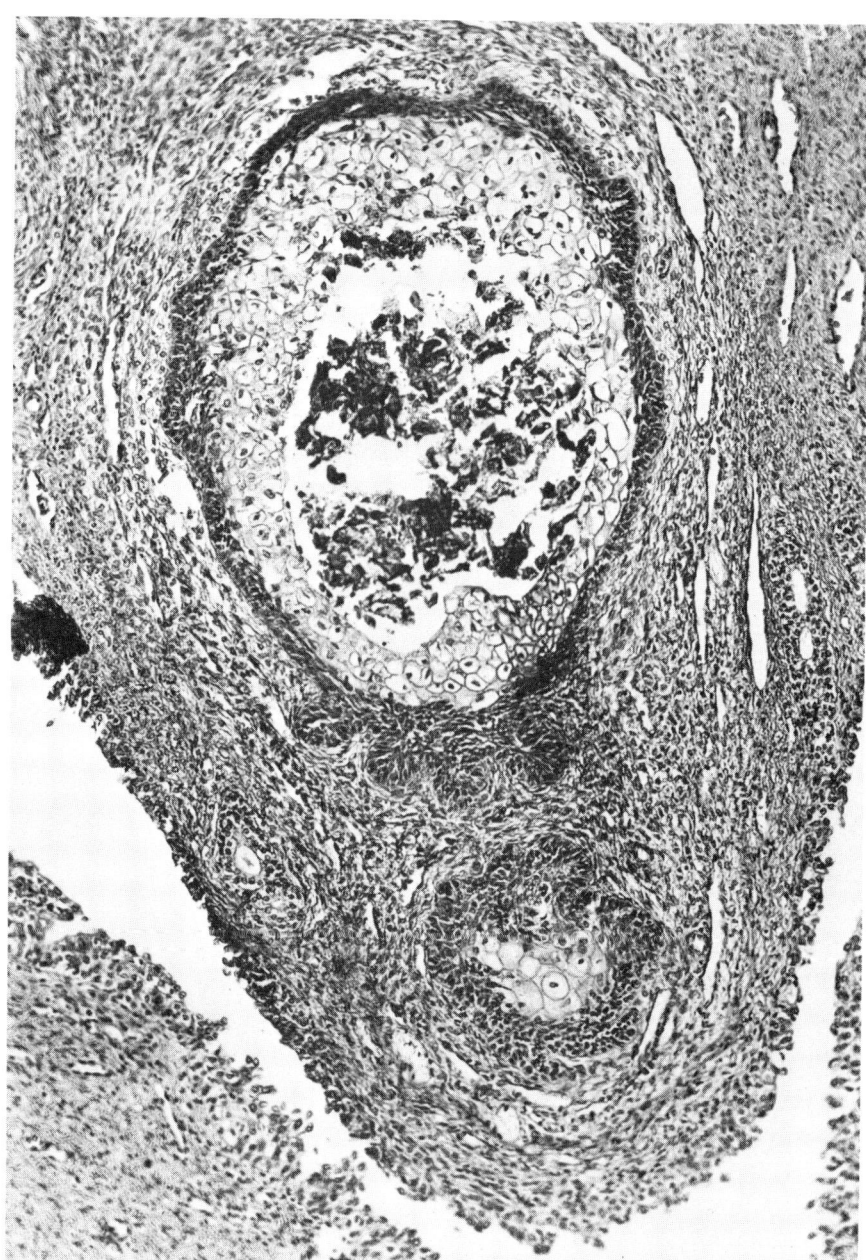

Figure 25–5

Figure 25–5. A section similar to Fig. 25–4, at higher magnification, from an infant of 835 grams. The stratified squamous epithelial lining is more clearly visible here.
Hematoxylin and eosin stain. Mag. 142×.

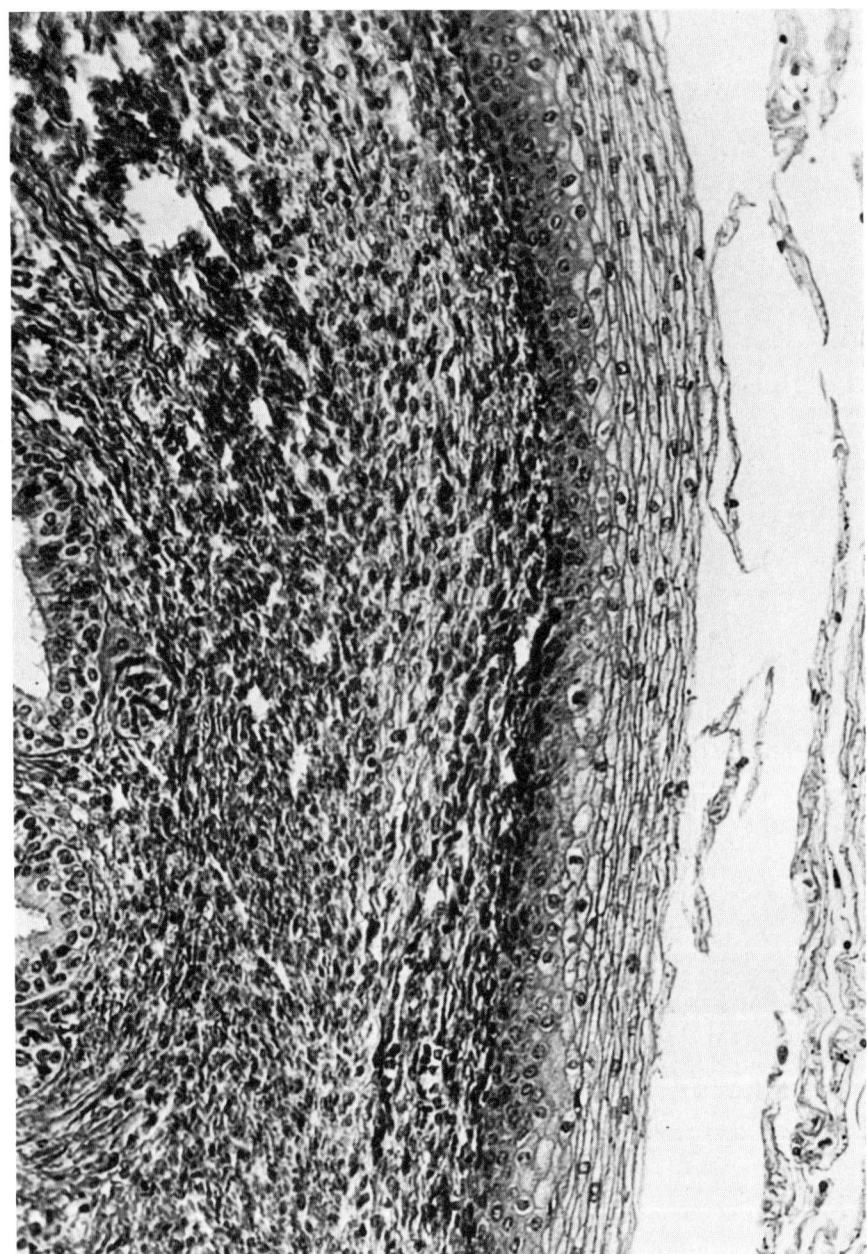

Figure 25-6

Figure 25-6. Higher magnification of the lining of the dilated utricle seen in Fig. 25-5. Hematoxylin and eosin stain. Mag. 243×.

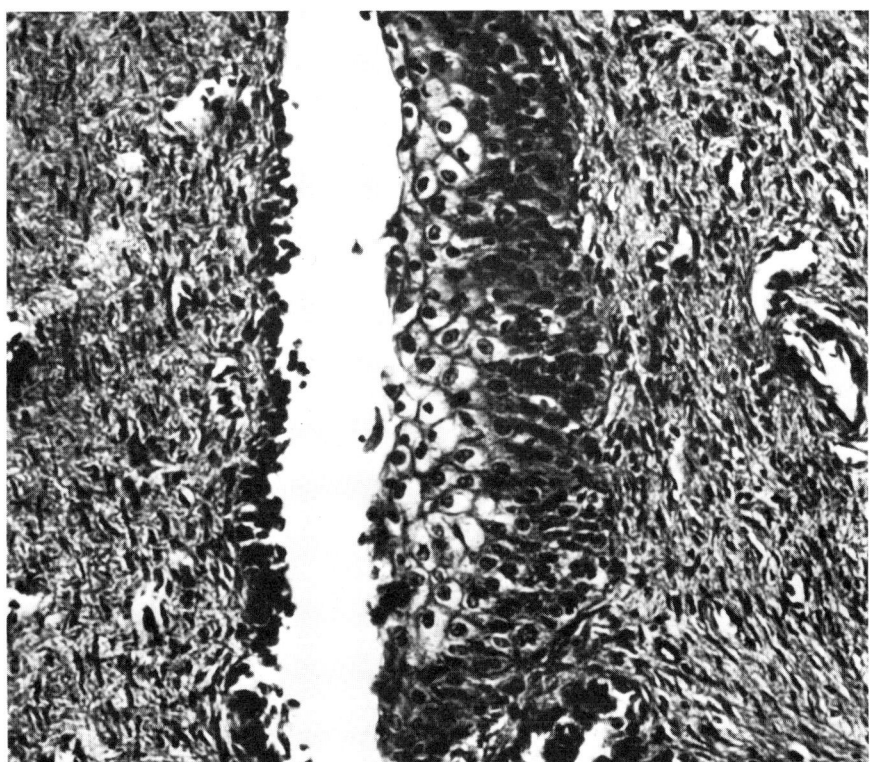

Figure 25–7

Figure 25–7. The lining of one of the major ducts of the prostate as it empties into the urethra. Only this segment was lined by stratified squamous epithelium; the remainder was lined by a kind of transitional epithelium. The infant weighed 2,290 grams and died at 8 hours of age.

Hematoxylin and eosin stain. Mag. 243×.

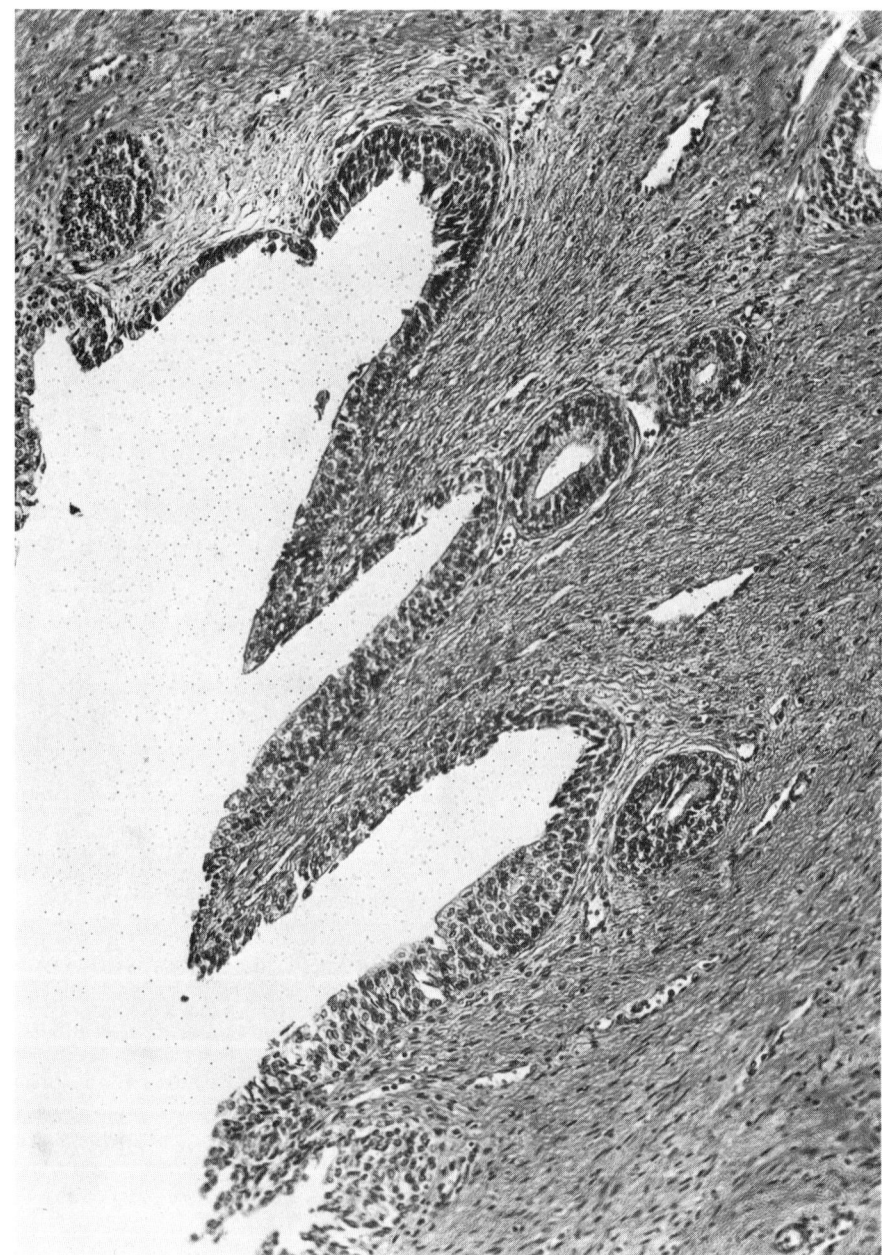

Figure 25-8

Figure 25-8. Major ducts at their point of entry into the urethra in the prostate of a one month old infant, who weighed 4,005 grams at death. Some of the epithelium is rather transitional, and some squamous.

Hematoxylin and eosin stain. Mag. 142×.

PROSTATE 425

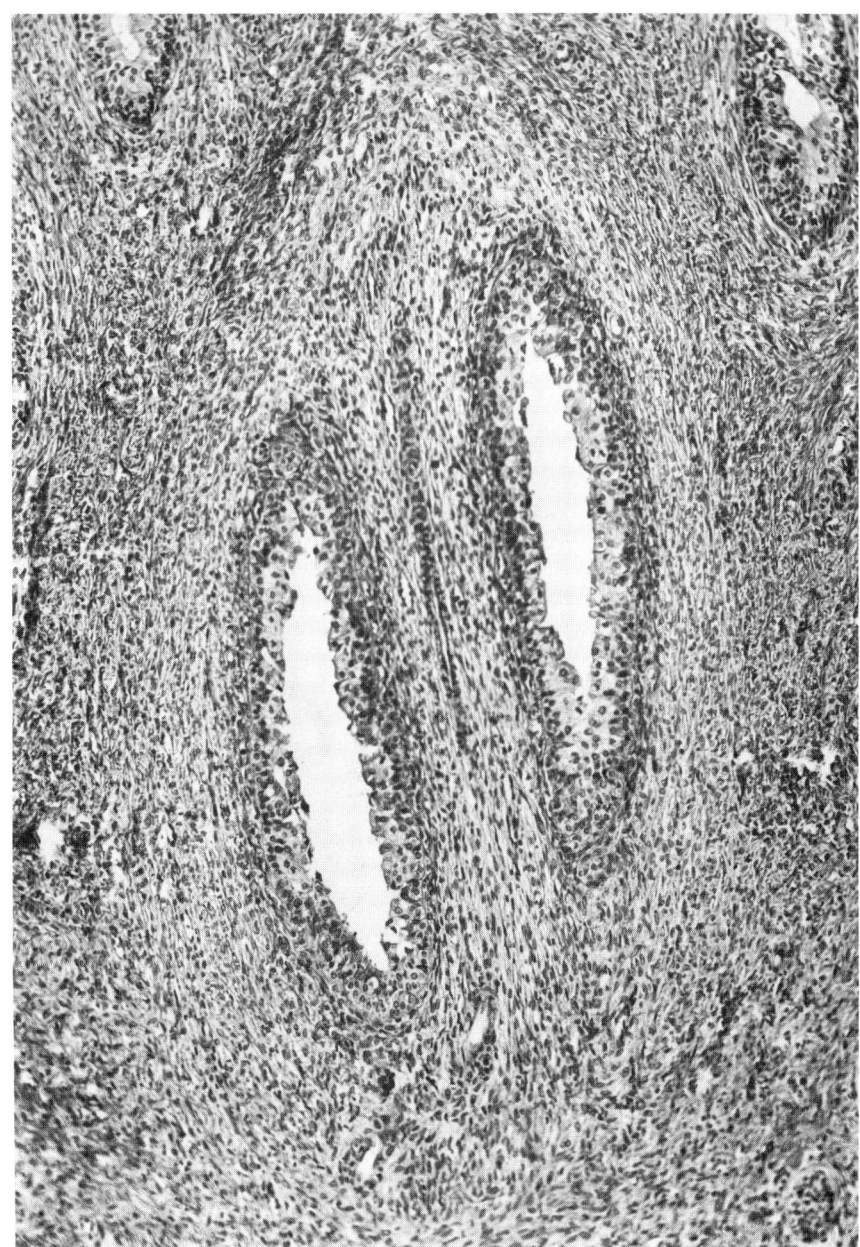

Figure 25–9

Figure 25–9. The paired ejaculatory ducts, near their point of entry into the urethra, in a section of the prostate of a 700 gram infant who survived for one hour after birth. The epithelium here is of a rather nondescript or mixed type.
Hematoxylin and eosin stain. Mag. 142×.

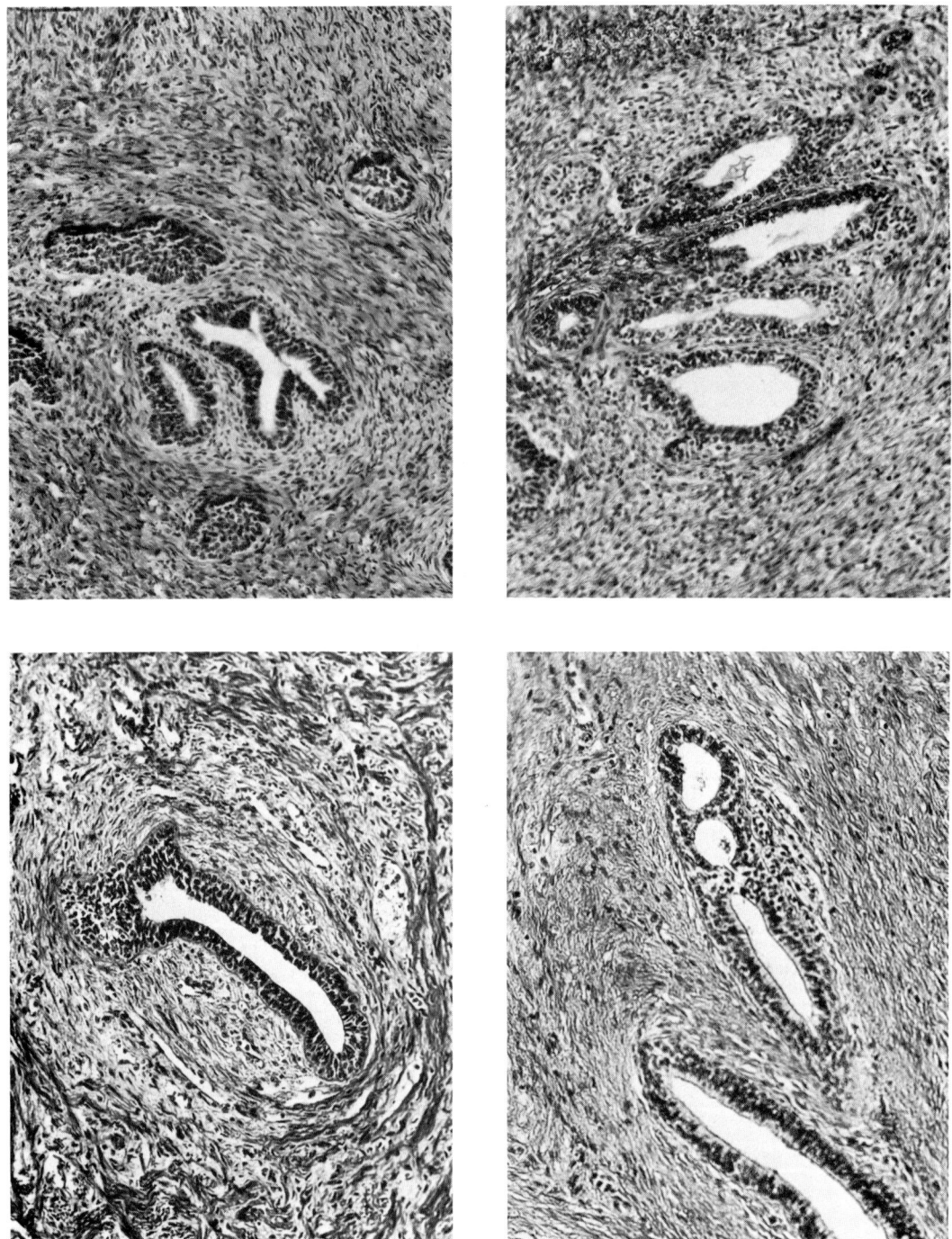

Figure 25–10

Figure 25–10. Larger ducts from within the body of the prostate, all at the same magnification, from infants with body weights of 430 grams (upper left), 700 grams (upper right), 1,720 grams (lower left), and 4,005 grams (lower right).
Hematoxylin and eosin stain. Mag. 142×.

PROSTATE 427

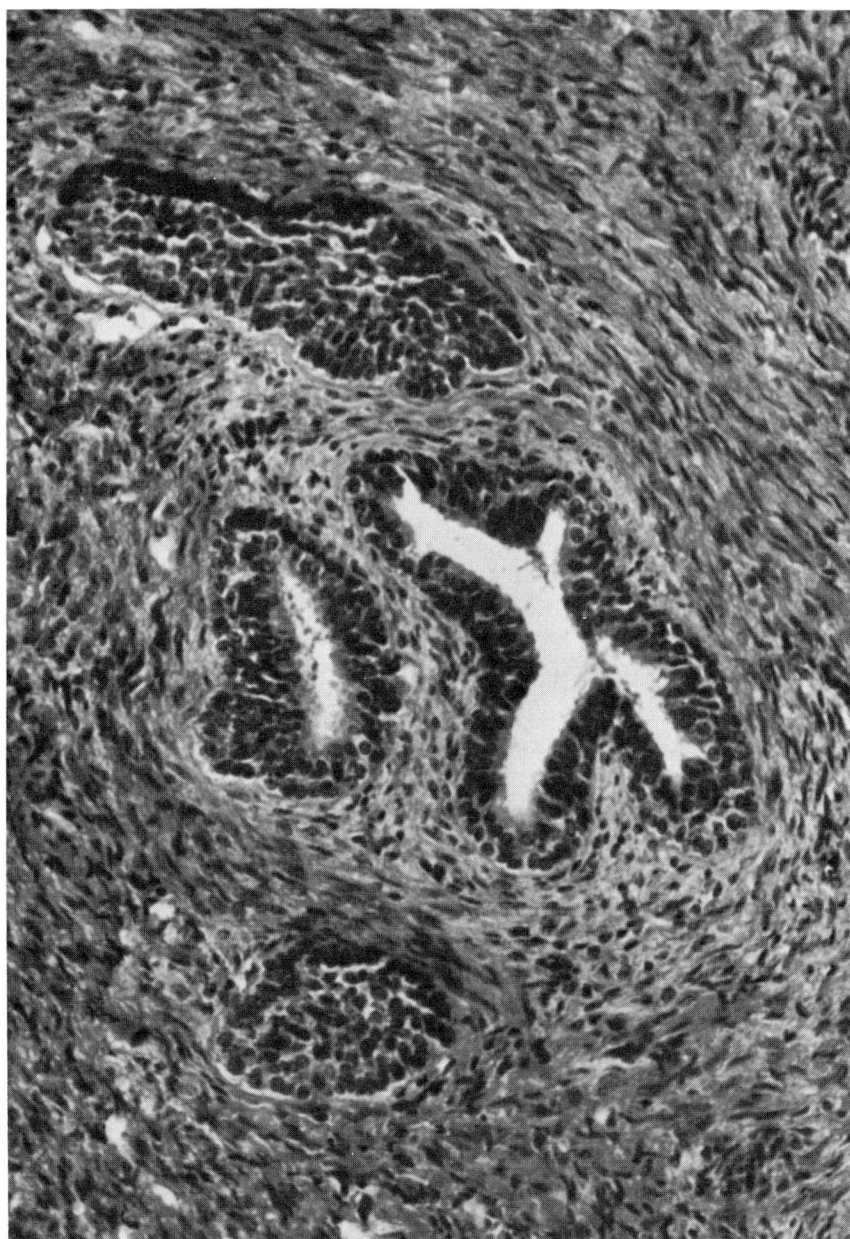

Figure 25–11

Figure 25–11. Higher magnification of the epithelial lining of the large duct depicted in the upper left section in Fig. 25–10.
Hematoxylin and eosin stain. Mag. 364×.

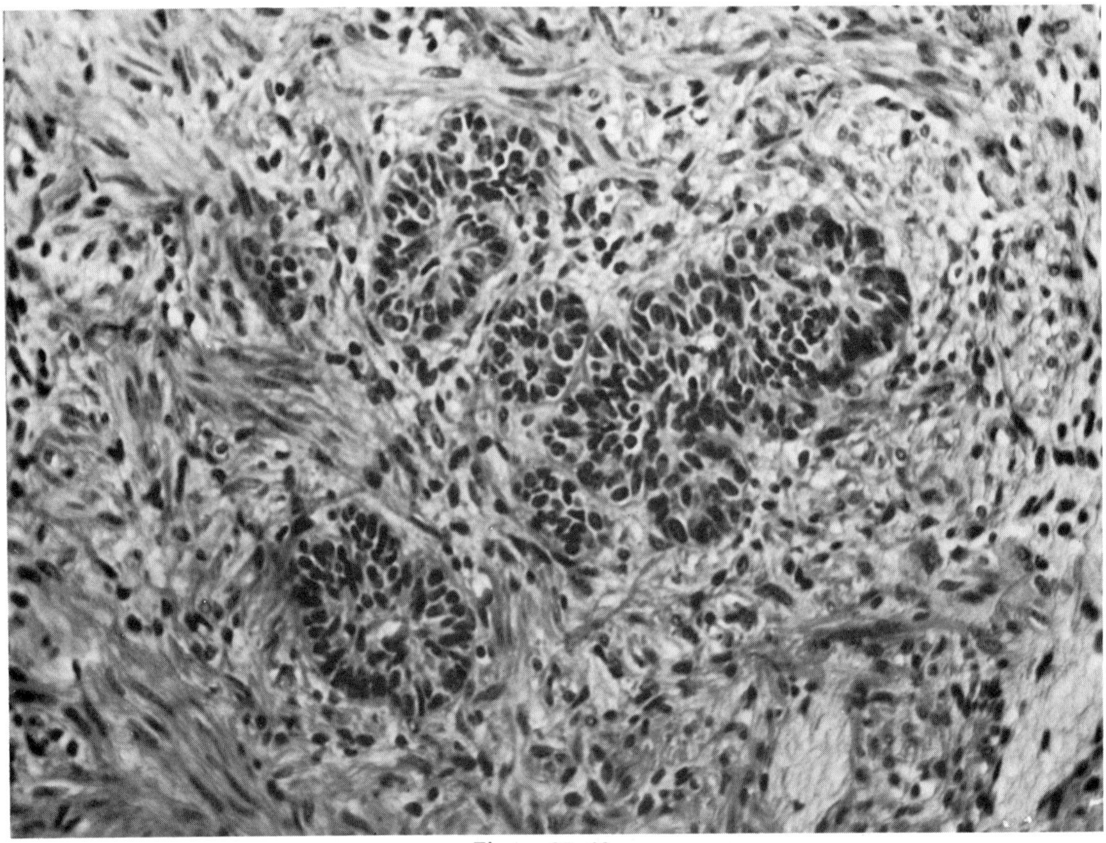

Figure 25–12a

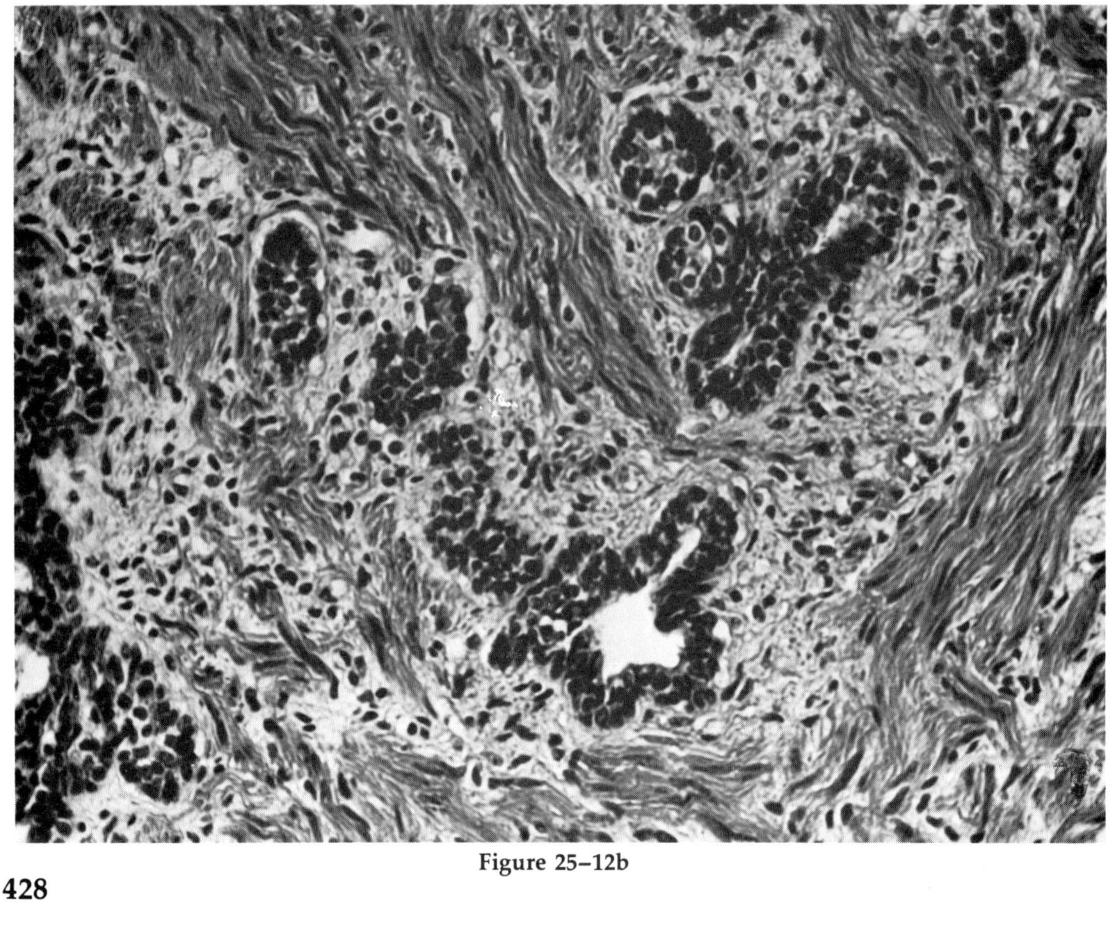

Figure 25–12b

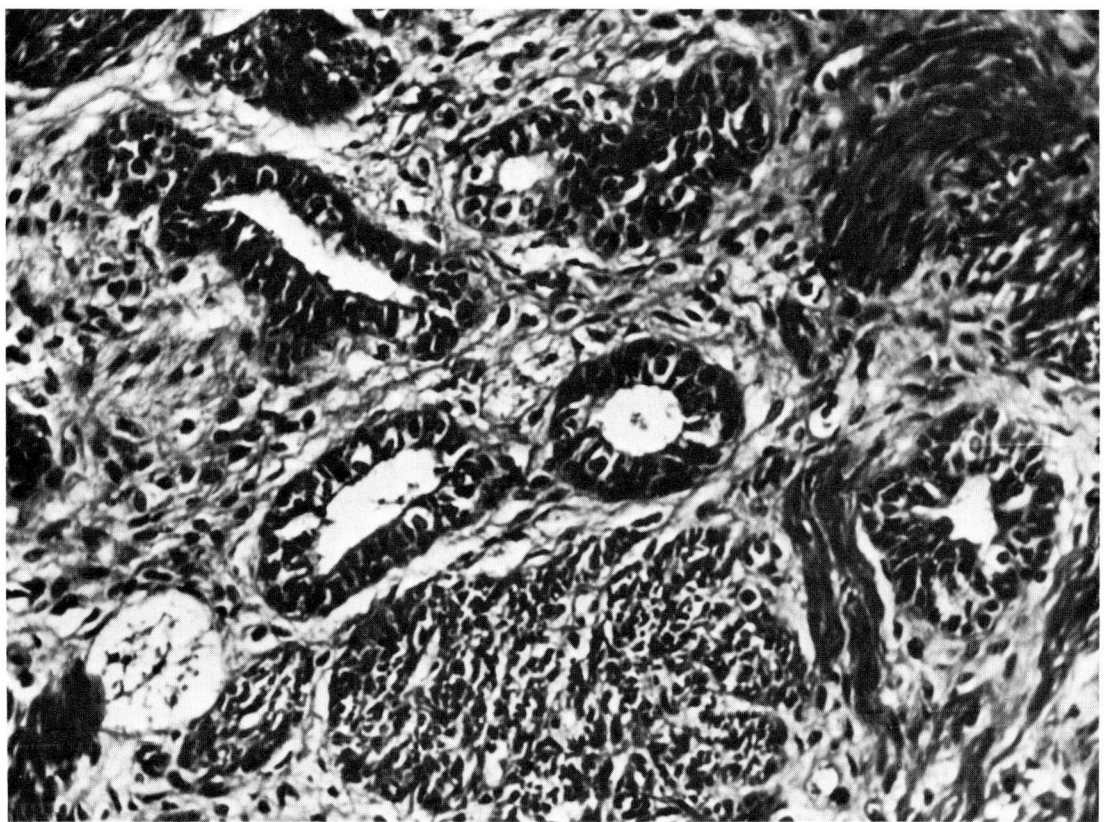

Figure 25–12c

Figure 25–12. The most peripherally placed tubuloalveolar glands of the prostate from three infants, whose respective body weights at death were (a) 700 grams, (b) 950 grams, and (c) 1,720 grams.
Hematoxylin and eosin stain. Mag. 304×.

Part 10

FEMALE REPRODUCTIVE SYSTEM

Chapter 26

OVARY

EMBRYOLOGY

That which is to be the ovary of the human first makes its appearance during the fifth week of embryonic life, when a thickened segment of the coelomic epithelium becomes the surface or germinal epithelium on the medial aspect of the urogenital ridge.[1] These cells proliferate and, as they do so, cells of the underlying mesenchyme also reproduce themselves to form a bulge on the medial aspect of each mesonephros known as the gonadal ridge. Soon thereafter, cords of small dark cells, the primary sex cords, grow down into the underlying mesenchyme.

The gonad, at this point in its development, is still indifferent, inasmuch as even histologically one cannot distinguish between the male and the female; the two are microscopically identical. The indifferent gonad consists, at this stage, of an outer cortex and an inner medulla. If the individual possesses an XX sex chromosome complex, the cortex differentiates into an ovary while the medulla regresses.

The primordial germ cells themselves originate in the fourth week in the wall of the yolk sac, actually outside the body of the fetus. During the fifth week they migrate, passively and actively, to the site of the gonad.[2] It is assumed that they are guided by chemical agents within the gonad.

As the ovary enlarges, connective tissue fibers and blood vessels penetrate the organ from its inner surface and divide it into compact strands, each made up of several clusters of germ cells derived from a common mother gonium, by repeated divisions. This pattern is most pronounced at about 12 weeks of gestation as some germ cells begin to mature. Such nests of oocytes (Fig. 26–8a) presage the cessation of multiplication.

Between the beginning of this process at about 11 weeks and its completion (with all gonia transformed into oocytes) at about 15 weeks, the total number of gonocytes increases from approximately one million to five or six million.

In the transfer of some gonia into the medulla, the sex cords serve as carriers.[3]

Following this stage, the fertile part of the cortex becomes separated from the germinal epithelium by the development of the mesenchymal albuginea; that layer eventually becomes quite thick (by 7 to 10 years) but is not remarkably so during neonatal life.

Following the fifteenth week, primary and secondary follicles emerge, with granulosa and theca cell differentiation (Fig. 26–8).

ANATOMY

The ovary in late fetal life and early infancy is elongate, thin, and rather flat and is of light flesh color. In near term infants this fundamental shape may be altered by the presence of a few thin-walled, translucent, fluid-filled cysts ranging in size from pin-head to 1 cm. in greatest diameter. There may be one or several cysts in one or both ovaries.

HISTOLOGY

During the perinatal period, 90 per cent of the ovarian cortex consists of crowded primitive oocytes. There is little visible supporting stroma between them; there is, however, a thin mantle of stroma located just beneath the covering germinal epithelium (Figs. 26–1 to 26–5).

At this time of life the supporting reticular fibers are arranged predominantly at right angles to the surfaces of the organ[4] (Fig. 26–3).

The Development of the Oocyte and Follicle

Perhaps the most striking characteristic of the infant ovary is the presence of oocytes and follicles in all stages of growth and atresia. The occurrence of antral follicles (both microscopic and macroscopic) from 7 months of gestation onward has been reported repeatedly.[5]

According to the classification of Lintern-Moore et al.[5] oocytes and follicles in fetal life and infancy pass through the following stages.

Class A Oocytes. These cells (9 to 25 μ in diameter) are in the transition stage of meiotic prophase (Fig. 26–8a). They are found in tight clusters either in the extreme outer cortex or in the medullary region. By six months of age (post-partum), all of these have disappeared.

Class B Oocytes. The nucleus has entered the resting stage of diplotene. Class B follicles are surrounded by a single layer of flattened granulosa cells with highly basophilic nuclei (Fig. 26–8b). These follicles form the major portion of the oocyte population at all stages of growth and constitute the resting pool from which further follicular development occurs. During the perinatal period they are abundant in the outer cortex (Figs. 26–1 to 26–3). This is the so-called *primitive follicle*.

Class BC Follicles. These follicles (Fig. 26–8c) differ from Class B in only one respect; approximately half of the surrounding granulosa cells are cuboidal while the other half remain flattened. Whether the cuboidal cells are derived from the flattened cells or represent a different cell population is unknown.

Class C Follicles. A Class C oocyte is completely surrounded by a single layer of cuboidal granulosa cells and a complete basement membrane separating the granulosa cells from adjacent stroma (Fig. 26–8d). Although no theca is present, surrounding stroma forms a halo of connective tissue fibers and fibroblast-like cells. Class C follicles are deeper in the cortex than Classes B or BC.

Class CD Follicles. One side of the oocyte is surrounded by a single layer of cuboidal granulosa cells while the other is covered by two or more layers.

Class D1 Follicle. This follicle contains a growing oocyte surrounded by two to seven layers of rounded granulosa cells (Fig. 26–8e). A zona pellucida is present. These follicles are located deeper in the cortex than any of the preceding classes. A theca layer is present and remains in further stages.

This is the equivalent of what is known as a *primary follicle*.

Class D2 Follicle. The only difference between this and the D1 follicle is the presence of fluid-filled spaces in the midst of the crowded granulosa cells (Fig. 26–8f) and occasional Call-Exner vacuoles (Fig. 26–11).

Class E Follicle. This type of follicle is the least common of the group thus far. It is characterized by the presence of a definite crescent-shaped antrum (Fig. 26–8g).

Class F Follicle. These follicles represent the ultimate stage of follicular growth in the infant ovary; they are the secondary follicles (graafian follicles). They are located deep in the medullary region. Each is characterized by a large fluid-filled antrum and an eccentrically placed oocyte nestled within the cumulus oophorus (Figs. 26–8h and 26–9). In some instances the theca layer is not only prominent but also strikingly luteinized.

Disappearance of Oocytes and Follicles in Infancy

There seems to be a tremendous reduction in the number of oocytes during the latter months of gestation and in the first year of life. Although no one knows the fate of these thousands of gonocytes, it is likely that the majority regress directly without ever having undergone development into full-blown follicles.[4]

On the other hand, the stages of regression of the complete but unruptured follicle are well known. The oocyte dies in the first stage of this process. Morphologically it presents the appearance of having undergone coagulation necrosis. In the second stage the follicle collapses, losing its spherical shape; its wall becomes intricately infolded. The liquor folliculi diminishes in quantity, and fibrocytes from the inner aspect of the convoluted wall invade the remaining proteinaceous fluid; their inward growth resembles that of fibrocytes in a tissue culture.

Eventually the center of the collapsed structure is converted into a solid mass of fibrous tissue, the corpus fibrosum. Delicate fibrils of connective tissue radiate away from this solid center like slender spokes of a wheel, and between them are nestled little clusters of still recognizable lutein cells. In time, a thick, pink-staining homogeneous band of hyalin is deposited between the atrophying granulosa cells and the more peripherally arranged lutein cells. As the whole structure collapses and shrinks, this pink band becomes ever more prominent. In the corpus atreticum (Fig. 26–12) there is only the central core of connective tissue surrounded by an undulating pink ribbon. In the final stages of follicular atresia, only the convoluted pink-staining band remains, folded upon itself in what is called the corpus albicans or corpus candicans. Eventually, this too vanishes, leaving behind no mark of its prior existence.

The Germinal Epithelium

During the latter half of gestation and in early infancy, the covering germinal epithelium is made up of a continuous, rather prominent single layer of columnar to cuboidal cells (Figs. 26–13 and 26–14).

"Aberrations"

There are certain singular morphologic features, sometimes encountered in the ovaries of fetuses and newborn infants, which are neither entirely normal nor abnormal. These aberrations include the following.

Para-ovarian Remnants. Remnants derived from the Wolffian ducts can frequently be identified in the mesovarium, between the tube and the ovary (Fig. 26–15). Each such remnant consists of a single layer of columnar epithelial cells arranged about a small central lumen. The epithelial lining is, in turn, embraced by a fairly thick sheath of circumferentially arranged smooth muscle fibers. Often three to ten of these structures can be seen in a single histologic section; rarely, as many as 70 have been observed.

Hilus Cells. These small, discrete, non-encapsulated nests of large pale-staining cells are sometimes encountered in or near the hilus of the ovary of the fetus or newborn infant (Fig. 26–16). The component cells have abundant pink-staining vaculated cytoplasm; they resemble their embryologic equivalent in the male, the interstitial cells of Leydig in the testis.

Adrenal Cortical Rests. Adrenal cortical rests are uncommon in direct relation to the ovary of the fetus and the newborn. They are sometimes encountered adjacent to the fallopian tube or in the mesosalpinx, mesovarium, and broad ligament.[6] The cortical cells are arranged in cords with intervening sinusoids, as in the adrenal itself (Fig. 26–17). Most if not all of these spherical nodules are encapsulated, unlike the nests of hilus cells.

Excessive Luteinization of Theca with Eosinophils. In infants of diabetic, prediabetic, and toxemic mothers there is apt to be excessive hyperplasia of the theca interna (Fig. 26–18), forming a single solitary nodule which, at times, may be as great as two-thirds the breadth of the ovary itself. This is, in a way, like the hyperplasia of the islets of Langerhans in the pancreas in infants of diabetic and prediabetic mothers; both lesions are occasionally the site of striking infiltration by eosinophils.

Multiovular Follicles. Multiovular follicles (Fig. 26–19) are numerous in the ovaries of fetuses and newborns.[7] One frequently sees two oocytes in one primordial follicle; three are less commonly observed, and rarely as many as five or six are seen. There is apparently some feature of the ambience that promotes their presence and persistence, for if one or two such follicles are found many more will be discovered to be present in both ovaries in that same individual, whereas in other infants of the same degree of maturity, none will be found.

Multinuclear Oocytes. Although oocytes having two or more nuclei are often seen in the ovaries of immature guinea pigs, mice, and rats, there are few binuclear oocytes (and apparently none which are trinuclear) in the ovaries of humans infants[7] (Fig. 26–20).

Follicular Cysts. Follicular cysts are relatively common in the ovaries of newborn infants (Figs. 26–21 and 26–22). Occasionally they are so large at birth as to interfere with the delivery of the infant.[8] When the pressure of the contained fluid is so great as to cause atrophy of the lining granulosa cells so that they are no longer recognizable, lutein cells, deeper in the wall, may remain intact and identifiable.

References

1. Moore, K. L.: The Developing Human. Clinically Oriented Embryology. Philadelphia, W. B. Saunders Co., 1973, pp. 207–212.
2. Witschi, E.: Embryology of the ovary. *In* The Ovary, International Academy of Pathology No. 3. Baltimore, The Williams and Wilkins Co., 1962.
3. Witschi, E.: Migration of the germ cells of human embryos from the yolk sac to the primitive gonadal folds. Contrib. Embryol., 32:67–80, 1948. Carnegie Inst. Wash. Publ. No. 575.
4. Valdes-Dapena, M. A.: The normal ovary of childhood. Ann. N. Y. Acad. Sci., *142*:597–613, 1967.
5. Lintern-Moore, S., Peters, H., Moore, G. P. M., and Faber, M.: Follicular development in the infant human ovary. J. Reprod. Fert., 39:53–64, 1974.
6. Willis, R. A.: The Borderland of Embryology and Pathology. London, Butterworth and Co., Ltd., 1958.
7. Bacsish, P.: Some observations on near-term human foetal ovaries. J. Endocrin. (Proc. Soc. Endocrinol.), 7:XIV–XVI, 1951.
8. Graves, G. Y., Mc Ilvoy, D. B., Jr., and Hudson, G. W.: Ovarian cyst in premature infant. Amer. J. Dis. Child., *81*:256–8, 1951.

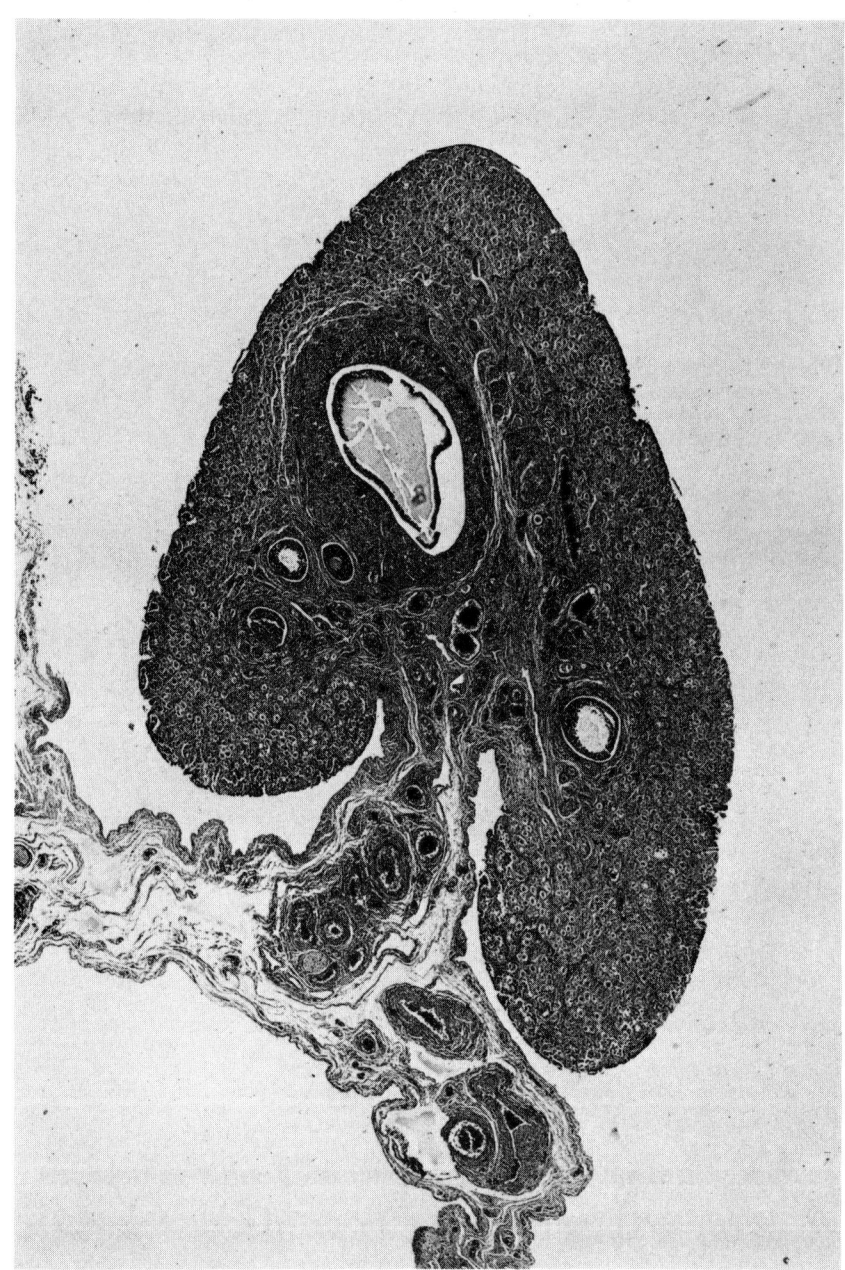

Figure 26–1

Figure 26–1. This is a survey view of the body of the ovary, sectioned in the sagittal plane. This infant, a white female, lived for 23 hours. Her body weight at autopsy was 2,560 grams.

Note the number of vessels in the mesovarium and hilus of the ovary, the crowding of the primitive follicles in the scanty stroma, and the obvious follicular cysts, the largest of which is surrounded by a halo of theca cells.

Hematoxylin and eosin stain. Mag. 30×.

OVARY 439

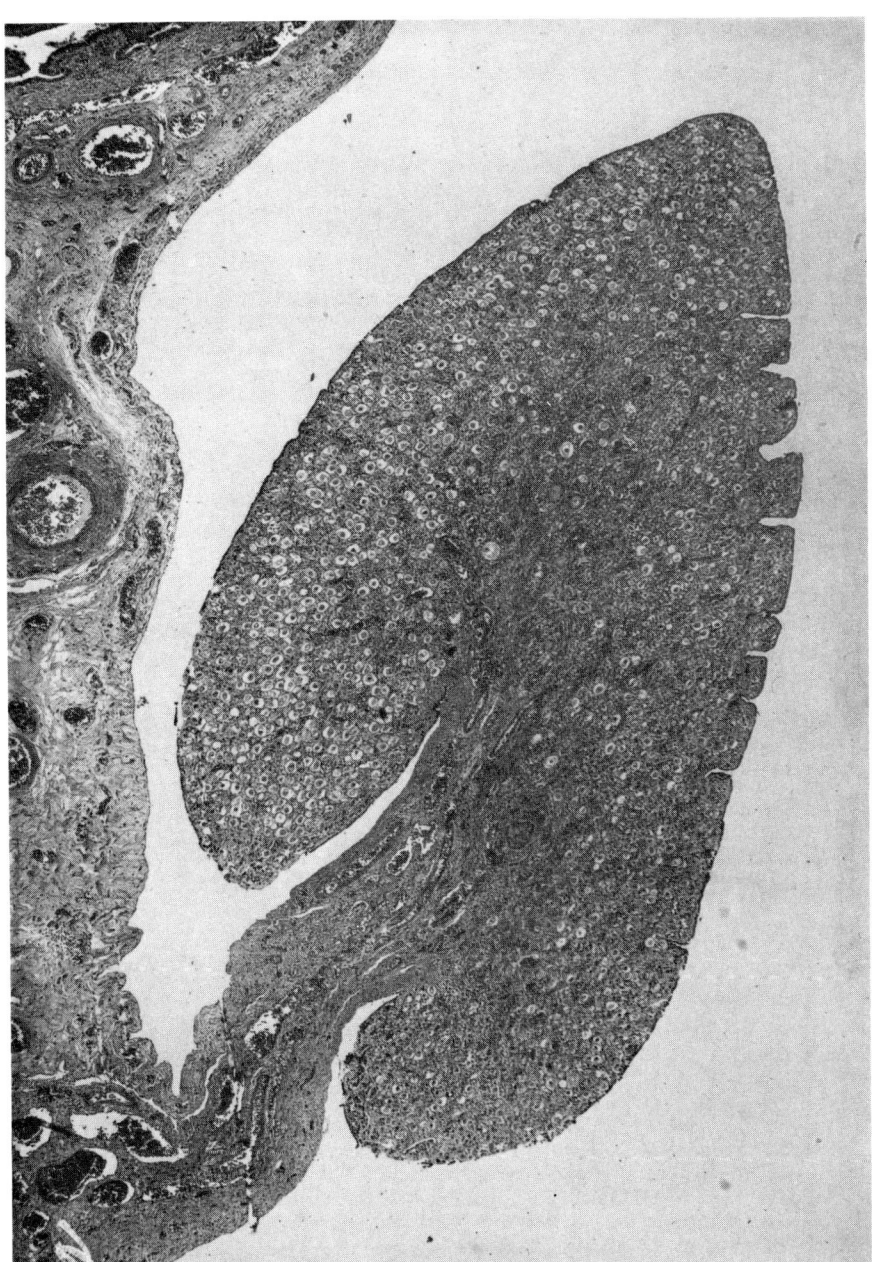

Figure 26–2

Figure 26–2. Survey view of the body of the ovary, again sectioned in the sagittal plane. This infant, born at term, weighed 2,700 grams and died at three minutes of age. Although there is scanty stroma and crowding of oocytes or primitive follicles, no sex cords are visible.
Hematoxylin and eosin stain. Mag. 42×.

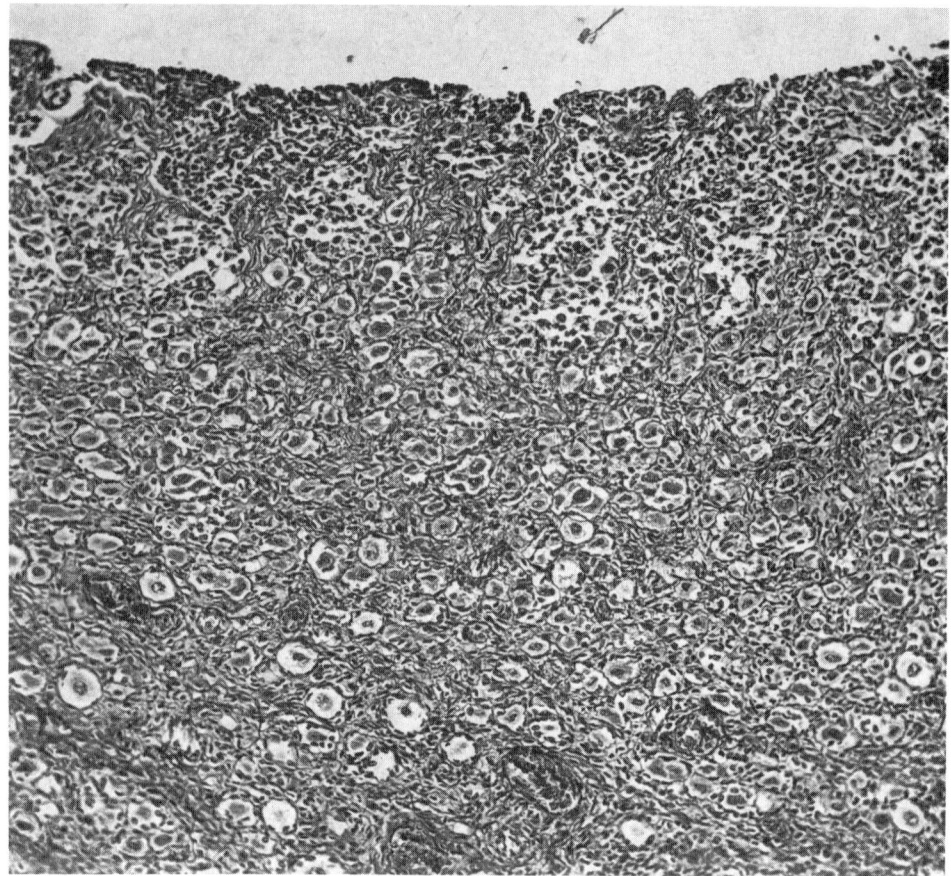

Figure 26-3

Figure 26-3. Superficial cortex of the ovary of a one-day old prematurely born infant (37 weeks gestation) with a body weight of 1,480 grams. Notice the scanty stroma and, peripherally, orientation of reticular fibers predominantly at right angles to the surface of the organ.

Wilder's stain for reticulum. Mag. 142×. (From Valdés-Dapena, M. A.: The Normal Ovary of Childhood. *Annals of the New York Academy of Sciences, 142*:597-613, 1967.)

OVARY 441

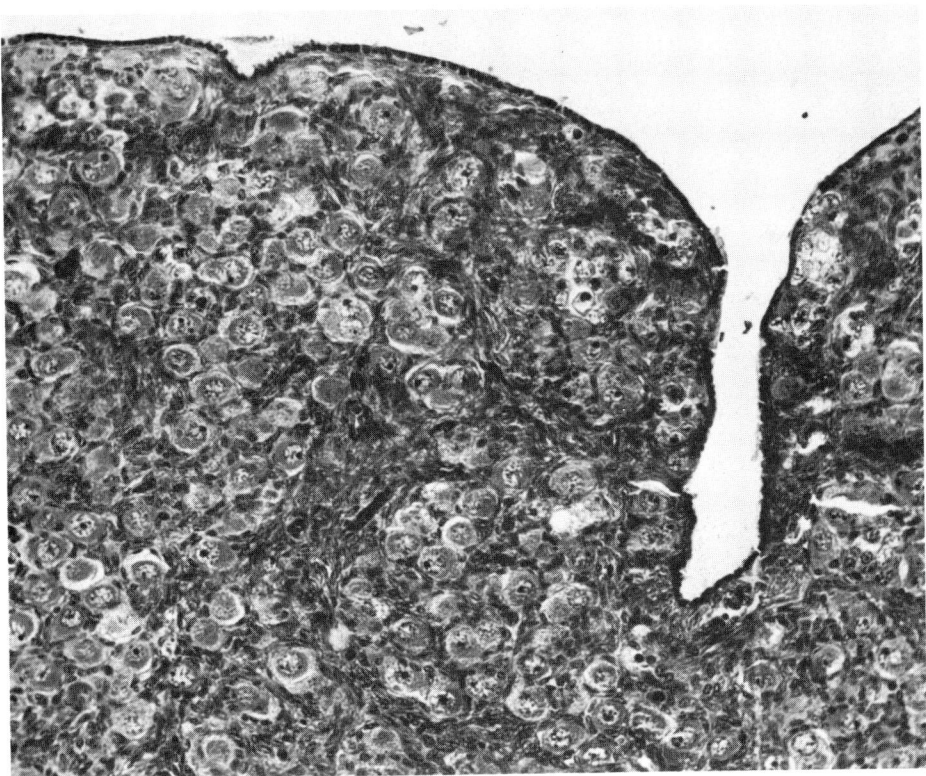

Figure 26–4

Figure 26–4. This is the superficial cortex of the ovary in a newborn white female infant who lived for one day. Body weight was 3,975 grams.
Notice that the oocytes are rather densely packed.
Periodic acid-Schiff stain. Mag. 175×.

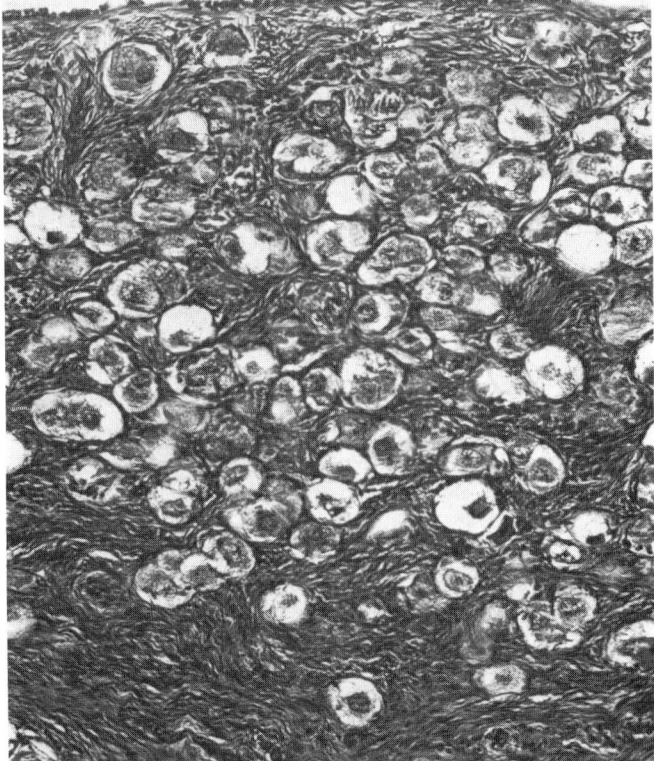

Figure 26–5. The cortex of the ovary at higher magnification. This infant, born at 24 weeks of gestation, weighed 650 grams and died at three hours of age. Note that there is very little visible stroma, as in the preceding figure. Oocytes, all in primitive follicles, are densely packed.
Hematoxylin and eosin stain. Mag. 255×.

Figure 26–5

Figures 26–6 and 26–7. This set of three illustrations, taken at progressively increasing magnification, depicts the so-called sex cords or ovigerous cords, unique to the ovary of the fetus and the premature infant. In the past it was thought that oogonia were actually produced within and by these distinct bands of primitive cells.

See illustration on the opposite page.

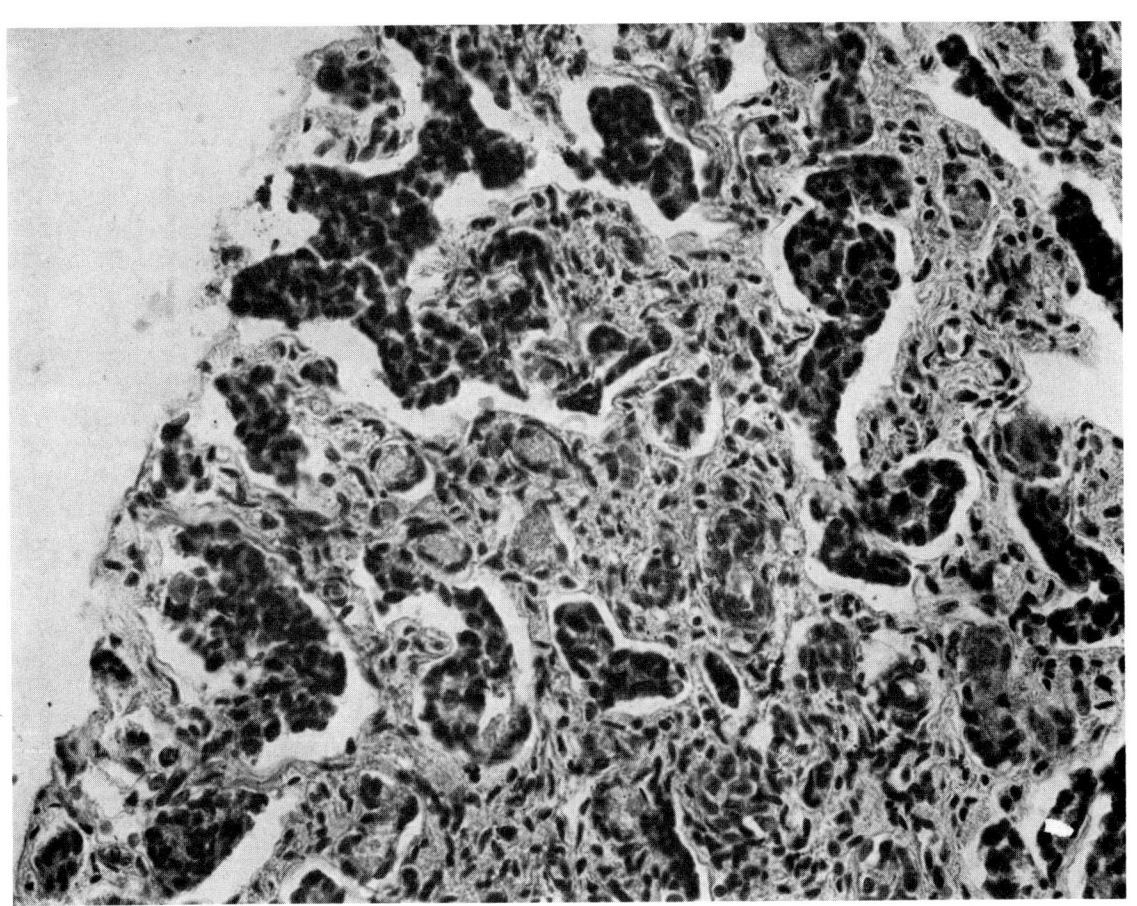

Figure 26–6

Figure 26–6. This is a section of the ovarian cortex of a 36 hour old black female whose body measured 33 cm. crown to rump and 44 cm. crown to heel. (Estimated gestational age: 33 weeks.) Hematoxylin and eosin stain. Mag. 310×.

444 OVARY

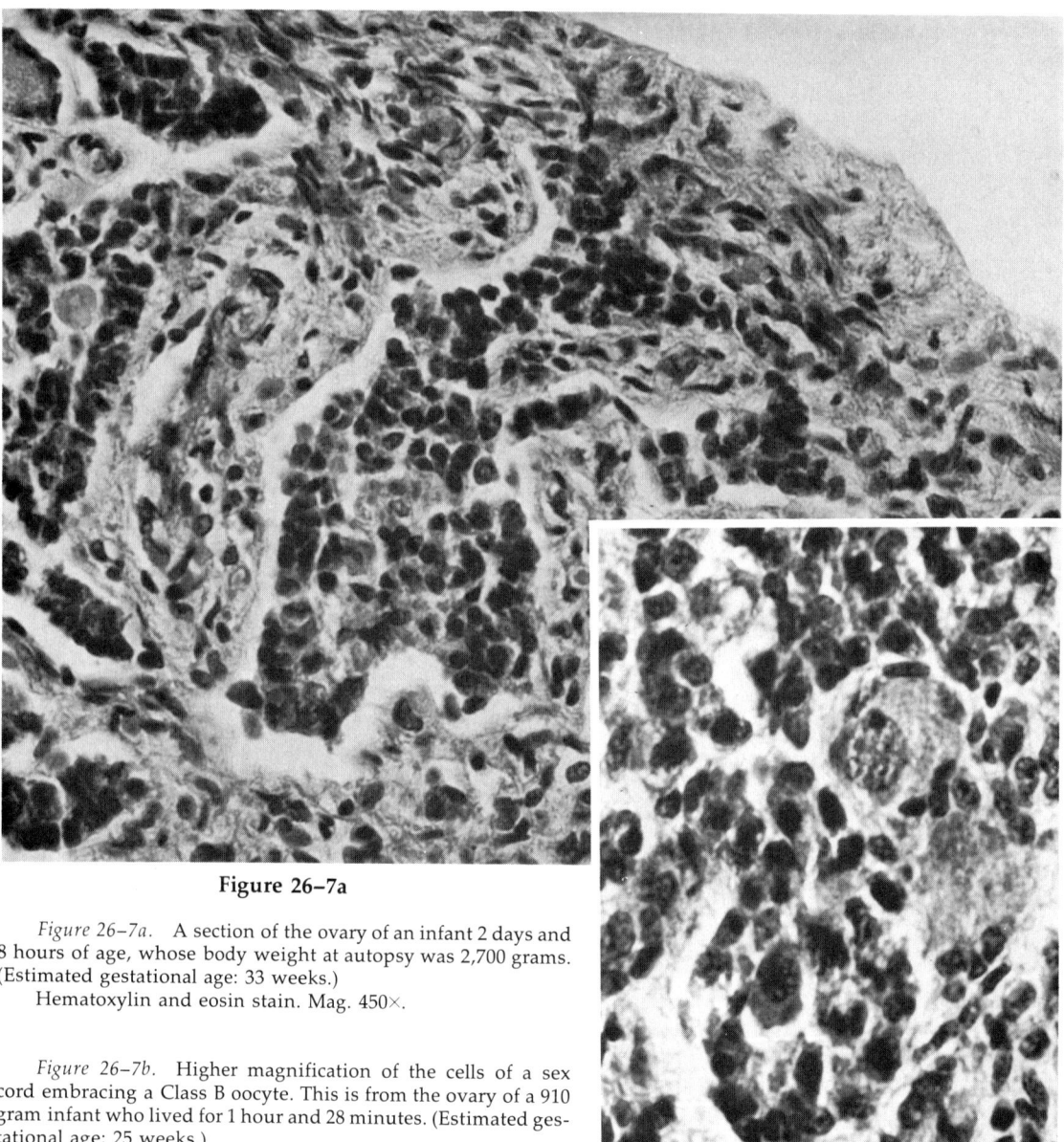

Figure 26–7a

Figure 26–7a. A section of the ovary of an infant 2 days and 8 hours of age, whose body weight at autopsy was 2,700 grams. (Estimated gestational age: 33 weeks.)
Hematoxylin and eosin stain. Mag. 450×.

Figure 26–7b. Higher magnification of the cells of a sex cord embracing a Class B oocyte. This is from the ovary of a 910 gram infant who lived for 1 hour and 28 minutes. (Estimated gestational age: 25 weeks.)
Hematoxylin and eosin stain. Mag. 534×.

Figure 26–7b

Figure 26–8. This series of nine photomicrographs depicts the growth of the human oocyte and ovarian follicle from the earliest stages to their full flowering in the form of antral follicles, all within the ovary of the newborn. In this set, the classification of Lintern-Moore et al.[5] has been employed; it is based on the diameter of the oocyte, the number of granulosa cells in the widest cross section, and the development of a fluid-filled antrum.

Figs. 28–8a, d, e, f, g, and h were taken from a white female infant with Down's syndrome, probably born of a diabetic mother. She lived one day and had a body weight at autopsy of 3,975 grams. Figs. 26–8b and c were taken from a term infant who lived for 21 hours and who weighed 3,080 grams. (From Valdés-Dapena, M. A.: Development of the Ovary in Childhood. American Registry of Pathology, Armed Forces Institute of Pathology. Washington, D.C., 1975.)

Figure 26–8a. Class A oocytes: The nuclei of at least five oocytes are seen here in a single cluster located, characteristically, just beneath the surface of the ovary. Hematoxylin and eosin stain. Mag. 660×.

Figure 26–8b. Class B oocyte: This single oocyte is surrounded by a single layer of flattened granulosa cells. These oocytes form the major portion of the population of the ovary at this stage. Hematoxylin and eosin stain. Mag. 660×.

Figure 26–8c. Class BC oocyte: Half of the perimeter is surrounded by flattened cells, inferiorly and to the left, and half by cuboidal cells, superiorly and to the right. Hematoxylin and eosin stain. Mag. 660×.

Figure 26–8d. Class C oocyte: This oocyte, which is still larger than that seen in Fig. 26–8c, is surrounded by a single complete layer of cuboidal granulosa cells and a complete basement membrane separating the granulosa layer from adjacent stroma. The stroma surrounding the follicle constitutes a halo of connective tissue fibers and fibroblast-like cells. Periodic acid-Schiff stain. Mag. 660×.

Figure 26–8e. Class D1 follicle: The growing oocyte is surrounded by two to, in this instance, five layers of granulosa cells, forming a solid cuff. These follicles appear deeper in the cortex than do those of the preceding classes. Note the presence of a clear theca cell layer inferiorly. Periodic acid-Schiff stain. Mag. 597×.

Figure 26–8f. Class D2 follicle: This follicle is like that in Fig. 26–8e except for the appearance of fluid-filled spaces among the granulosa cells. Note the complete clear theca cell layer. Hematoxylin and eosin stain. Mag. 440×.

Figure 26–8g. Class E follicle: This follicle, least numerous of the set up to this point, is characterized by the presence of a definite crescent-shaped antrum. The oocyte has ceased to grow. Hematoxylin and eosin stain. Mag. 390×.

See illustration on the next page.

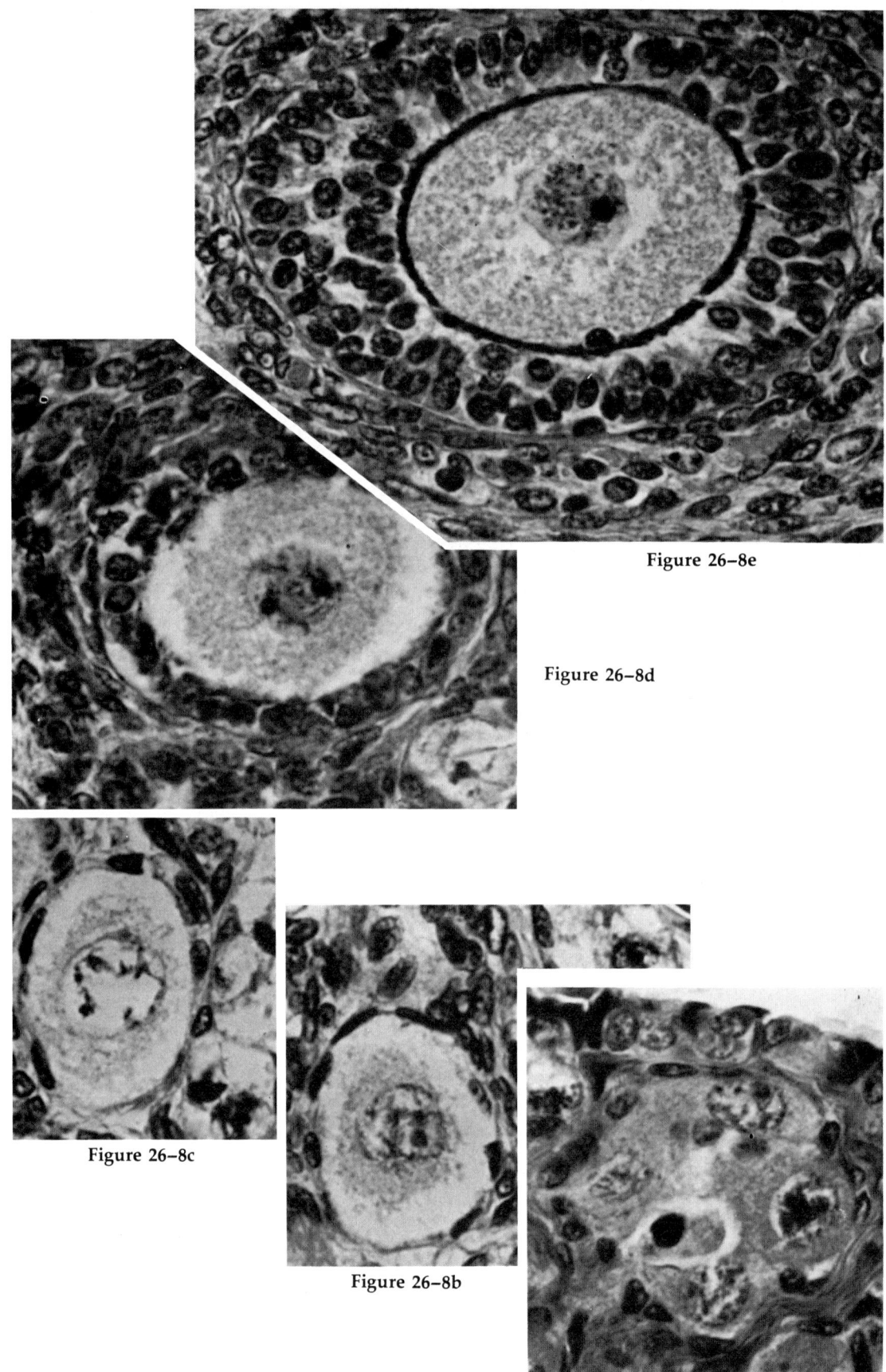

Figure 26–8e

Figure 26–8d

Figure 26–8c

Figure 26–8b

Figure 26–8a

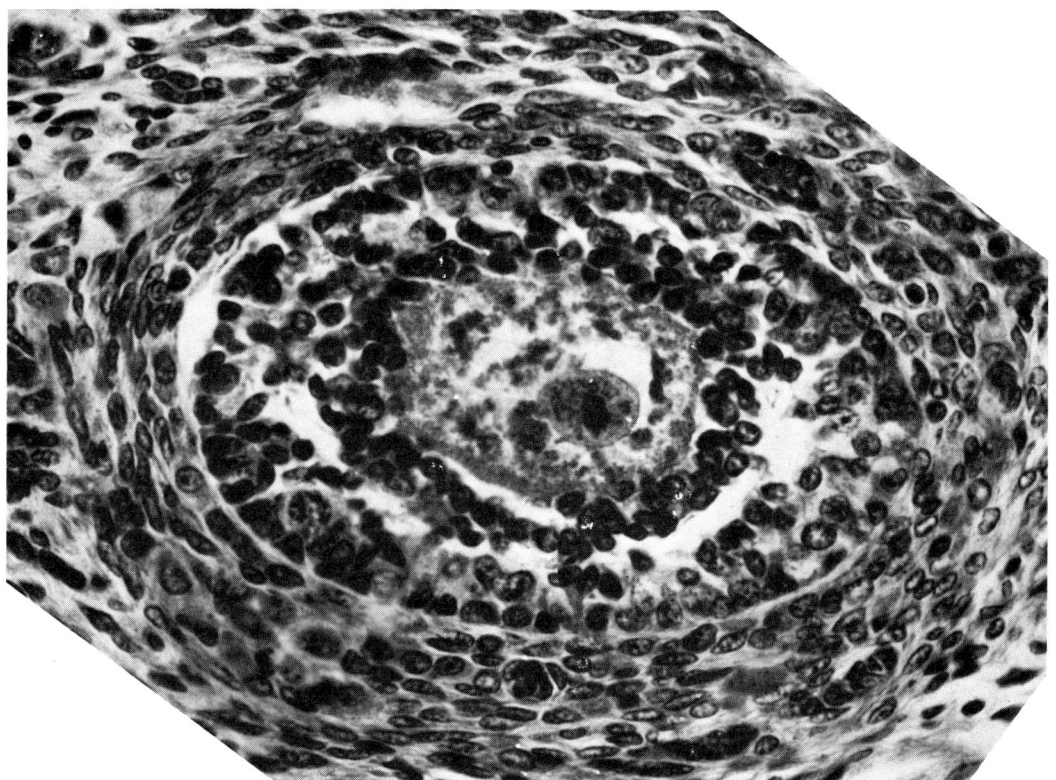

Figure 26–8f

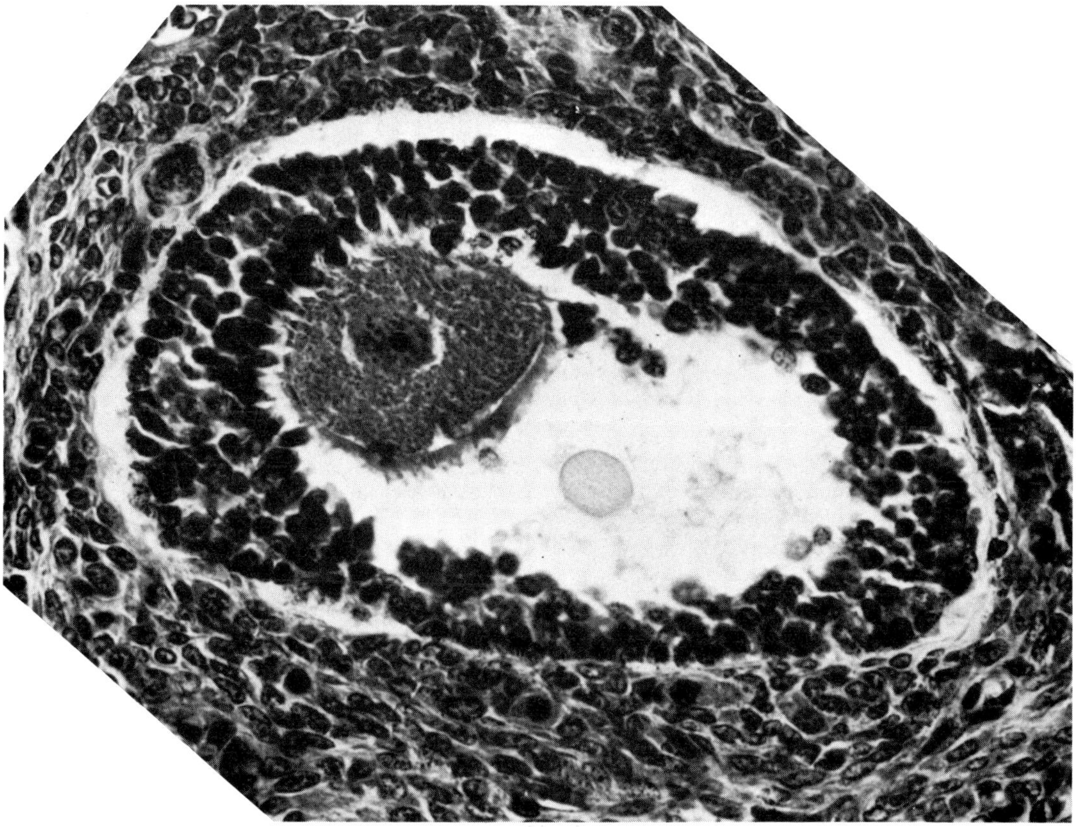

Figure 26–8g

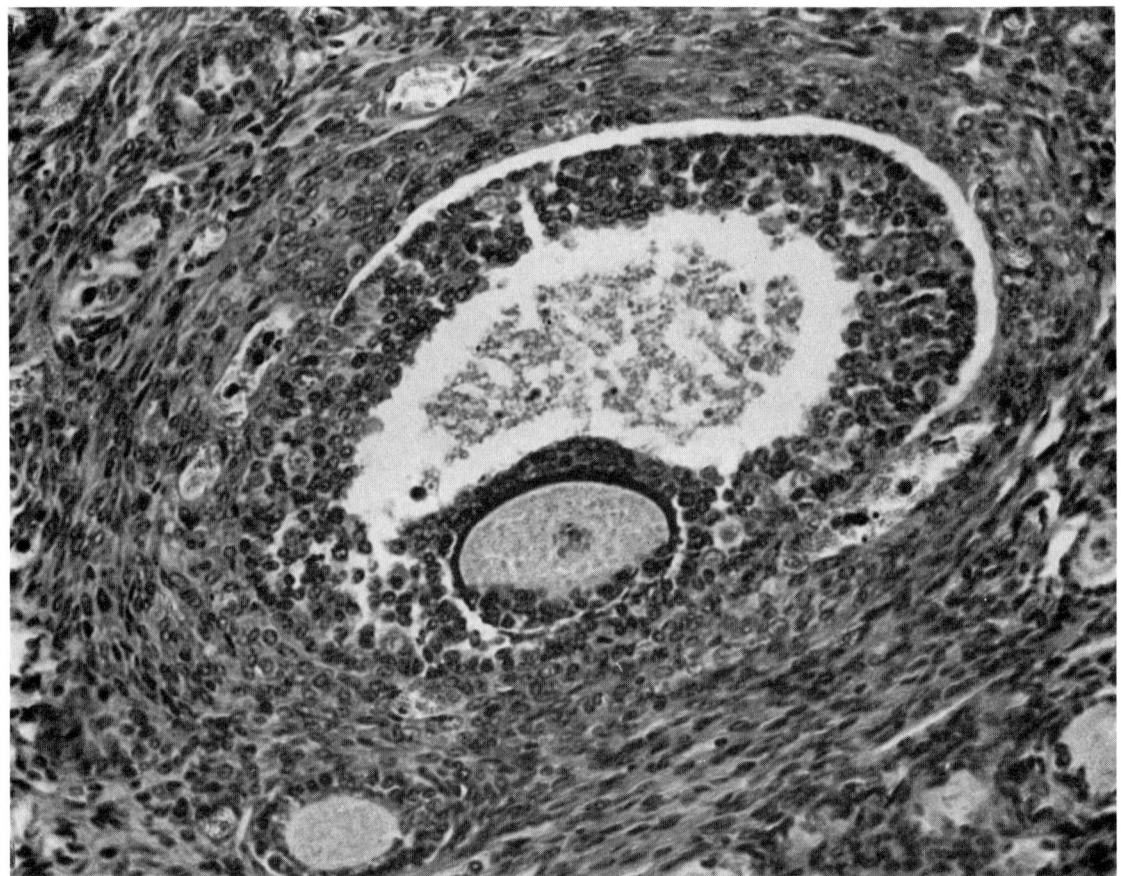

Figure 26–8h

Figure 26–8h. This is a full-blown Class F follicle or graafian follicle. These lie deep in the ovary and represent the final stage of follicular growth in the infant ovary. It is characterized by the presence of a large, rounded, fluid-filled antrum and the oocyte, which is no longer growing, embedded in a cumulus of granulosa cells. In some instances, as here, theca lutein cells are prominent. Periodic acid-Schiff stain. Mag. 255×.

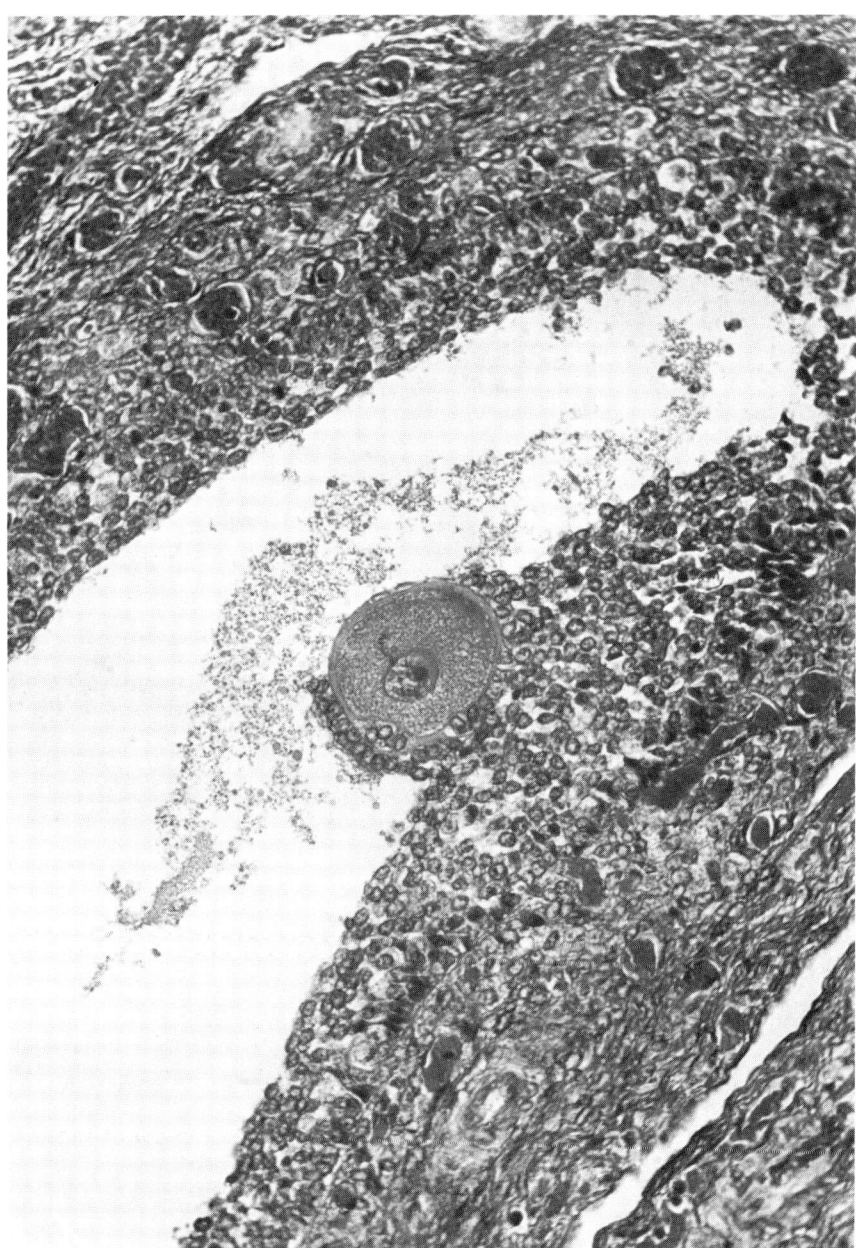

Figure 26–9

Figure 26–9. Class F follicle: The oocyte is nested in the cumulus oophorus. The liquor-filled antrum is surrounded by multiple layers of granulosa cells.

The subject, a female infant weighing 3,080 grams, was born at term and lived for 21 hours. Hematoxylin and eosin stain. Mag. 250×.

Figure 26–10. This photograph of the peripheral portion of a secondary or graafian follicle, Class F, illustrates the striking difference between the darker staining, centrally placed granulosa cells and the plump, paler staining cells of the theca interna. This infant weighed 2,320 grams and died at six hours of age.

Hematoxylin and eosin stain. Mag. 369×.

See illustration on the opposite page.

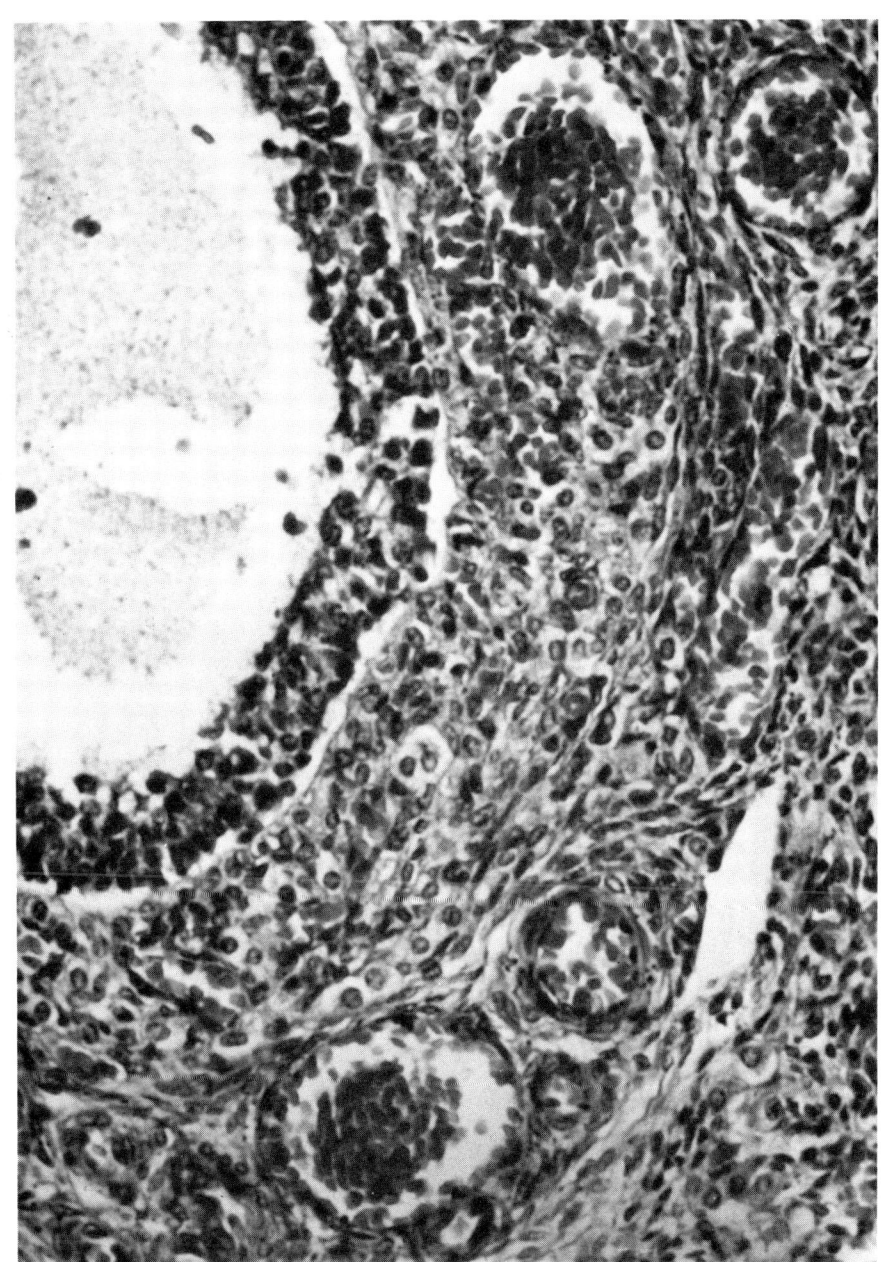

Figure 26-10

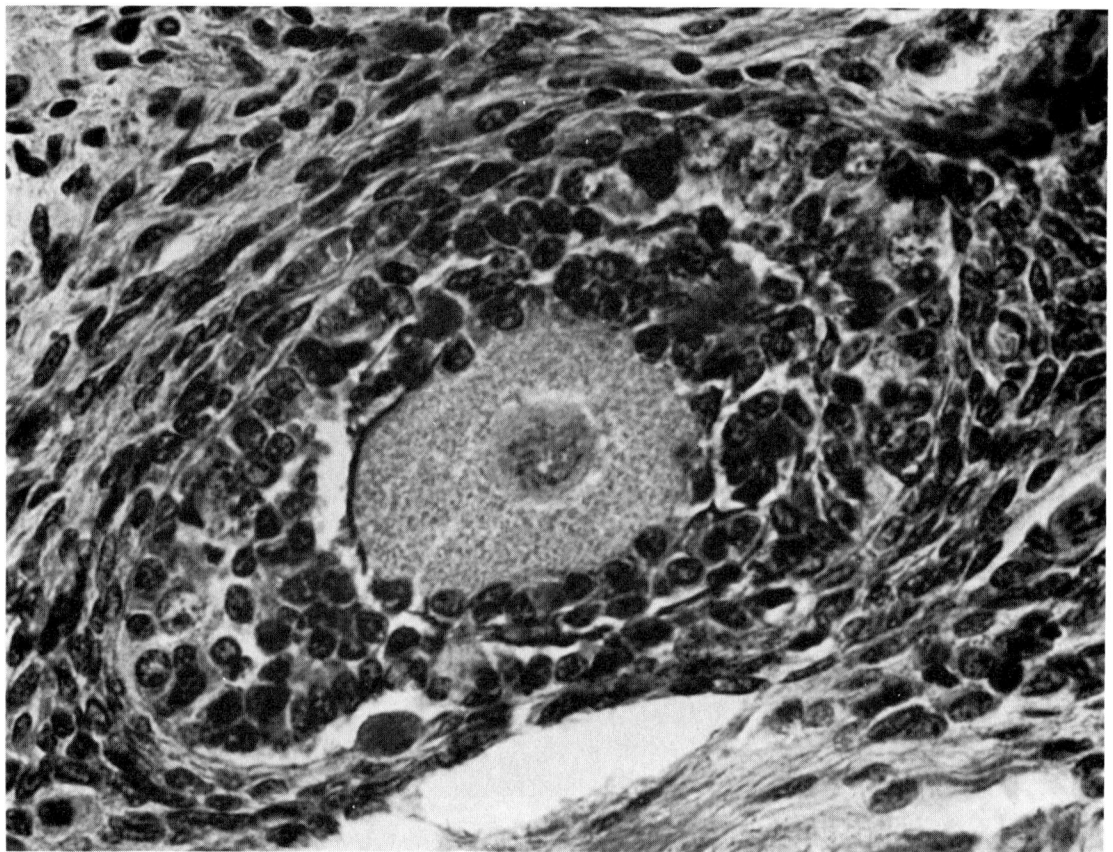

Figure 26–11

Figure 26–11. Even in the follicles of newborn infants, Call-Exner bodies are observed. This is a Class D2 follicle exhibiting, as they often do, the beginning of a space along the granulosa cells to the left of the oocyte and two darkly stained Call-Exner vacuoles to the right.

This subject was a white female infant with Down's syndrome whose mother was probably either diabetic or pre-diabetic. The infant lived for one day, and her body weight at autopsy was 3,975 grams.

Hematoxylin and eosin stain. Mag. 534×.

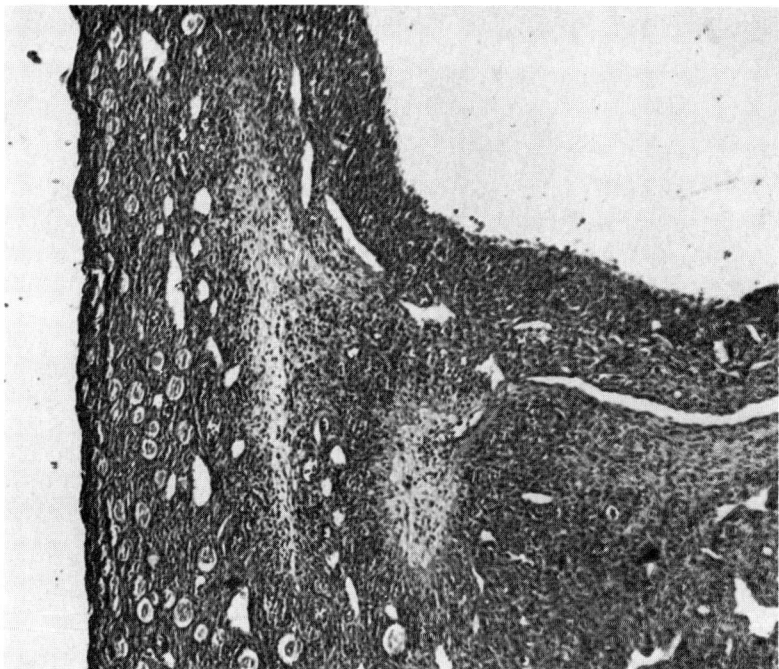

Figure 26–12

Figure 26–12. This photograph includes two corpora atretica within the cortex of an ovary. The infant, who died at one month of age, weighed 4,445 grams.
Hematoxylin and eosin stain. Mag. 45×. (From Valdés-Dapena, M. A.: The Normal Ovary of Childhood. *Annals of the New York Academy of Sciences, 142*:597–613, 1967.)

454 OVARY

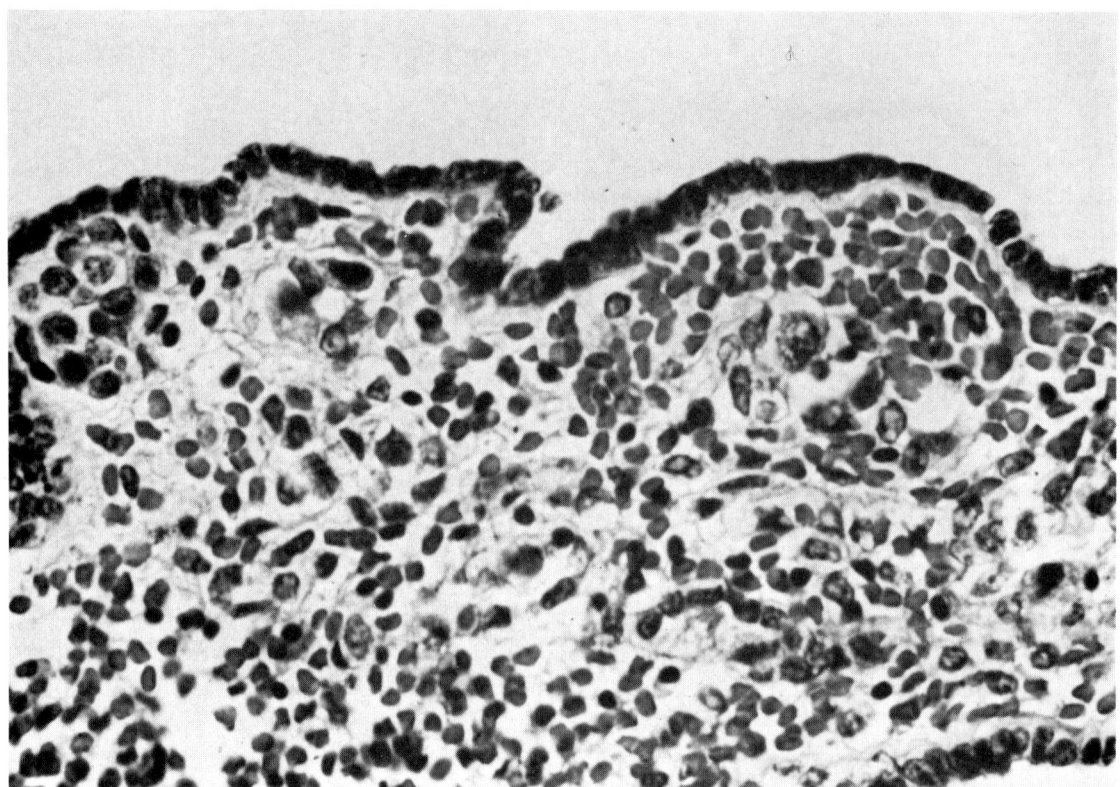

Figure 26–13

Figure 26–13. Depicted here is the covering, the so-called germinal epithelium, characteristic of the ovary of the premature infant. It consists of a single continuous layer of prominent columnar to cuboidal cells.

This infant was 2 hours of age at death. Her body weight at post-mortem examination was 930 grams. (Estimated gestational age: 25 weeks.)

Hematoxylin and eosin stain. Mag. 513×. (From Valdés-Dapena, M. A.: The Normal Ovary of Childhood. *Annals of the New York Academy of Sciences,* 142:597–613, 1967.)

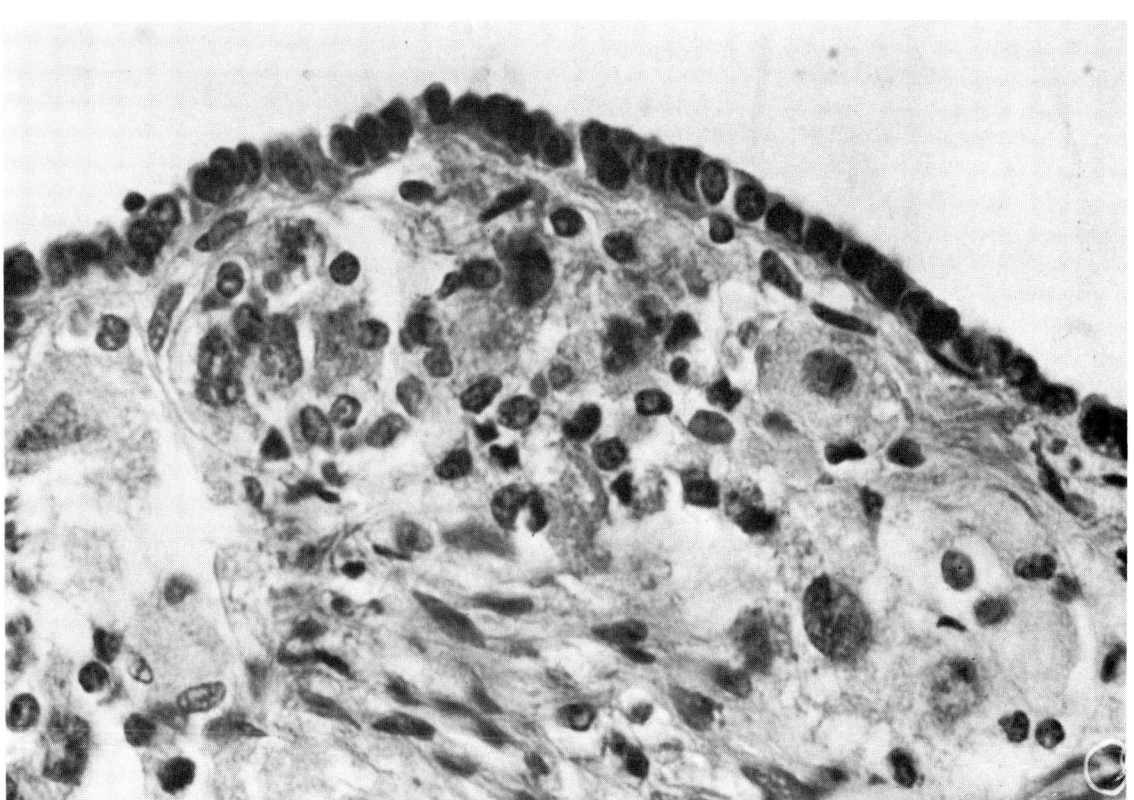

Figure 26-14

Figure 26-14. As is apparent from the stroma of this ovary, compared to that in the preceding figure, this infant was considerably more mature although still not at term. Yet the germinal epithelium here maintains its very prominent appearance.

This patient survived for 8 days and weighed 1,950 grams at autopsy. (Estimated gestational age: 31 weeks.)

Hematoxylin and eosin stain. Mag. 639×.

OVARY

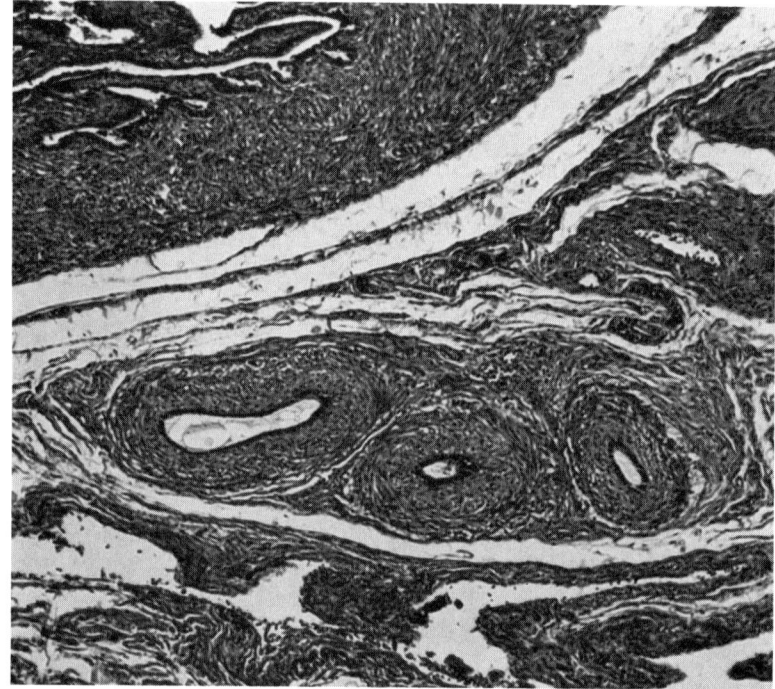

Figure 26–15a

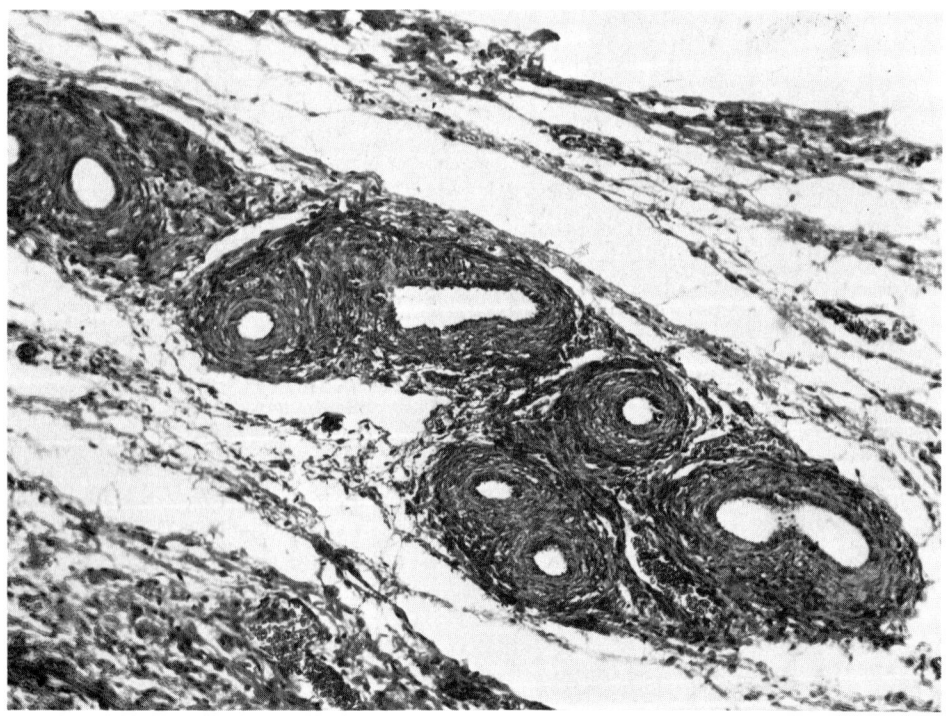

Figure 26–15b

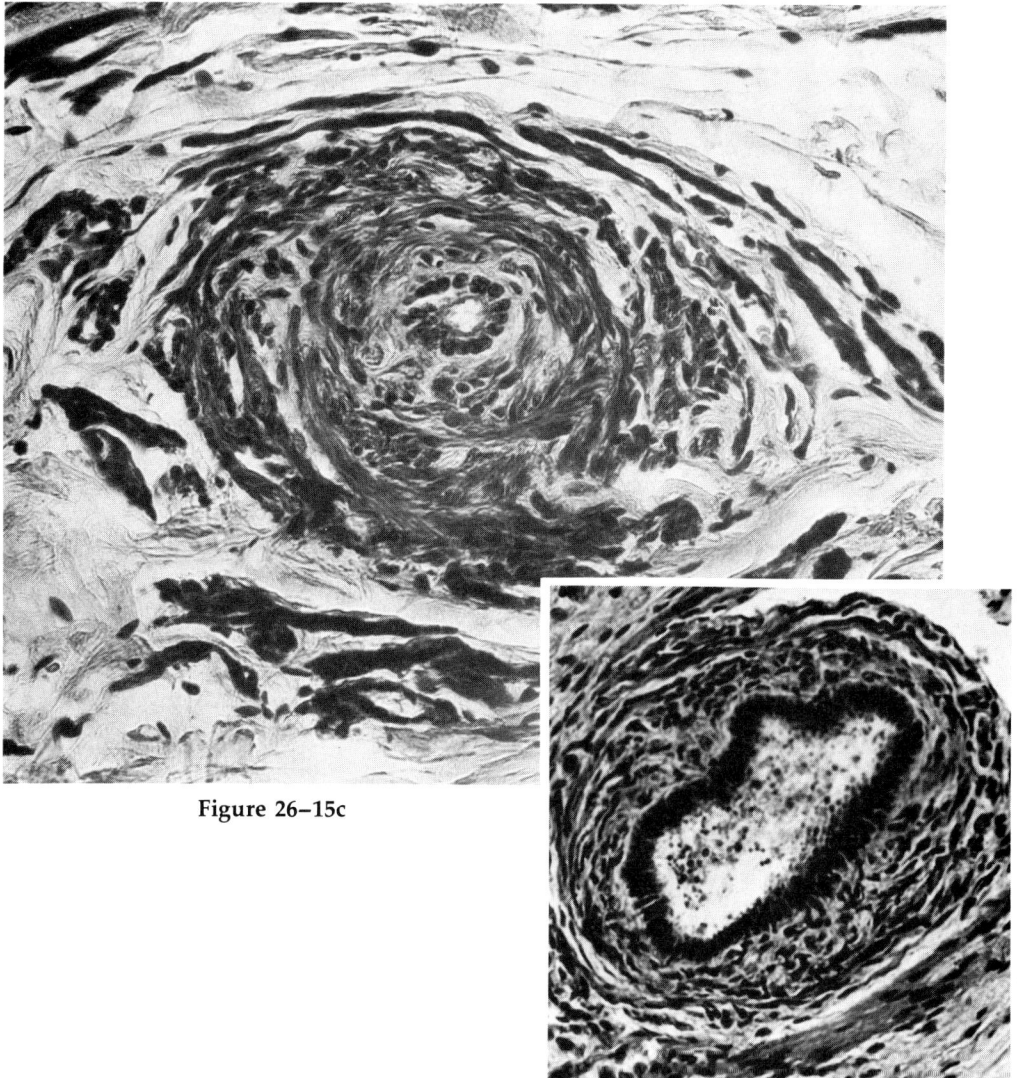

Figure 26–15c

Figure 26–15d

Figure 26–15. These four are illustrations of Wolffian duct or para-ovarian remnants, often encountered in cross sections taken through the neonatal ovary and fallopian tube together; the remnants lie about midway between the two in the mesovarium. Although they may appear singly, they are more often multiple.
Hematoxylin and eosin stain.

Figure 26–15a. In the lower half of this photomicrograph, three para-ovarian remnants appear. The fallopian tube is seen in the left upper corner. Section is from a 15 month old girl. Mag. 65×. (From Valdés-Dapena, M. A.: The Normal Ovary of Childhood. *Annals of the New York Academy of Sciences, 142*:597–613, 1967.)

Figure 26–15b. Here, at slightly higher magnification, eight separate lumina are seen. Note that the wall of each is rather stout. This is from a six day old infant weighing 2,041 grams. Mag. 142×.

Figure 26–15c. The typical para-ovarian remnant is characterized by a lining of columnar to cuboidal epithelial cells and concentric lamina of smooth muscle in the wall, both of which are clearly visible in this section taken from an eight year old girl. Mag. 310×. (From Valdés-Dapena, M. A.: The Normal Ovary of Childhood. *Annals of the New York Academy of Sciences, 142*:597–613, 1967.)

Figure 26–15d. At times, as in this section, the epithelial lining is quite tall. This is from a seven month old child. Mag. 208×.

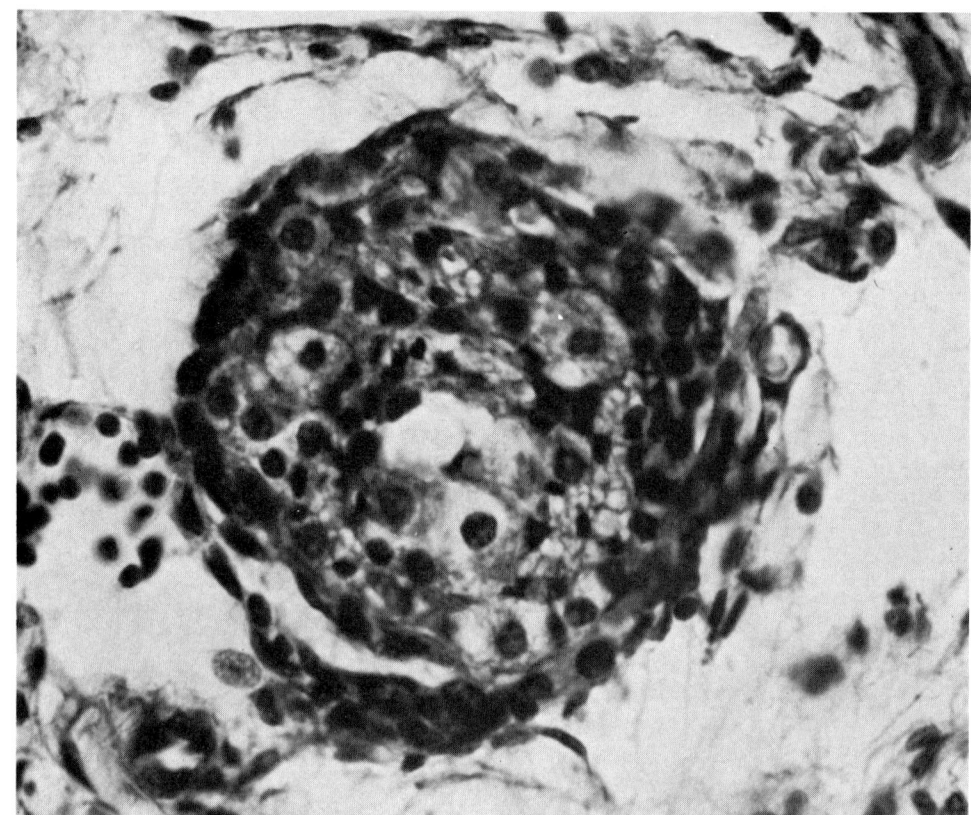

Figure 26-16a

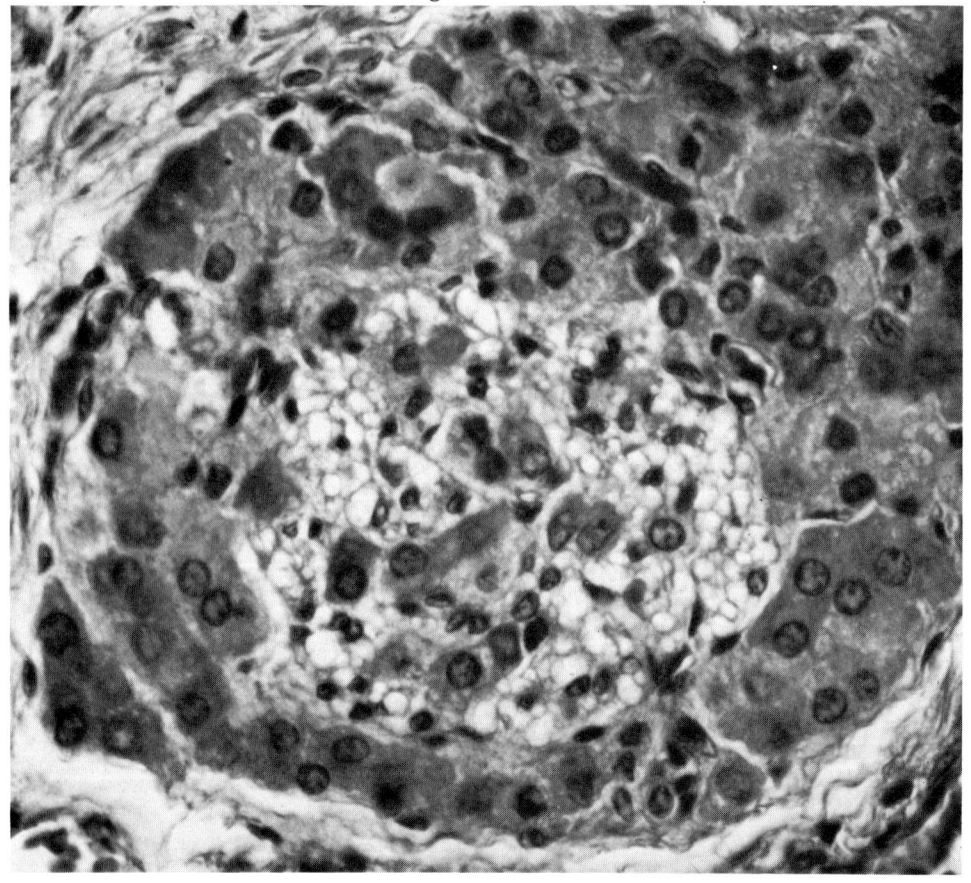

Figure 26-16b

OVARY 459

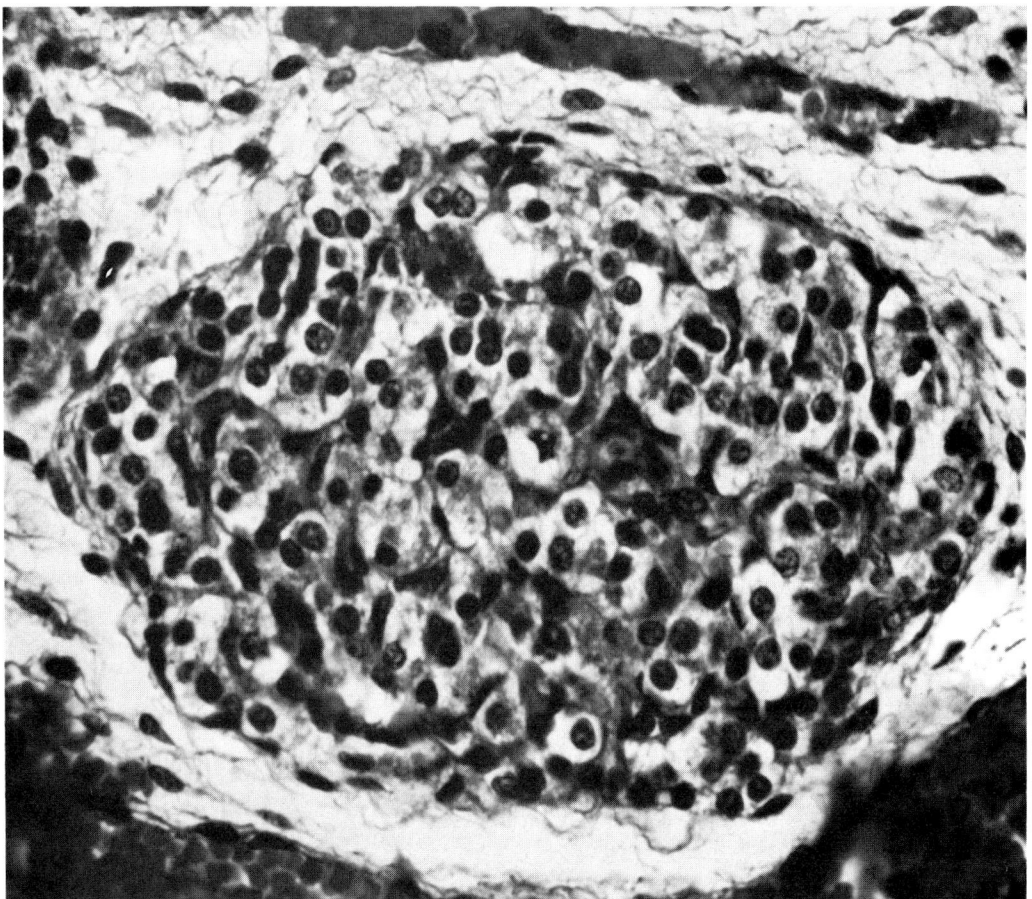

Figure 26–16c

Figure 26–16. These are three pictures of nests of hilus cells, occasionally encountered in the loose areolar connective tissue adjacent to the hilus of the ovary in the newborn infant. Like the Leydig cells of the testis, their embryologic counterpart in the male, they are present at birth and disappear within the first year of life, to re-appear at adolescence.

Figure 26–16a. The smallest of the three is derived from a term infant who survived for 19¾ hours. Note the vacuolated quality of the cytoplasm of many of the cells, especially those that are more centrally placed. Mag. 555×. (From Valdés-Dapena, M. A.: The Normal Ovary of Childhood. *Annals of the New York Academy of Sciences,* 142:597–613, 1967.)

Figure 26–16b. Mag. 534×.

Figure 26–16c. Mag. 534×.

All three are from hematoxylin and eosin stained sections.

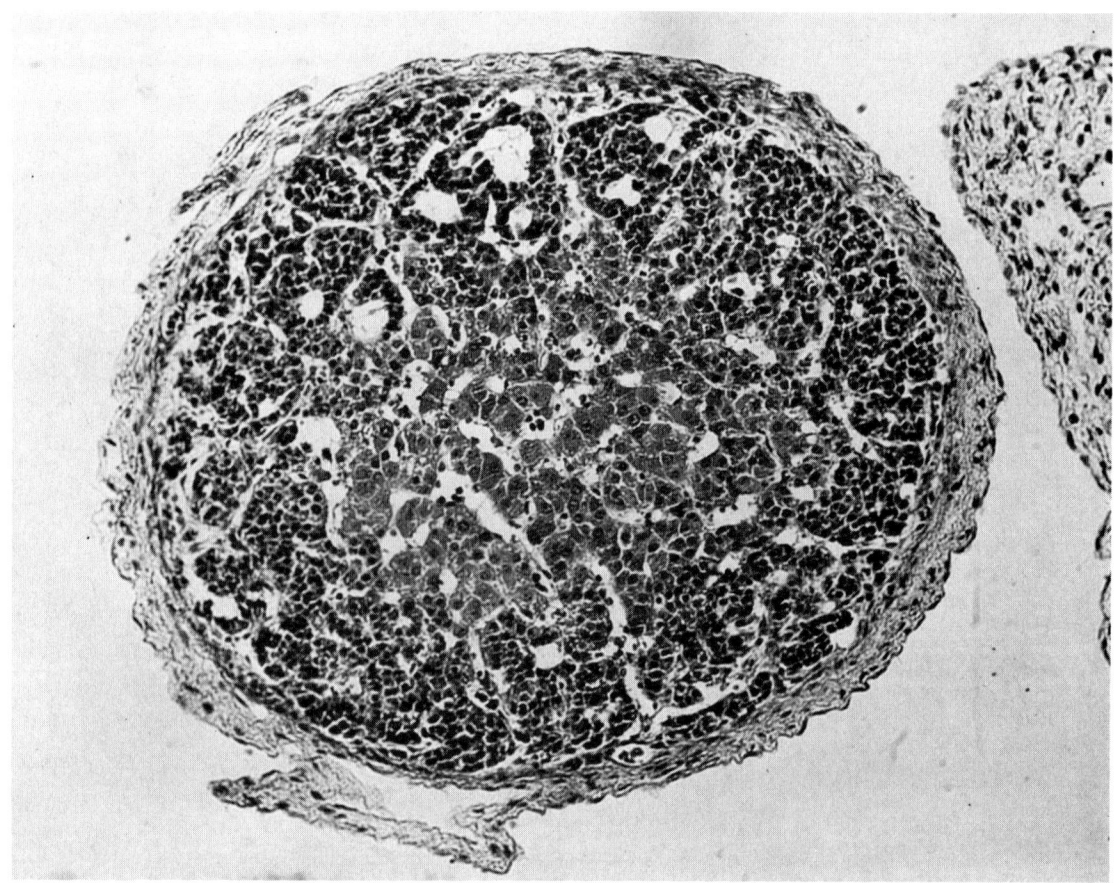

Figure 26–17

Figure 26–17. One of the aberrations of the human infant ovary is the presence of nodules of adrenal cortical tissue, which may be encountered, although not commonly, in the vicinity of the ovarian hilus. They can be distinguished from clusters of hilus cells by their capsules, if nothing else. They are the equivalent of adrenal cortical rests so commonly found near the hilus of the testis and along the course of the vas deferens. Similar nodules may occur in relation to the fallopian tube, mesosalpinx, mesovarium, or broad ligament.[4]

Hematoxylin and eosin stain. Mag. 243×.

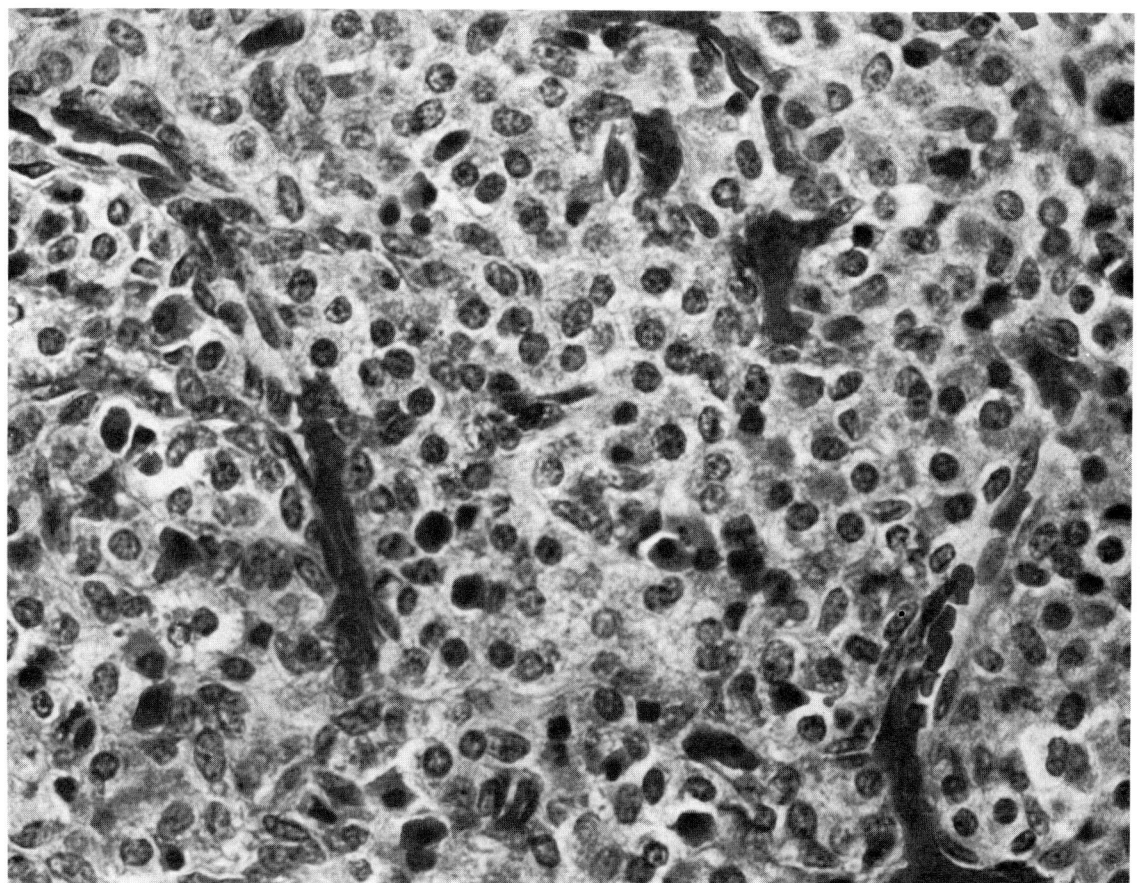

Figure 26–18

Figure 26–18. This photomicrograph illustrates the character of the cells of the theca interna in the state of over-proliferation. Such "over-development" is apt to be seen in the ovaries of infants of diabetic, pre-diabetic, and toxemic mothers. In some instances, large masses of these lutein cells are diffusely "peppered" with eosinophils. This change is comparable to the hyperplasia of the islets of Langerhans in the infants of diabetic or pre-diabetic mothers, that hyperplasia also frequently being the site of abundant infiltration of eosinophils.

This infant was a white female weighing 3,348 grams, born at 38 weeks of gestation, who lived for 1 day.

Hematoxylin and eosin stain. Mag. 400×. (From Valdés-Dapena, M. A.: The Normal Ovary of Childhood. *Annals of the New York Academy of Sciences,* 142:597–613, 1967.)

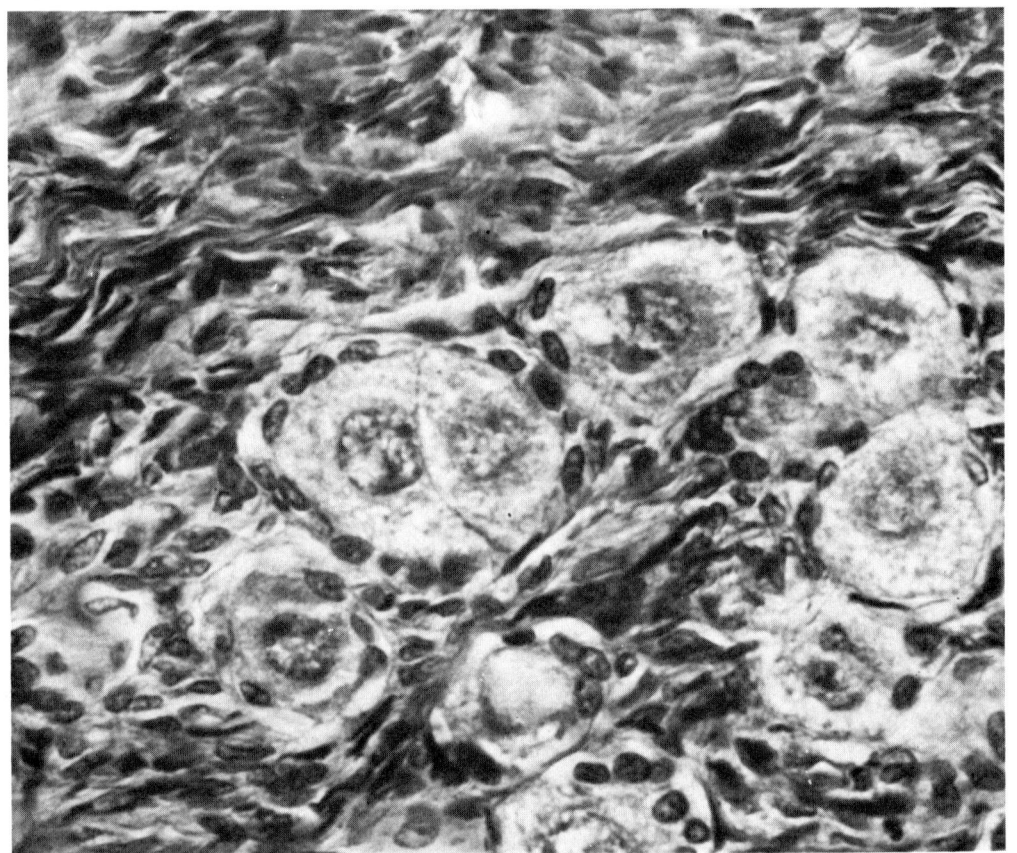

Figure 26–19a

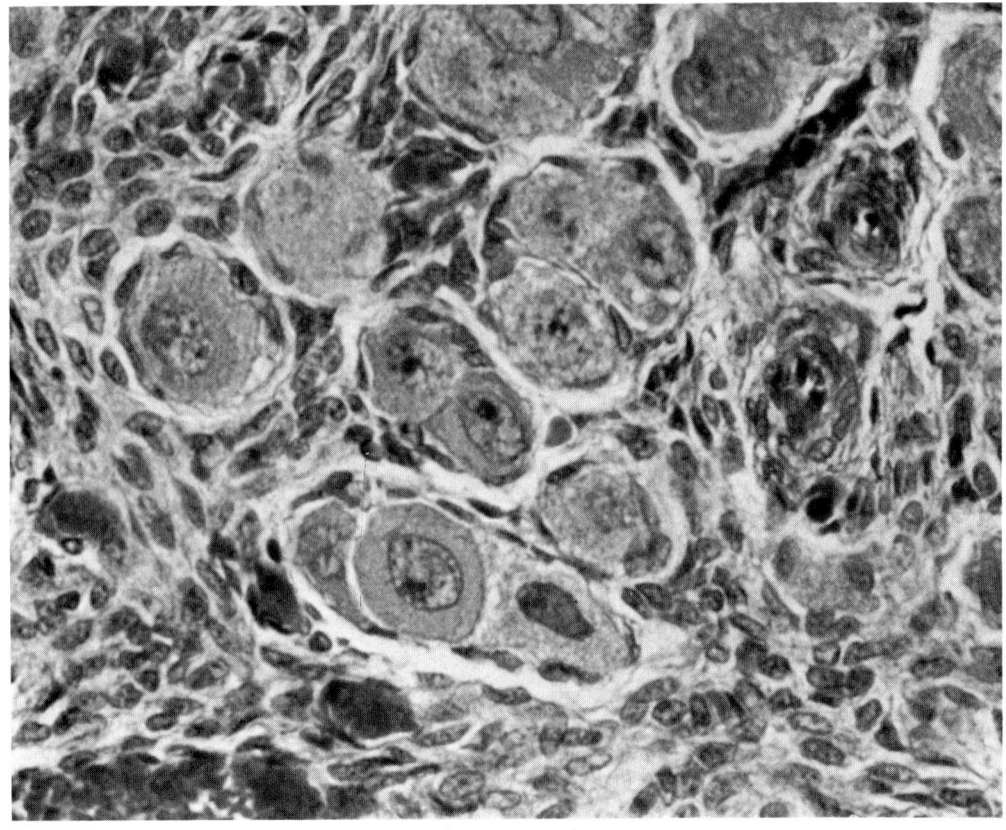

Figure 26–19b

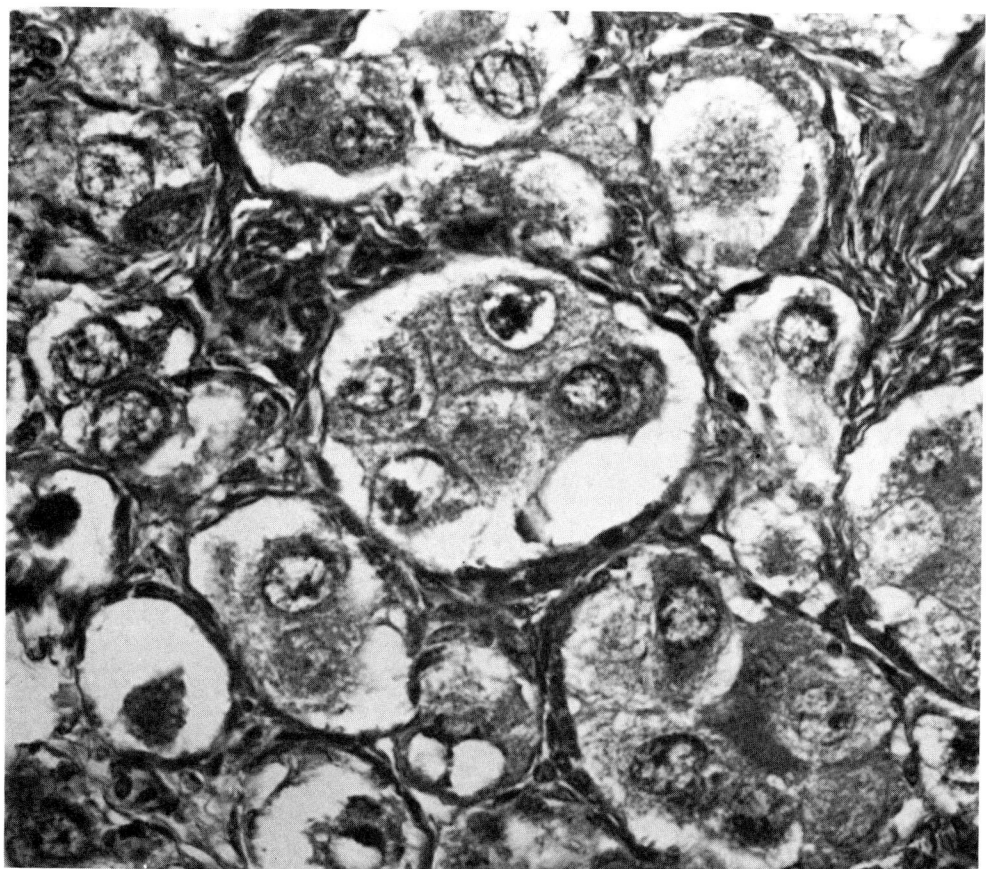

Figure 26–19c

Figure 26–19. Multiovular follicles, common in the ovary of the newborn, are illustrated in this set of three photomicrographs.

Figure 26–19a. Although not from the ovary of an infant but from an eight year old girl, this photograph depicts quite clearly a biovular follicle which is, as one might expect, the type most frequently encountered. Mag. 555×.

Figure 26–19b. In this photograph there are two triovular follicles separated from each other by a single biovular follicle. This is from the ovary of a six year old girl. Mag. 492×. (From Valdés-Dapena, M. A.: The Normal Ovary of Childhood. *Annals of the New York Academy of Sciences, 142*: 597–613, 1967.)

Figure 26–19c. This also is not from a neonate but an infant of fourteen months. It illustrates at least two follicles that contain five visible oocytes each (and probably others not visible in this plane of section). Mag. 450×. (From Valdés-Dapena, M. A.: Development of the Ovary in Childhood. American Registry of Pathology, Armed Forces Institute of Pathology. Washington, D.C., 1975.)

All three are hematoxylin and eosin stained sections.

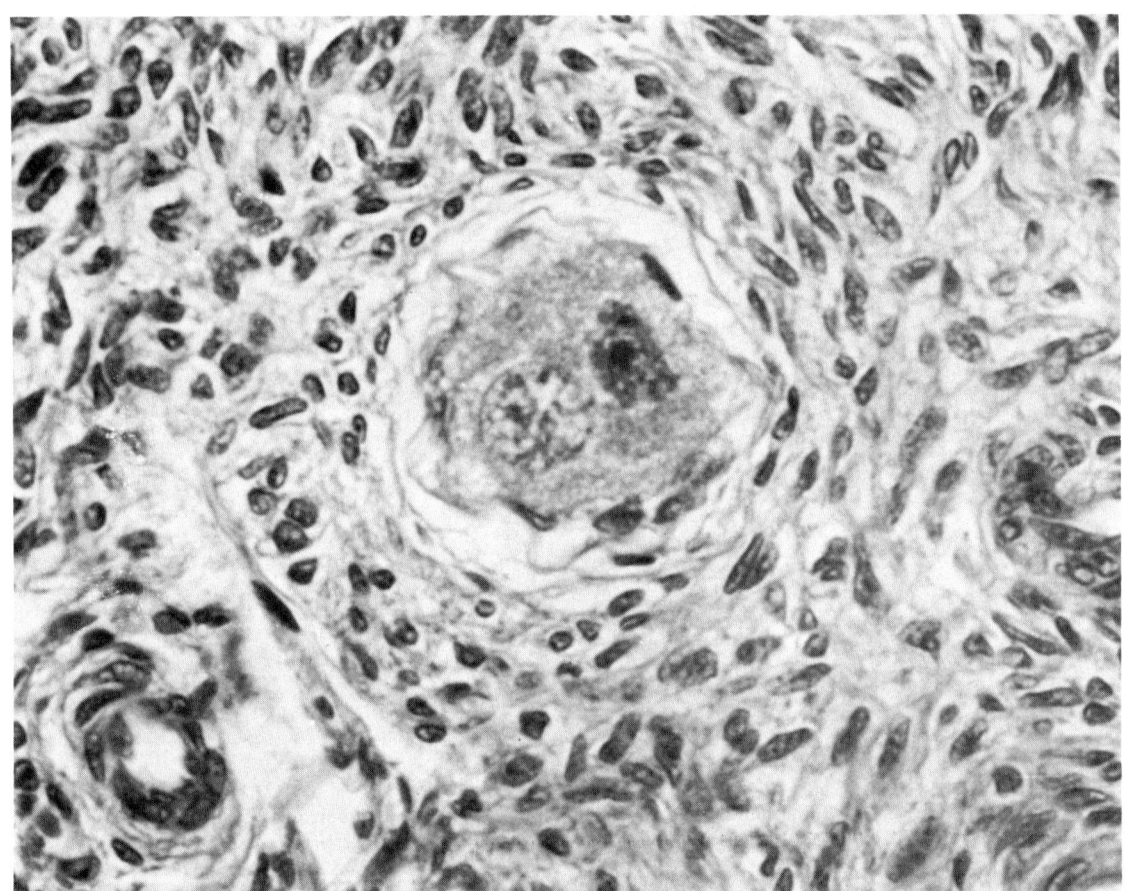

Figure 26–20a

Figure 26–20. Both of these photomicrographs were taken from a single ovary from an infant who had come to autopsy at the Office of the Medical Examiner in New York City. (We have no knowledge of the age or race of the infant, nor the length of life.)

They depict binuclear oocytes, not uncommonly encountered in the ovaries of neonates. Hematoxylin and eosin stain. Mag. 660×.

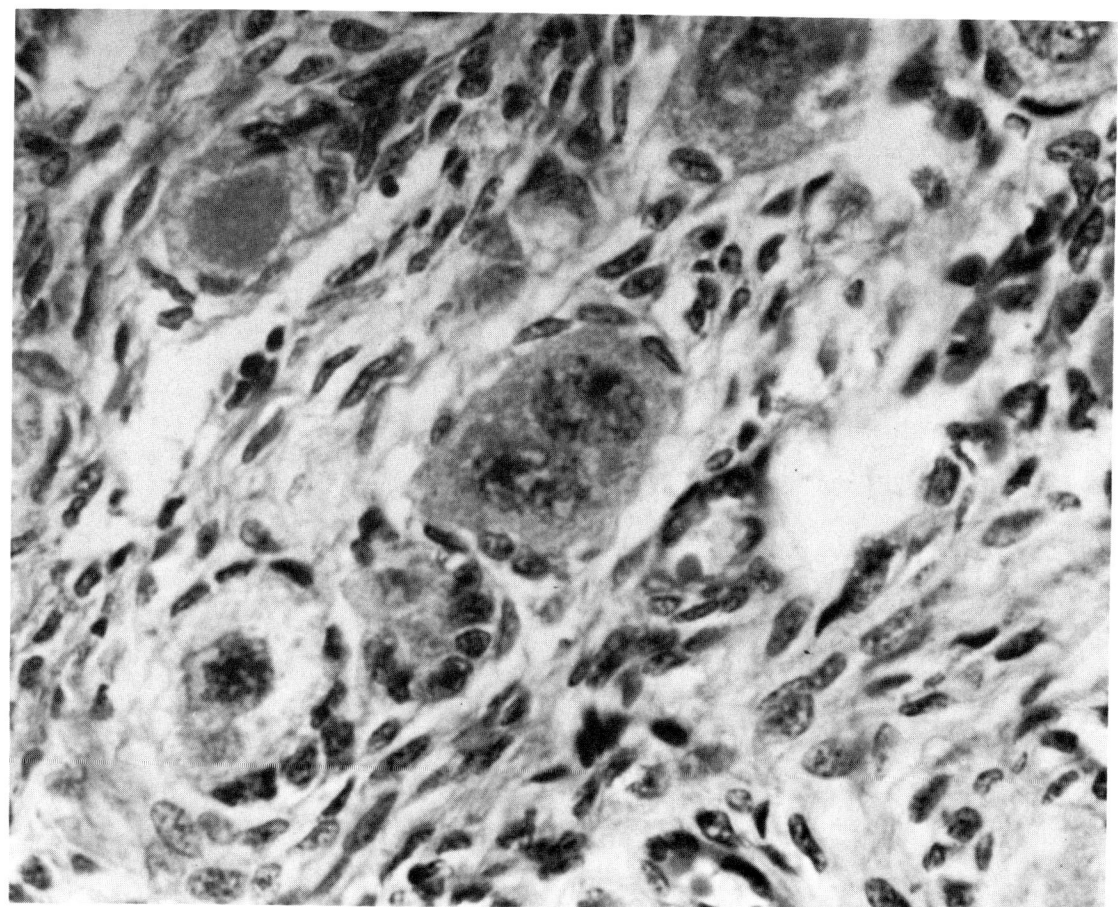

Figure 26-20b

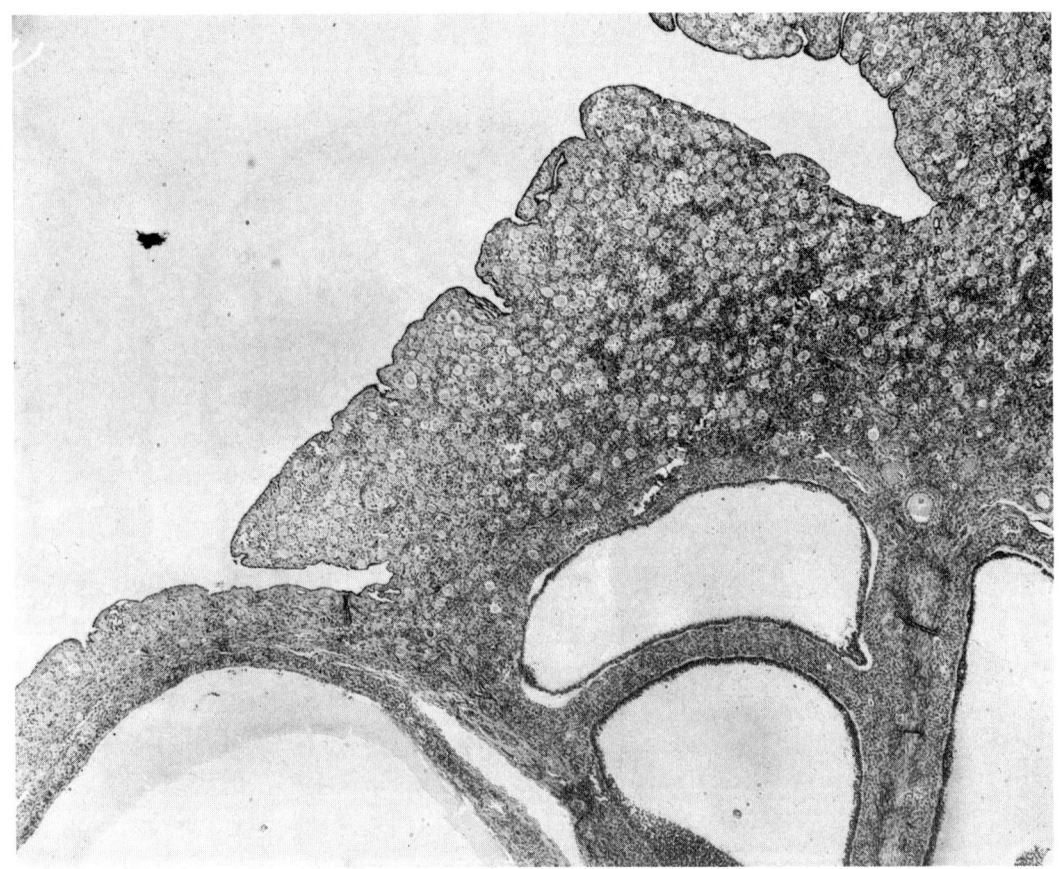

Figure 26–21

Figure 26–21. This is a survey view of the ovary of an infant born at term. She weighed 3,080 grams and lived for 21 hours.

Note the considerable number of follicular cysts. Granulosa cells are seen lining the two in the center, and theca cells about the two in the lower corners.

Hematoxylin and eosin stain. Mag. 41×.

OVARY 467

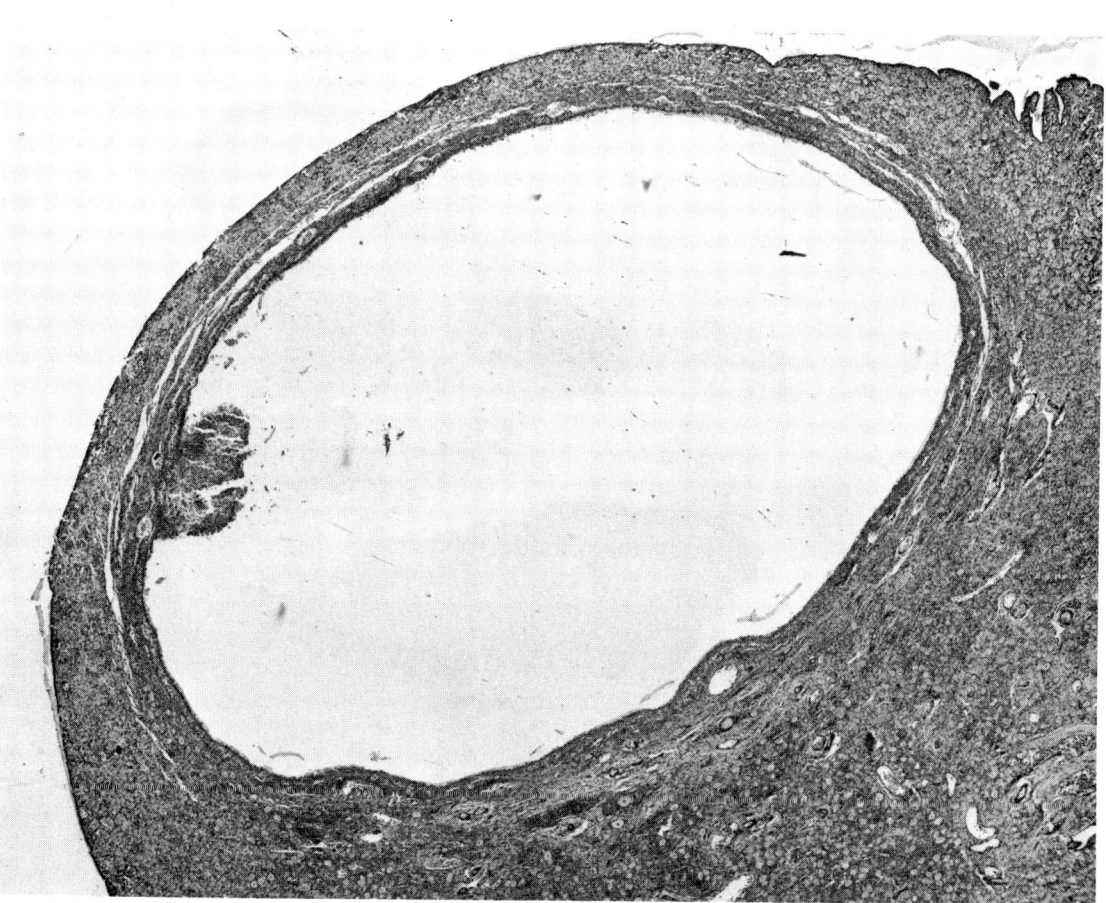

Figure 26–22

Figure 26–22. A rather large follicular cyst seen at very low magnification. The cyst is surrounded by both granulosa cells and theca cells.

The patient was a one day old white female, the infant of a woman who was probably diabetic. Body weight at necropsy was 3,975 grams.

Periodic acid-Schiff stain. Mag. 26.5×.

Chapter 27

FALLOPIAN TUBES

EMBRYOLOGY

In embryos with ovaries, the mesonephric ducts regress and the paramesonephric (Müllerian) ducts develop into the female genital tract. The cranial unfused portions of these latter ducts become the fallopian tubes, with their funnel-shaped cranial ends opening into the coelomic or peritoneal cavity.[1]

ANATOMY

Each tube is situated in the upper margin of the broad ligament of the uterus. The uterine tubes of infants tend to be quite convoluted in their course from the uterus itself to the fimbriated end (Fig. 27–1). The diameter of the tube increases progressively from the proximal to the distal extremity; at the level of the infundibulum, near the lateral end, it may be twice what it is at the uterine ostium (Fig. 27–1).

The most medial portion of the tube, that which is intramural, is called the *uterine part*. The adjacent free, round, slender cord-like segment is spoken of as the *isthmus*, with a rather stout wall and slender lumen. This portion is succeeded by the *ampulla*, which is thin-walled and tortuous and forms more than half of the length of the oviduct (Fig. 27–1). The ampulla, in turn, opens into the *infundibulum*, the trumpet-shaped expansion opening into the peritoneal cavity by way of the fimbriated end.

HISTOLOGY

The following coats are identifiable in sections of the wall of the fallopian tube: the mucosa, the muscular coat, and the serosa (Fig. 27–3).

The mucosa consists of an epithelium and an underlying layer of connective tissue bearing mucosal blood and lymph vessels and nerve fibers (Fig. 27–8).

The epithelium is composed of a single layer of columnar cells joined at their bases to an incomplete basement membrane.[1] At least three kinds of cells constitute this epithelium, only one of which is ciliated.

The mucosa is invaginated into the lumen of the tube in a series of plicae or folds, each of which exhibits secondary and teritary branching (Fig. 27–7). Thus, in transverse sections, especially those taken rather laterally (or distally), the lumen appears to be almost completely occupied by plicae (Fig. 27–5).

The muscular coat consists of external longitudinal and internal circular layers of smooth muscle. The muscular coat is thickest in the isthmic portion and become remarkably thinner as it proceeds laterally (compare Figs. 27–4 and 27–5).

The serosa is a layer of peritoneum with subjacent areolar tissue. In infants it is often quite prominent (Figs. 27–3 and 27–4).

Reference

1. Warwick, R., and Williams, P. L.: Gray's Anatomy, 35th British Ed. Philadelphia, W. B. Saunders Co., 1973, pp. 1354–1355.

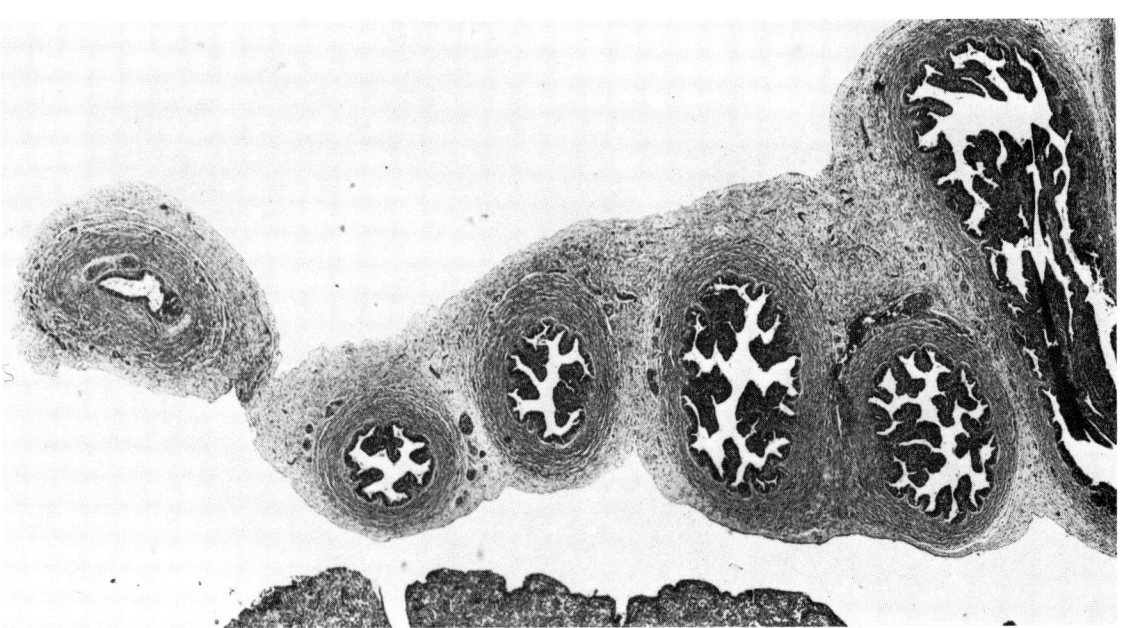

Figure 27–1

Figure 27–1. A series of cross sections of the markedly convoluted fallopian tube of a 450 gram infant (born at six months gestation) who survived for two days. The simplest and most proximal portion of the tube is represented on the left, and the infundibulum on the right. A tiny segment of the ovary appears at the lower margin of the photograph.

Hematoxylin and eosin stain. Mag. 28.5×.

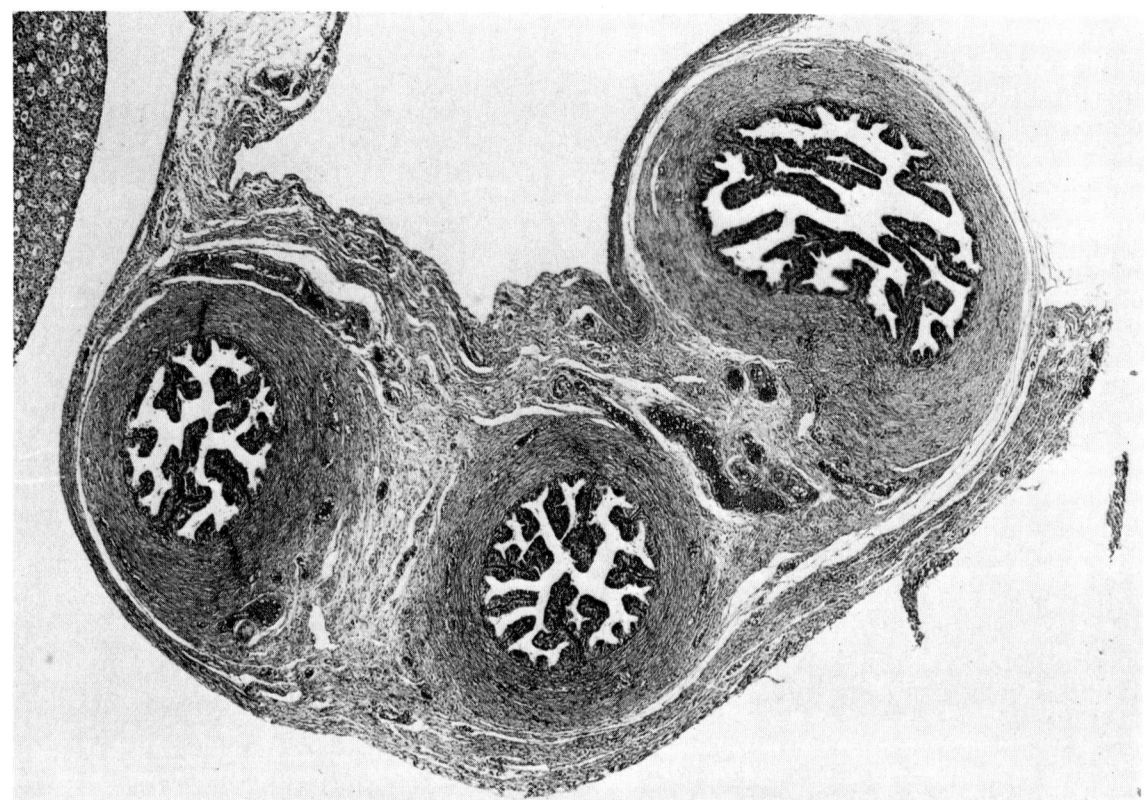

Figure 27–2

Figure 27–2. By contrast with Fig. 27–1, taken at the same magnification, this photomicrograph depicts a series of cross sections of the fallopian tube of a more mature and larger infant who weighed 2,930 grams at autopsy. In this instance the visible segment of ovary appears on the left-hand margin of the illustration.

Hematoxylin and eosin stain. Mag. 28.5×.

FALLOPIAN TUBES 473

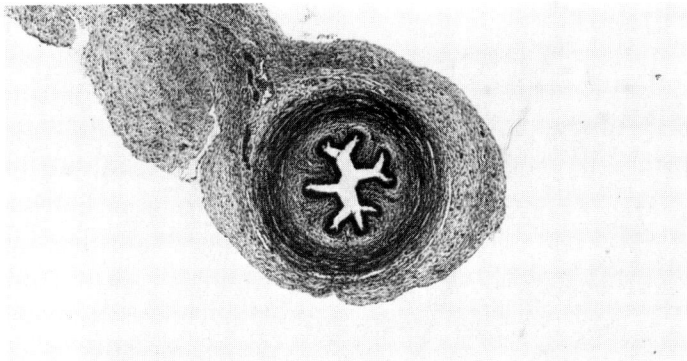

Figure 27–3

Figure 27–3. This is a single cross section of the uterine tube of a prematurely born 520 gram infant (24 weeks gestation) who lived for four hours. Clearly visible here are the rather thick serosa, the muscular coat, and the mucosa.
Hematoxylin and eosin stain. Mag. 45×

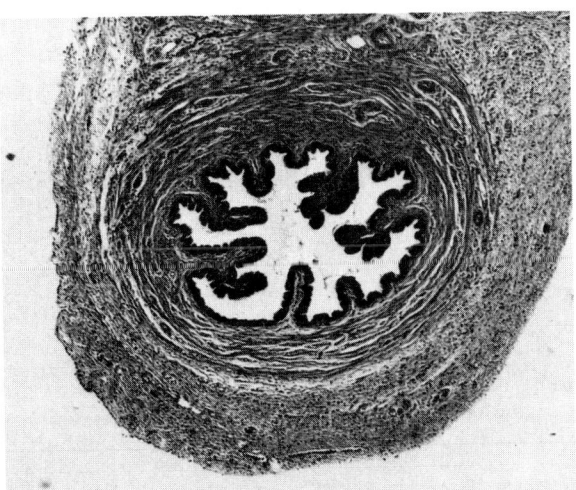

Figure 27–4

Figure 27–4. Cross section of the uterine tube of a much more mature infant who weighed 2,360 grams (38 weeks gestation) and who survived for 59 hours.
Hematoxylin and eosin stain. Mag. 45×.

474   FALLOPIAN TUBES

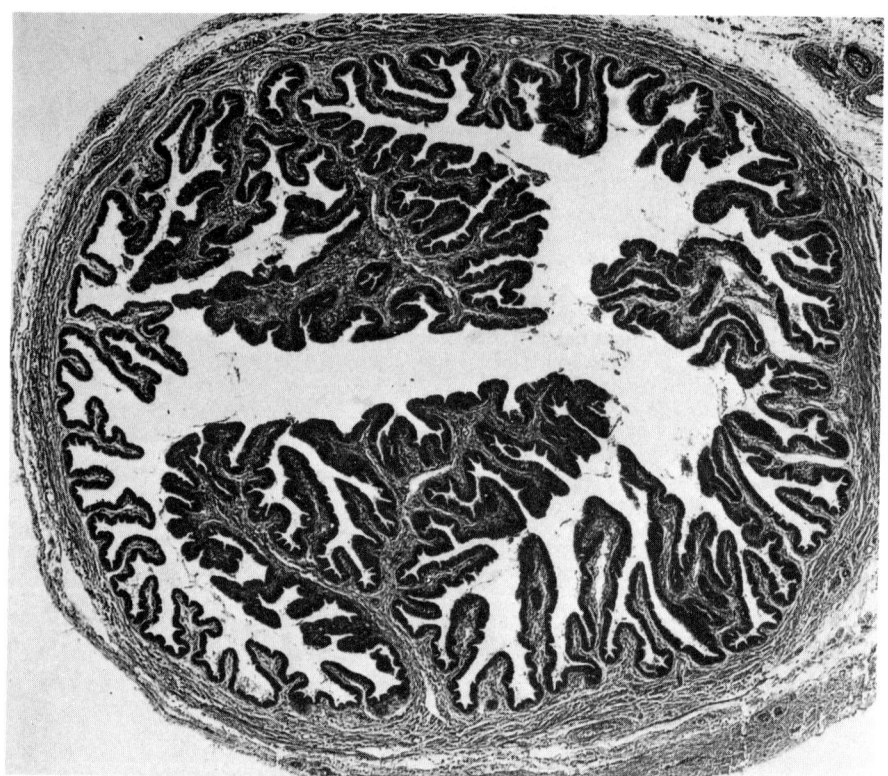

Figure 27–5

Figure 27–5. This is a cross section of the fallopian tube of the same infant as is represented in Fig. 27–4. Taken at the same magnification, it serves to illustrate the marked difference which exists in the diameter of the tube from one end to the other and the difference in size and complexity of the mucosal folds. Proximally the folds are few, short, stout, and simple, whereas distally they are numerous, tall, slender, and branching with secondary and even tertiary projections.
Hematoxylin and eosin stain. Mag. 45×.

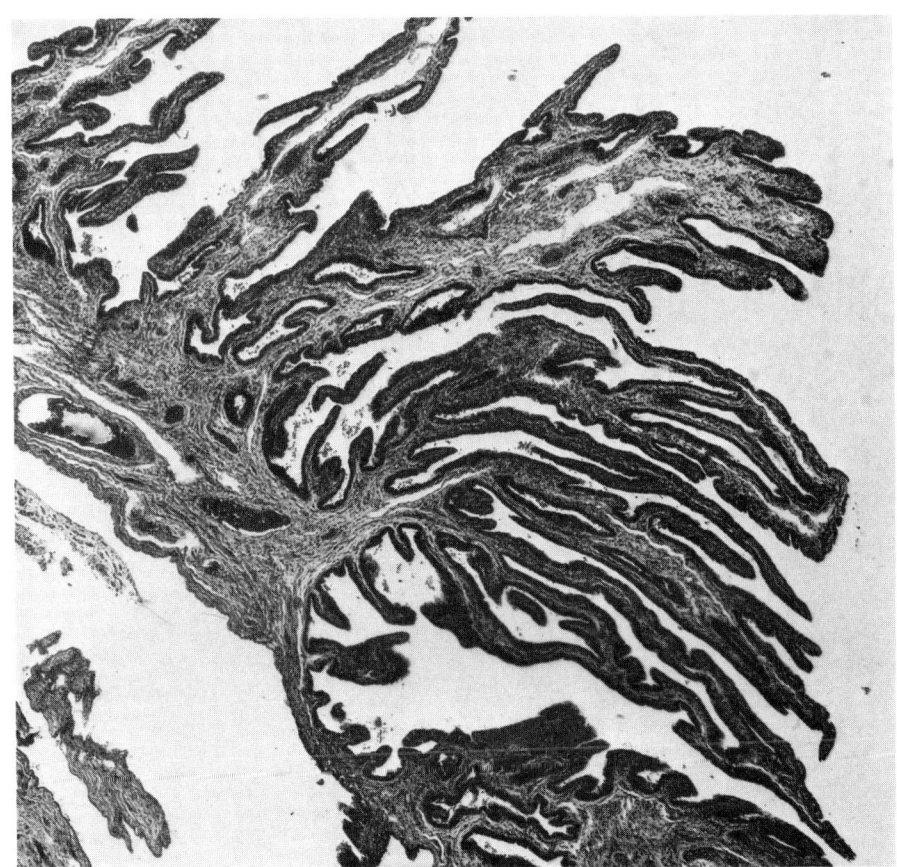

Figure 27-6

Figure 27-6. Depicted here is the junction of the infundibulum and the fimbriated end of the uterine tube of a 3,940 gram infant born at term (40 weeks gestation) who lived for 25 days. The large longitudinal folds of the infundibulum are continuous with similar folds in the larger fimbriae. Hematoxylin and eosin stain. Mag. 31×.

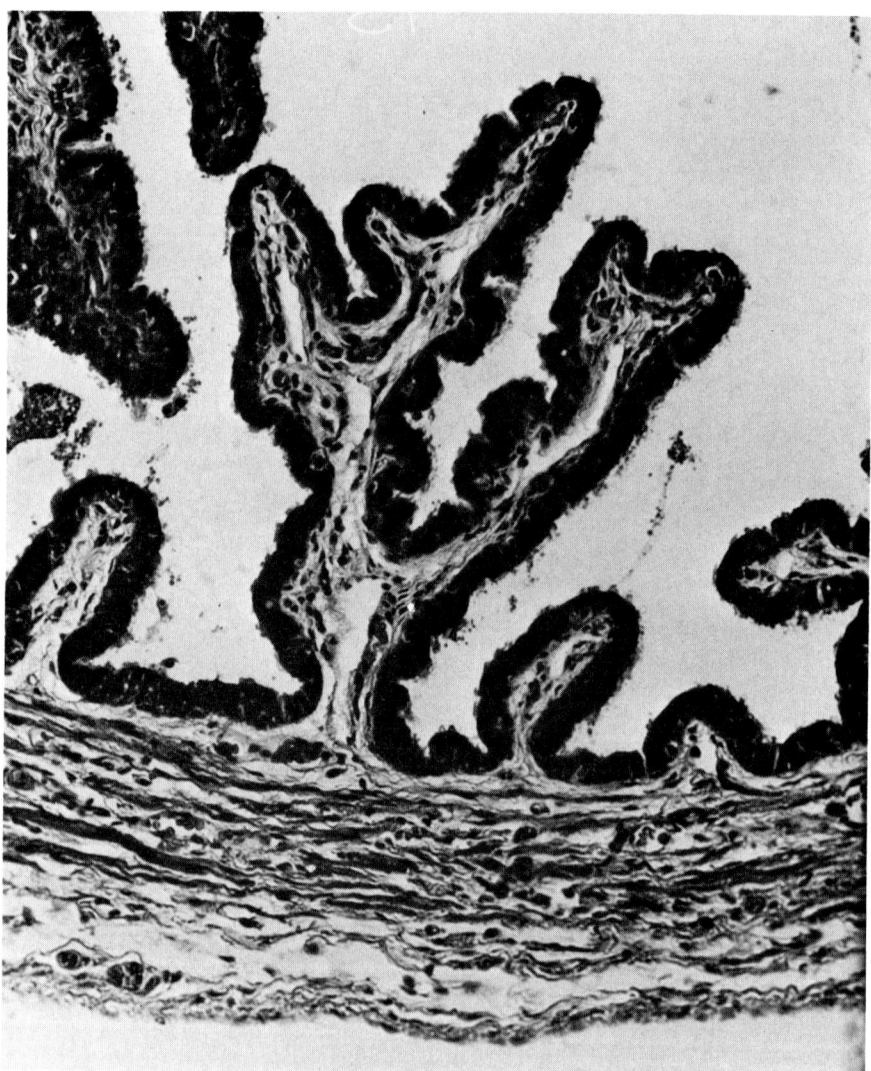

Figure 27-7

Figure 27-7. Seen here at higher magnification is a single moderately complex branching fold of the mucosa. Secondary and tertiary projections are evident. The remainder of the wall, including the muscular coat and the serosa (both of which are seen here in their entire breadth), is quite thin. The subject is the same as that represented in Figs. 27-4 and 27-5.

Hematoxylin and eosin stain. Mag. 208×.

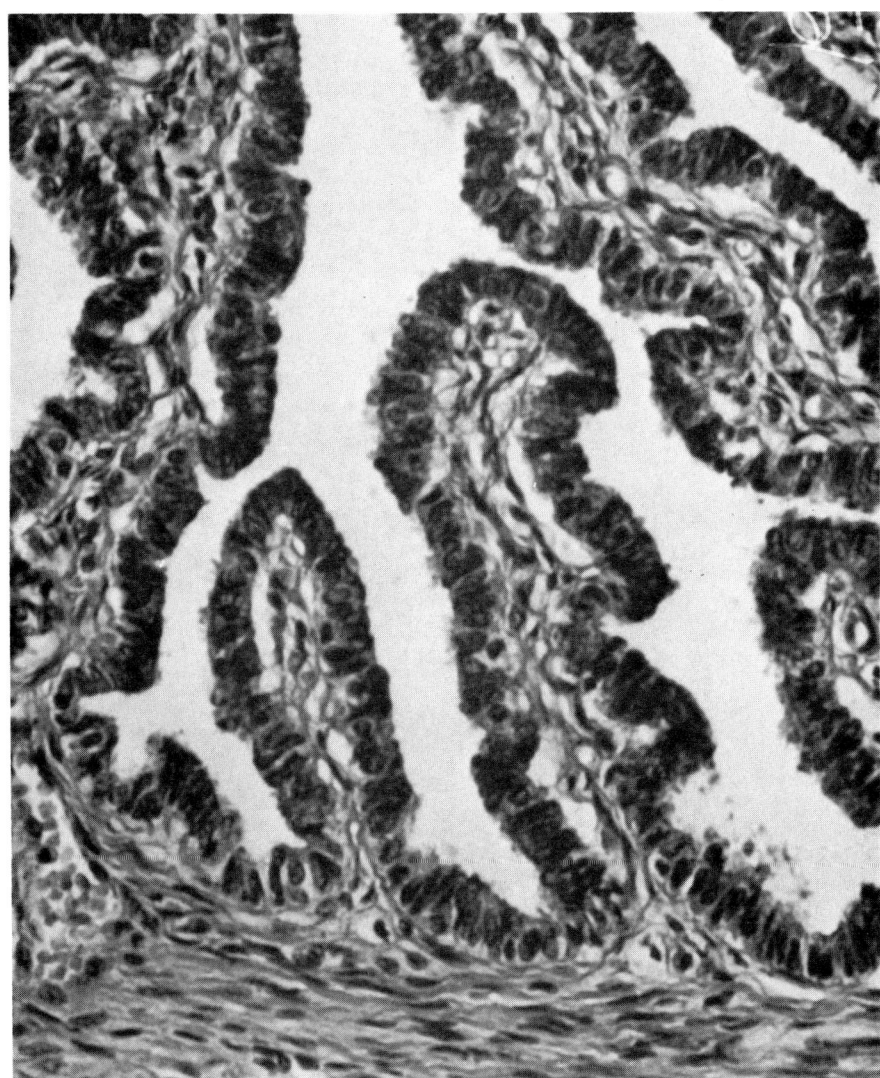

Figure 27–8

Figure 27–8. The mucous membrane of the uterine tube consists of an epithelium, a single layer of columnar cells, some of which are ciliated, and an underlying connective tissue stratum containing, as is evident here, blood and lymph vessels and nerve fibers. The patient was an infant who died at the age of 16 hours and whose body weight at autopsy was 3,075 grams.

Hematoxylin and eosin stain. Mag. 382×.

Chapter 28

UTERUS AND VAGINA

EMBRYOLOGY

In all placental animals the Müllerian ducts fuse at their caudal ends, to varying degrees.[3] In primates, complete caudal union produces a common uterus as well as a common vagina; but only in the highest primate, the human, does the union reach its fullest expression.

As the urogenital ridges are crowded laterally by the growing adrenals and kidneys, the Müllerian ducts are also displaced. As a result, each duct makes two bends in its course, thus establishing roughly three different regions: (1) the cranial, which will become the fallopian tube, (2) the middle, which will give rise to the uterine fundus and corpus, and (3) the caudal, which fuses with its fellow to produce a common tube, the uterine cervix and the upper part of the vagina.

Originally the future middle part, fundus-corpus, is represented by two transverse limbs. After a time the cranial walls of those two tubes bulge in a cranial direction so that their original angular junction becomes a convex dome, the fundus.[3]

It has traditionally been held that the cervix arises from the primary fusion of the Müllerian ducts. Some contend, however, that its original epithelium is replaced, as in the vagina, by invading entoderm from the urogenital sinus.

ANATOMY

The uterus of the infant, like that of the adult, is a relatively thick-walled muscular organ. The vagina is lightly adherent to the posterior aspect of the urinary bladder, and the uterus rises up into the peritoneal cavity above that, most of the cervix and body being covered by mesothelium.

During the perinatal period the organ is tiny, often less than one centimeter in overall length. In very immature infants its shape is the reverse of the pear-shape of the adult, the large prominent bulging portion below representing the cervix and the diminutive portion at the top being the body and fundus. The latter together equal roughly one-third the size of the former.

The serosa is shiny and pale pink, as is the smooth muscle beneath it. The consistency is firm. The central lumen, flattened from before backwards, is only a potential space, the walls being in close apposition to one another. The endometrium is smooth and pale pink. The lining of the prominent cervix, however, displays a completely characteristic and striking internal configuration sometimes referred to as the "tree of life," or arbor vitae, made up of numerous, delicate interweaving mucosal folds. It is into these that the cervical glands open.

The cervix projects prominently into the vagina. Its external os is usually linear, side to side.

Not uncommonly there will be a brighter pink patch of mucosa adjacent to the os, spreading out over one or two "lips" of the cervix, and very sharply demarcated; this is the so-called "congenital erosion" which is really nothing more nor less than replacement of stratified squamous epithelium there with a single layer of tall columnar mucus-producing epithelium through which one can see the light red color of underlying capillaries. The vagina, relatively speaking, has a spacious lumen and rather rough or wrinkled white mucosa.

HISTOLOGY

As the uterus increases in size during late fetal life and early infancy, the various component parts of it increase in complexity, too. Figures 28-1 to 28-3 represent sagittal sections of the entire organ including the fundus, body, and cervix as well as the upper part of the vagina, from fetuses in the sixth, seventh, and eighth months of gestation respectively. Even at this very low magnification, it is apparent that in the smallest of them there are neither endometrial nor cervical glands. Just a little difference between mucosa and muscularis begins to become apparent in the uterus in the seventh month of gestation (Fig. 28-2); only a few cervical glands can be seen. In the eighth month, however, both cervical and endometrial glands are visible; both are still simple and relatively widely separated.

Figure 28-3 illustrates well the relatively large size of the cervical portion of the uterus in this phase of growth and development;[1] measuring from the lowermost extremity of the portio vaginalis or the cervical os upward, 7/10 of the length of the uterus consists of the cervix and only the darker 3/10 at the top represents the body.

Figures 28-4 to 28-6 illustrate the changing pattern of the endometrium during late fetal life and early infancy. In Figure 28-4, a section taken from the body of the uterus of a 400 gram fetus, the endometrium is solid and blank. It is covered by a single layer of epithelium and bears no glands. In Figure 28-5, at the same magnification, is seen the endometrium of a fetus weighing 550 grams. A few glands have begun to appear, but this certainly does not resemble adult endometrium. In Figure 28-6, from a fetus in the seventh month of gestation weighing 1,470 grams, the endometrial glands seem not very different, either in number, size, or complexity, from those in Figure 28-5. The definitive histological character of the endometrium begins to take shape near the time of term birth.

In the three portions of Figure 28-7, the changing intimate morphology of the endometrial gland itself is apparent. In Figure 28-7a, from a fetus of 600 grams, no endometrial glands appear. In Figure 28-7b, from a fetus of 940 grams, only a single gland is depicted; it is straight, short, and simple. In Figure 28-7c, from a premature infant weighing 1,280 grams, the glands appear to be not only more numerous but also longer.

The four parts of Figure 28-8 illustrate the changing pattern of contrast between endometrium and myometrium. In the fifth month of gestation, as illustrated in parts a and c, the endometrium being above (a) and the myometrium below (c), there is really little contrast between the pattern of endometrial stroma and the weave of the myometrium. On the other hand, in parts b and d (sections taken from an infant weighing 1,925 grams), the difference is clear; the cells of the endometrial stroma above (b) are rounded whereas those of the myometrium (d) are not only spindle-shaped but also clearly arranged in interweaving bundles.

During this phase of human life, as previously mentioned, the cervix is the dominant segment of the uterus. Its changing histologic morphology is depicted in Figures 28–9 to 28–11, all of which are sagittal sections. In the first of these, taken from a fetus of 700 grams, the simplicity of the structure is obvious. There are almost no glands present; there are none at the junction of the canal and portio vaginalis. In a fetus of twice that weight, 1,390 grams (Fig. 28—10), cervical glands are well formed, especially near the os. Near term (Fig. 28–11a), the portio vaginalis is still larger, and glands are seen not only at the os but also throughout the length of the canal; the glands are large, long, and branching.

From their very first appearance, the glands of the cervical canal are slanted in parallel fashion, with the fundus directed upward and the ostium downward[2] (Fig. 28–12). In later stages of development, as the glands themselves evolve and become more complex, this parallel slant persists (Fig. 28–13).

As regards the production of mucus by the cervical glands, none is apparent in fetuses with a body weight less than 1,000 grams (Fig. 28–14). In the latter months of gestation, more and more mucus is produced until finally, at term, the cytoplasm of all of the cells contains some and a few cells are swollen with their burden (Fig. 28–15).

Islands of apparently aberrant squamous epithelium (? squamous metaplasia) are commonly encountered in the lining of the infantile cervical glands, especially those near the external os (Fig. 28–16). The smallest infant in whom I have observed it weighed 1,910 grams.

Another relatively common morphologic variant of the infantile cervix is the so-called "cervical erosion," which is really only replacement of the stratified squamous epithelial covering of the portio vaginalis by a single layer of columnar cells, often mucus-producing. Such replacement can be seen in infants weighing slightly more than 1,000 grams. From that point in development forward, throughout late fetal life and infancy, about 4 to 6 per cent of cervices exhibit this variant. In Figure 28–17 the columnar epithelium extends halfway across the convexity of the portio vaginalis, whereas in Figure 28–18 it covers the convexity almost completely and in Figure 28–19 it clothes all of the vaginal portion of the cervix. In the last of these it is accompanied by branching glands.

References

1. Valdés-Dapena, M. A.: The development of the uterus in late fetal life, infancy and childhood. Chap. 3 in "The Uterus," H. J. Norris and A. T. Hertig, eds. Baltimore, The Williams and Wilkins Co., 1973, pp. 40–67.
2. Fluhman, C. G.: The nature and development of the so-called glands of the cervix uteri. Am. J. Obstet. Gynecol., 74:753-766, 1957.
3. Arey, L. B.: Developmental Anatomy. A Textbook and Laboratory Manual of Embryology. Philadelphia, W. B. Saunders Co., 1974, pp. 326–327.

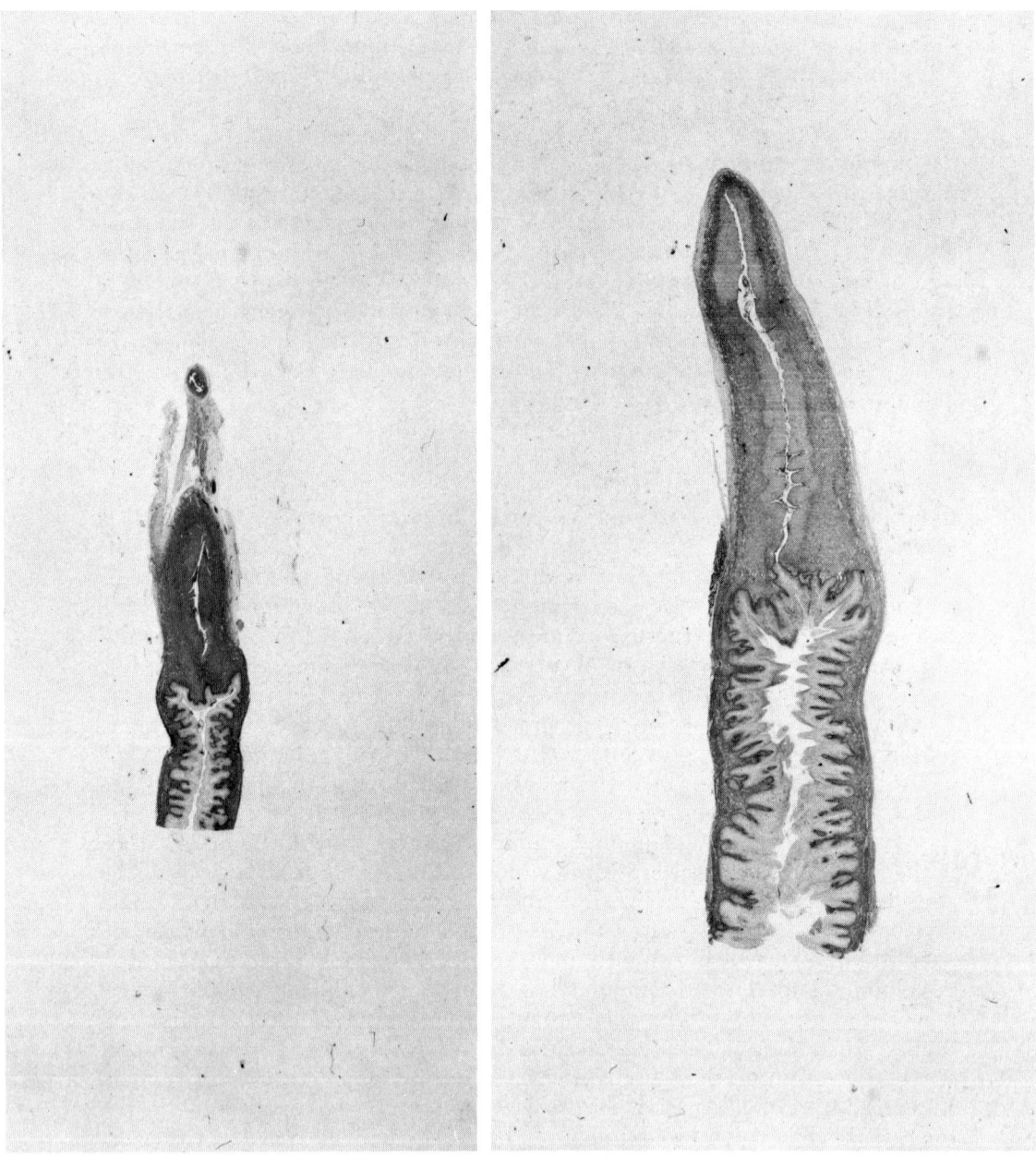

Figure 28-1

Figure 28-2

Figure 28-1. Sagittal section of the uterus of a fetus weighing 500 grams (6th month of gestation). Masson's trichrome stain. Mag. 4.5×. (From Valdés-Dapena, M. A., in "The Uterus," Norris, H. J., and Hertig, A. T., eds. Monograph, International Academy of Pathology. Baltimore, The Williams and Wilkins Co., 1973.)

Figure 28-2. Sagittal section of the uterus of a fetus weighing 625 grams (7th month of gestation). Masson's trichrome stain. Mag. 4.5×. (From Valdés-Dapena, M. A., in "The Uterus," Norris, H. J., and Hertig, A. T., eds. Monograph, International Academy of Pathology. Baltimore, The Williams and Wilkins Co., 1973.)

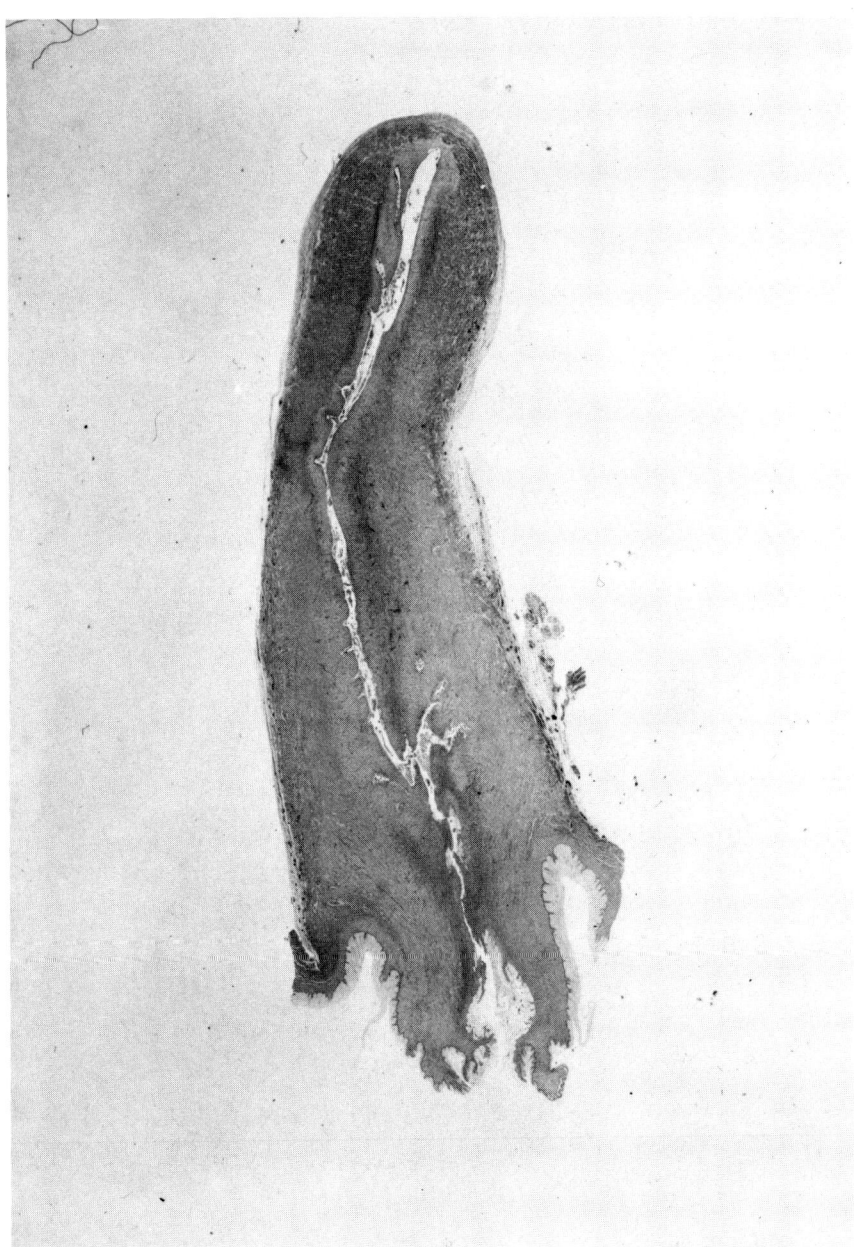

Figure 28-3

Figure 28-3. Sagittal section of the uterus of a premature infant born in the eighth month of gestation, weighing 1,935 grams. Masson's trichrome stain. Mag. 4.5×. (From Valdés-Dapena, M. A., in "The Uterus," Norris, H. J., and Hertig, A. T., eds. Monograph, International Academy of Pathology. Baltimore, The Williams and Wilkins Co., 1973.)

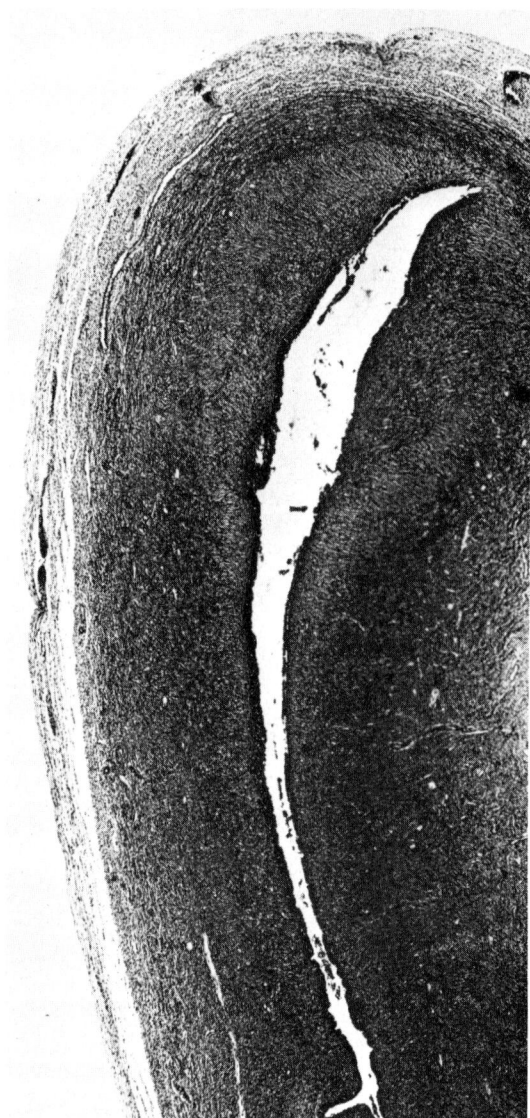

Figure 28–4

Figure 28–4. The endometrium of a fetus weighing 400 grams. There are no glands present. Hematoxylin and eosin stain. Mag. 31×.

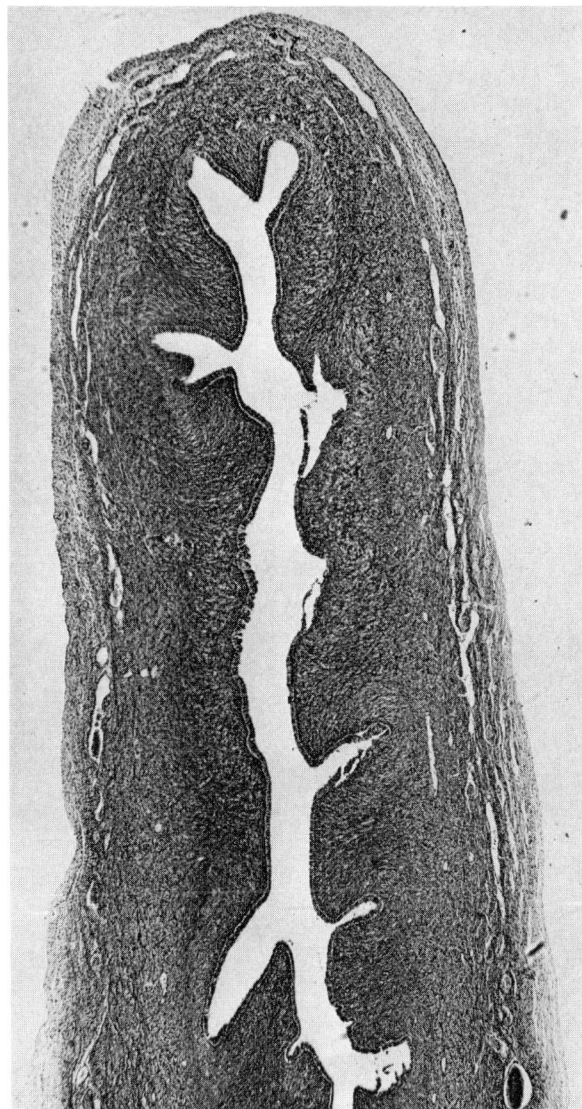

Figure 28–5

Figure 28–5. In this infant, whose body weight was 550 grams, endometrial glands show the beginnings of their development. The "glands" are few, short, straight and wide-mouthed. Hematoxylin and eosin stain. Mag. 31×.

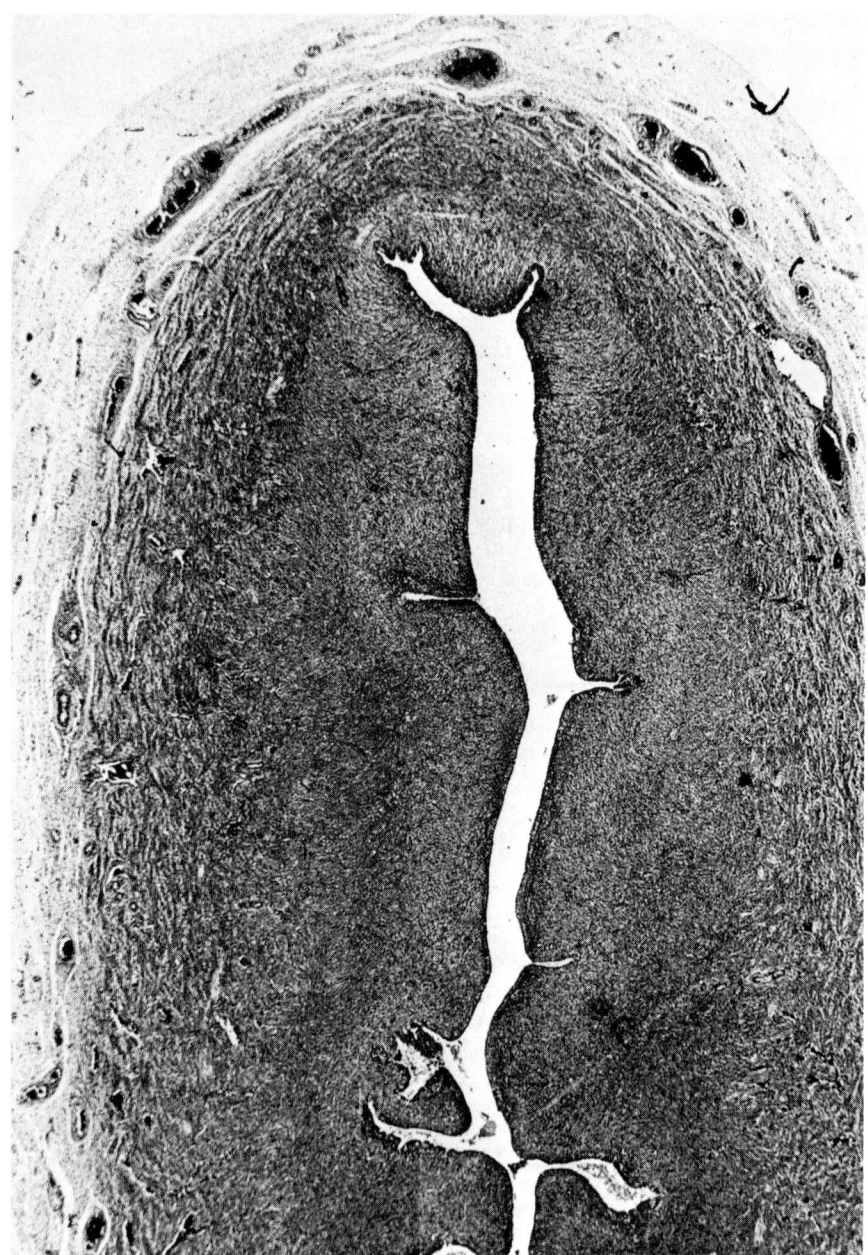

Figure 28–6

Figure 28–6. The endometrium of a fetus in the seventh month of gestation, weighing 1,470 grams.
Hematoxylin and eosin stain. Mag. 31×. (From Valdés-Dapena, M. A., in "The Uterus," Norris, H. J., and Hertig, A. T., eds. Monograph, International Academy of Pathology. Baltimore, The Williams and Wilkins Co., 1973.)

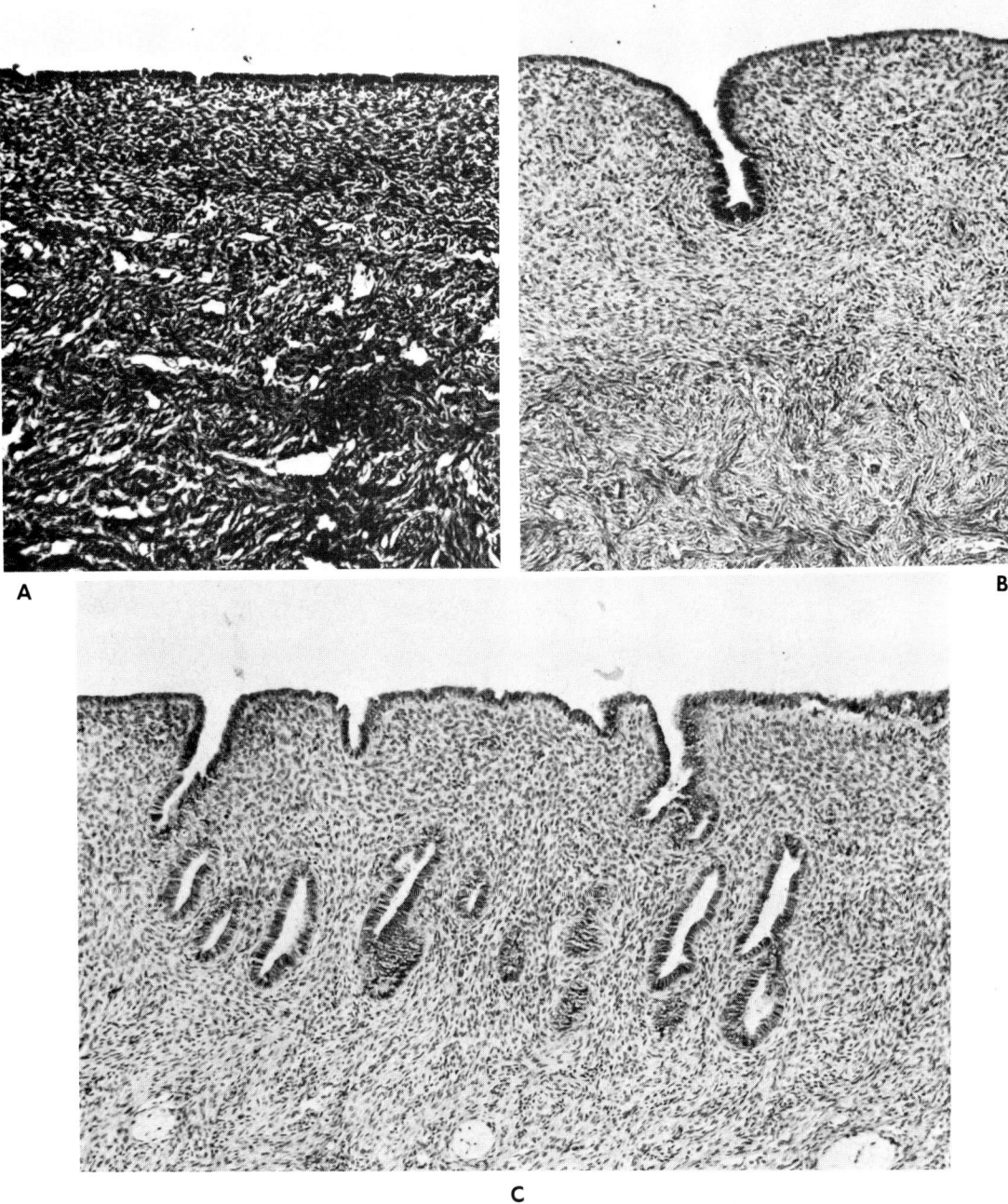

Figure 28–7

Figure 28–7. The changing morphology of the endometrial glands in fetal life and infancy is depicted in this set of three photomicrographs. In the infant of 600 grams (a) there are no glands. In the infant of 940 grams, the few glands are short, straight, and simple (b). In the infant of 1,280 grams (c), they are longer and more numerous.

Hematoxylin and eosin stain. Mag. 124×. (From Valdés-Dapena, M. A., in "The Uterus," Norris, H. J., and Hertig, A. T., eds. Monograph, International Academy of Pathology. Baltimore, The Williams and Wilkins Co., 1973.)

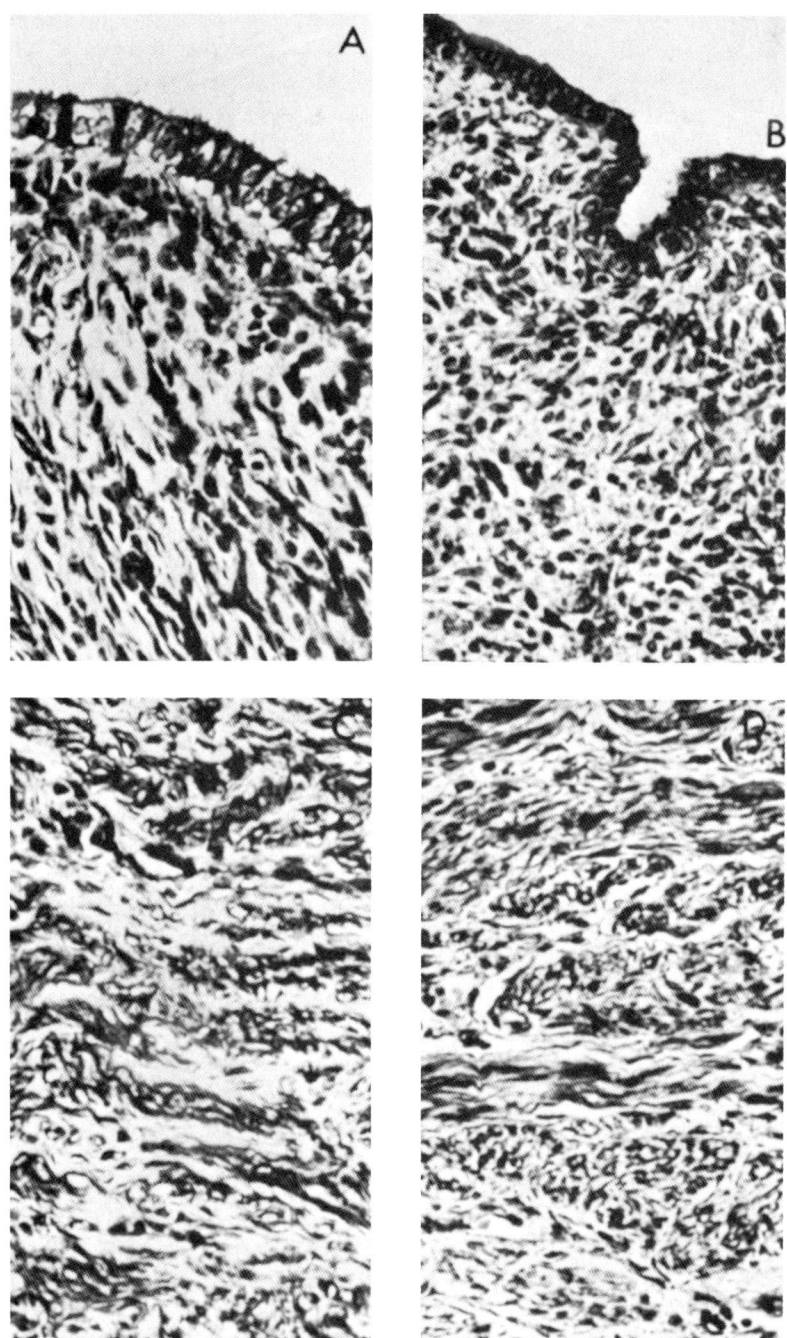

Figure 28–8

Figure 28–8. The minimal contrast between the endometrial stroma (a) and the myometrium (c) in a fetus of 550 grams in the fifth month of gestation is apparent in the two photographs on the left. By comparison, there is marked contrast between the endometrial stroma (b) and the myometrium (d) in a premature infant weighing 1,925 grams seen in the two illustrations on the right.

All are Masson's trichrome stain. Mag. 343×. (From Valdés-Dapena, M. A., in "The Uterus," Norris, H. J., and Hertig, A. T., eds. Monograph, International Academy of Pathology. Baltimore, The Williams and Wilkins Co., 1973.)

UTERUS AND VAGINA 489

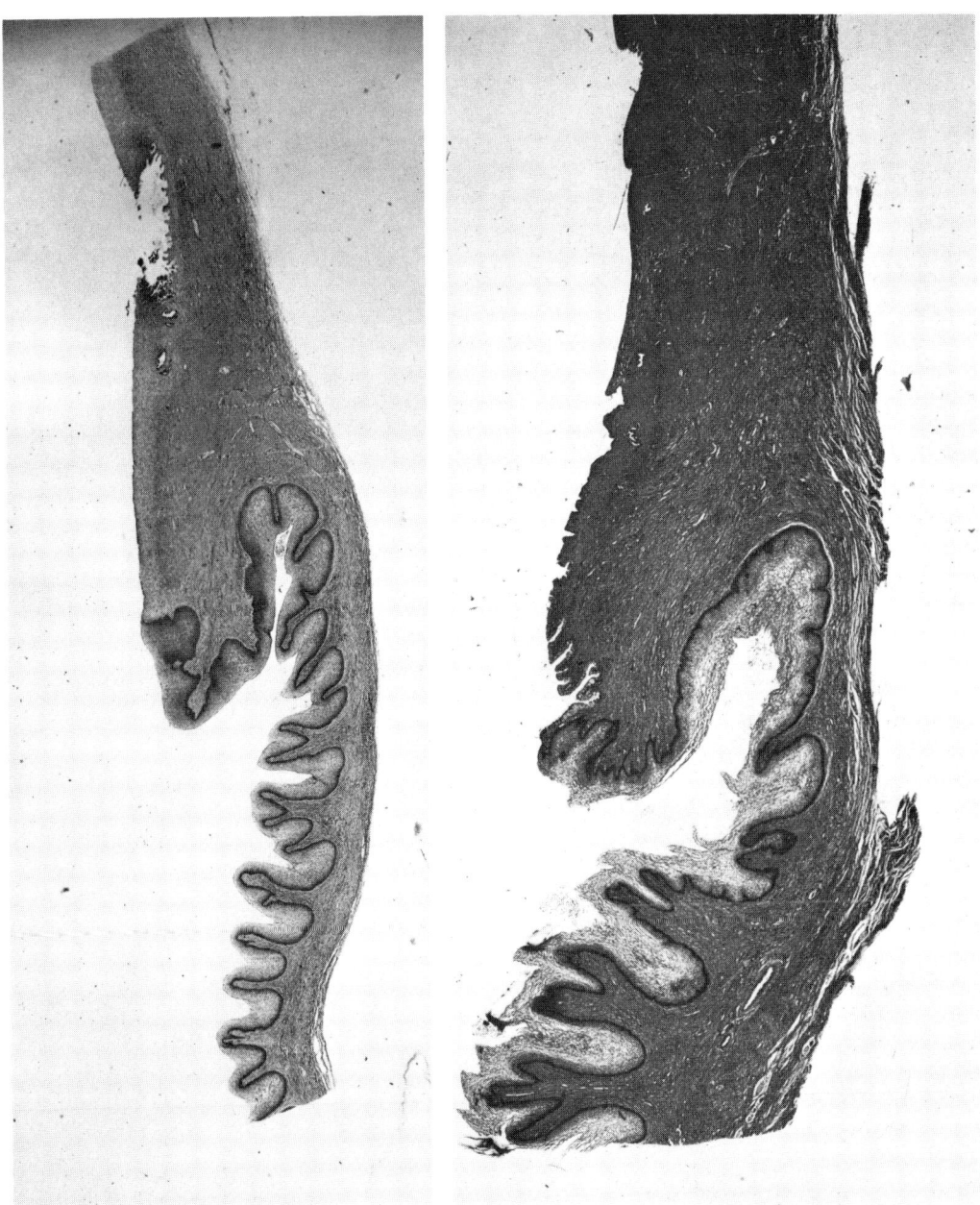

Figure 28–9   Figure 28–10

Figure 28–9. A longitudinal section of the cervix and upper vagina from a 700 gram fetus (6th month of gestation). Hematoxylin and eosin stain. Mag. 11×. (From Valdés-Dapena, M. A., in "The Uterus," Norris, H. J., and Hertig, A. T., eds. Monograph, International Academy of Pathology. Baltimore, The Williams and Wilkins Co., 1973.)

Figure 28–10. The same section from a fetus of 1,390 grams. Hematoxylin and eosin stain. Mag. 11×.

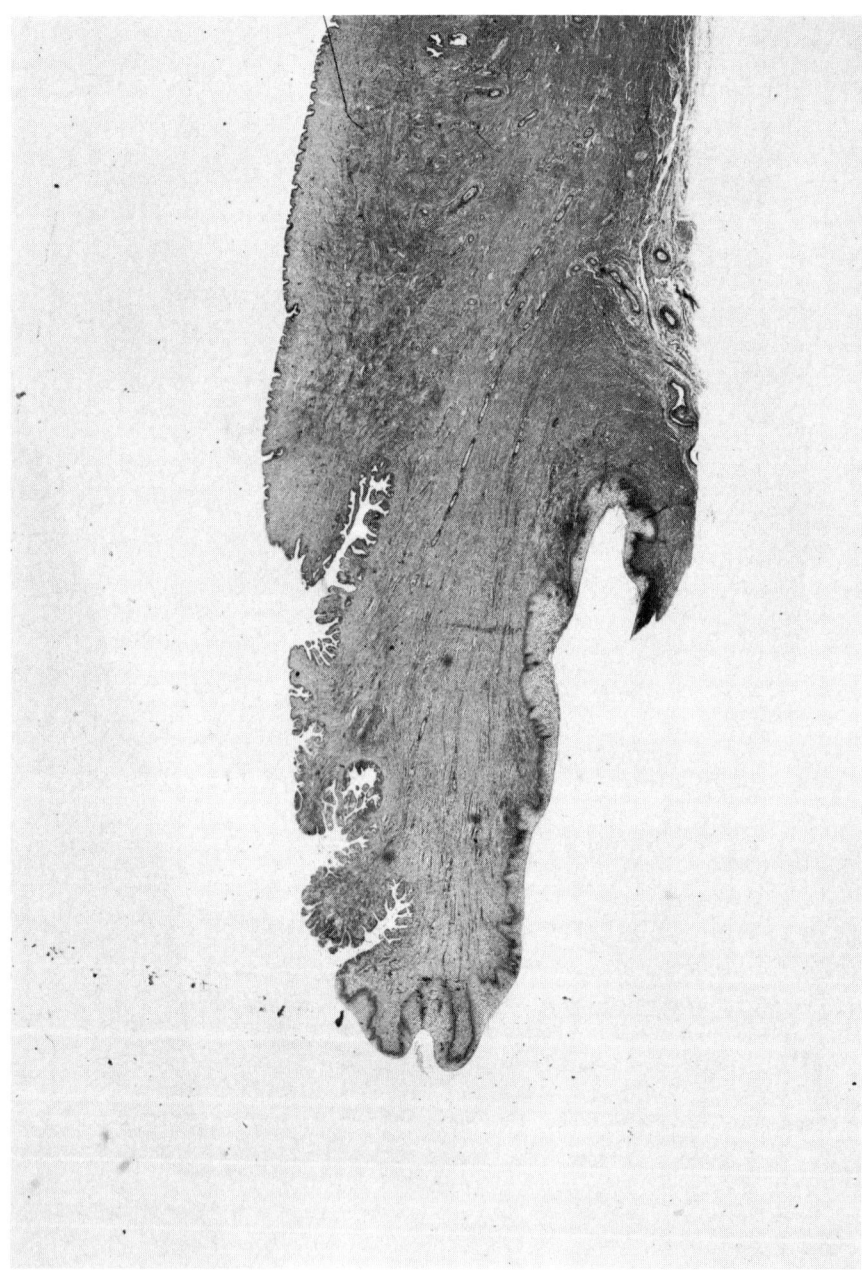

Figure 28–11a

Figure 28–11a. In this longitudinal section of the cervix, the wall of the vagina is to the right and the cervical canal is to the left. This is from an infant of 2,390 grams. Cervical glands are quite well formed.

Hematoxylin and eosin stain. Mag. 11×. (From Valdés-Dapena, M. A., in "The Uterus," Norris, H. J., and Hertig, A. T., eds. Monograph, International Academy of Pathology. Baltimore, The Williams and Wilkins Co., 1973.)

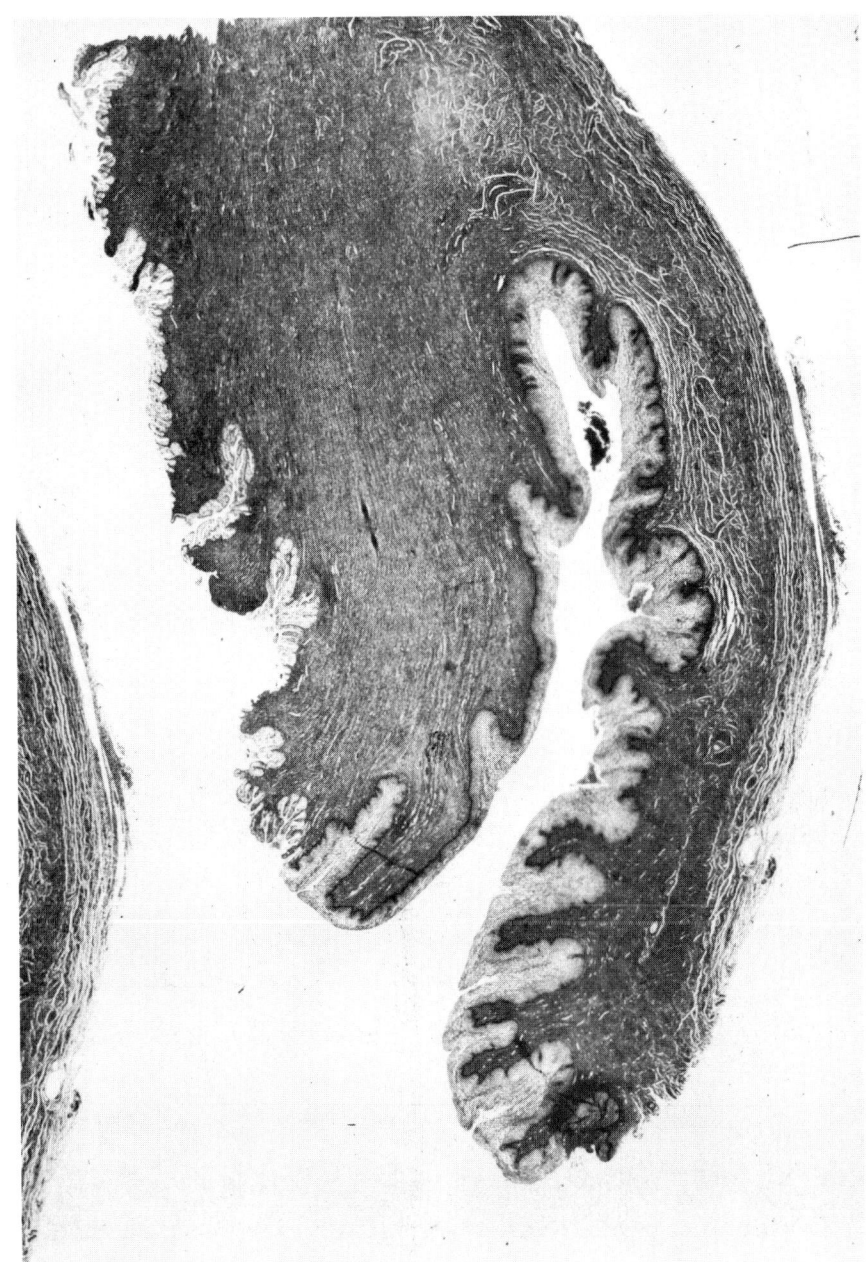

Figure 28–11b

Figure 28–11b. A longitudinal section of the cervix from an infant weighing 3,300 grams. Note the large size of the mucus-producing glands in the cervical canal.

Hematoxylin and eosin stain. Mag. 11×. (From Valdés-Dapena, M. A., in "The Uterus," Norris, H. J., and Hertig, A. T., eds. Monograph, International Academy of Pathology. Baltimore, The Williams and Wilkins Co., 1973.)

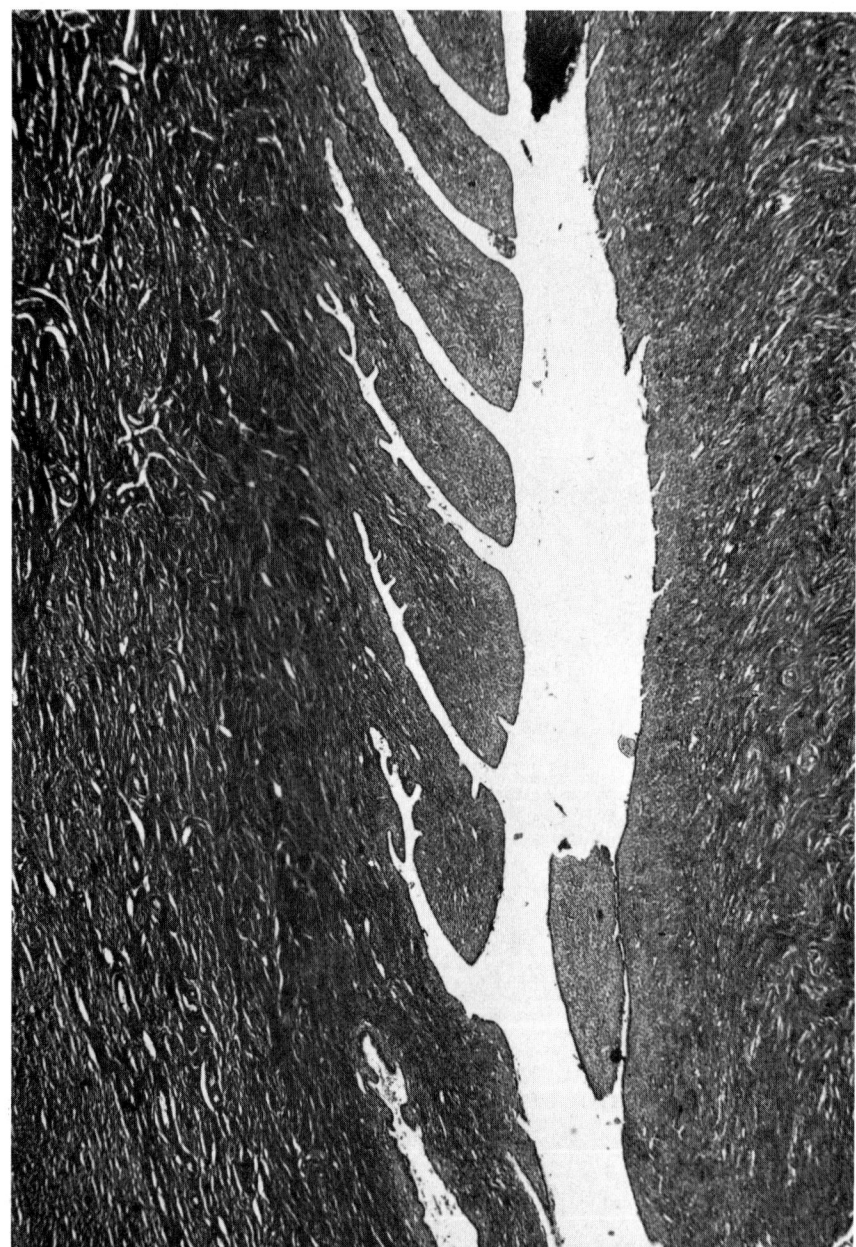

Figure 28–12

Figure 28–12. A sagittal section of the lining of the cervical canal from a premature infant. Note the parallel arrangement of the cervical glands and their distinctive orientation, with fundus directed upward and ostium downward.

Hematoxylin and eosin stain. Mag. 31×. (From Valdés-Dapena, M. A., in "The Uterus," Norris, H. J., and Hertig, A. T., eds. Monograph, International Academy of Pathology. Baltimore, The Williams and Wilkins Co., 1973.)

UTERUS AND VAGINA 493

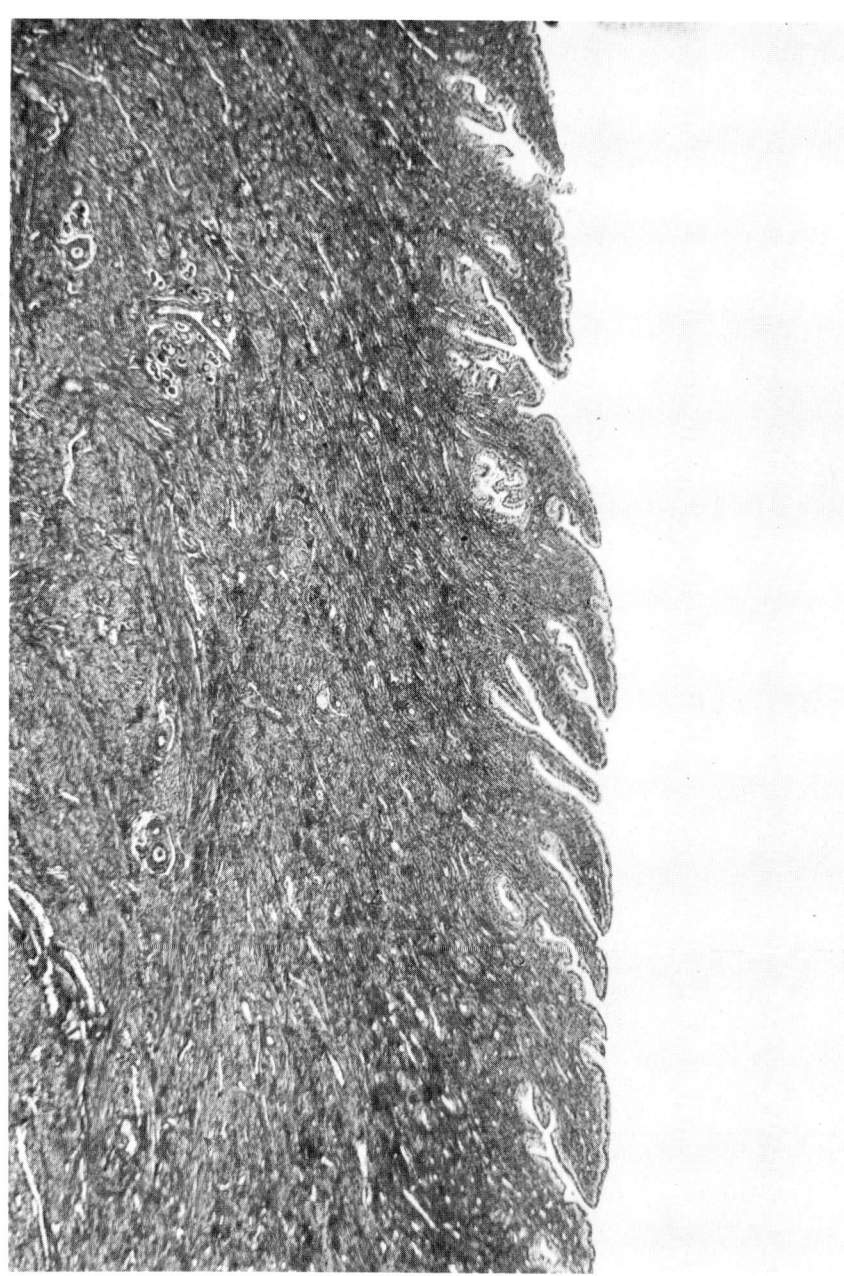

Figure 28–13

Figure 28–13. Sagittal section of the lining of the cervical canal in a later stage of its development; this is from an infant weighing 4,155 grams. Even though the glands are branching and mucus-producing, their parallel arrangement is maintained.
Hematoxylin and eosin stain. Mag. 31×.

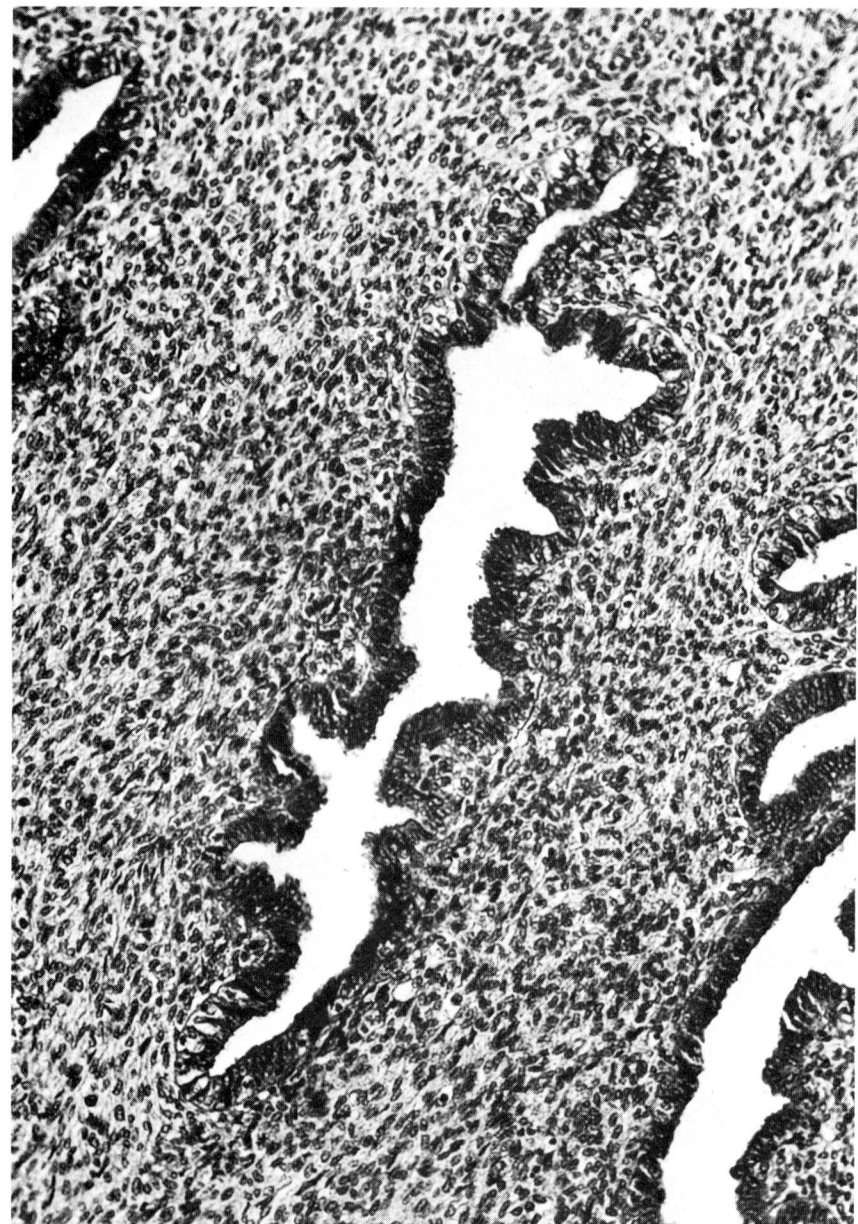

Figure 28–14

Figure 28–14. Cervical glands from a fetus weighing 1,245 grams (7th month of gestation). Note the absence of mucus production by the lining epithelial cells.

Hematoxylin and eosin stain. Mag. 19×. (From Valdés-Dapena, M. A., in "The Uterus," Norris, H. J., and Hertig, A. T., eds. Monograph, International Academy of Pathology. Baltimore, The Williams and Wilkins Co., 1973.)

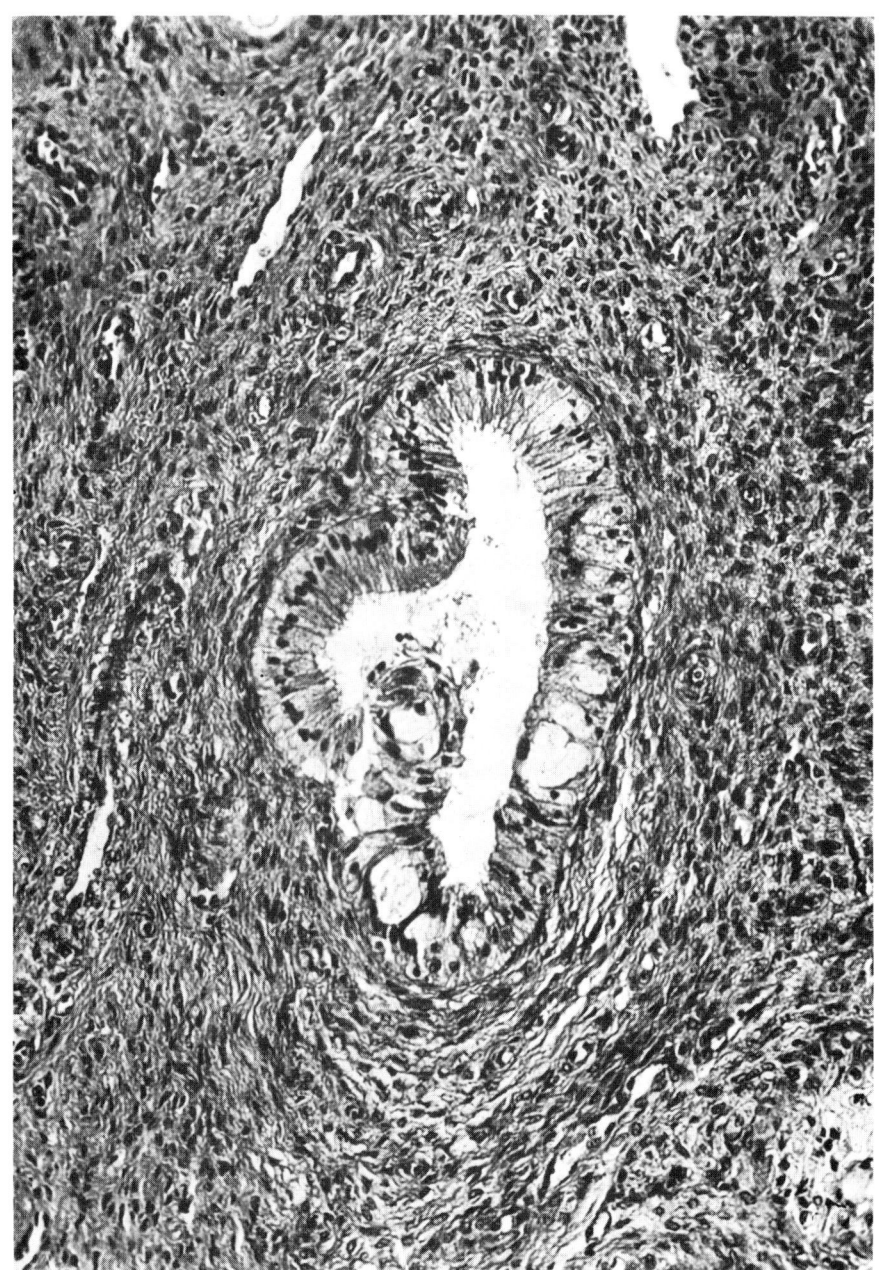

Figure 28–15

Figure 28–15. The cervical gland of an infant born at term, weighing 3,100 grams. The production of mucus by these lining epithelial cells is obvious. Some of the cells have even assumed a spherical shape.

Hematoxylin and eosin stain. Mag. 197×. (From Valdés-Dapena, M. A., in "The Uterus," Norris, H. J., and Hertig, A. T., eds. Monograph, International Academy of Pathology. Baltimore, The Williams and Wilkins Co., 1973.)

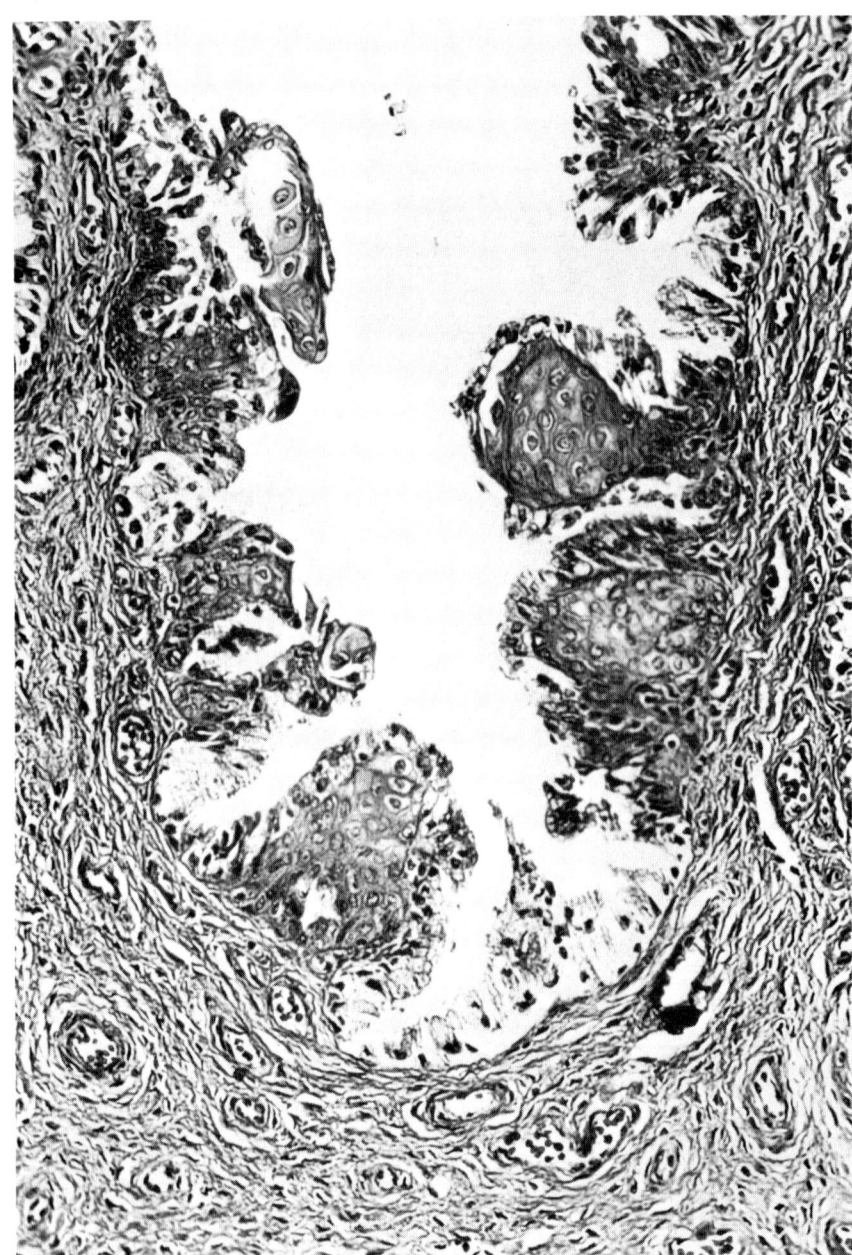

Figure 28–16

Figure 28–16. Apparently aberrant islands of squamous epithelium in the midst of columnar cells lining a cervical gland. This section is from an infant weighing 2,555 grams, born at term. Hematoxylin and eosin stain. Mag. 219×. (From Valdés-Dapena, M. A., in "The Uterus," Norris, H. J., and Hertig, A. T., eds. Monograph, International Academy of Pathology. Baltimore, The Williams and Wilkins Co., 1973.)

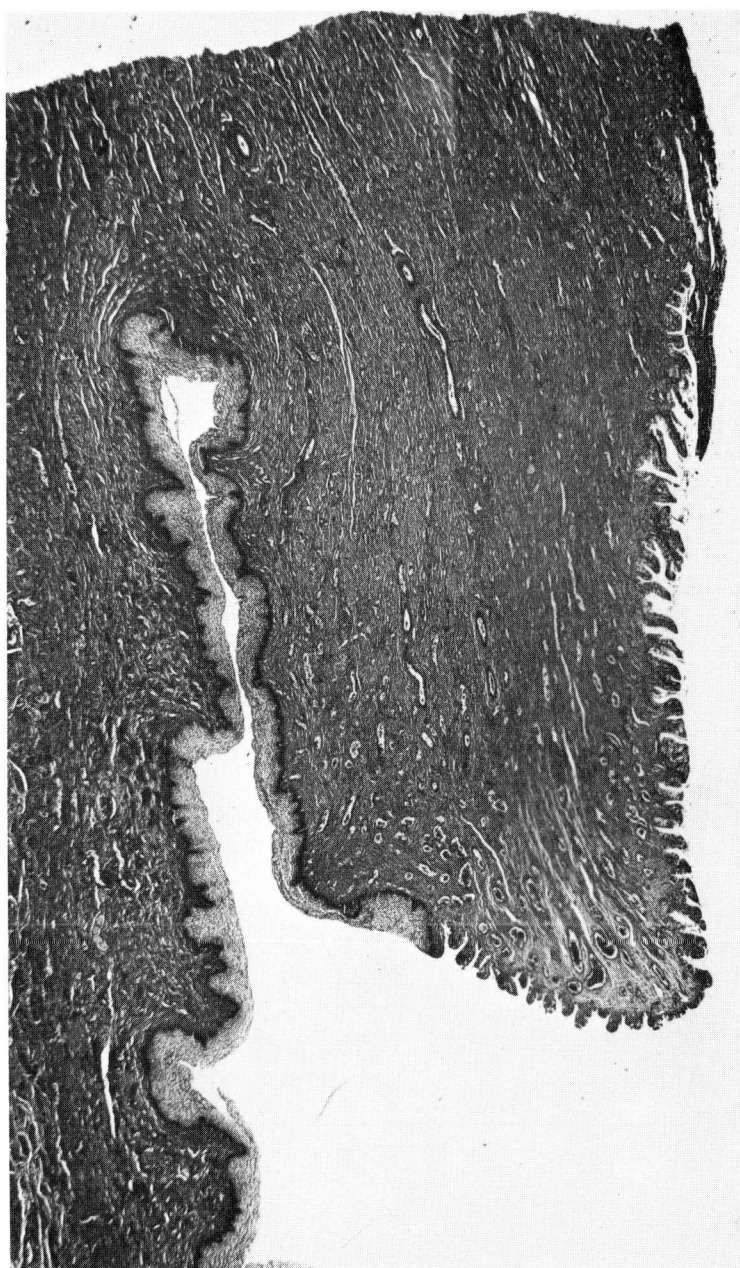

Figure 28–17

Figure 28–17. Sagittal section of the cervix from an infant weighing 3,550 grams, born at term. Columnar epithelium extends down the canal and out over the exposed portio vaginalis to cover half of it as a replacement for the usual stratified squamous epithelial covering.

Hematoxylin and eosin stain. Mag. 18.2×. (From Valdés-Dapena, M. A., in "The Uterus," Norris, H. J., and Hertig, A. T., eds. Monograph, International Academy of Pathology. Baltimore, The Williams and Wilkins Co., 1973.)

498 UTERUS AND VAGINA

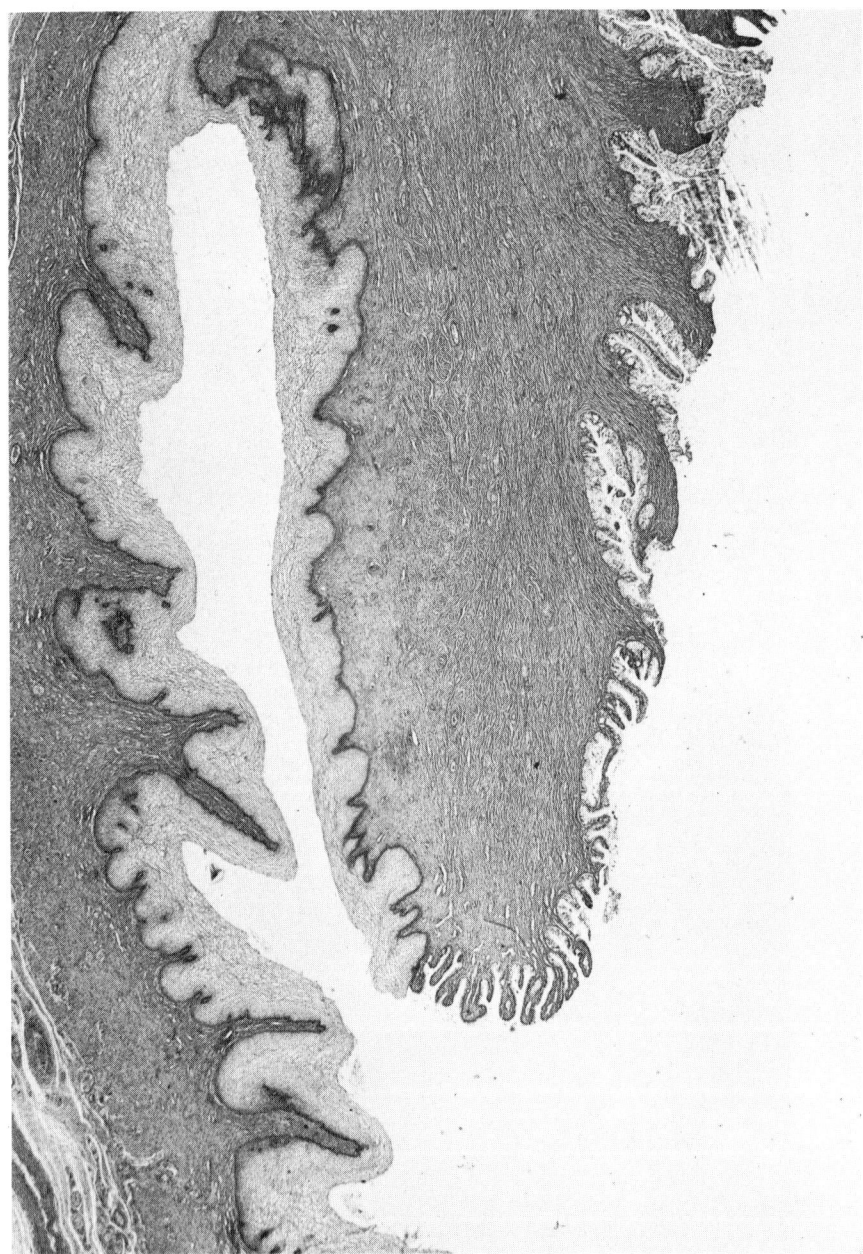

Figure 28–18

Figure 28–18. Sagittal section of the cervix from an infant, weighing 3,965 grams, who was stillborn. The columnar epithelium covers all of the convexity of the portio vaginalis, extending out to its most lateral margin.

Hematoxylin and eosin stain. Mag. 18.2×.

UTERUS AND VAGINA 499

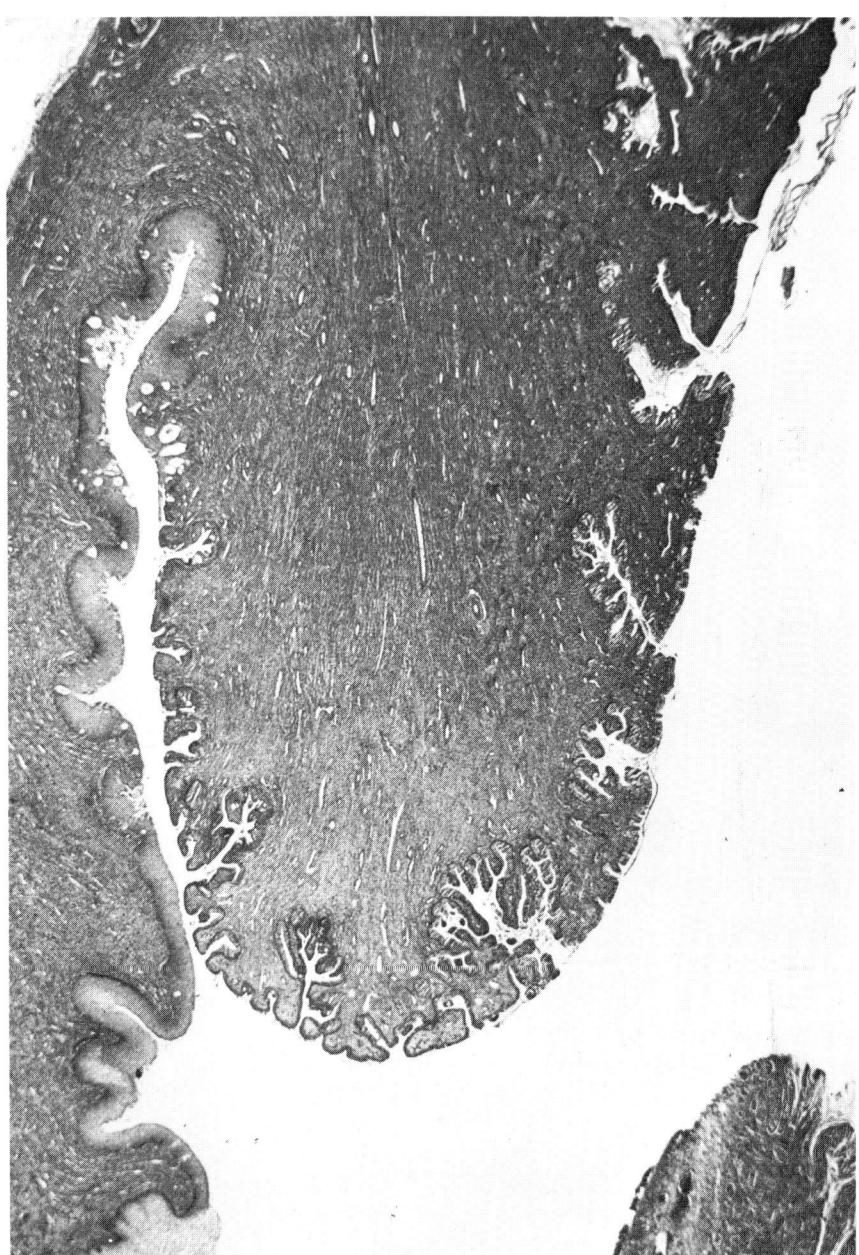

Figure 28–19

Figure 28–19. Sagittal section of the cervix from an infant weighing 3,150 grams. Note that the columnar epithelium replacing stratified squamous over the portio vaginalis extends outward almost to the vaginal wall.
Hematoxylin and eosin stain. Mag. 18.2×.

Part 11

BREAST

Chapter 29

BREAST

EMBRYOLOGY

The mammary glands are considered to be much modified sudoriferous glands, as they are basically ingrowths of the ectoderm that gives rise to their ducts and alveoli.

In the first stage of human mammary development, in the sixth week of gestation, an altered area of skin, the milk streak, is identifiable on either side of the trunk of the embryo, extending from the upper limb bud caudally. This milk line, histologically, consists of a thickened ridge of four or five layers of transitional cells in the epidermis. As it migrates ventrally, a little later, it is accompanied by increased cellularity in underlying mesenchyme.[1]

In the second stage, in the ninth week of gestation, the milk line atrophies except in the pectoral region. While the cells of the milk line elsewhere all but disappear, there is a downward proliferation of a mass of basal cells at the site of the nipple bud. Epidermal cells of the nipple differentiate and increase in number as the underlying mesenchyme continues to proliferate.

Toward the end of the third month, in the third stage of the development of the human breast, squamous cells on the surface invade the nipple bud and line a central tubular canal. The adjacent basal cells multiply to form a series of 15 to 20 down-growing sprouts, the mammary buds, which become the permanent mammary ducts. This process continues as the ducts progressively invade surrounding connective tissue and are canalized (in the last two months) to form milk channels. Their distal ends are embraced by caps of loose vascular mesenchyme (Fig. 29–4). The epidermis, at the point of original development of the gland, forms a small mammary pit into which the milk ducts open (Fig. 29–1).

In the last stages of embryonic development (about the 36th week of gestation) the milk ducts form a series of branching channels with definite lumina, lined by two or three layers of cells (Figs. 29–3 and 29–4). At their distal ends are small aggregates of basal cells, the future buds of mammary lobules. The nipple is usually everted (Fig. 29–1) by the gradual growth of subepidermal connective tissue.

The lobular buds from which clusters of acini develop do not appear until puberty.

At birth the mammary glands are alike, in their stage of development, in both sexes;[2] in both, some transient secretory activity (Fig. 29–5) may be observed, presumably caused by circulating prolactin from the mother.[3] In males, thereafter, the mammary glands remain at this stage in their evolution; in females, by contrast, further changes develop at puberty.

ANATOMY

In the immature infant the breast, whether in the male or the female, is scarcely recognizable grossly. There seems, usually, to be no substance to it but only the areola and nipple, which are tiny. In fact, there is little present except connective tissue supporting a few major ducts which emerge at the nipple.

Later, however, in the infant born at term (Fig. 29–5), there may be a visible and palpable "button" of tissue beneath the areola, usually bilaterally. The plaque of breast tissue may be as much as one centimeter in diameter and up to about three millimeters in thickness. Although not encapsulated, it is rather discrete. It is, however, normally tightly adherent to overlying skin. The color is white and the consistency firm.

At times, so-called "witch's milk" can be expressed from the major ducts at the nipple with the exertion of little pressure on the body of the gland (Fig. 29–5).

HISTOLOGY

Histologically, the nipple is traversed by 15 to 20 lactiferous or milk ducts, which open by minute orifices at its irregular tip (Figs. 29–1 and 29–2). It contains, within connective tissue, numerous smooth muscle fibers (Fig. 29–2) arranged circularly and longitudinally.

As previously mentioned, the major ducts of the breast, in the perinatal period, are lined by stratified squamous epithelium in the vicinity of the surface of the nipple (Fig. 29–2). More distally, this type of lining gives way to a cuboidal form, two to three layers in thickness (Figs. 29–3 and 29–4). In the more mature neonate near term, the major ducts, at their distal ends, re-branch to produce numerous ductules (Fig. 29–5) that are similarly lined.

When, as was mentioned above, the infant breast responds to maternal hormones by producing its own secretion, the ducts and ductules tend to stretch and their epithelial lining tends to flatten as in Figure 29–6.

The connective tissue of the breast, in the perinatal period, is rather sharply demarcated from surrounding adipose tissue, sometimes with a prominent curvilinear margin as in Figure 29–5.

The connective tissue that immediately surrounds the ducts, especially in the last two months of gestation, may be of a very loosely woven pale-staining character (Figs. 29–3 and 29–4). Not uncommonly, extramedullary hematopoiesis may be seen there (Fig. 29–4).

References

1. Geschickter, C. F.: Diseases of the Breast. 2nd ed. Philadelphia, J. B. Lippincott Co., 1945, pp. 5–11.
2. Warwick, R., and Williams, P. L.: Gray's Anatomy, 35th British ed. Philadelphia, W. B. Saunders Co., 1973, pp. 126 and 1365–1367.
3. Smith, C. A.: The Physiology of the Newborn Infant. 3rd ed. Springfield, Charles C Thomas, 1959.

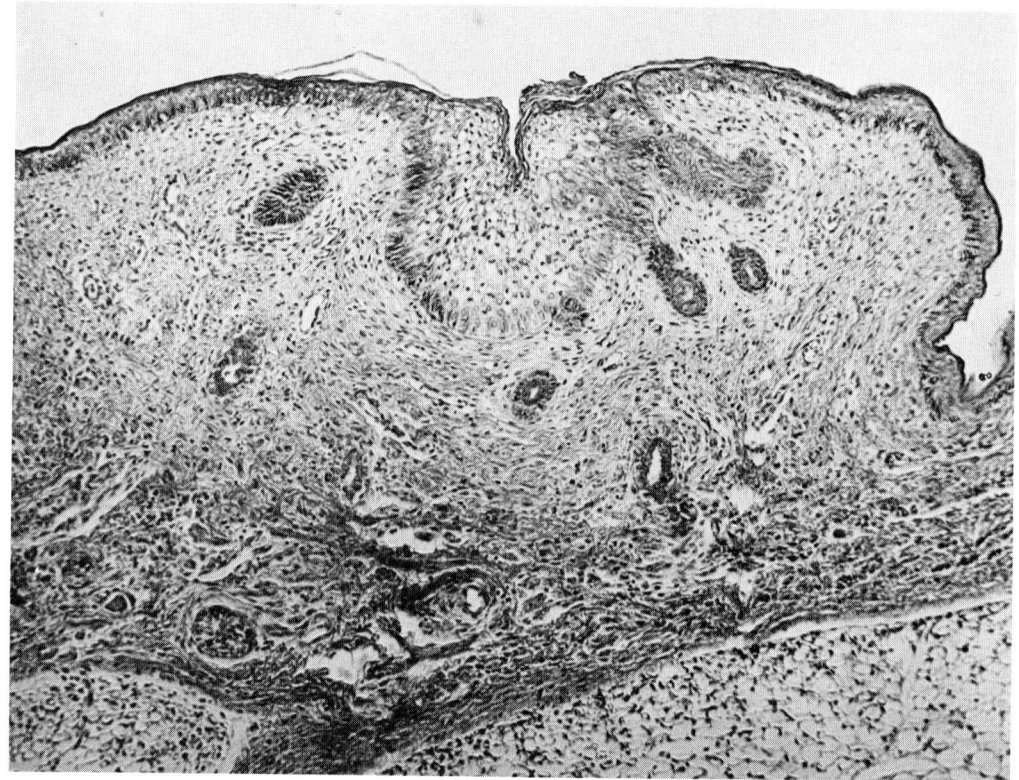

Figure 29–1

Figures 29–1 and 29–2. These two photographs, taken at very different magnifications, illustrate the differences in the microscopic appearance of the breast in the premature (Fig. 29–1) and in the term infant (Fig. 29–2). Each is a sagittal section taken through the nipple and the body of the breast. Although both breasts are quite simple structurally, the organ is considerably larger in every dimension in the more mature infant; the ducts are longer, more dilated, and more numerous. (One very dilated duct appears in the left lower corner of the second photograph.)

The male and female breasts are indistinguishable at this age, histologically.

Figure 29–1. This is a sagittal section through the nipple and the breast of an 880 gram black male who lived for 5 days and 20 hours. The gestational age was 28 weeks.

Hematoxylin and eosin stain. Mag. 132×.

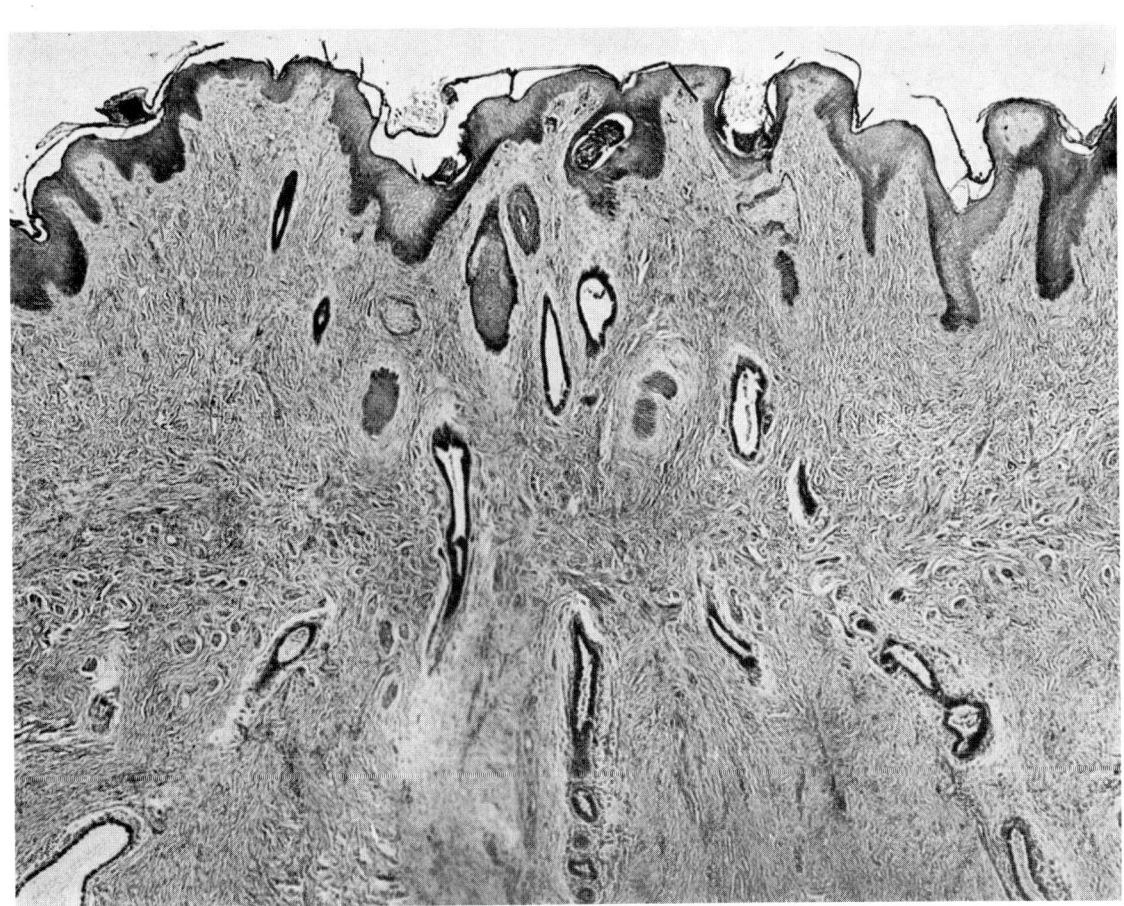

Figure 29-2

Figure 29-2. This, too, is a sagittal section through the nipple and the breast of a 3,540 gram white male infant who lived for 31 hours.
Hematoxylin and eosin stain. Mag. 45×.

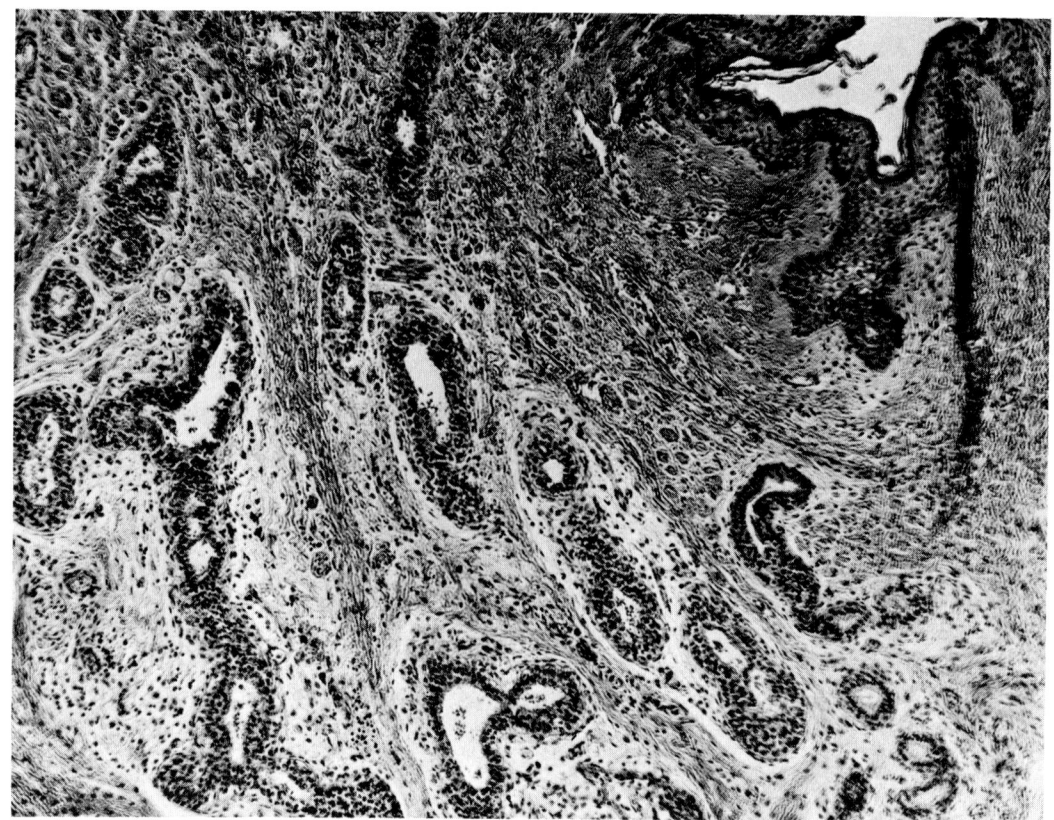

Figure 29–3

Figure 29–3 and 29–4. Seen here at low and then high magnification are the ducts and the supportive connective tissue of the breast of two neonates.

The epithelial lining of the ducts, in each instance, is lush and composed of crowded cuboidal to low columnar cells.

In both sections, extramedullary hematopoiesis is apparent in the form of cuffs or arcs of dark round cells within the looser connective tissue immediately surrounding many of the individual ducts. This is a common observation among premature neonates.

Figure 29–3. This is a sagittal section through the nipple and the breast of a 1,560 gram black female infant born after a 34 week gestation, who survived for 16 hours.

Hematoxylin and eosin stain. Mag. 116×.

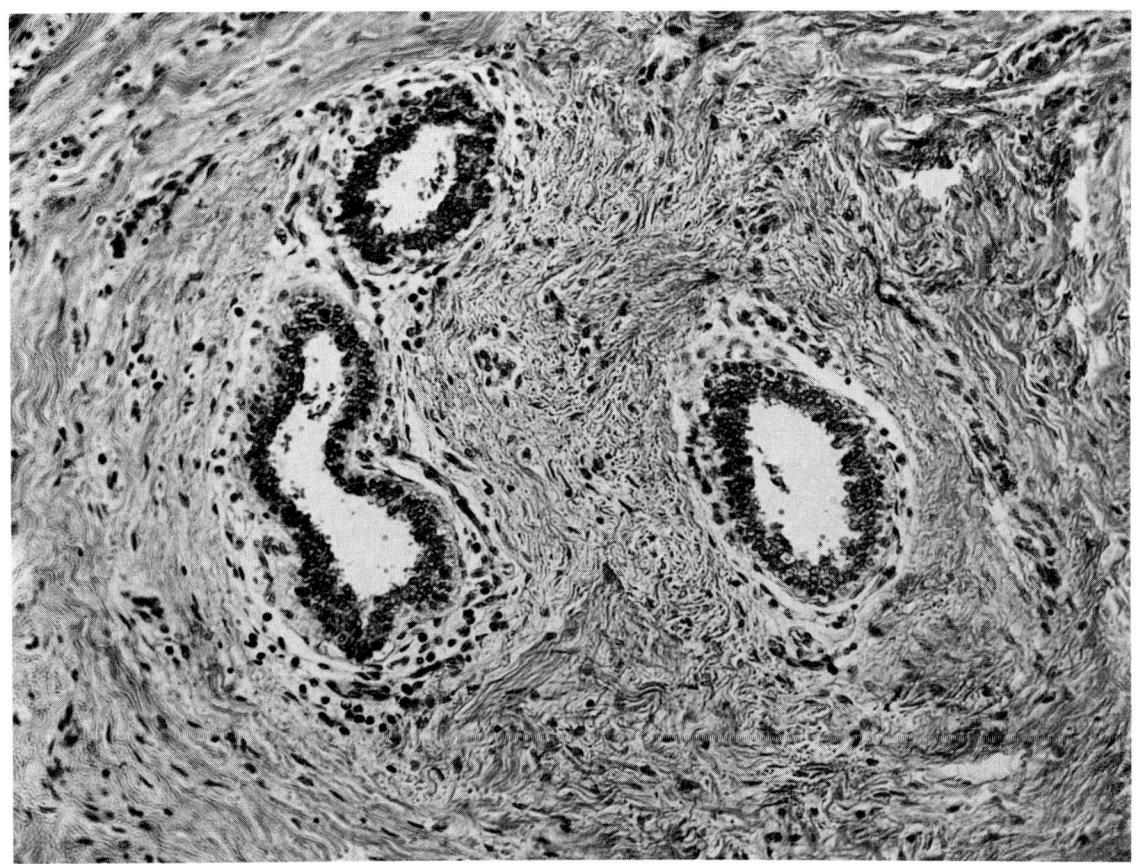

Figure 29-4

Figure 29-4. This is a section through the breast of a two week old black male infant whose body weight and gestational age are not recorded.
Hematoxylin and eosin stain. Mag. 175×.

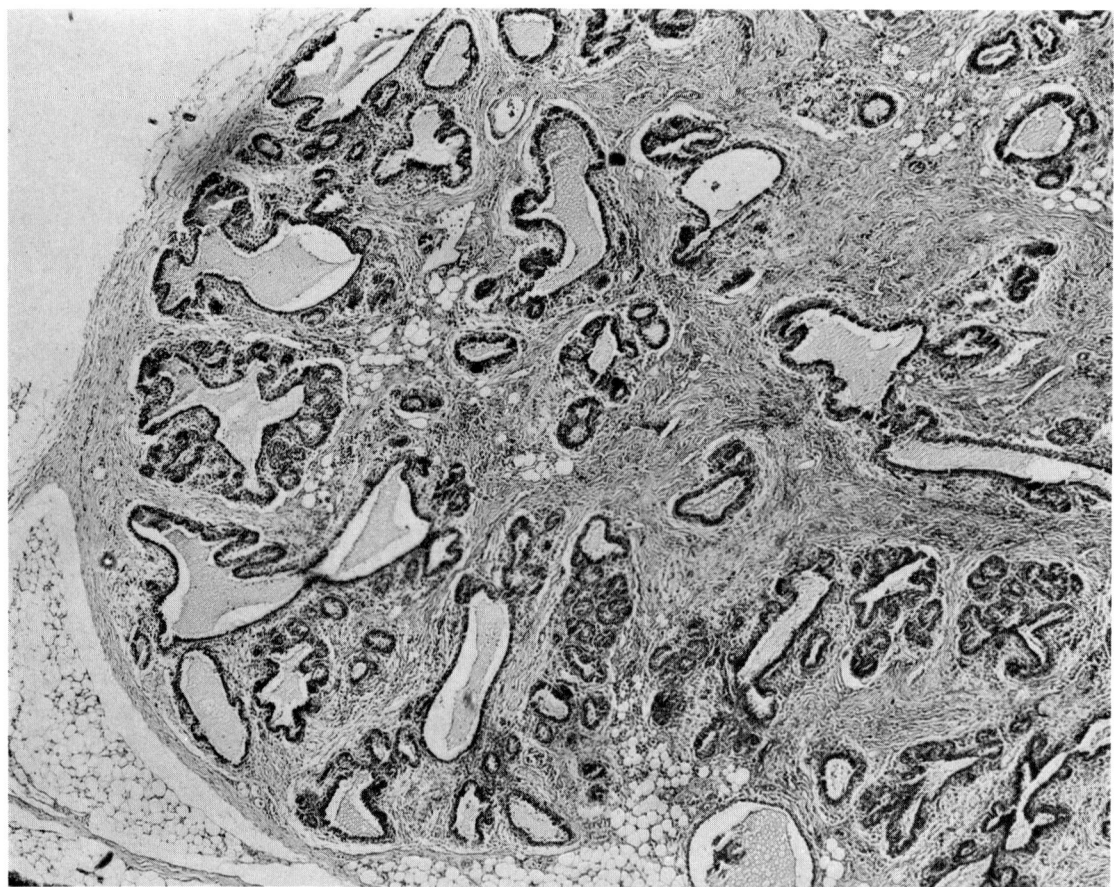

Figure 29–5

Figure 29–5 and 29–6. These two photomicrographs depict, at low and high magnification respectively, the relatively advanced degree of development of the breast that may be seen in the infant at term, and the rather striking degree of dilatation of ducts not uncommonly encountered during the neonatal period.

Figure 29–5. This illustration includes one peripheral margin of the body of this breast. The lumina of major ducts and their ramifications contain the proteinaceous secretion produced by the epithelial lining cells, the so-called "witch's milk" characteristic of the newborn.

This is a section from a 31 hour old white male infant whose weight at autopsy was 3,540 grams.

Hematoxylin and eosin stain. Mag. 45×.

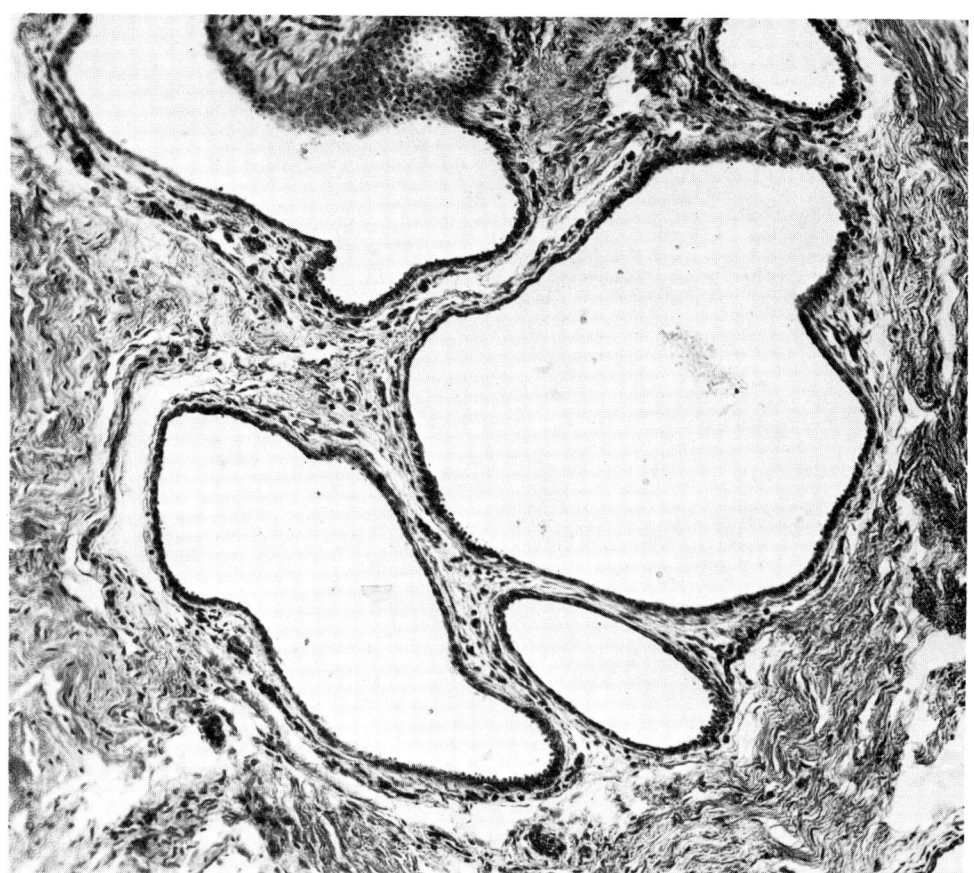

Figure 29–6

Figure 29–6. When the ducts of the neonatal breast become markedly dilated, as they are in this illustration, the epithelial lining cells tend to become quite flattened.

This is a section from the breast of a 4,100 gram white male infant, born at term, who died at 16 days of age.

Hematoxylin and eosin stain. Mag. 142×.

Part 12

EYE

Chapter 30

EYE

EMBRYOLOGY

The eye develops from three sources: surface ectoderm, mesoderm, and neuroectoderm. The first evidences of its development appear during the fourth week in the form of a pair of optic grooves in the neural folds at the cranial end of the embryo. Each groove evaginates to form a hollow diverticulum, the optic vesicle, which projects laterally from the side of the forebrain into adjacent mesenchyme just deep to the forming lens placode in the ectoderm. As the vesicle grows laterally, its distal end expands, while its proximal connection with the forebrain becomes constricted as the optic stalk. The central part of the thick lens placode invaginates to form the lens pit; the edges of the pit then approach each other and fuse to form the lens vesicle. While the lens vesicle is enlarging, the optic vesicle invaginates to become the double-layered optic cup. The lens vesicle then separates from the surface ectoderm and lies within the optic cup. A groove then develops along the caudal aspect of the optic cup and stalk; this groove is called the optic fissure, and through it blood vessels emerge. As the edges of this fissure ultimately close, they embrace the artery and vein within the optic nerve; these become the central artery and vein of the retina.[1]

The retina develops from the optic cup; the outer layer gives rise to the pigment epithelium and the inner to the neural layer. During embryonic and early fetal periods these two are separated by a space, the cavity of the optic vesicle; this disappears as the retina forms. Finally the cells of the inner layer become the rods and cones, bipolar cells, and ganglion cells.

The pigmented portion of the epithelium of the ciliary body is derived from the outer layer of the optic cup and thus is continuous posteriorly with the pigment epithelium of the retina. The non-pigmented portion of the ciliary epithelium is the anterior extension of the retinal neural layer. Ciliary muscle and connective tissue are derived from mesenchyme at the edge of the optic cup.[1]

The iris develops from the rim of the optic cup partly covering the lens. Both layers of the optic cup contribute epithelium to the iris, which is often deeply pigmented. The muscles of the iris are derived from neuroectoderm of the outer layer of the optic cup. Mesenchyme anterior to the rim of the optic cup gives rise to the vascular connective tissue of the iris.

The lens evolves from the lens vesicle. Its anterior low columnar epithelial covering becomes the anterior epithelium of the lens. Cells of the posterior wall become the lens fibers, which gradually invade and obliterate the cavity. The capsule of the lens is produced by underlying epithelial cells.

The vitreous body forms within the optic cup, derived partly from neuroectoderm and partly from mesenchyme.[1]

The anterior chamber develops from a space in the mesenchyme between the lens and the surface. Mesenchyme superficial to the space forms the posterior portion of the cornea. Surface ectoderm gives rise to the epithelium of the cornea and conjunctiva.

The sclera and the choroid are derived from the mesenchyme surrounding the optic cup.[1]

ANATOMY

The eyeball comprises three tunics and the contents enclosed by them. From without inwards, they are: (1) the fibrous tunic, consisting of the sclera behind and the cornea in front; (2) the vascular, pigmented tunic, comprising, from behind forwards, the choroid, ciliary body, and iris (together these are the uveal tract); and (3) the neural layer, the retina.

The sclera is so named because of its hardness; it is a firm membrane, which when distended by intraocular pressure serves to maintain the form of the eyeball. Around its anterior rim, its anterior surface is covered by the conjunctival epithelium, which is reflected onto it from the deep surfaces of the eyelids. It is continuous anteriorly with the epithelium covering the cornea. The internal surface is brown. Posteriorly the sclera is pierced by the optic nerve; it is continuous with the fibrous sheath of that nerve and, beyond that, with the dura mater.[2]

The cornea is the anterior projecting and transparent part of this fibrous external tunic. It is responsible for refraction of light entering the eye. It is convex anteriorly and projects as a flattened dome in front of the sclera. As the curvature of the cornea is greater than that of the rest of the eyeball, a slight furrow called the sulcus sclerae marks the junction of the cornea and the sclera. The cornea is dense, and its anterior surface is somewhat elliptical, its transverse diameter being slightly greater than the vertical.

The choroid lines the inner surface of the sclera and extends as far forward as the ora serrata of the retina. From its anterior margin, the ciliary body continues forward to the circumference of the iris. The iris is a circular diaphragm behind the cornea, with a rounded aperture near its center known as the pupil.[2]

The choroid is a thin, highly vascular membrane of dark brown color, lining a little less than the posterior five-sixths of the eyeball. It is pierced posteriorly by the optic nerve and is firmly adherent there to the sclera. Its internal surface is firmly attached to the pigmented layer of the retina.

The ciliary body is a direct anterior continuation of the choroid, and the iris is a further extension of the ciliary body. The ciliary body suspends the lens and controls accommodation. This accounts for the muscle within it which causes it to bulge toward the interior of the eyeball. It is also involved in the production of aqueous fluid into the anterior segment of the eye, with which its anterior aspect is related. Posteriorly it is directly contiguous with the vitreous humor, and it is probable that it secretes some of the vitreous mucopolysaccharides.[2]

The iris is the delicate and adjustable diaphragm which surrounds the pupil, its central orifice (slightly medial to the true center). It exerts considerable control over the amount of light entering the eye. In the iris of the newborn there is not very much pigment, and therefore the color is apt to be light blue.

The shape of the iris is not a discoid diaphragm; the anterior convexity bulges a little so that it is more accurately described as a very shallow cone, truncated by the pupillary aperture. It is situated between the cornea and the lens, immersed in the aqueous fluid, and it partially divides the anterior segment of the eye into an anterior chamber (enclosed by the cornea and the iris) and a posterior chamber (between the iris and the lens). Peripherally, in the latter cavity, the ciliary processes protrude a little. It is here that most of the aqueous fluid is formed, to find its way through the pupil into the anterior chamber and finally to its exit into the scleral venous sinus at the iridocorneal angle or filtration angle.

The retina is the neural, sensory stratum of the eyeball. It is very thin. Its external surface is in contact with the choroid, its internal with the vitreous body. Posteriorly it is continuous with the optic nerve. It gradually diminishes in thickness from the optic disc to the ciliary body. Its anterior margin is crenated and is known as the ora serrata; here its neural elements end. Only a thin extension of the membrane proceeds from this point forward. The retina is soft, translucent, and of purple color in the fresh state. Near the center of the posterior part there is an oval yellow area named the macula lutea; it bears a central depresison, known as the fovea centralis, where visual resolution is greatest. Very near the nasal side of the macula, the optic nerve pierces the retina at the optic disc. The circumference of the disc is slightly elevated and the central portion slightly depressed. Through the ophthalmoscope the disc appears to be pink but, in fact, it is either grey or almost white.[2]

The lens of the neonate is 6.5 mm. in diameter; its anteroposterior dimension is 3.5 to 4.0 mm. at birth. The lens of the fetus (Fig. 30–10) is nearly spherical; it is soft and breaks readily under pressure. A small branch of the central artery enters it from the vitreous body; this disappears about six weeks before birth.

HISTOLOGY

Fibrous Tunic. The fibrous outer layer of the eyeball consists of an opaque posterior part, the sclera, and a transparent anterior part, the cornea.

The sclera consists of white fibrous tissue admixed with fine elastic fibers. Slender connective tissue cells, some of which are pigmented, lie in lacunae between the fibers. The fibers are arranged in bundles, the patterns of which are characteristic for different parts of the sclera[2] (Fig. 30–1).

The cornea comprises five layers which, from before backward, are these: (1) the corneal epithelium (Fig. 30–4), which is continuous with that of the conjunctiva; (2) the anterior limiting membrane of Bowman (Fig. 30–

4); (3) the substantia propria; (4) the posterior limiting lamina of Descemet; and (5) the endothelium of the anterior chamber.[2]

Vascular Tunic. The vascular tunic or uveal tract comprises the choroid posteriorly, the ciliary body laterally, and the iris anteriorly.

The choroid is made up of an external layer composed of arteries, veins, and supporting connective tissue with scattered pigment cells; an intermediate layer bearing capillaries; and a thin, internal, basal lamina, the membrane of Bruch, made up of elastic tissue between collagenous layers.[2]

The ciliary body is a highly vascular structure that supports the lens by virtue of its musculature. The physical arrangement of the various component parts of the ciliary body is exceedingly complex, but basically it is a circular rim surrounding and supporting the lens, which it holds by means of many slender suspensory ligaments. It comprises (1) an epithelial clothing (Fig. 30–2), (2) connective tissue and vessels, and (3) an annular mass of non-striated muscle arranged in a variety of directions.[2]

The iris (Fig. 30–3) is an unusual structure; its anterior surface, the posterior boundary of the anterior chamber, is not covered by epithelium but is merely a modified anterior border of the general stroma. The stroma contains vessels and nerves and, directly around the pupil, an aggregation of smooth muscle fibers, forming a sphincter. The posterior surface is a continuation of the epithelial covering of the ciliary body.[2]

Neural Layer. The innermost, neural layer of the eyeball is the retina. In the retina (except for the fovea, the papilla, and the ora serrata), ten parallel layers can be distinguished from without inward (Figs. 30–5 and 30–6): (1) the pigment epithelium; (2) the layer of rods and cones; (3) the outer limiting membrane; (4) the outer nuclear layer; (5) the outer plexiform layer; (6) the inner nuclear layer; (7) the inner plexiform layer; (8) the layer of ganglion cells; (9) the layer of optic nerve fibers; and (10) the inner limiting membrane.[3]

The aqueous humor fills the anterior and posterior chambers.

The vitreous body occupies the vitreous chamber, filling the concavity of the retina. It is 99 per cent water, with some salts and a little mucoprotein and hyaluronic acid. Fibrils about 16 mm. in diameter and an interfibrillary substance (vitreous humor) can be appreciated within it by electron microscopy. A narrow canal, the hyaloid canal, runs through it from the optic disc to the center of the posterior aspect of the lens. In the fetus this canal is occupied by the hyaloid artery, a branch of the central artery.[2]

The lens is made up of a soft cortical substance and a firm central part. Faint sutural lines radiate through it from the poles to the equator. In the fetus there are only three such lines, arranged in the shape of a Y; on the anterior surface the Y is upright. These lines correspond to septa. The lens consists of a series of concentrically arranged laminae, each of which is interrupted at the septa; each is made of fibers with serrated interdigitating edges.[2]

The optic nerve (Figs. 30–7 to 30–9) is an evagination of the prosencephalon, rather than a peripheral nerve like other cranial nerves. It consists of about 1200 bundles of nerve fibers whose myelin sheaths are produced by oligodendroglial cells.

The meninges and the intermeningeal spaces of the brain continue along the optic nerve. The dura fuses with the sclera and the pia also, at the entrance of the optic nerve into the globe. The pia sends blood vessels and connective tissue into the nerve.

The central artery and vein reach the eyeball through the optic nerve.[3]

References

1. Moore, K. L.: The Developing Human. Clinically Oriented Embryology. Philadelphia, W. B. Saunders Co., 1973, pp. 335–341.
2. Warwick, R., and Williams, P. L.: Gray's Anatomy, 35th British ed. Philadelphia, W. B. Saunders Co., 1973, pp. 1095–1122.
3. Bloom, W., and Fawcett, D. W.: A Textbook of Histology, 10th ed. Philadelphia, W. B. Saunders Co., 1975, pp. 917–963.

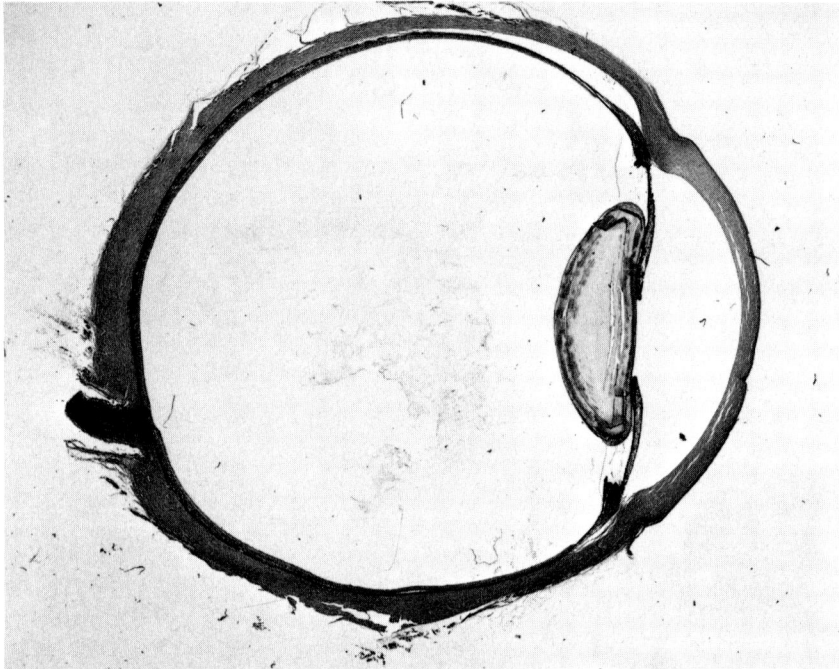

Figure 30–1

Figure 30–1. This is a sagittal section of the eye of an infant. The lens is on the right and the optic nerve is on the left. The grey band rimming the entire globe is the sclera, consisting of fibrous tissue, posteriorly, and the cornea, consisting of epithelium and supporting substantia propria, anteriorly.

Hematoxylin and eosin stain. Mag. 5×.

Courtesy of Dr. William R. Green, Wilmer Institute, Johns Hopkins Hospital, Baltimore, Md.

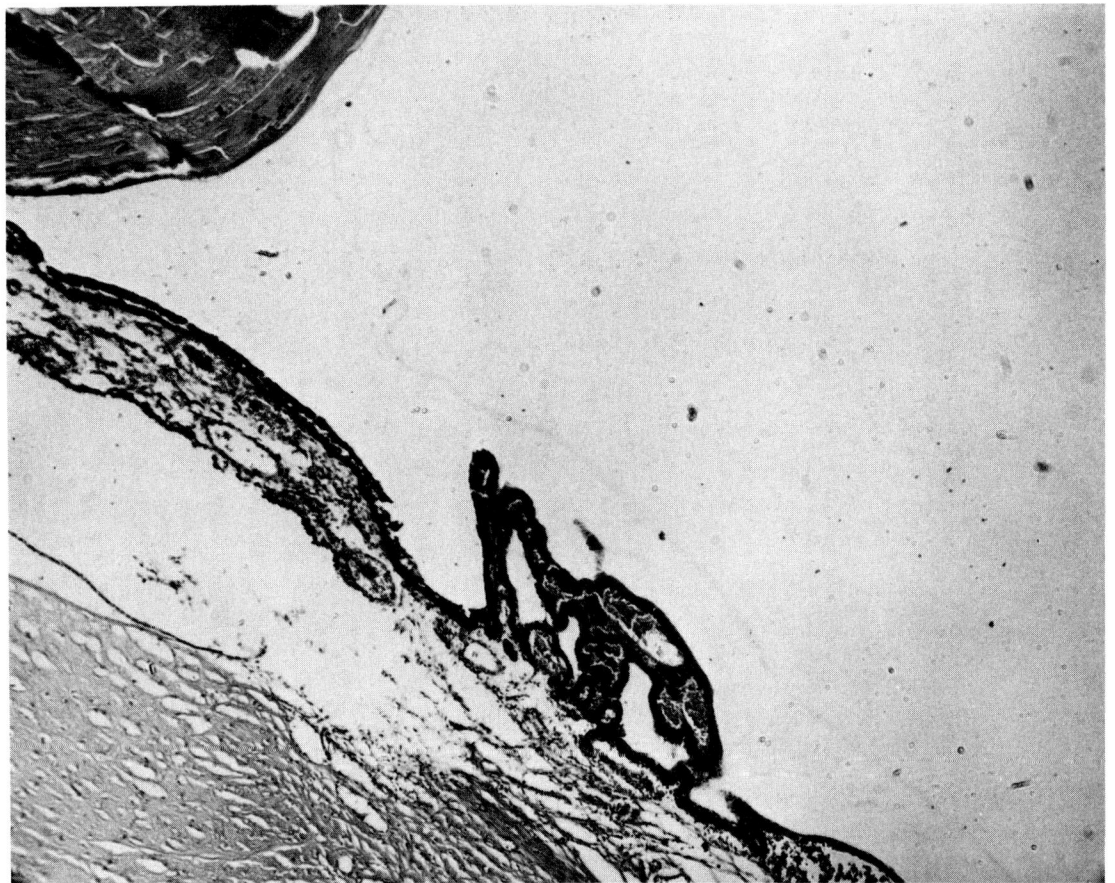

Figure 30–2

Figure 30–2. This is a section of the angle of the eye including, in the left upper corner, a bit of the lens and, in the inferior central portion, ciliary processes projecting into the posterior chamber. The ciliary epithelium consists of two layers of cells, an inner, non-pigmented one bounding the chamber and an outer pigmented one resting on the stroma of the ciliary body.

This infant was a stillborn black male whose body, at autopsy, weighed 2,100 grams.
Hematoxylin and eosin stain. Mag. 55×.

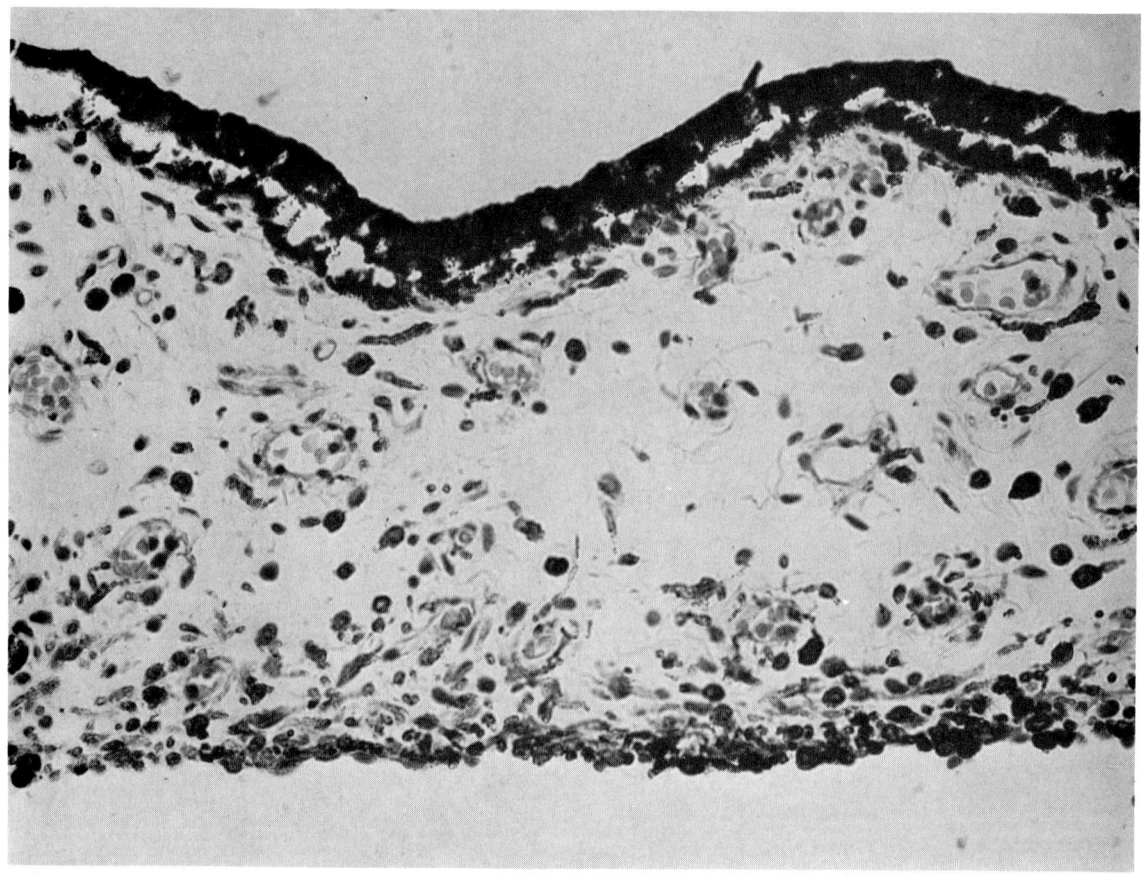

Figure 30–3

Figure 30–3. This is a section of the iris. The lower pigmented margin represents the posterior aspect and the upper, the anterior. Between the two is a mass of loosely woven, pigmented, highly vascular connective tissue. The anterior covering is said to be a discontinuous layer of fibroblasts and melanocytes. The posterior surface is covered by a double layer of heavily pigmented epithelium, the iridial portion of the retina.

This infant was a 2,125 gram black female, born post-term to a 17 year old mother. The baby lived for 11 hours.

Hematoxylin and eosin stain. Mag. 330×.

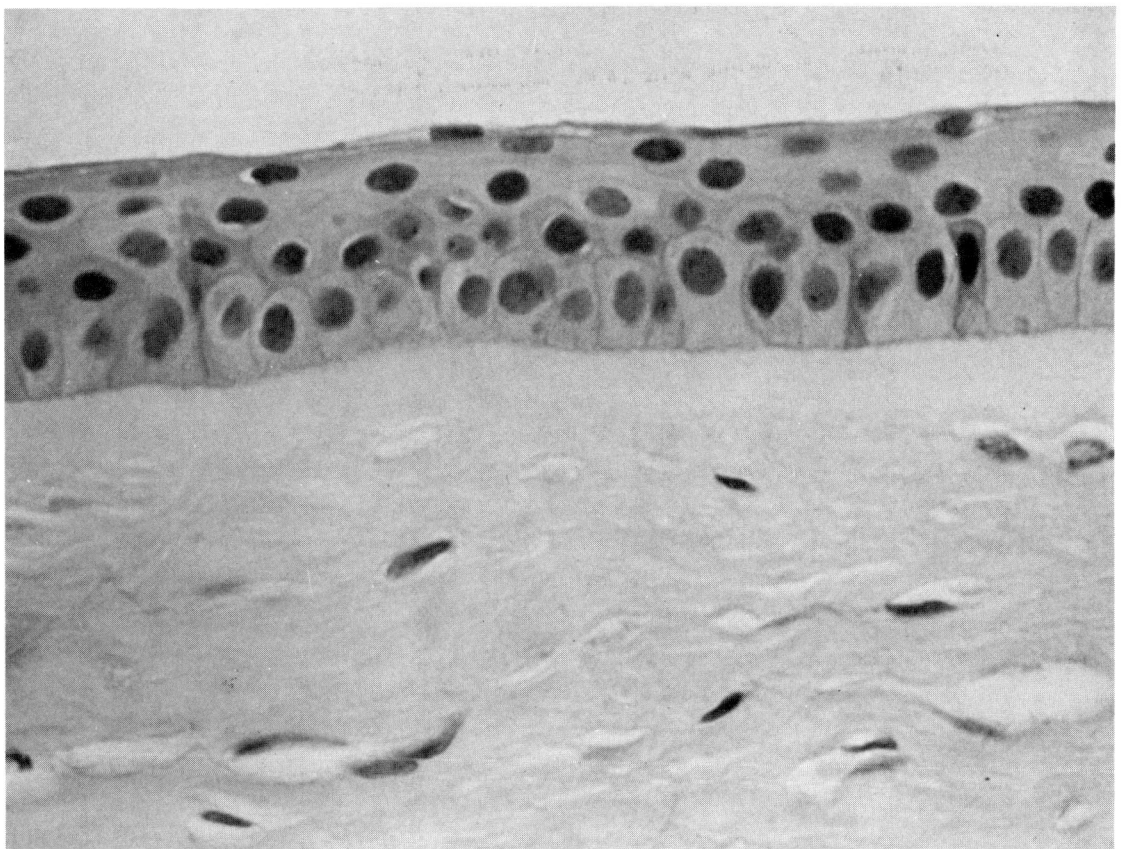

Figure 30-4

Figure 30-4. At very high magnification, this illustration depicts the corneal epithelium, overlying the membrane of Bowman, the stroma, and the substantia propria of the cornea. The epithelium is stratified squamous and consists of five layers of cells. The outer surface is smooth and is made up of large squamous cells. The cells of this epithelium are interconnected by short interdigitating processes that adhere to one another at desmosomes.

The infant is that described in the legend for Fig. 30-3.

Hematoxylin and eosin stain. Mag. 660×.

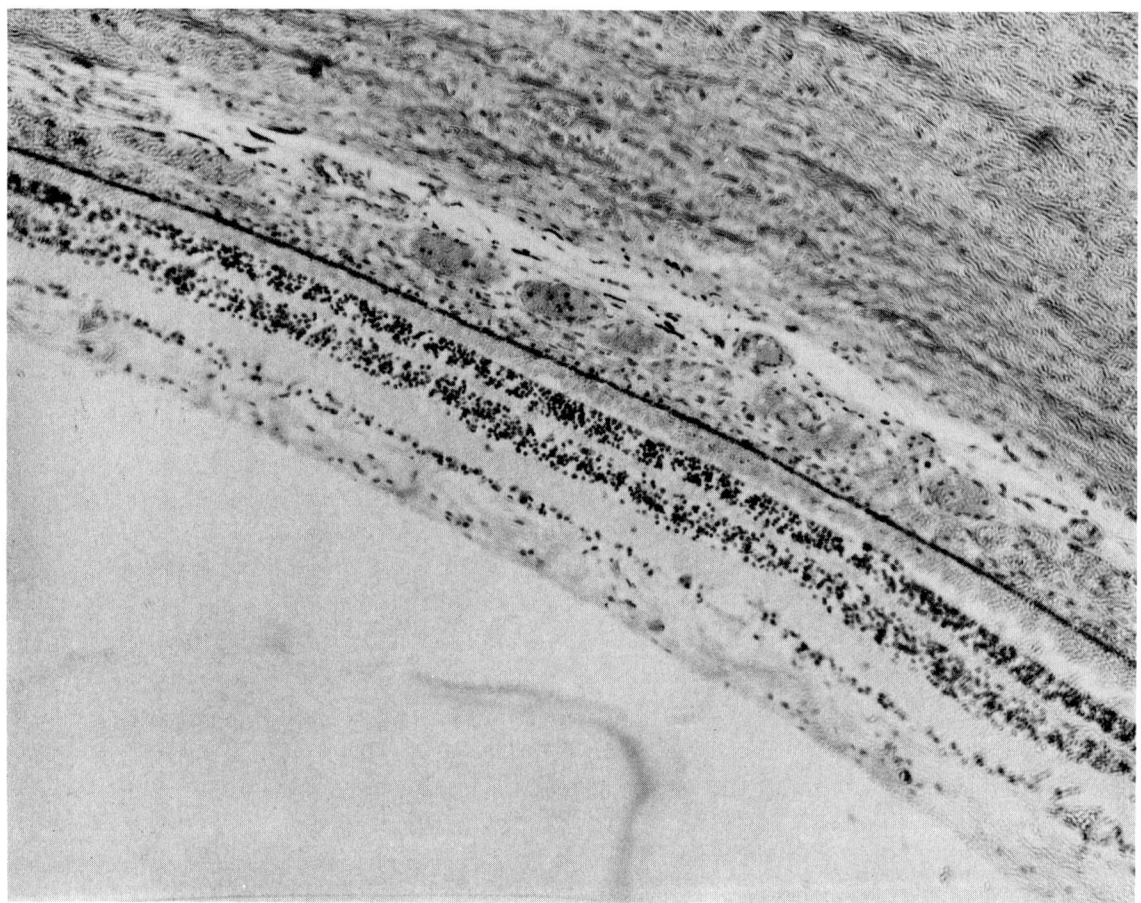

Figure 30–5

Figure 30–5. This is a photograph of the retina of the eye of a newborn infant. The slender dark line extending from the upper left portion to the lower right represents the pigment epithelium. The granular band below that is the outer nuclear layer. The broad speckled stripe below that is the inner nuclear layer. The fine stippled line inferior and parallel to that is the layer of ganglion cells. The supporting structure deep to the retina is the choroid.

The infant is the same as that described in the legend for Figure 30–3.

Hematoxylin and eosin stain. Mag. 132×.

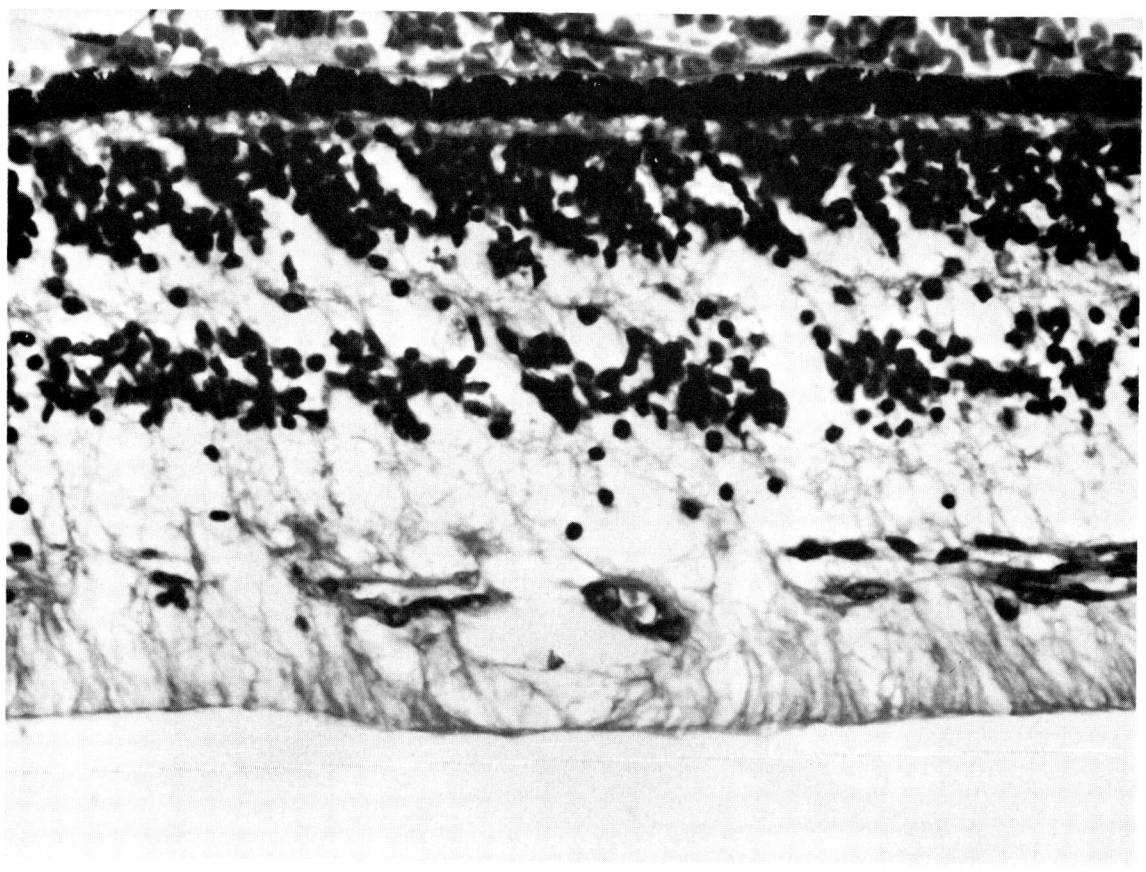

Figure 30-6

Figure 30-6. Seen here at considerably higher magnification is the retina of another newborn infant.

This baby, a black male, was born at 8½ months of gestation. He lived for one day and three hours. His body weight at autopsy was 1,780 grams.

Hematoxylin and eosin stain. Mag. 450×.

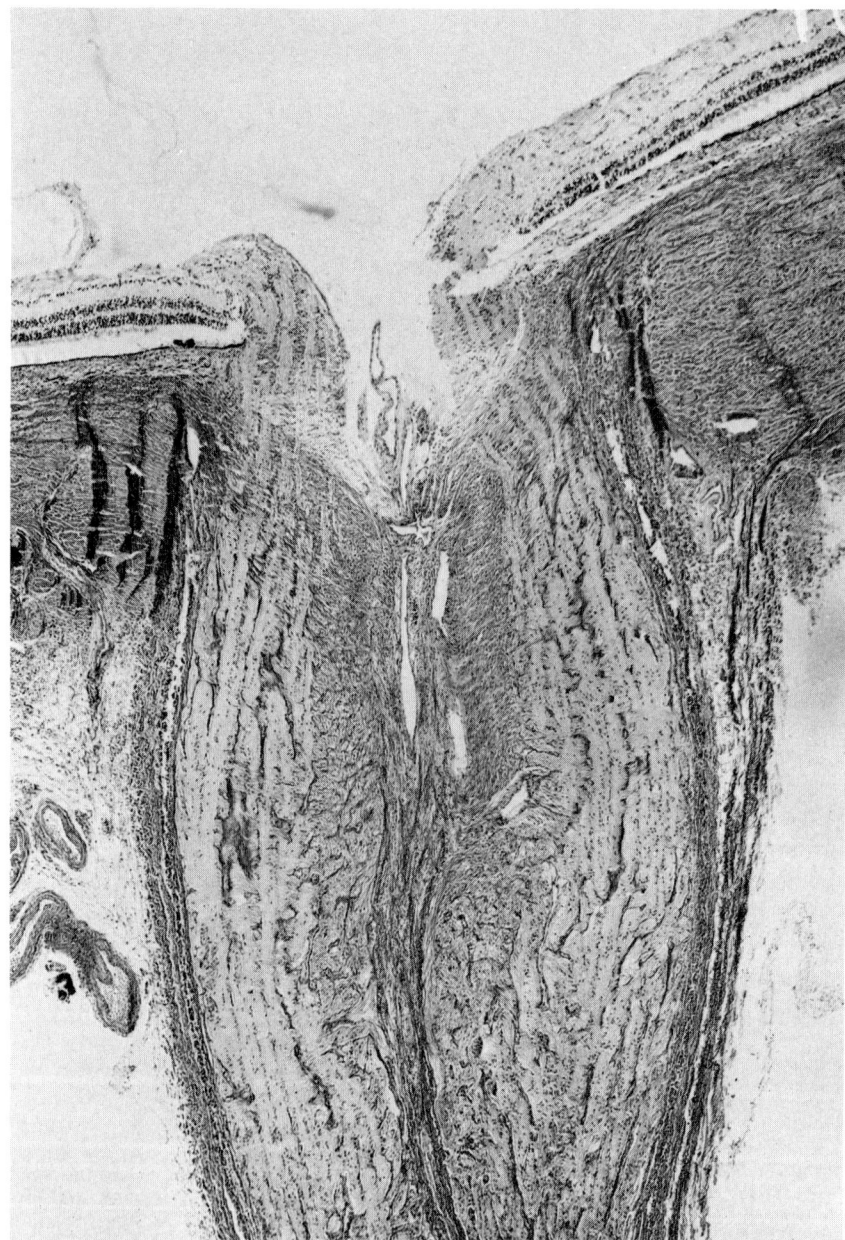

Figure 30-7

Figures 30–7 and 30–8. These two photographs depict the entrance of the optic nerve into the eye. In both, the layers of the retina, as described in the legend for Fig. 30–6, can be seen quite distinctly: the pigment layer most inferiorly, above that the outer and inner nuclear layers, respectively, and above those, the layer of ganglion cells. Particularly in Fig. 30–7, a pale nerve fiber layer is heaped up on both sides of the central excavation, forming a kind of shoulder at the edges of the precipice. The delicate pial sheath is directly adherent to the nerve; external to it, as seen best in Fig. 30–8, is the stouter dural sheath.

Hematoxylin and eosin stain. Mag. 45×.

Figure 30–7. This infant is the same as that described in the legend for Fig. 30–3.

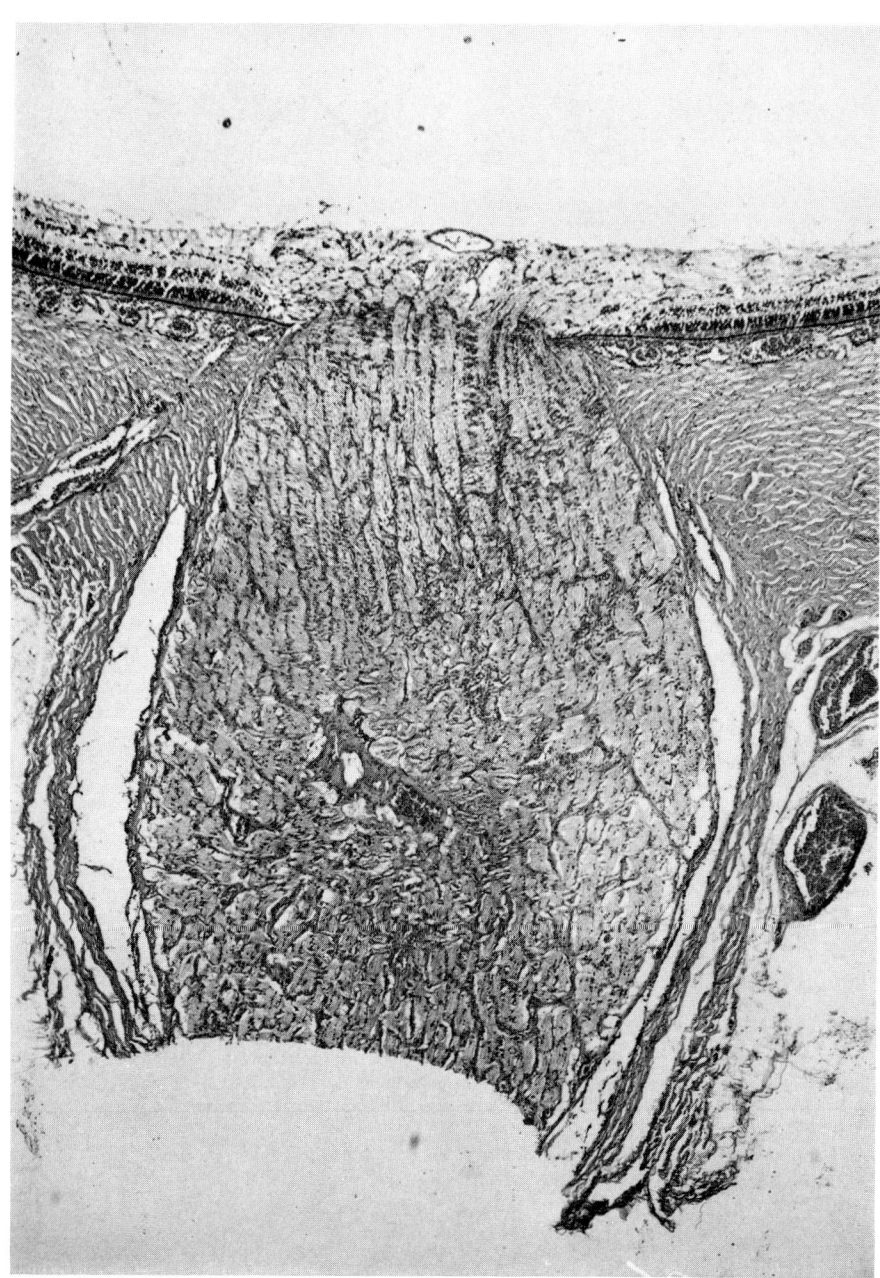

Figure 30-8

Figure 30-8. This infant is the same as that described in the legend for Fig. 30-6.

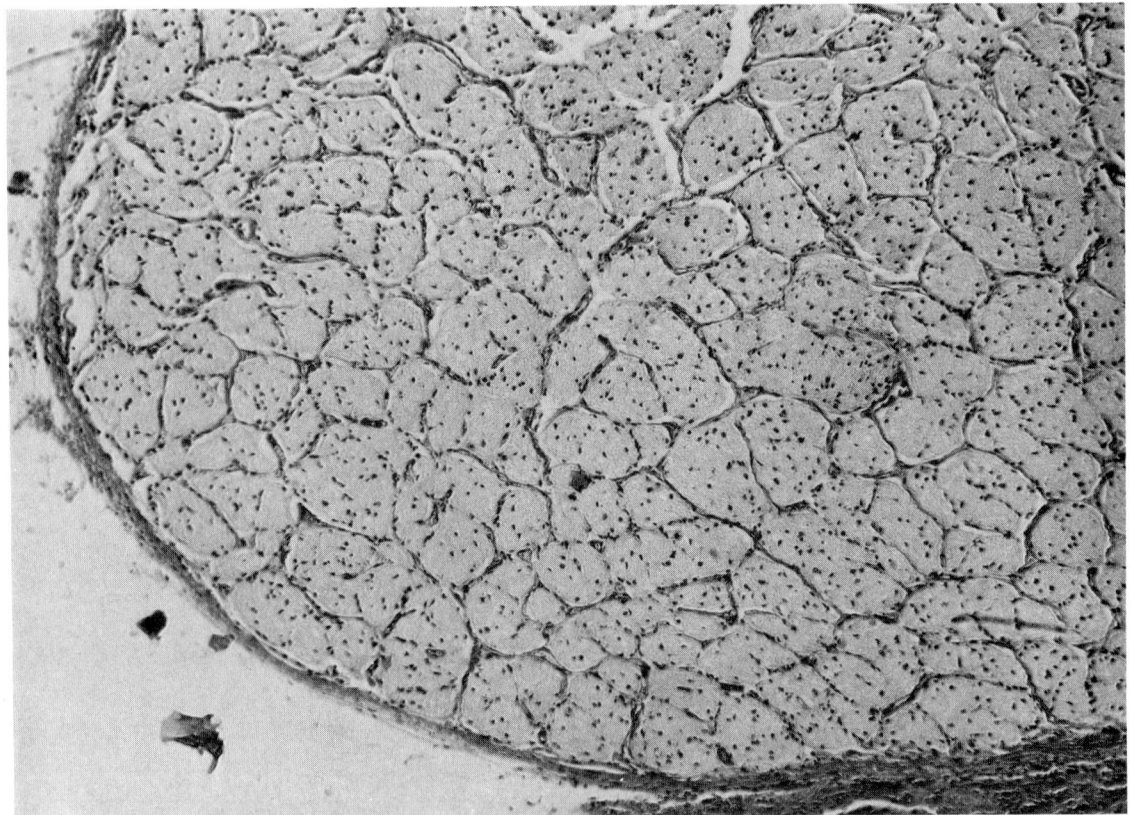

Figure 30–9

Figure 30–9. This is a cross section of the optic nerve not far from the globe.
Wrapped around the nerve is the pia mater, which forms a connective tissue layer closely adherent to the surface of the nerve. As is apparent here, it sends connective tissue partitions and tiny blood vessels into the nerve.
The infant is the same as that described in the legend for Fig. 30–3.
Hematoxylin and eosin stain. Mag. 108×.

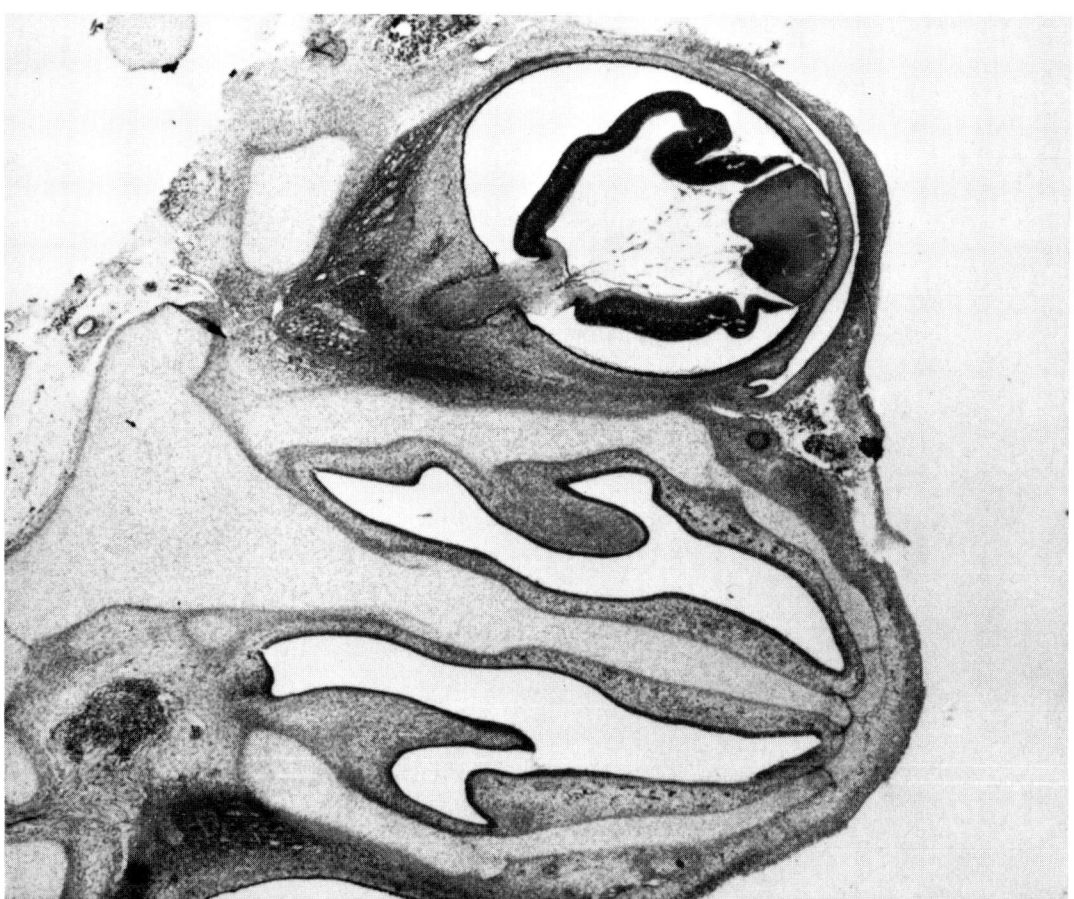

Figure 30–10

Figure 30–10. This section is made almost in the horizontal plane. The eye appears near the midline just above the nasal passages.

Internal layers are somewhat convoluted because of artifact. The nerve is seen posteriorly (on the left, in the photograph) and the lens anteriorly (on the right).

This embryo was of 10 weeks gestation.

Hematoxylin and eosin stain. Mag. 1.75×.

Part 13

NEURAL TISSUES

Chapter 31

CENTRAL NERVOUS SYSTEM

EMBRYOLOGY

Before the neural tube closes, the neural folds expand in the region of the head as the first evidence of the developing brain. Later these enlarged folds form three distinct vesicles separated from one another by constrictions; they are the forebrain, the midbrain, and the hindbrain (or prosencephalon, mesencephalon, and rhombencephalon, respectively). The last is continuous with the spinal cord. Because they grow at different rates, these parts flex in relation to one another. First, the forebrain bends ventrally until its floor is almost parallel with that of the hindbrain. The second bend occurs at the junction of the hindbrain and the spinal cord; this is another ventral bend and results in the hindbrain being at nearly a right angle to the cord. The third bend, between the other two, and in the vicinity of the future pons, is in the opposite direction, that of dorsiflexion.[1] These are known respectively as the midbrain flexure, the neck flexure, and the pontine flexure.

Forebrain. Early in the development of the embryo, a transverse section through the forebrain reveals thick lateral walls connected by thin floor and roof plates. Each lateral wall is divided into a dorsal and a ventral area, the two being separated internally by the hypothalamic sulcus.

Early on, two lateral vesicles appear, one on each side of the forebrain. These are the optic vesicles. Ultimately they expand distally (see Chapter 30) and their proximal parts constrict to become the optic stalks. Then the forebrain grows ventrally and two more diverticula expand from it to form two large pouches, one on each side; these subsequently become the cerebral hemispheres and their cavities, the lateral ventricles. They communicate with the central portion of the forebrain by wide openings that are later to be the foramina of Luschka. The anterior part of the roof plate is a thin sheet called the lamina terminalis. It stretches from the foramina of Luschka to the recess at the base of the optic stalk. This anterior part of the forebrain, including the rudiments of the two cerebral hemispheres, is the telencephalon, while the posterior part is the diencephalon. Both contribute to the formation of the third ventricle, but the latter predominates.

The telencephalon consists of the two lateral diverticula mentioned above and the connecting median region. From the latter develops the anterior part of the cavity of the third ventricle, closed anteriorly and below by the lamina terminalis. The large lateral diverticula become the lateral ventricles, and their thick walls become the substance of the cerebral hemispheres. The roof plate of the telencephalon is thin and continuous with that of the diencephalon. In the floor plate and lateral walls of the prosencephalon ventral to the two interventricular foramina, the anterior parts of the hypothalamus are developed; these include the optic chiasm and optic recesses.

As the cerebral hemispheres grow, they enlarge forward, upward, and backward and become oval. The medial surfaces are then separated from each other by a longitudinal fissure, the floor of which is the epithelial roof plate of the telencephalon. The cranial end of each hemisphere becomes the frontal pole. As the cerebral hemisphere grows, the original posterior pole curves caudally and ventrally to become the temporal pole, and the new posterior part becomes the definitive occipital pole.[1] The great expansion of the growing cerebral hemispheres causes them to overlap the diencephalon, the midbrain, and the cerebellum, successively, while the temporal lobes grow around the sides of the brain stem.

About the fifth week a diverticulum appears anteriorly and medially in the floor of each lateral ventricle; the diverticulum grows forward and then loses its cavity to become the olfactory bulb. Its stalk becomes the olfactory tract.

The pia mater over the roof of the third ventricle is covered with loose mesenchyme, in which many blood vessels develop on each side of the midline; these invaginate the roof of the ventricle to form the choroid plexus of the third ventricle.

Most of the wall of each hemisphere remains thick, forming the pallium. However, the lower part medially adjoining the roof of the foramen remains thin, consisting only of pia mater and ependyma. This thin part is invaginated by vascular tissue, continuous in front with that of the third ventricle; it constitutes the choroid plexus of the lateral ventricle.

Early growth in the hemisphere proceeds rapidly in the floor and adjacent portion of the lateral wall; as a result, elevations develop there which encroach on the lumen of the lateral ventricle. These protrusions are the corpus striatum and the caudate nucleus.

The first part of the cortex to differentiate is that which borders the interventricular foramen or foramen of Luschka. Below and in front of that circular strip the cells of the cortex, where the stalk of the olfactory tract is attached, constitute part of the piriform area. In that part which is to become the hippocampus, cells of the cortex proliferate and the wall of the lateral ventricle thickens to produce still another internal elevation.

When they appear, the two cerebral hemispheres are connected to each other by the median part of the telencephalon. The roof plate of that part remains thin and epithelial, while the floor is invaded by the decussating fibers of the optic nerves. Thus the roof and floor are not available for fibers that connect the two hemispheres, crossing the midline. Those fibers therefore pass through the lamina terminalis. Fibers of the olfactory tracts cross in the ventral part together with fibers from other areas to form the anterior commissure. The two hippocampi become interconnected by fibers crossing from fornix to fornix in the upper part; this is the commissure of the fornix. Commissures of the neopallium develop later and lie on the dorsal surface of the commissure of the fornix. They increase tremendously in number, and this bundle thus outgrows its neighbors to become the corpus callosum. The rostrum of the corpus callosum develops later; the backward growth of its trunk creates a new floor for the longitudinal fissure.

Growth of the neocortex and its enormous expansion are associated with the appearance of projection fibers late in the third month. They extend downward and medially to divide the corpus striatum into a lateral part, the lentiform nucleus, and a medial part, the caudate nucleus.

At the end of the third month, a slight depression appears on the superolateral surface of each cerebral hemisphere corresponding to the underlying site of the corpus striatum; its presence is the result of more rapid growth of adjoining cortical regions. This lateral cerebral fossa gradually becomes overlapped and submerged and is converted into the lateral cerebral sulcus; its floor becomes the insula. This process of submersion and overlapping is not completed in its most anterior part until after birth.

Except for the shallow hippocampal sulcus and the lateral cerebral fossa, the surfaces of the hemispheres remain smooth and uninterrupted until about the beginning of the fourth month of gestation.[1] The parietooccipital sulcus appears at about that time on the medial surface, and at the same time the posterior portion of the calcarine sulcus forms. During the fifth month the cingulate sulcus appears on the medial aspect. It is not until the sixth month that sulci appear on the inferior and superolateral aspects. By the end of the seventh month all of the important sulci can be recognized.[1]

An excellent review of the stages of development of the primary fissures and of the cerebral lobes was published by Chi, Dooling, and Gilles in 1977.[2]

At about the sixth week of gestation, the wall of the hemisphere, or pallium, consists of a thin outer or marginal layer, an intermediate mantle, and an inner thick ependymal layer. Beginning in about the seventh week in the paleopallium, medially and inferiorly, and later in the neopallium, cells from the ependymal and mantle zones migrate into the marginal zone to form the cerebral cortex. In the neopallium, further differentiation transforms that into the six-layered pattern characteristic of the adult neocortex by the eighth month. All the cortical cells are initially derived from the ependymal layer.[1]

Midbrain. The midbrain is derived from the intermediate primary cerebral vesicle, which persists for a time as a thin-walled tube enclosing a cavity, which communicates with those of the fore- and hindbrains. Its own lumen later becomes reduced in diameter to form the cerebral aqueduct. The ventral laminae increase in thickness to become the cerebral peduncles.

Hindbrain. At the time that the head fold or midbrain flexure occurs, the hindbrain is longer than the forebrain and midbrain combined. At its cranial end it is constricted in the isthmus rhombencephali. Ventrally it is separated from the pharynx by the notocord and the two dorsal aortae. Its thin epithelial roof becomes stretched and widened during the flexure. The lateral walls become separated, especially dorsally, and the cavity of the hindbrain (destined to become the fourth ventricle) becomes flattened and rather triangular in cross section. As the pontine flexure becomes more acute, at the end of the second month, the laminae of the cranial and caudal slopes become opposed to each other and the lateral angles of the cavity stretch out to form the lateral recesses of the fourth ventricle. The lateral walls differentiate into dorsal and ventral laminae, with a limiting sulcus between. The cells of the hindbrain, like those of the developing cerebral hemisphere, are arranged for a time in three layers, the inner or ependymal, the intermediate mantle, and the outer or marginal layer.

The cranial slope of the hindbrain is the metencephalon, and from it both the pons and the cerebellum are developed. Before the formation of the pontine flexure, the dorsal laminae of the metencephalon are parallel to one another. Subsequently they lie obliquely and are close together at the cranial end of the fourth ventricle, but are widely separated in the vicinity of the lateral angles. Accentuation of the pontine flexure brings the cranial and caudal angles of the ventricle adjacent to one another, and the dorsal laminae then lie almost horizontally.

Meanwhile, cells in the rhombic lip and dorsal part of the dorsal laminae proliferate to form the rudiment of the cerebellum. Two rounded swellings are formed which first project partly into the ventricle; they are the rudimentary cerebellar hemispheres. The most cranial part of the roof of the metencephalon originally separates the two swellings, but it becomes invaded by cells which form the rudiment of the vermis. At a later stage, known as extroversion of the cerebellum, there is reduction of its intraventricular projection and increasing prominence of dorsal projection. The growing cerebellum then consists of a dumbbell shaped swelling stretched across the cranial part of the fourth ventricle. As it grows, a number of transverse grooves appear on its dorsal aspect, precursors of the definitive fissures of the adult.

The remainder of the metencephalon becomes the pons, which, like the rudimentary cerebellum, begins by having the same basic three layers (epedymal, mantle, and marginal); apparently, however, little else is known about the stages of its transformation.[1]

The caudal slope of the hindbrain is known as the myelencephalon; it becomes the medulla oblongata. As the walls of the hindbrain spread outward, the so-called rhombic lip, at the upper edge of the dorsal lamina, becomes characteristically folded over laterally just below the junction with the roof plate.

The lower part of the myelencephalon does not participate in the formation of the fourth ventricle; its development resembles that of the spinal cord.[1]

Spinal Cord. Recent investigation regarding the histogenesis of the spinal cord indicates that the early neural epithelium, including the deep, paraluminal mitotic zone, consists of a homogeneous population of pluripotent cells,[1] the different appearances of which reflect merely different phases in their proliferative cycle. The ependymal layer is considered to be populated by a single basic type of matrix cell which, in passing through a complete mitotic and intermitotic cycle, appears to move up and down, progressively approaching and receding from the internal limiting membrane. While some daughter cells start another cycle, others migrate outward and differentiate into neuroblasts as they approach and enter the mantle layer. Eventually neuroblast formation wanes and the mitotic activity of the remaining matrix cells declines as they differentiate into ependymal cells.

The roof plate and the floor plate of the oval neural tube do not participate in the cellular proliferation of the lateral walls, and hence they remain thin. Their cells contribute only to the formation of the ependyma.

At first the lumen of the neural tube is narrow and slit-like. As the lateral walls thicken, the lumen widens dorsally and becomes rather diamond-shaped in cross section. As it does so, a longitudinally oriented sulcus, the sulcus limitans, develops on each side, dividing the ependymal and mantle layers in each lateral wall into ventral and dorsal laminae. The cells of the ventral lamina become the motor cells of the anterior and lateral grey columns, while those of the dorsal lamina form intercalated neurons, some of which receive the terminals of primary sensory neurons. At its caudal end the central canal of the spinal cord becomes dilated to form the terminal ventricle.

In early embryonic life the spinal cord occupies the entire length of the vertebral canal, and the spinal nerves pass away from it at right angles. After the embryo attains a length of 30 mm., in the seventh week, the vertebral column grows more rapidly than the spinal cord, the caudal end of which gradually becomes more cranial in the vertebral canal. Most of this migration occurs during the first half of intrauterine life. By the twenty-fifth week the terminal ventricle has moved from the second coccygeal vertebra to the third lumbar, and only two segments remain for further migration before the adult position is reached. As the change in level cranially begins, the caudal end of the terminal ventricle, adherent to overlying ectoderm, remains in place and the walls of the intermediate part of the ventricle and its covering pia mater become drawn out to form the delicate filum terminale. The distal part of the terminal ventricle disappears before birth as a rule, but it may occasionally give rise to congenital cysts in the neighborhood of the coccyx.

ANATOMY

The brain is described as consisting of a number of parts, the prosencephalon or forebrain, the mesencephalon or midbrain, and the rhombencephalon or hindbrain. The forebrain is divided into the telencephalon, comprising the two cerebral hemispheres or cerebrum, and the diencephalon ("between brain"), which is the central connecting part, corresponding roughly to the thalamus and hypothalamus.

The hindbrain includes the cerebellum, pons (metencephalon), and medulla oblongata (myelencephalon).

The midbrain, pons, and medulla oblongata together are spoken of as the brain stem, connecting the forebrain and the spinal cord.

Forebrain. The cerebrum is the most cranial part of the brain and is responsible for the greatest part of the volume. It occupies the anterior and middle cranial fossae and is in direct contact with almost the whole concavity of the vault of the skull. Each cerebral hemisphere, which is not truly hemispherical in shape, is roughly the equivalent of a quarter of a sphere. Each contains a large, crescentic lateral ventricle, continuous medially with the third ventricle in the diencephalon. Each hemisphere has an external layer of grey matter (the cerebral cortex) and a central core of white matter, in which are several large masses of grey matter, the basal ganglia.

The hemispheres are incompletely separated by a deep median cleft, the longitudinal cerebral fissure, which contains the falx cerebri, a sickle-shaped extension of the dura mater, and the anterior cerebral vessels. Anteriorly and posteriorly this fissure completely separates the hemispheres from each other; centrally it extends down only to the central commissure called the corpus callosum, which connects the hemispheres across the median plane.

Each cerebral hemisphere presents three surfaces, the superolateral, medial, and inferior. The superolateral surface is convex and corresponds to half of the vault of the cranium. The medial surface is flat and vertical, and is separated from that of the opposite hemisphere by the longitudinal fissure and the falx cerebri. The inferior surface is irregular and may be divided into two parts, the orbital and the tentorial. The former is concave and in contact with the roofs of the orbits and the nose. The latter is the inferior surface of the temporal and occipital lobes; anteriorly it corresponds to the middle cranial fossa, and posteriorly it rests on the tentorium cerebelli. The anterior end of each hemisphere is called the frontal pole; the posterior part is the occipital pole; and the anterior end of each temporal lobe is the temporal pole.

The surfaces of the hemispheres are arranged in a number of irregular elongate eminences called gyri or convolutions, which are separated from one another by furrows termed the sulci or fissures. Each sulcus corresponds to an infolding of the cortex; thus, the total amount of grey matter is about three times as much as it might be were the surface of the brain smooth. Some sulci exist along lines which separate entire areas from one another, those areas differing in microscopic structure and in function. These are called limiting sulci.

The gyri and intervening sulci are rather constant in their arrangement but vary within limits, not only in different individuals but also in the two hemispheres of the same brain.[1]

The superolateral surface of the cerebral hemisphere bears two major sulci, the lateral and the central. The lateral is a deep cleft located inferolaterally. It is oriented roughly anteroposteriorly, extending slightly upward and curving to its end under the parietal eminence. The central sulcus is more vertically oriented, arising near the superomedial border just posterior to the midpoint between the frontal and occipital poles, running downward and forward to end a little above the lateral sulcus.

The frontal lobe is the anterior part of the hemisphere. On the superolateral surface it is bounded posteriorly by the central sulcus. Superolaterally it is traversed by four gyri separated from one another by three sulci. The gyri are the precentral and the superior, middle, and inferior frontal gyri.

The temporal pole is inferior to the lateral sulcus. Its lateral surface is divided into three parallel gyri by two sulci. The gyri are the superior, middle, and inferior temporal gyri.

The parietal lobe is bounded anteriorly by the central sulcus and posteriorly by a line joining the pre-occipital incisure to the superomedial margin at the point where it is cut by the parieto-occipital sulcus. Its inferior limit is the posterior ramus of the lateral sulcus and a line drawn to the posterior boundary from the point where the ramus ascends. The lateral aspect of the parietal lobe can be divided roughly into three major portions, the postcentral gyrus and the superior and inferior parietal lobules.

The occipital lobe bears, superiorly and laterally, three principal gyri: the superior and inferior occipital gyri and behind them, the vertically oriented gyrus descendens.

The insula is deep in the floor of the lateral sulcus. It is overlapped by overgrowth of the cortical areas adjacent to it, and can be seen only when the lips of the lateral sulcus are separated.

The medial surface of the hemisphere can be examined only after its separation from its mate by division of the commissures which connect them and the roof, floor, and anterior and posterior walls of the third ventricle. The most conspicuous commissure is the corpus callosum, which forms a broad arched band lying in the floor of the central part of the longitudinal fissure. Even in small infants it is readily seen. Its down-curved anterior end is the genu, which is continuous inferiorly with the rostrum and, beyond that, the lamina terminalis. The main body of the commissure arches up and back to end in a rounded posterior extremity, the splenium. The concave aspects of the genu, trunk or main body, and rostrum are attached below to the laminae of the septum pellucidum, which occupies the space between them and the fornix inferiorly. Curving around the arch of the corpus callosum is the cingulate gyrus, which begins below the rostrum anteriorly and follows the curve posteriorly. Above that, on the medial aspect, are (from front to back) the medial frontal gyrus, the paracentral lobule, the precuneus, and the cuneus.

The inferior surface of the cerebral hemisphere is divisible into a smaller anterior part and a larger posterior. The anterior part is the concave orbital surface. Medially it presents the gyrus rectus. The remainder bears a number of orbital gyri; four can usually be identified, called the anterior, medial, posterior, and lateral gyri. The large posterior region is the tentorial part. Here there is a parahippocampal gyrus immediately below the attachment of the cerebral peduncle, and it continues posteriorly directly into the lingual gyrus, which proceeds from that point to the occipital pole. Below the parahippocampal gyrus are the medial occipitotemporal gyrus and the lateral occipitotemporal gyrus.

Along the developmental junction of the superolateral surfaces of the diencephalon with the central areas of the inferomedial surfaces of the cerebrum, there is a series of structures in the wall of the hemisphere which compose the limbic lobe, or bordering lobe, or limbic system. Included in it are: (1) the olfactory nerves, bulbs and tracts, (2) the anterior olfactory nucleus, (3) the olfactory striae and gyri, (4) the olfactory trigone, (5) the piriform lobe, (6) the amygdaloid complex of nuclei, (7) the septal areas, (8) the hippocampal formation, (9) the fornix, (10) the stria terminalis, (11) the stria habenularis, and (12) the cingulate and parahippocampal gyri.

The two lateral ventricles are irregular cavities in the lower and medial parts of the cerebral hemispheres, one on each side of the median plane. Each communicates with the third ventricle and indirectly with the other, by way of the foramen of Luschka. Each is lined by ependyma (Figs. 31–20 and 31–21) and contains cerebrospinal fluid. Each consists of a central part and three horns, the anterior, posterior, and inferior.

In a coronal section of the cerebral hemisphere, the internal capsule (Figs. 31–8 and 31–9) is a broad band of white fibers passing obliquely downward and medially, posteriorly between the lentiform nucleus and the caudate. It can be divided into an anterior limb, a genu, a posterior limb, a retrolentiform part, and sublentiform part.

Within each cerebral hemisphere is a series of subcortical nuclear masses of grey matter loosely grouped under the general term basal nuclei. The individual units included vary from one anatomist to another, but there is generally agreement upon the following set: the amygdaloid complex, the claustrum, the caudate nucleus, and the lentiform nucleus. (They are a heterogeneous group with regard to structure, function, and phylogenetic history.) The lentiform nucleus consists of a larger darker portion, the putamen, and a smaller portion of lighter color, the globus pallidus.

The external capsule is a thin layer of white matter situated lateral to the lentiform nucleus.

The hippocampus consists of the complex interfolded layers of the dentate gyrus and the cornu ammonis. The name of the structure is derived from its resemblance, in coronal section, to the profile of a sea-horse (Figs. 31–28 to 31–31). It forms a curved elevation extending throughout the length of the floor of the inferior horn of the lateral ventricle.

The choroid plexus of the lateral ventricle is a highly vascularized fringe composed of pia mater and the ependymal lining of that cavity (Figs. 31–22 to 31–27). The choroid plexus of each lateral ventricle is an extension of the tela choroidea of the third ventricle, a triangular fold at the level of the interventricular foramina.

The third ventricle is a median cleft between the two thalami, which communicates anteriorly with the two lateral ventricles by way of the interventricular foramina, and posteriorly with the fourth ventricle by way of the aqueduct of Sylvius. It has a roof, lined by the tela choroidea, from the inferior surface of which the choroid plexuses of the third ventricle project downward, one on each side of the midline. Inferiorly is the hypothalamus; anteriorly, the lamina terminalis; and posteriorly, the pineal body.

Midbrain. The midbrain occupies the hiatus of the tentorium cerebelli and connects the forebrain with the pons and cerebellum. It is the shortest segment of the brainstem. On each side it is bounded by the parahippocampal gyrus, which hides part of it from view when the inferior aspect of the brain is examined. It is composed of two halves, the right and left cerebral peduncles, each of which has a ventral portion, the crus cerebri, and a dorsal portion, the tegmental part. The crus cerebri and tegmental part are separated by a lamina of pigmented grey matter, the substantia nigra. The crura are separate; the tegmental parts are united and are traversed longitudinally by the cerebral aqueduct, connecting the third and fourth ventricles.[1] That part of the tegmentum dorsal to the aqueduct is called the tectum, and it comprises the four colliculi.

Hindbrain. The cerebellum is the largest part of the hindbrain. It lies posterior to the pons and medulla and is separated from them by the cavity of the fourth ventricle. It is ovoid but constricted in the midline and somewhat flattened from above downward. Its greatest diameter is from side to side. The ratio of weights of cerebellum to cerebrum, in the infant, is 1:20.[1] The cerebellum consists of two hemispheres joined by a narrow median strip, the vermis. On the inferior surface the hemispheres are separated from each other by a deep hollow known as the vallecula.

The surface of the cerebellum is universally marked by closely set transverse curved fissures which give it a laminated appearance; these fissures or grooves separate the folia from one another (Fig. 31–35). Some of the fissures are deeper than others and divide the organ into several lobules.

On section it is apparent that the grey matter or cortex covers the whole surface, dipping inward to line the fissures (Fig. 31–36). In addition, there are aggregates of grey matter interiorly, within the white matter that forms the central core. One of these is the dentate nucleus (Figs. 31–42 to 31–45), which is situated rather medially in the white matter.

The fourth ventricle (Figs. 31–70 to 31–76) is a somewhat tent-shaped space situated ventral to the cerebellum, and dorsal to the pons and cranial half of the medulla. There are three openings in the caudal part of the roof of the fourth ventricle. The median aperture, or foramen of Magendie, is large and funnel-shaped, and faces the cerebellomedullary cistern. The two lateral apertures are located at the extremities of the lateral recesses and contain extensions of the choroid plexus which protrude through them into the subarachnoid space.

Two vascular processes of the tela choroidea contain the choroid plexuses of the fourth ventricle (Figs. 31–72 to 31–74). They invaginate the caudal part of the roof of the fourth ventricle and are covered by ependyma.

The pons (Figs. 31–46 to 31–56) is ventral to the cerebellum. Cranial to it is the midbrain. Inferiorly it is continuous with the medulla oblongata, from which it is separated, anteriorly and on each side, by a transverse furrow. The anterior surface of the pons is markedly convex from side to side, and less so from above down. The dorsal surface is hidden by the cerebellum.

Internally, the ventral or basilar part is characterized by a striking and unique pattern of alternating groups of fibers, the transverse fibers of the pons and the various longitudinally oriented groups including the corticopontine, corticonuclear, and corticospinal fibers (Figs. 31–48 through 31–53).

The medulla oblongata (Figs. 31–57 to 31–69) extends from the lower margin of the pons caudally to a transverse plane just above the first pair of cervical nerves. In fact, there is no clear line of demarcation, and the internal structures of the medulla change gradually into those of the spinal cord.

The medulla oblongata is rather piriform, its broad extremity being directed upward to blend with the pons while its narrow lower end is continuous with the spinal cord. The lower half of the cavity of the fourth ventricle occupies its upper half, while the lower half contains only a slender central canal like that of the spinal cord. Its anterior and posterior surfaces bear median longitudinal fissures.

The anterior part of the medulla bulges downward prominently on each side of the midline between the anterior median fissure and the anterolateral sulcus, forming an elongate elevation known as the pyramid.

The olive (Figs. 31–63 to 31–69) is an oval elevation on each side of the midline of the medulla located between the anterolateral and posterolateral sulci and lateral to the pyramid.

The spinal cord is the elongate, roughly cylindrical part of the central nervous system which occupies most of the vertebral canal. It narrows caudally to a sharp tip, the conus medullaris. In transverse width it varies from level to level but, in general, tapers gradually from its cranial to its caudal extremity. It is not exactly cylindrical, being, for the most part, greater in its transverse dimension than in its vertical. Fissures and sulci mark the external surface of the cord throughout most of its length. There is an anterior median fissure and a posterior median sulcus; between the two the cord is divided into two halves, a right and a left, joined in the middle by a band of neural tissue in which the central canal is located. The anterior median fissure is very deep and contains a little of the pia mater.

At every level of the cord there are central (dorsal and ventral) columns of grey matter and a commisural grey mass, all surrounded by a sheath of white matter.

Meninges. The brain and spinal cord are enveloped by three membranes, the meninges, named (from without inwards) dura mater, arachnoid, and pia mater. The most external, the dura mater, is tough, tightly adherent to overlying bone, and inelastic. The arachnoid or middle layer is thin and cobweb-like, formed of delicate interlacing reticular fibers. The most internal, the pia mater, is very like the arachnoid, being thin and delicate. It is intimately attached to all of the contours of the brain and spinal cord. Because the last two are so similar anatomically, because they are, for the most part, in close approximation, and because it is likely that they are developed from the same embryonic layer, they are often regarded as a single structure, the leptomeninges (Fig. 31-77), of which the inner vascular layer is pia mater and outer membrane is the arachnoid.

The cerebral dura serves both as an investing sheath for the brain and as periosteum for the inner surface of the cranium. It comprises two layers, an inner fibrous layer and an outer vascular; between the two are the large venous sinuses of the brain. The cerebral dura gives rise to several septa which divide the cranial cavity into incomplete compartments. They are the falx cerebri, the median septum; the tentorium cerebelli, the transverse septum overlying the cerebellum; the falx cerebelli, incompletely separating the hemispheres of the cerebellum; and the diaphragma sellae, forming the fibrous roof of the pituitary fossa.[3]

The spinal dura extends as a closed tough sac from the margins of the foramen magnum above to the level of the second sacral vertebra below. (The spinal dura corresponds to only the *inner* layer of the cerebral dura, as the vertebrae have their own periosteum.)[3]

The arachnoid is nonvascular and passes over the sulci without dipping into them. It extends outward, on the other hand, along the roots of the cerebrospinal nerves and along the optic nerves.

The pia mater is not only adherent to underlying neural tissue but also sends fibrous septa into the spinal cord. In addition, at the points where blood vessels enter or leave the central nervous system, the pia is invaginated to form the outer wall of a perivascular space.[3]

HISTOLOGY

Cerebral Cortex. (Figs. 31-1 to 31-7) The size and type of cells found in the cerebral cortex in the adult vary at different depths from the surface; they are disposed in fairly definite layers. Likewise, many fibers are arranged in bands parallel to the surface. By means of cell and fiber lamination, Brodmann in 1909 initially identified the classical six layers of the cerebral cortex.[4] The arrangement varies in different parts of the cortex; in certain areas one or more of the strata may be reduced, enlarged, or subdivided. The six layers are as follows: (1) *The molecular layer,* which is the most superficial. It contains fibers, many neuroglia, and a few nerve cells. (2) *The external granular layer* of small pyramidal cells. It contains a large number of small nerve cells. (3) *The layer of pyramidal cells* which is divided into two strata, a superficial layer containing chiefly medium-sized pyramidal cells and a deeper one populated chiefly by larger cells. (4) *The internal granular layer* or layer of small stellate cells, characterized by the presence of many small multipolar cells with short axons. Scattered among them are small pyramidal cells. (5) *The ganglionic layer* or deep layer, containing the large pyramidal cells. The apical dendrites of these cells are very long and, like those of the more superficial pyramidal cells, reach and ramify within the molecular layer. (6) *The multiform layer,* which contains a considerable range of cell types; most of them are small and are considered to be modified pyramidal elements.

When the fetus reaches 80 mm. crown-rump length (about 12 weeks of gestation), the cortical layer begins to show signs of differentiation in its deeper portion.[5] The nature of this change is better characterized at 95 mm. crown-rump length (13 weeks gestation), when three layers are apparent; these are probably the precursors of layers 4, 5, and 6.[5] Differentiation beyond this time is extremely complex and varies in different regions of the brain. Streeter[6] states that it is during the *sixth* or *seventh* month of intrauterine life that these cells become grouped into the six layers mentioned above, those of the adult cortex.

Internal Capsule. The internal capsule is a broad band of white substance separating the lenticular nucleus laterally from the caudate nucleus and thalamus medially. In a coronal section taken at the level of the hippocampus (Figs. 31–8 and 31—9) it is C-shaped as it curves around the caudate and thalamus.

Caudate Nucleus. (Figs. 31–10 and 31–11) The caudate nucleus is an elongate mass of grey matter bent on itself, like a horseshoe. Throughout its length it is closely related to the lateral ventricle, into which it bulges. Its rounded anterior extremity is pear-shaped and protrudes into the anterior horn of the lateral ventricle. The remainder is drawn out into a long, slender, highly arched tail, which curves around into the roof of the inferior horn and then extends rostrally.

Lenticular Nucleus. The lenticular nucleus is situated deep in the white matter of the hemisphere between the insula laterally and the caudate nucleus and thalamus medially. Its shape resembles that of a biconcave lens. Its medial surface is closely applied to the internal capsule. It is divided into two parts; the more lateral and larger is the putamen, and the smaller and more medial is the globus pallidus with its internal and external divisions.

Especially in the anterior part of the internal capsule, bands of grey matter stretch across from the lenticular to the caudate nucleus, producing a striated appearance (Fig. 31–8 and 31–9). (This is the basis for the term *corpus striatum,* which applies to the entire mass formed by those two nuclei and the internal capsule separating them.)

The caudate and the putamen are both composed of small nerve cells, among which are interspersed a few of medium size (Figs. 31–10 and 31–11). Cells of the globus pallidus, on the other hand, are large. In the human it is now customary to group the caudate and putamen together as the striatum and to call the globus pallidus the pallidum.[4]

Lateral Ventricles and Their Walls. Developmentally, the pallium or primitive cerebral cortex consists at first of three zones, the ependymal, mantle, and marginal layers. During the third month, neuroblasts migrate outward from the ependymal and mantle layers into the marginal zone, where they give rise to the cerebral cortex. Fibers from those cells and others give rise to the white matter of the hemisphere. Hence, the more immature the infant, the broader the mantle zone will be (Fig. 31–12). In the sixth month of gestation (Figs. 31–14 and 31–15) that mantle is very prominent. It is in this area that so many grave primary hemorrhages occur in infants born prematurely. Even in the term infant one can often find discrete small aggregates of these neuroblasts in the vicinity of the ependymal lining of the lateral ventricle.

Although derived from neuroglia, the lining cells of the entire ventricular system have a distinctly epithelial character and are known as the *ependymal cells* (Figs. 31–20 and 31–21). These cells have long processes that extend out into and support the surrounding substance of the brain. During embryonic life the ependymal cells are ciliated, and even at the time of a term birth they may remain so (Fig. 31–20); some cilia persist into adult life.

Choroid Plexus. (Figs. 31–22 to 31–27) The choroid plexus is of basically the same histologic pattern in the two lateral ventricles and in the roof of the third and fourth ventricles. In each, it is much folded and invaginated into the chamber so that its exposed free surface is large. It is almost papillary in its microscopic appearance, with many branching tufts. Each branch is supported by a delicate fibrous stroma that is rich in capillaries (Figs. 31–23 and 31–24).

The epithelium is different from that of the ependymal lining cells. In the perinatal period the cytoplasm is often vacuolated because it contains abundant glycogen; such vacuolization is not seen in ependymal cells. In addition, these cells are arranged in a single, regular layer and do not appear crowded or heaped up as ependymal cells often do (Figs. 31–20 and 31–21). Each cell contains a distinct large, round nucleus (Fig. 31–27).

Hippocampus. (Figs. 31–28 to 31–34) The hippocampus is composed of highly specialized cortex rolled into the floor of the inferior horn of the lateral ventricle. It is covered on its ventricular surface by a thin coating of white matter. In Figure 31–30 its characteristic "sea-horse" configuration is especially well seen.

Cerebellum. (Figs. 31–35 to 31–45) The cerebellum, like the cerebral cortex, is a specialized accumulation of neurons. It is different from the spinal cord in that the relative positions of its grey and white matter are reversed. The grey matter forms the delicate cortex, and the white matter makes up the central body.

The white medullary body (Fig. 31–41) forms a compact mass in the interior, continuous from hemisphere to hemisphere through the vermis. It gives off many thick laminae that project out into the lobules and secondary and tertiary laminae (Fig. 31–36).

Supported by the white laminae, the cortex is spread in a thin, even layer forming long, narrow folds known as the folia, which are separated from one another by sulci (Figs. 31–35 to 31–40).

The denate nucleus is a crumpled purse-like lamina of grey matter within the white medullary body (Figs. 31–42 to 31–45) of each cerebellar hemisphere. Like the inferior olivary nucleus, which it resembles closely, it has a white center and a medially placed hilus. It contains large multipolar cells (Fig. 31–45).

Pons. (Figs. 31–46 to 31–56) The pons is made up of two portions that differ greatly in structure. The dorsal or tegmental part (Figs. 31–46 and 31–47) resembles the medulla oblongata, with which it is continuous. The ventral or basilar part (Figs. 31–48 to 31–56) contains the longitudinally oriented fibers that go to form the pyramids, but apart from those it is composed of structures peculiar to the level.[4]

On the dorsal surface of the tegmental part there is a thick layer of grey matter lining the rhomboid fossa or floor of the fourth ventricle (Figs. 31–46 and 31–47). Between that layer and the basilar portion of the pons is the reticular formation (Figs. 31–46 and 31–47), divided by a median raphe into two symmetric halves. This formation contains many longitudinal tracts as well as groups of neurons belonging to cranial nerve nuclei.

The basis pontis or basilar portion (Figs. 31–48 to 31–56) is the larger of the two divisions. It is made up of fascicles of longitudinal and transverse fibers and of irregular masses of grey substance, which occupy the spaces left among the bundles of nerve fibers and which are known as nuclei pontis. The nuclei pontis contain medium-sized rounded or polygonal cells. There are also small nerve cells.

Medulla Oblongata. (Figs. 31–57 to 31–69) The medulla oblongata, although not very long from above down, changes its shape and size remarkably in a series of cross sections. At the upper or rostral end it is large and vaguely rectangular (Fig. 31–57). At this level, near the caudal end of the pons, the inferior olivary nucleus is a conspicuous feature, and there is one on each side of the median raphe (Figs. 31–57 and 31–58). It is a broad, irregularly folded band of grey matter, curved in such a way as to enclose a white core, which extends into the nucleus from the medial aspect through an opening known as the hilus. The grey lamina consists of neuroglia and many rounded nerve cells beset with numerous short branching dendrites (Figs. 31–63 to 31–69). At the same level, on the dorsal aspect of the medulla, the floor of the fourth ventricle appears (Figs. 31–59 and 31–60). Ventrally, again on the two sides of the midline, are the pyramids, each creating a rounded bulge. Also located at this level, in the upper third of a cross section, not far from the median raphe or the floor of the fourth ventricle, are four important nuclei for the cranial nerves: the nuclei of the hypoglossal nerve, the nucleus ambiguous, the dorsal motor nucleus of the vagus, and the nucleus of the tractus solitarius.[4]

Slightly more caudally, a representative cross section is almost, but not quite, round; it is the pyramids projecting inferiorly that disturb that rounded contour slightly. At this level, there is no evidence of the fourth ventricle and instead, in the center of the section, a central canal appears (Fig. 31–62). The ependymal lining cells of the canal, even in an infant born at term, may be ciliated.

In successive sections taken in the same plane, passing caudally, the histologic morphology of the medulla oblongata becomes gradually but progressively more like that of the spinal cord (Fig. 31–78).

The Fourth Ventricle. (Figs. 31–70 to 31–76) The fourth ventricle is a diamond-shaped cavity lying between the pons and medulla oblongata ventrally and the cerebellum dorsally. It is continuous with the cerebral aqueduct above and the central canal of the closed portion of the medulla below. Laterally, on each side, the cavity extends into a pointed recess. It communicates with the subarachnoid space on each side through a lateral aperture, the foramen of Luschka, through which a small portion of the choroid plexus protrudes. There is also a median aperture, the foramen of Magendie, in the roof of the ventricle near the caudal extremity.

The floor of the fourth ventricle is known as the rhomboid fossa. It is formed by the dorsal surfaces of the pons and the open part of the medulla oblongata, which are continuous with each other. A midline sulcus divides the fossa into two symmetric lateral halves (Figs. 31–70 and 31–71). Suspended from the roof is the tela choroidea (Figs. 31–72 to 31–74). The cells of the ependymal lining, like those in the more rostral parts of the system, are often ciliated (Fig. 31–76).

Leptomeninges. (Fig. 31–77) The pia mater is very thin over the cerebral cortex, but thicker over the brain stem.[4] The blood vessels of the brain ramify within it, and as they enter the brain substance they are accompanied for a short distance by a pial sheath.

The arachnoid, which lies directly upon the external surface of the pia, is avascular. Because the pia and arachnoid are bound together by fibrous trabeculae (bridging the subarachnoid space), the two together are referred to as the pia-arachnoid.

Spinal Cord. (Figs. 31–78 to 31–84) White matter forms the outer portion of the spinal cord, and grey matter forms the central part. Grey matter forms a continuous fluted vertical column throughout the length of the cord. In cross section it is roughly the shape of the letter H; it is as though there were two comma-shaped structures, mirror-images of each other and back-to-back, joined to each other in the midline by means of a transverse bar known as the grey commissure.

In a cross section of the cord the posterior columns are directed backward and laterally, opposite or away from the anterior median fissure. In the cervical portion of the cord the posterior columns are long and narrow, constricted proximally and distally with an expanded part in between known as the caput. In the thoracic portion the posterior column does not come so close to the surface, and in the lumbosacral segments it is much thicker.

The anterior columns are relatively short and thick and project anterolaterally. They contain the cells of origin of the fibers of the ventral roots (Figs. 31–80 and 31–82 to 31–84).

The grey commissure contains the central canal (Fig. 31–81). It is lined with ependymal epithelium. It is narrowest in the thoracic region.

Ganglion. (Fig. 31–85) The ganglion is a collection of nerve cells and fibers bound together by a covering of fibrous connective tissue and well supplied with blood vessels.[4] The cell bodies are irregularly spherical.

References

1. Warwick, R., and Williams, P. L.: Gray's Anatomy, 35th British ed. Philadelphia, W. B. Saunders Co., 1973, pp. 127–144, 746–1169.
2. Chi, J. G., Dooling, E. C., and Gilles, F. H.: Gyral development of the human brain. Ann. Neurol., 1:86–93, (Jan.) 1977.
3. Truex, R. C., and Carpenter, M. B.: Human Neuroanatomy. Baltimore, The Williams and Wilkins Co., 1969, pp. 12–17.
4. Ranson, S. W., and Clark, S. L.: The Anatomy of The Nervous System. W. B. Saunders Company, Philadelphia, 1959, p. 622.
5. Lemire, R. L., Loeser, J. D., Leech, R. W., and Alvord, E. C.: Normal and Abnormal Development of The Human Nervous System. Hagerstown, Md., Harper and Row, Publishers, 1975, p. 238.
6. Streeter, G. L.: The cortex of the brain in the human embryo during the fourth month with special reference to the so-called "Papillae of Retzius." Am. J. Anat., 7:337–344, 1907.

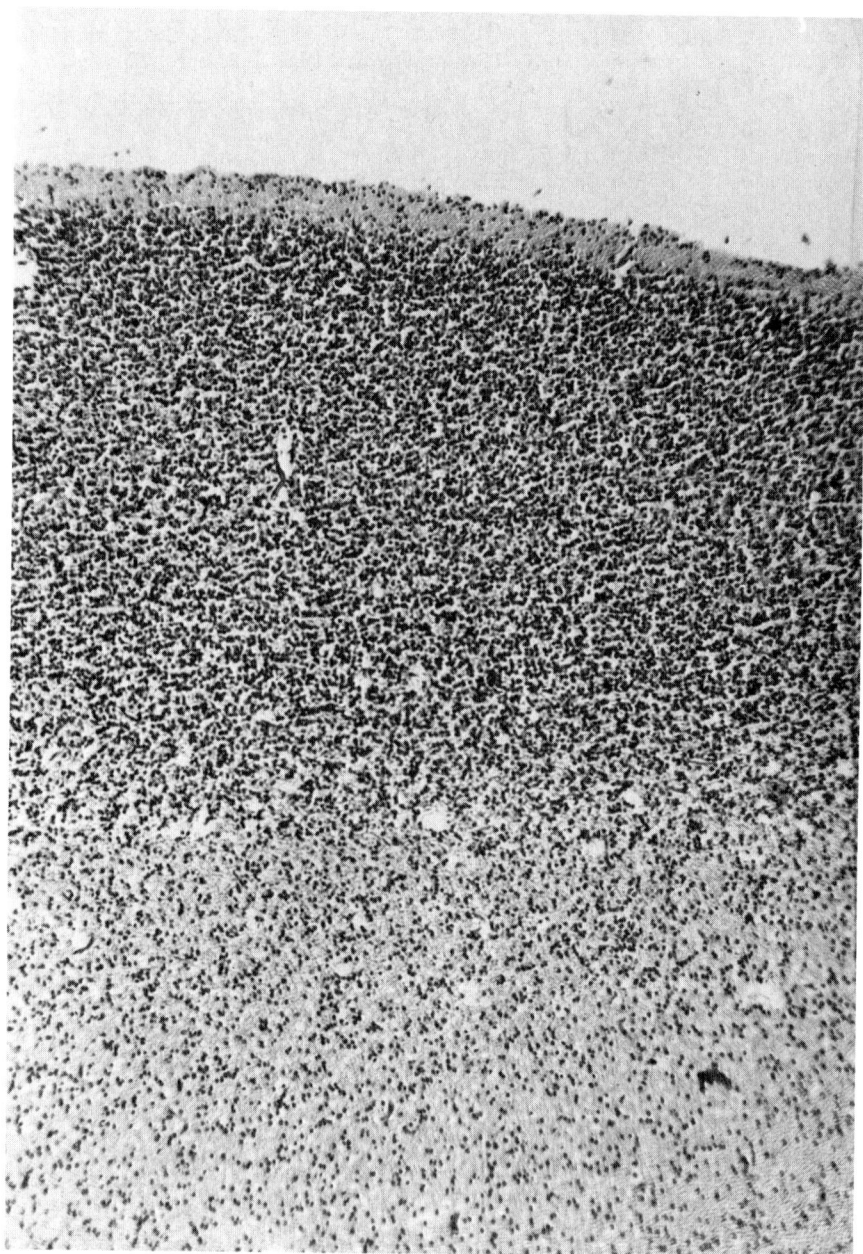

Figure 31-1

Figure 31-1. This is a section of the entire thickness of the cortex of the cerebral hemisphere in a very immature infant. Note the density or crowding of nuclei. (The leptomeninges have been stripped away.) At this magnification and with this stain, the population of cells appears to be remarkably homogeneous.

The patient was a 251 gram female infant who survived for one hour and 18 minutes.
Hematoxylin and eosin stain. Mag. 142×.

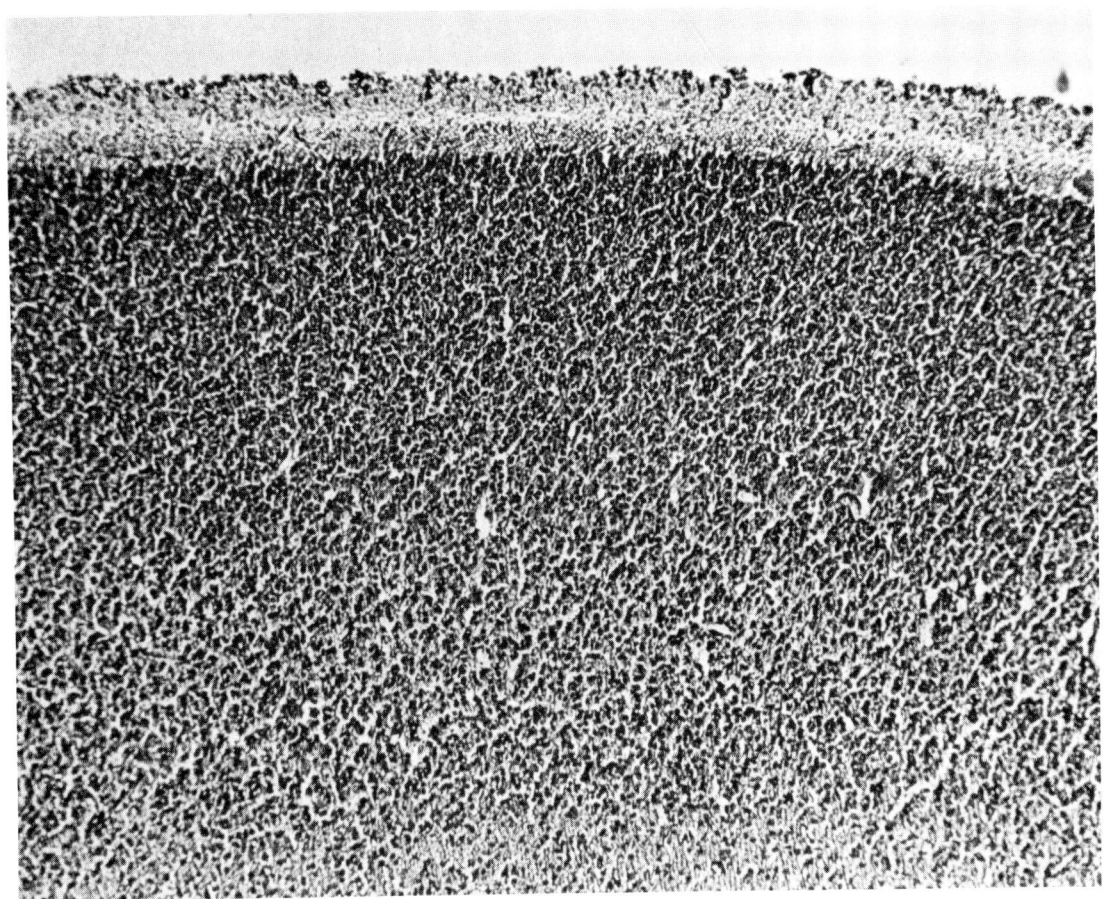

Figure 31–2

Figure 31–2. This is also the cerebral cortex of a very small and prematurely born infant with striking homogeneity of the cell population deep to the surface.
The patient was a 475 gram infant about whom no other details are recorded.
Hematoxylin and eosin stain. Mag. 132×.

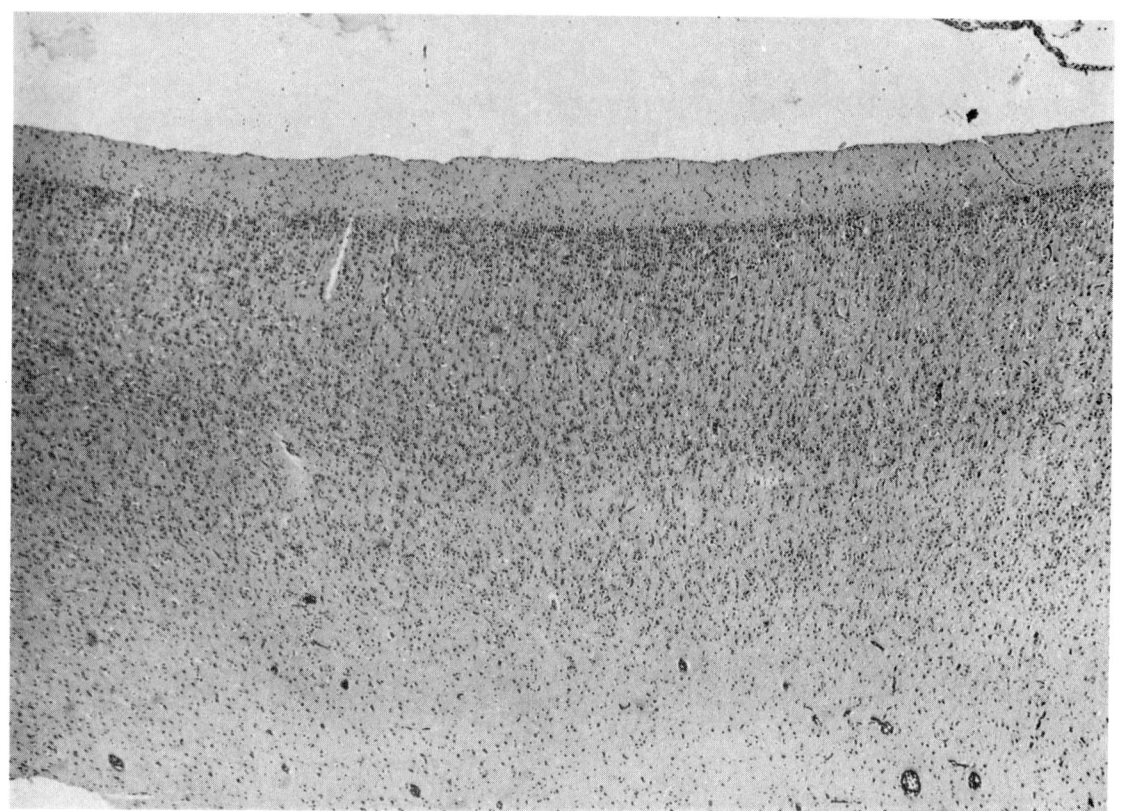

Figure 31-3

Figures 31-3 to 31-5. By contrast with Figs. 31-1 and 31-2, these three photomicrographs illustrate the remarkable differences between the cerebral cortex of the immature infant and that of the infant born at term. There are clear-cut layers here, most easily differentiated from one another in Figure 31-3 at lowest magnification.

Hematoxylin and eosin stain.

Figure 31-3. A stillborn white female with body weight of 3,120 grams. Mag. 45×.

Figure 31-4. A stillborn black male with body weight of 3,470 grams. Mag. 72×.

Figure 31-5. A stillborn black male with body weight of 3,470 grams. Mag. 132×.

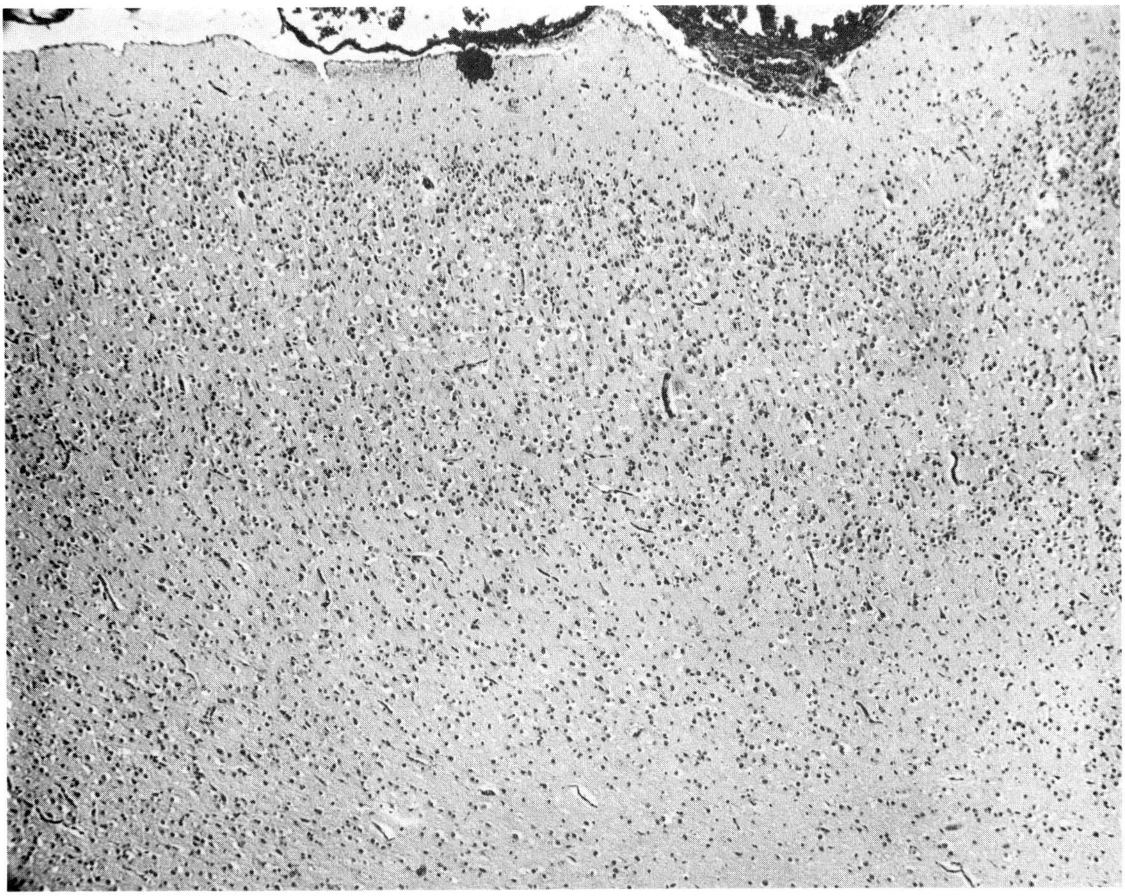

Figure 31–4

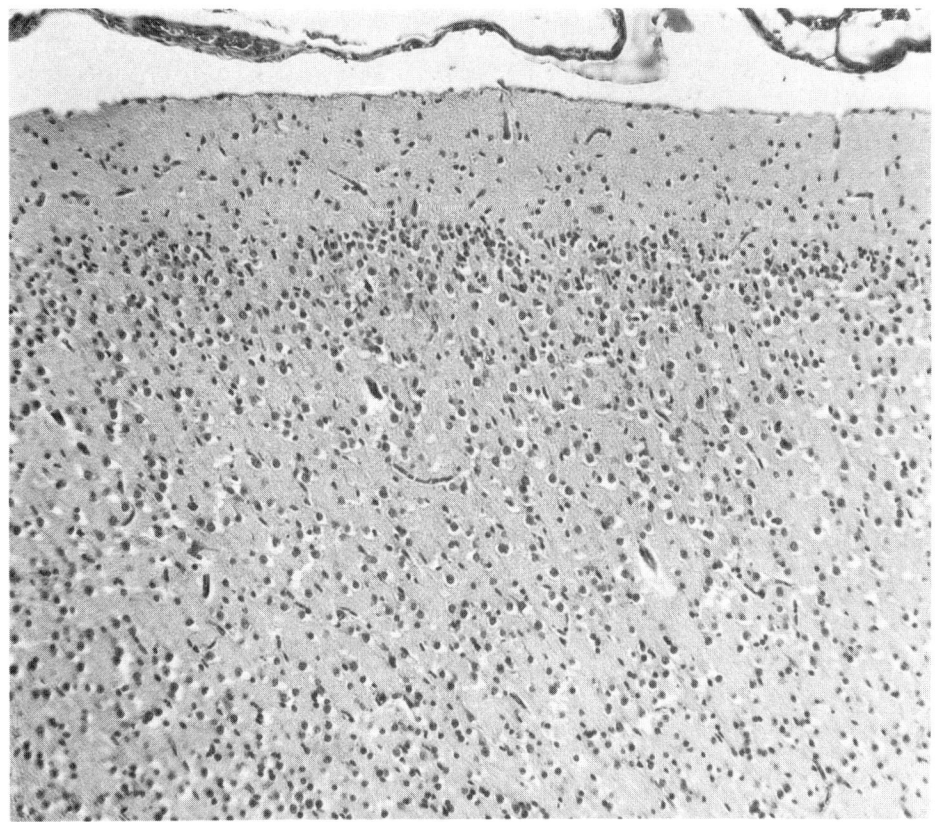

Figure 31–5

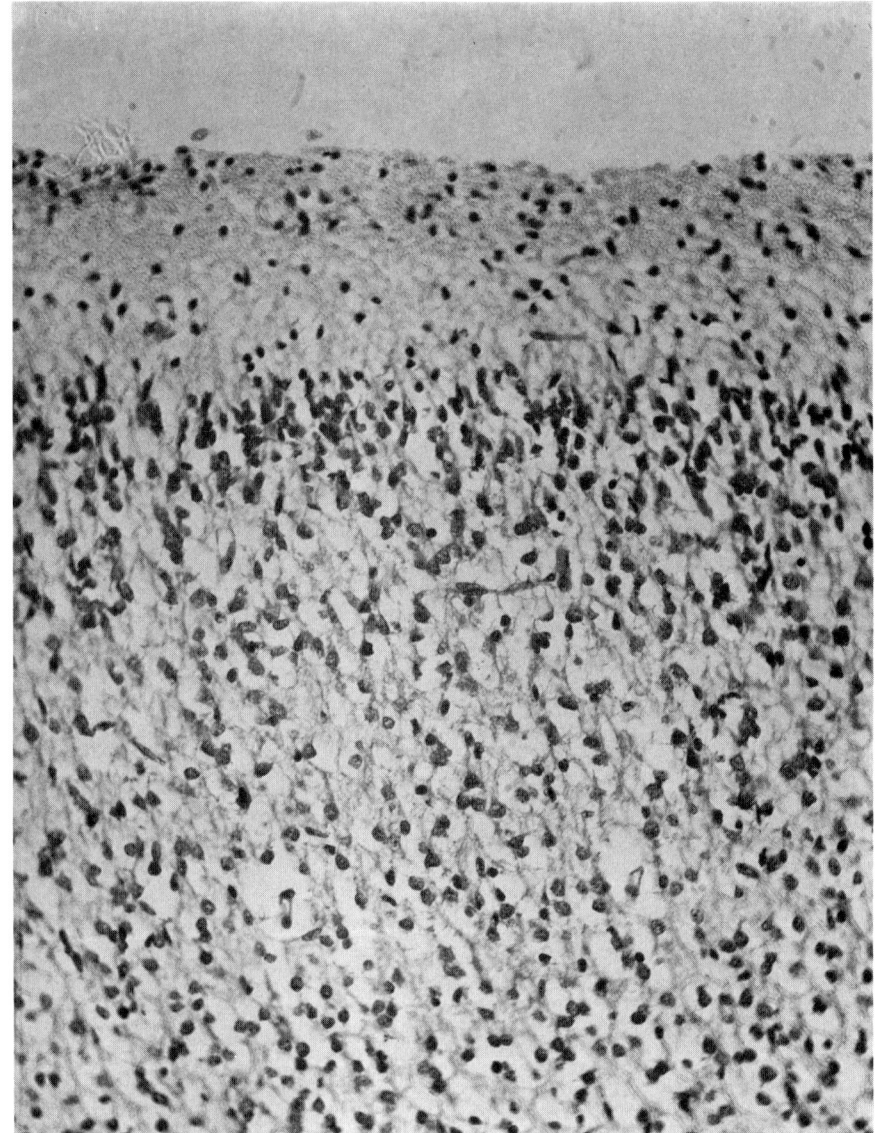

Figure 31-6

Figures 31-6 and 31-7. These two illustrations show clearly the differences in the superficial part of the cerebral cortex in infants of different gestational ages. Both were taken at the same magnification.

Figure 31-6. This infant was a female born at approximately 32 weeks of gestation. She survived for one hour and 15 minutes. At autopsy her body weighed 2,020 grams.

Hematoxylin and eosin stain. Mag. 250×.

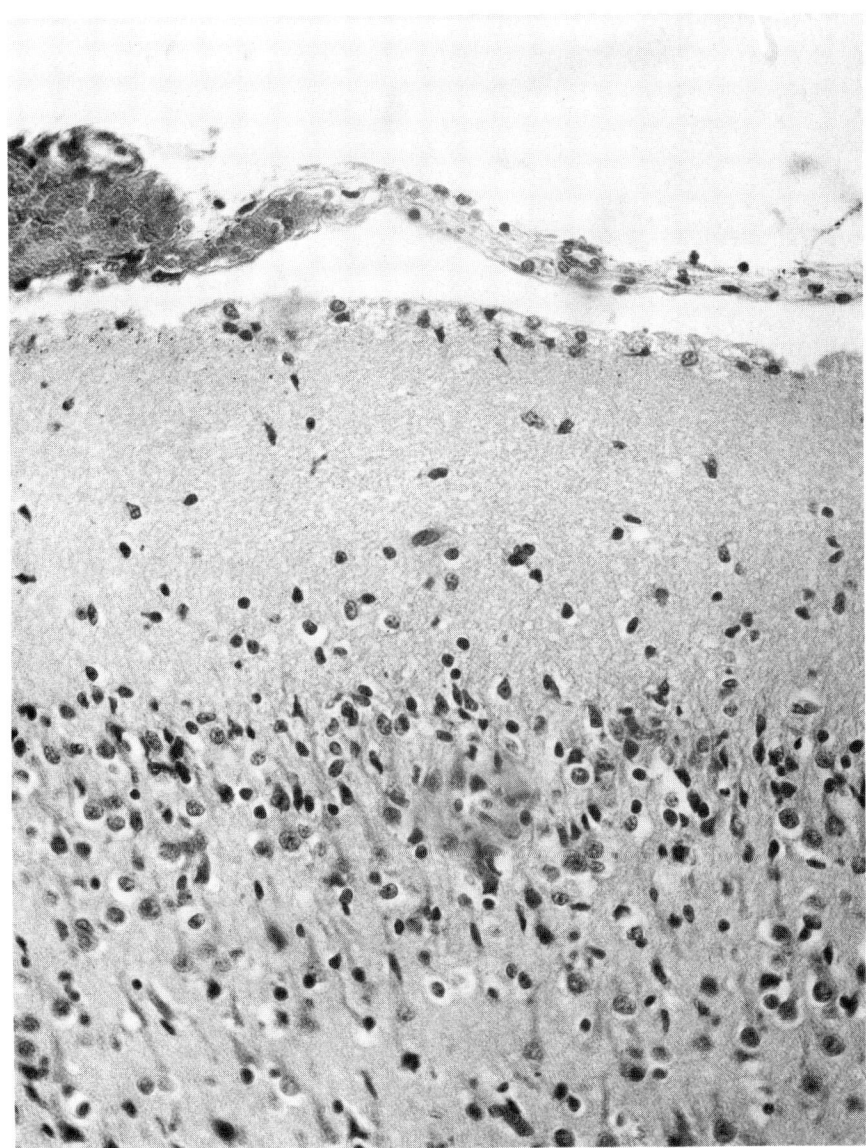

Figure 31-7

Figure 31-7. The infant from whom this photograph was taken was a stillborn white female delivered at about 38 weeks of gestation. At autopsy her body weight was 3,120 grams.
Hematoxylin and eosin stain. Mag. 250×.

554 CENTRAL NERVOUS SYSTEM

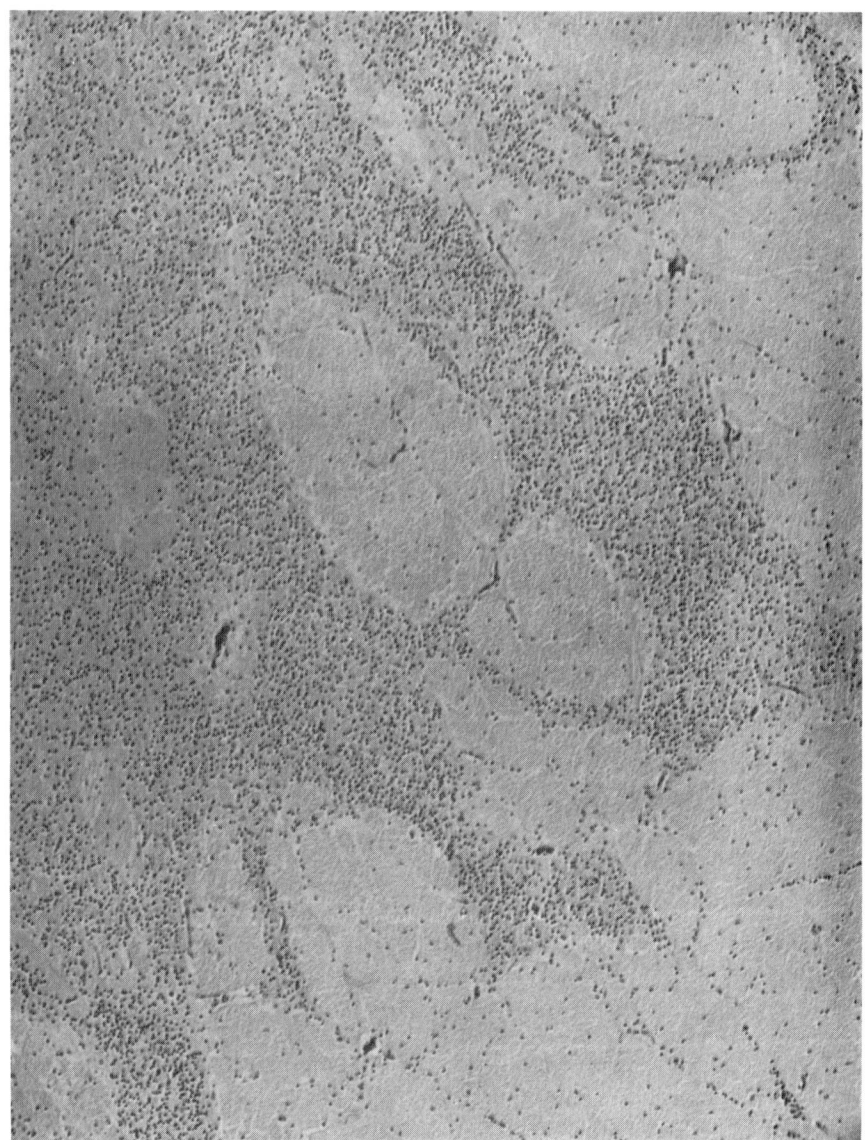

Figure 31–8

Figures 31–8 and 31–9.   Taken at approximately the same magnification, these two photographs show the internal capsule in two infants at different stages of intrauterine development, the first at roughly five months and second at roughly six months of gestation.

Figure 31–8.   Here the elements of the internal capsule appear in the lower right. This infant was born at 16 weeks of gestation. She was a 512 gram black female who lived for 27 hours.
Hematoxylin and eosin stain. Mag. 55×.

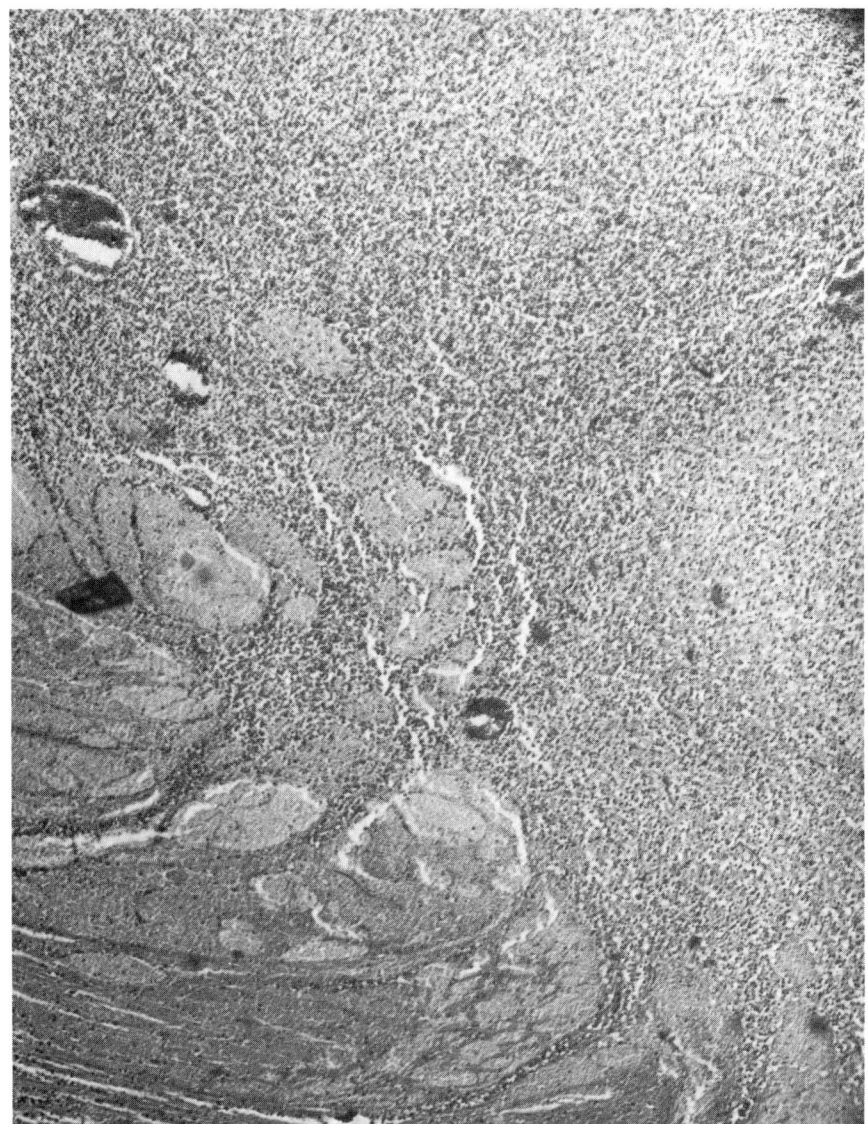

Figure 31–9

Figure 31–9. Pictured here, in the lower left, is the internal capsule of a 750 gram black male infant born at 26 weeks of gestation. He survived for 13 hours and 42 minutes.
Hematoxylin and eosin stain. Mag. 55×.

556 CENTRAL NERVOUS SYSTEM

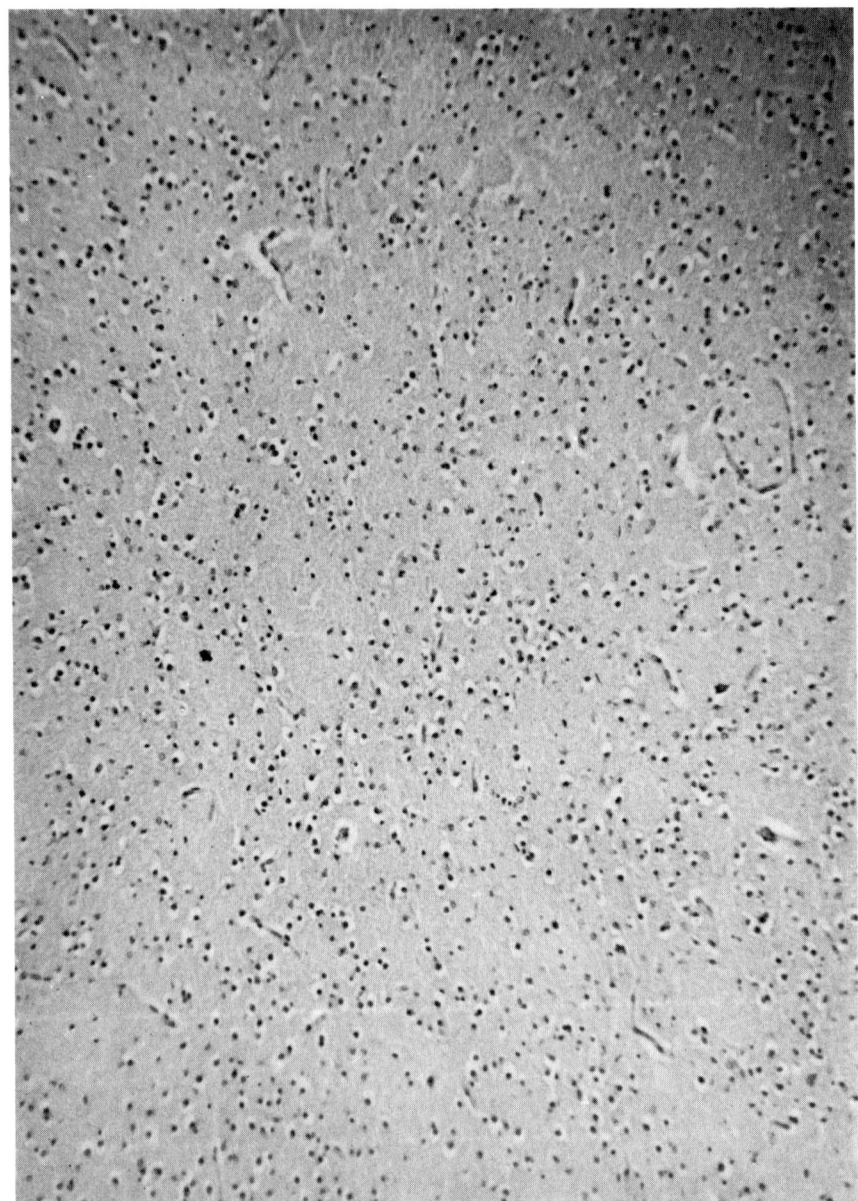

Figure 31–10

Figures 31–10 and 31–11. This set of two photographs shows, at relatively high magnification, the nature of the population of cells in the caudate nucleus in a very immature baby and in one born in the last trimester.

Figure 31–10. This section is from a 730 gram infant whose gestational age was probably about six months.
Hematoxylin and eosin stain. Mag. 132×.

CENTRAL NERVOUS SYSTEM 557

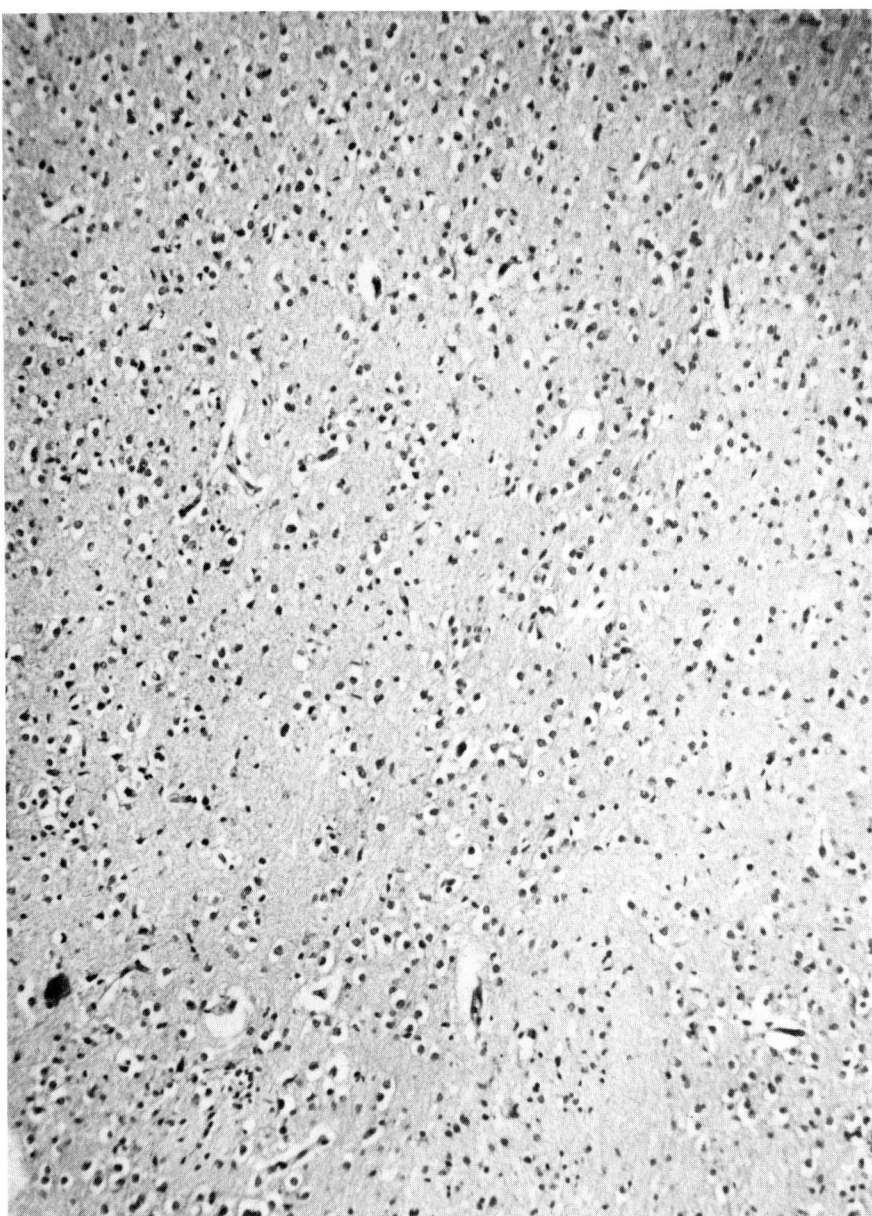

Figure 31–11

Figure 31–11. The infant from whom this section was taken was a female weighing 2,020 grams who lived for one hour and 15 minutes. The gestational age is unknown but was probably about 8 months.
Hematoxylin and eosin stain. Mag. 132×.

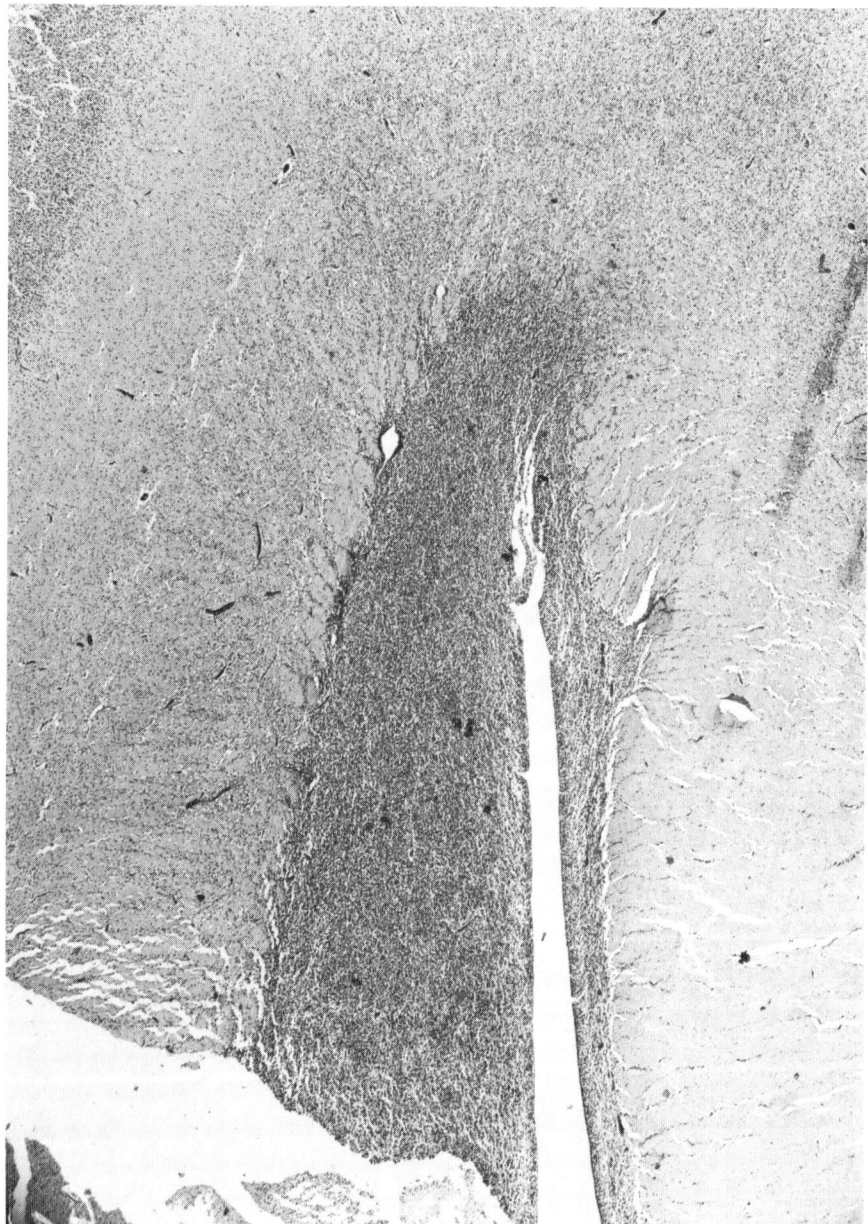

Figure 31–12

Figures 31–12 and 31–13. These two photomicrographs depict the typical glial mantle of the immature infant. It is a densely populated zone immediately adjacent to the lining of the lateral ventricle. The cells are predominantly glial cells that have not yet migrated away from that site into their definitive positions in the cerebral hemisphere.

CENTRAL NERVOUS SYSTEM 559

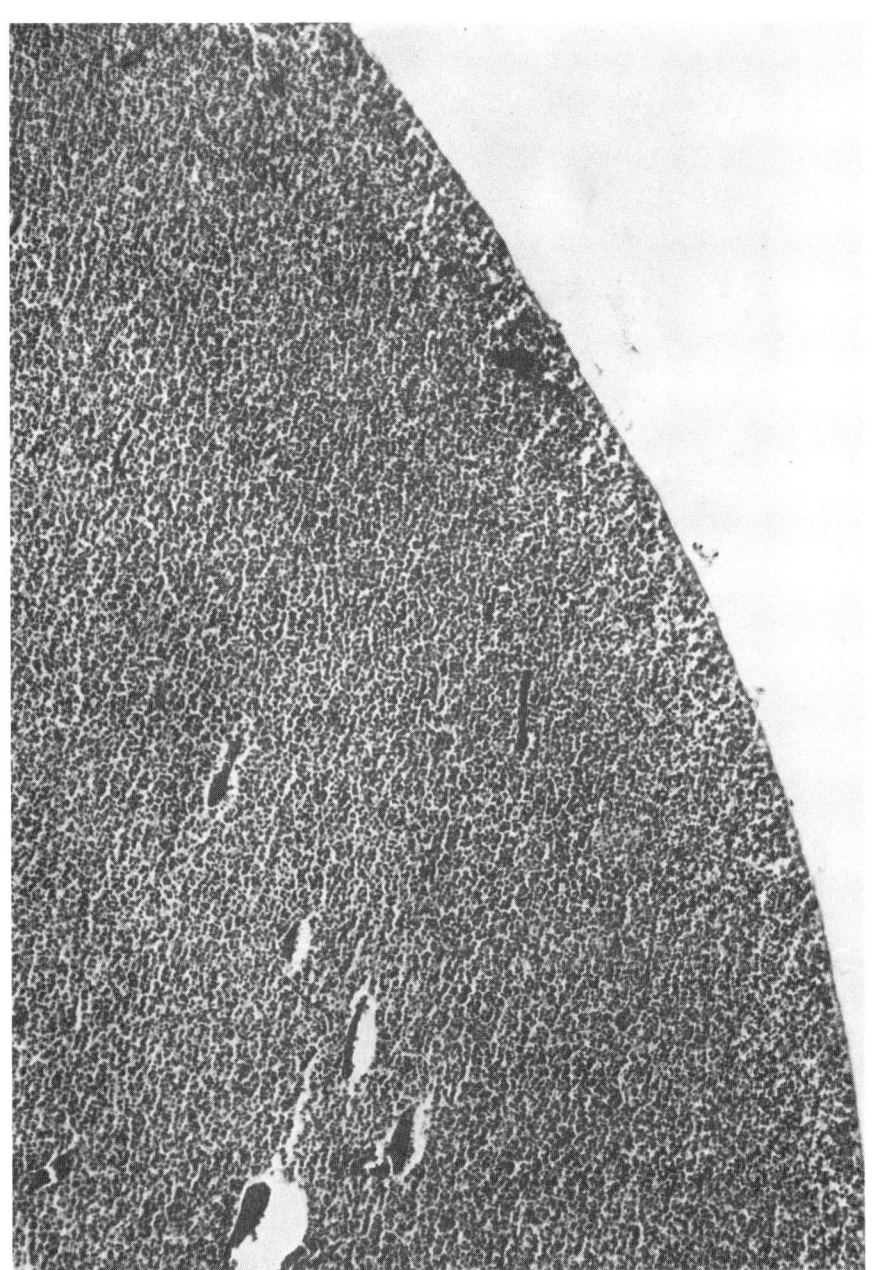

Figure 31–13

This infant was a black female weighing 340 grams at postmortem examination. She lived for two hours. Gestational age was 21–22 weeks.

Hematoxylin and eosin stain. Fig. 31–12: Mag. 45×.
Fig. 31–13: Mag. 132×.

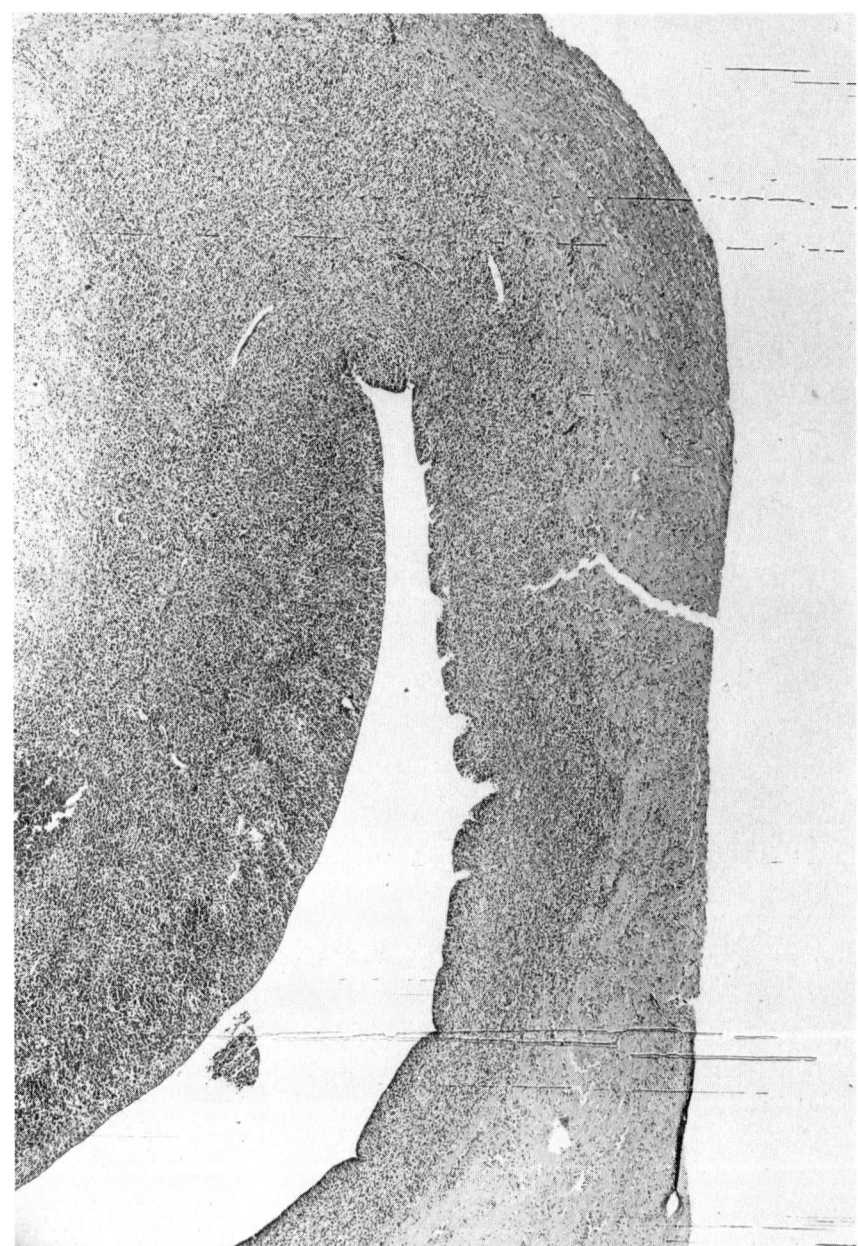

Figure 31–14

Figures 31–14 to 31–16. These three pictures illustrate the changing morphology in the immediate vicinity of the lateral ventricle during this period of life. The numbers of glial cells diminish as the infant matures.

Fig. 31–14 is from a 720 gram black male born in the sixth month of gestation, who lived for three hours and 30 minutes. Figs. 31–15 and 31–16 are from a 17 day old black female weighing 1800 grams, born in the 35th week of gestation.

Hematoxylin and eosin stain.
Fig. 31–14: Mag. 45×.
Fig. 31–15: Mag. 72×.
Fig. 31–16: Mag. 142×.

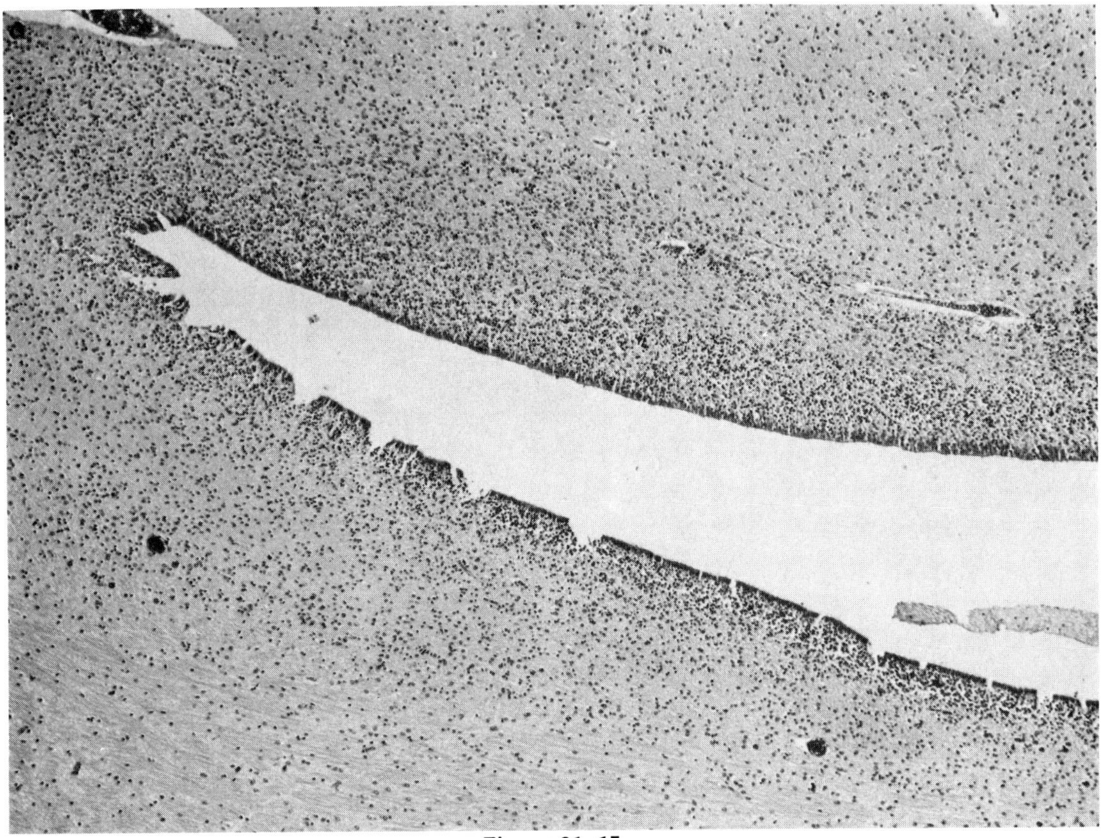

Figure 31–15

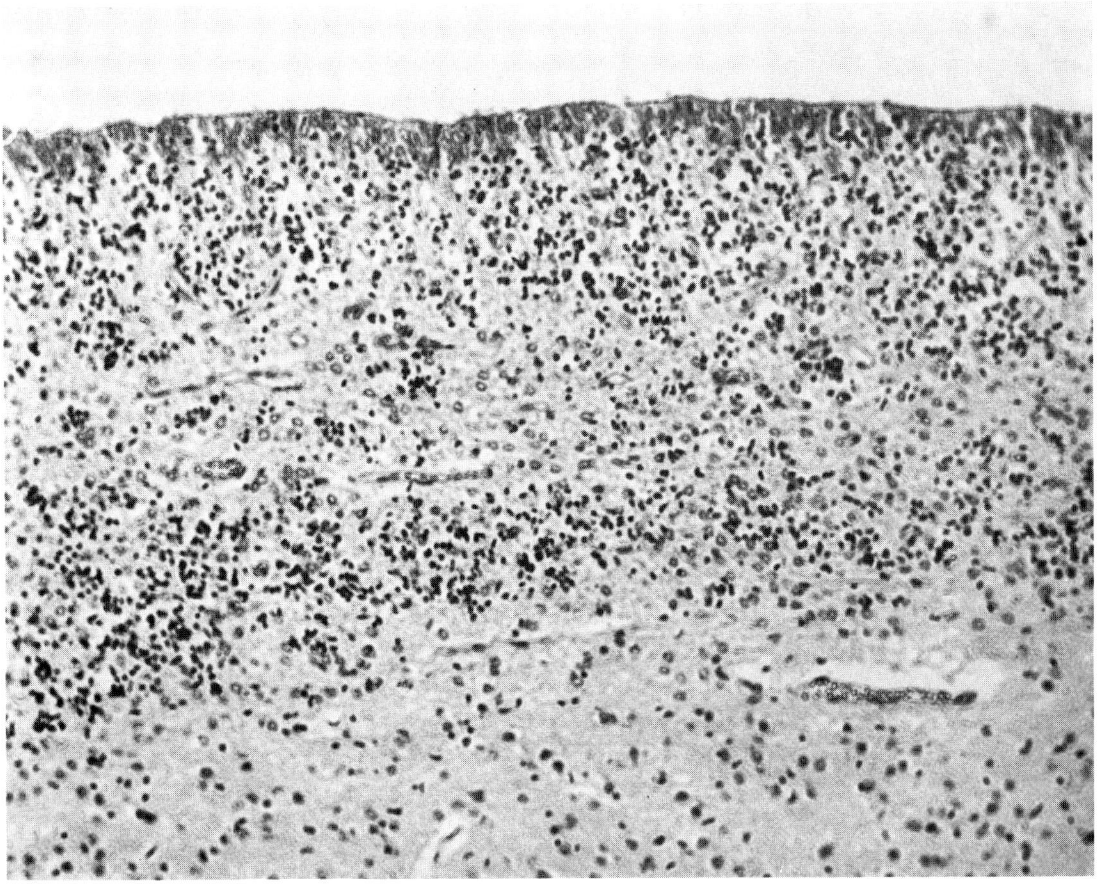

Figure 31–16

562 CENTRAL NERVOUS SYSTEM

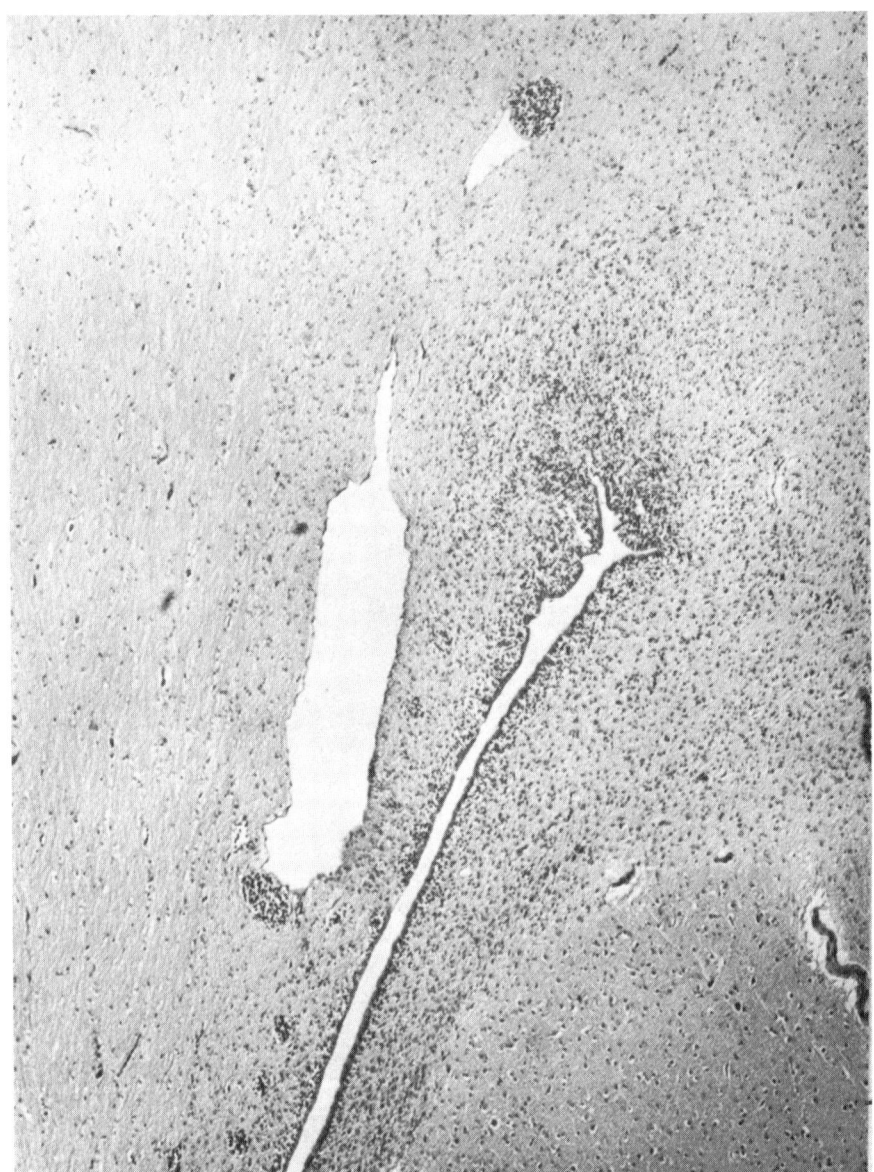

Figure 31–17

Figures 31–17 to 31–19. These three sections, taken in the coronal plane, illustrate the angle of the lateral ventricle in three progressively more mature infants. Fig. 31–17 is from an immature infant, and it shows dark clusters of glial cells that have not yet migrated away from that vicinity; two such aggregates are adjacent to vessels and others are nestled near the angle itself. No such clusters are seen in the ensuing two photographs.

Figure 31–17. Black female, 1 hour old; 40 weeks of gestation; 3,200 grams. Mag. 45×.

Figure 31–18. Black male, 5 days old; 43 weeks of gestation; 3,460 grams. Mag. 45×.

Figure 31–19. Black female, 2 hours 35 minutes old; 40 weeks of gestation; 4,815 grams. Mag. 18×.
Hematoxylin and eosin stain.

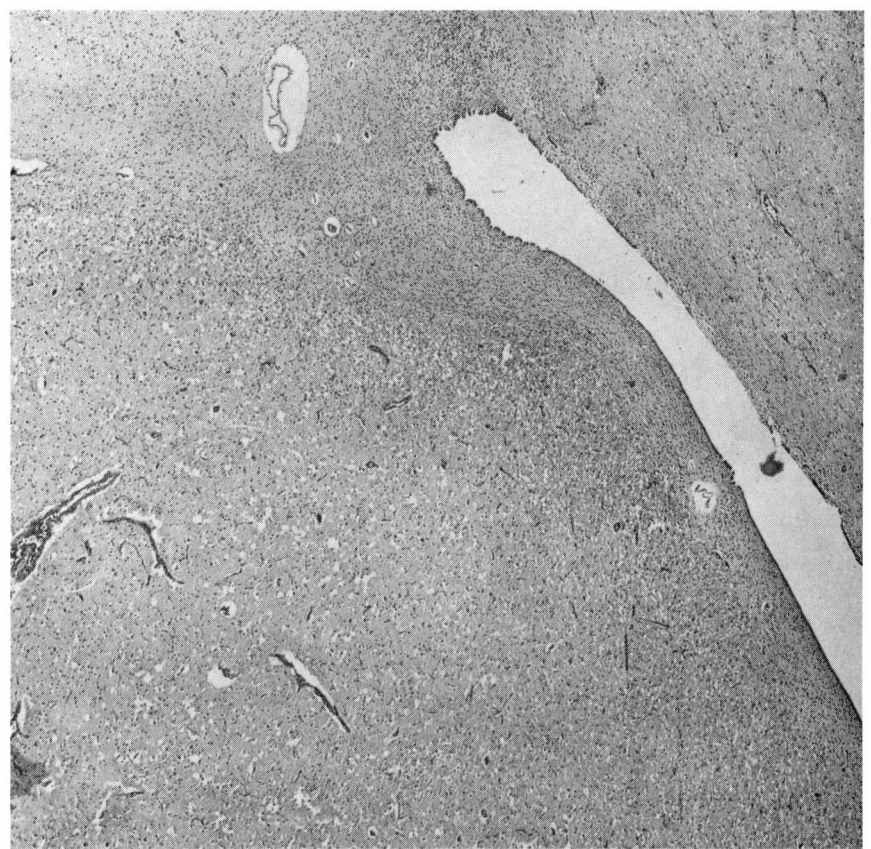

Figure 31–18

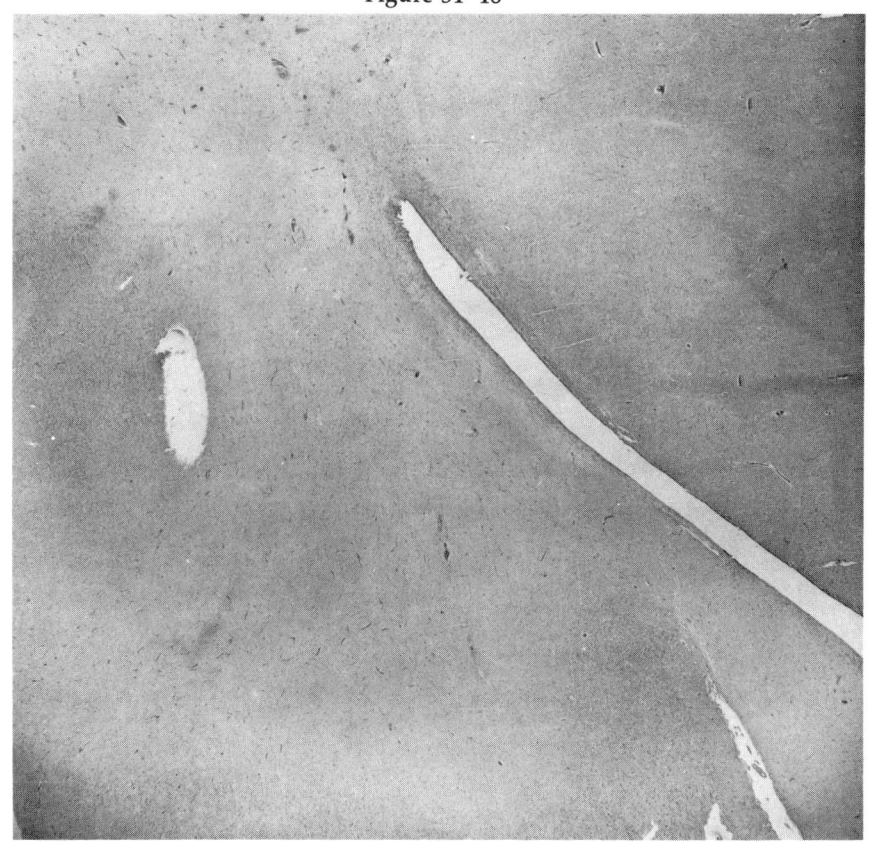

Figure 31–19

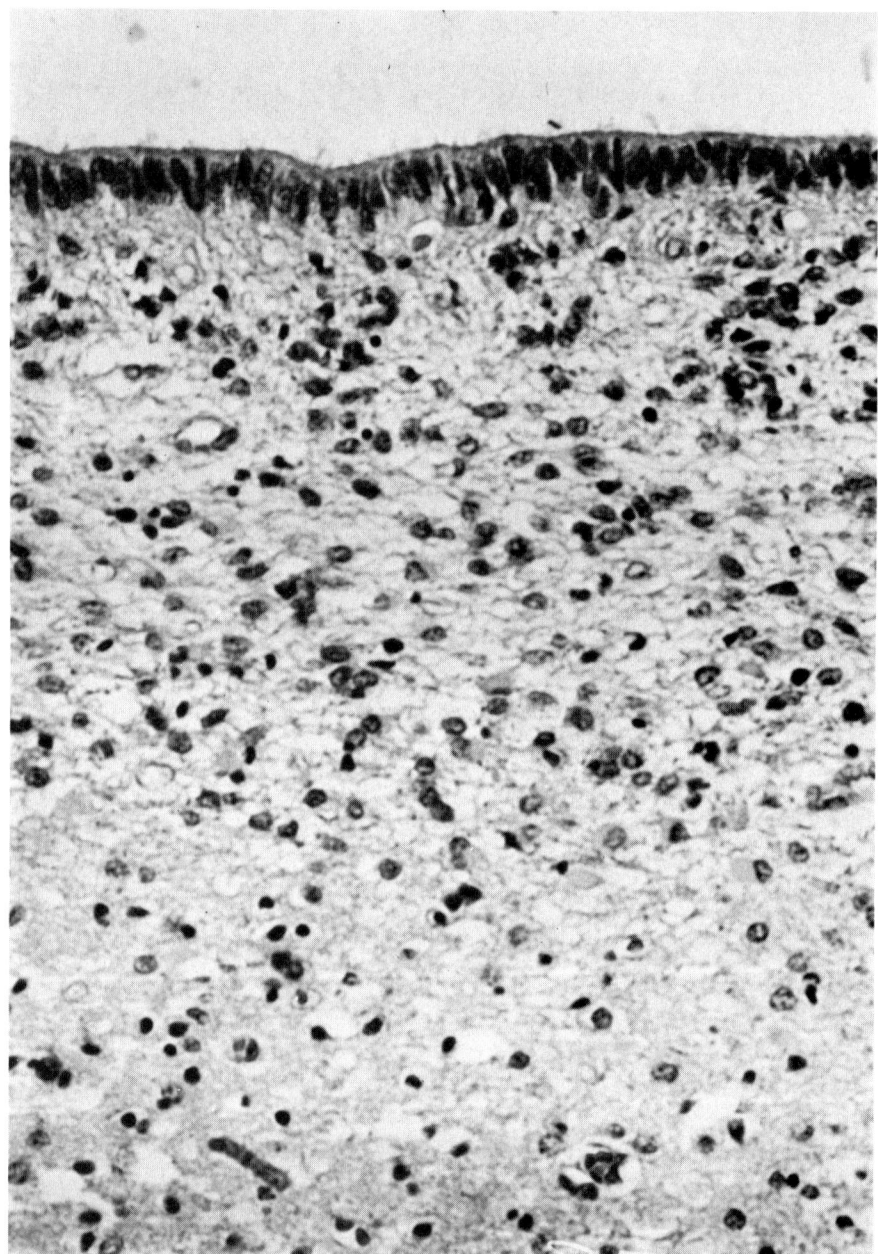

Figure 31–20

Figure 31–20. This figure illustrates, at high magnification, the nature of the ependymal cells lining the lateral ventricle. The cilia are quite evident.

This patient was a five day old black male whose body at autopsy weighed 3,460 grams. He was said to have been born in the 43rd week of gestation.

Hematoxylin and eosin stain. Mag. 660×.

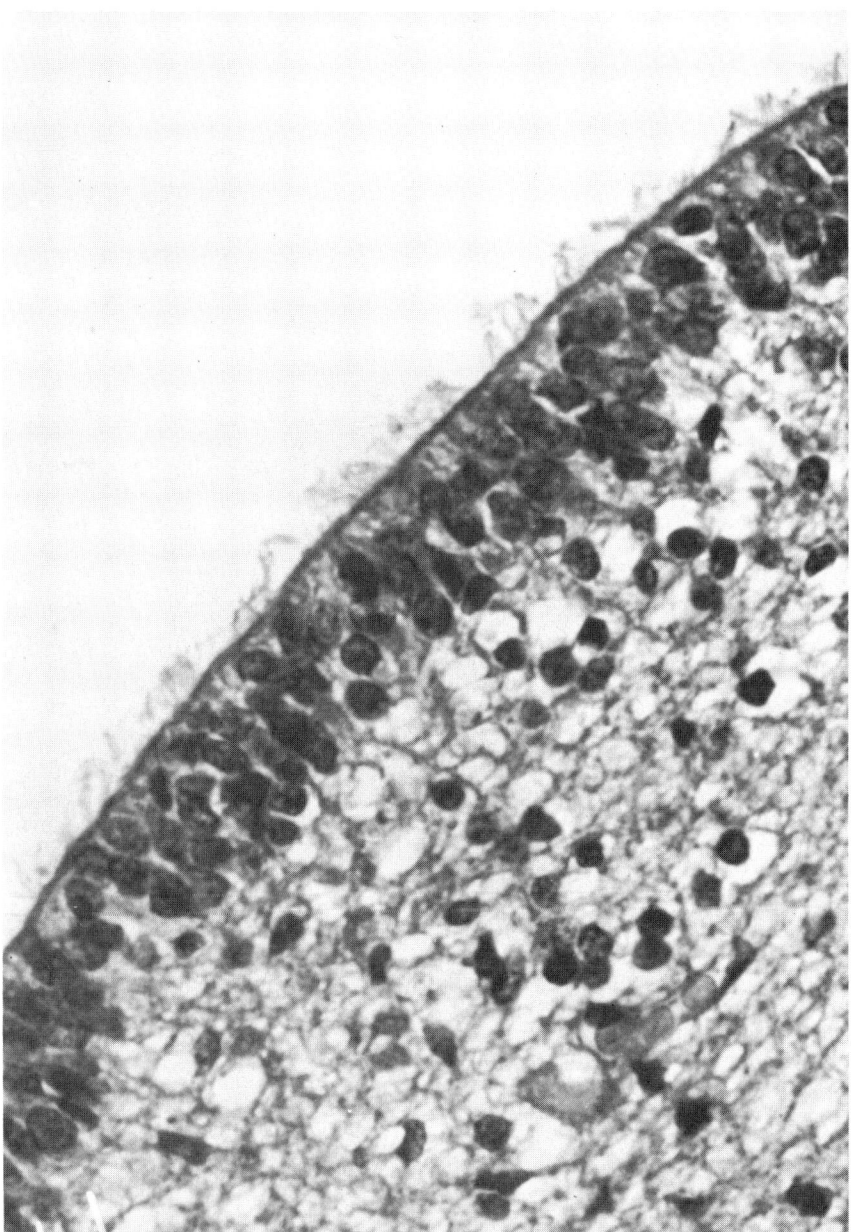

Figure 31-21

Figure 31-21. This illustration depicts the ependymal lining and the wall of the lateral ventricle in an infant born at term. It was taken from the same patient described in Fig. 31-20. Hematoxylin and eosin stain. Mag. 382×.

566 CENTRAL NERVOUS SYSTEM

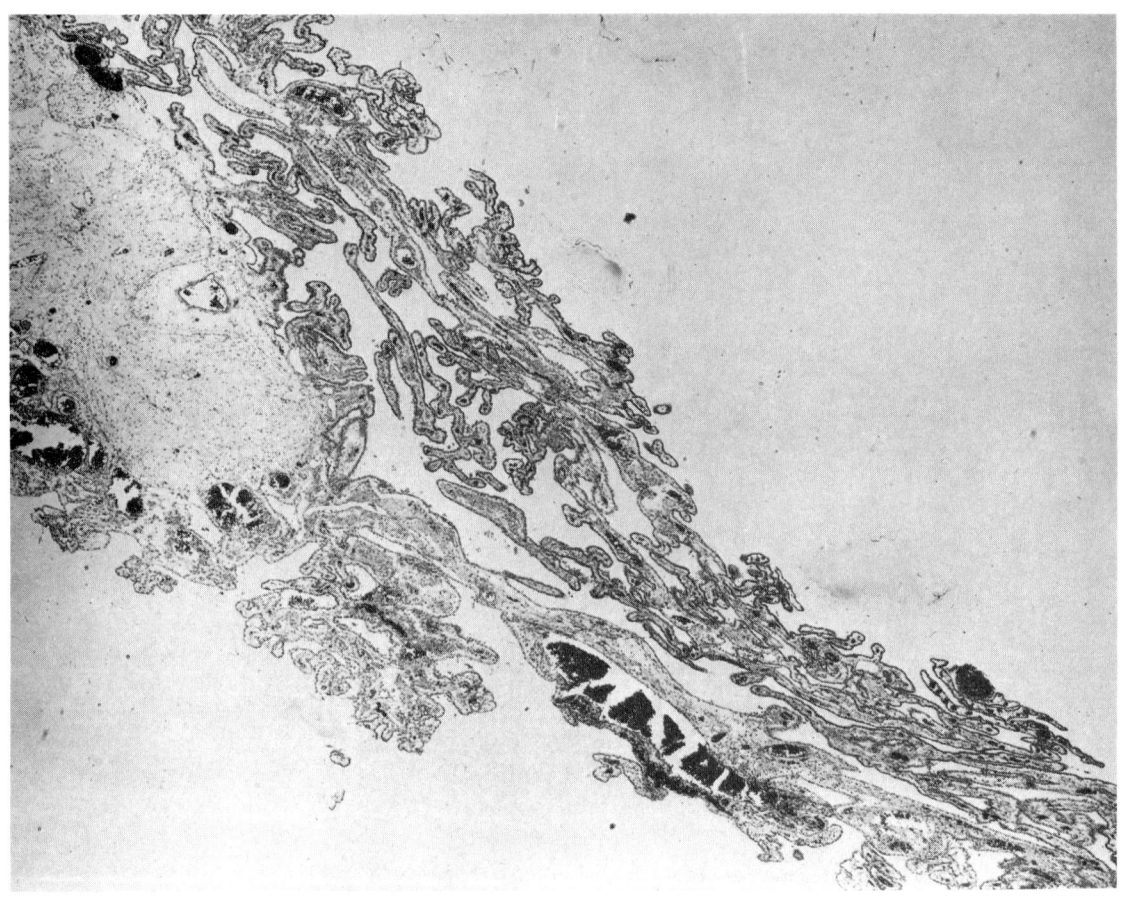

Figure 31–22

Figures 31–22 to 31–24. At low, medium, and high magnification, these three illustrations show the morphologic characteristics of the choroid plexus of the premature infant.

Figure 31–22. The choroid plexus from the lateral ventricle of a 710 gram male infant who lived for 2 days and 17 hours. Mag. 43×.

Figure 31–23. The choroid plexus of a 720 gram black male who survived for 3 hours and 30 minutes. Mag. 76×.

Figure 31–24. Specimen from a stillborn 200 gram female infant. Mag. 132×.

Hematoxylin and eosin stain.

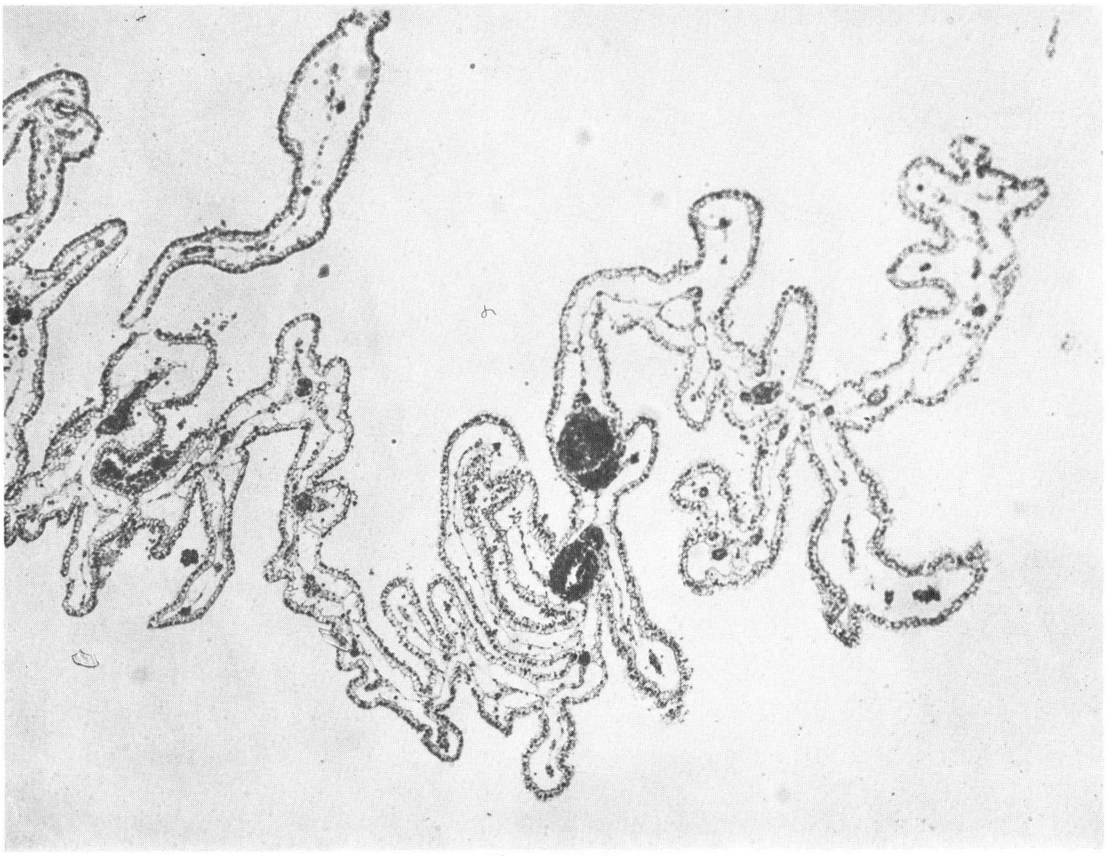

Figure 31-23

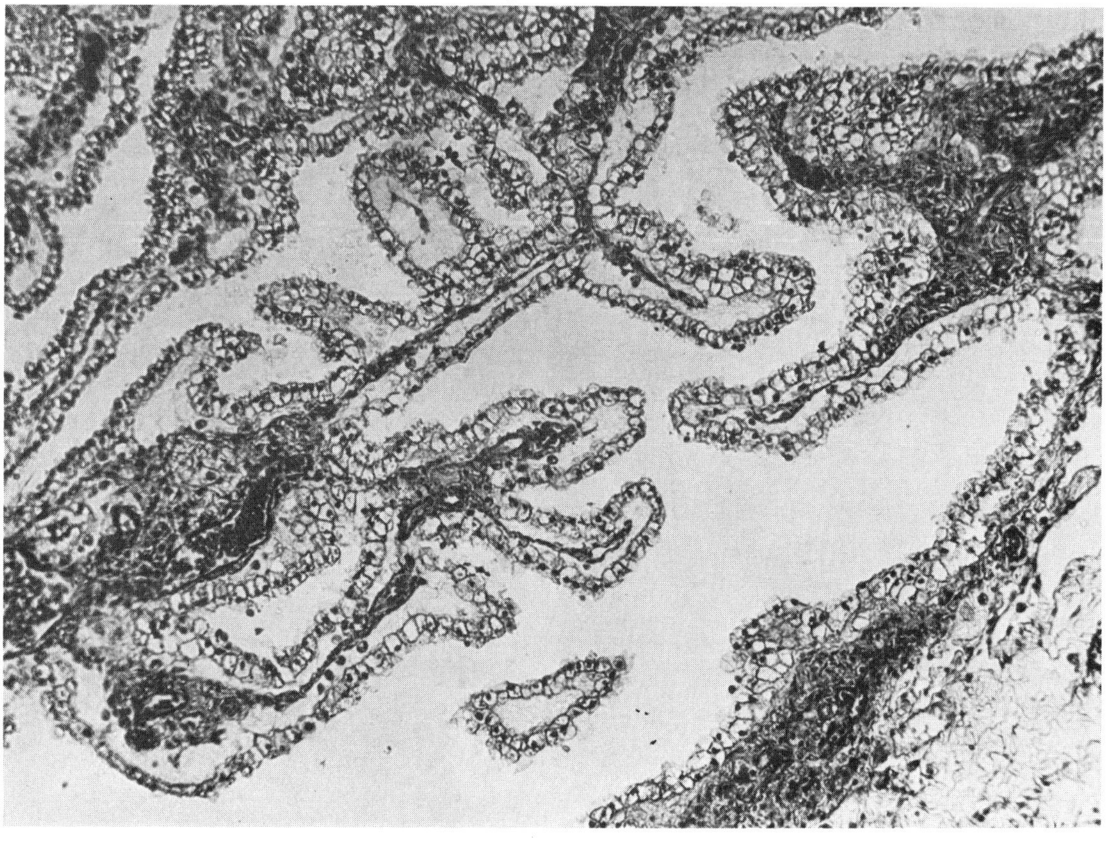

Figure 31-24

568 CENTRAL NERVOUS SYSTEM

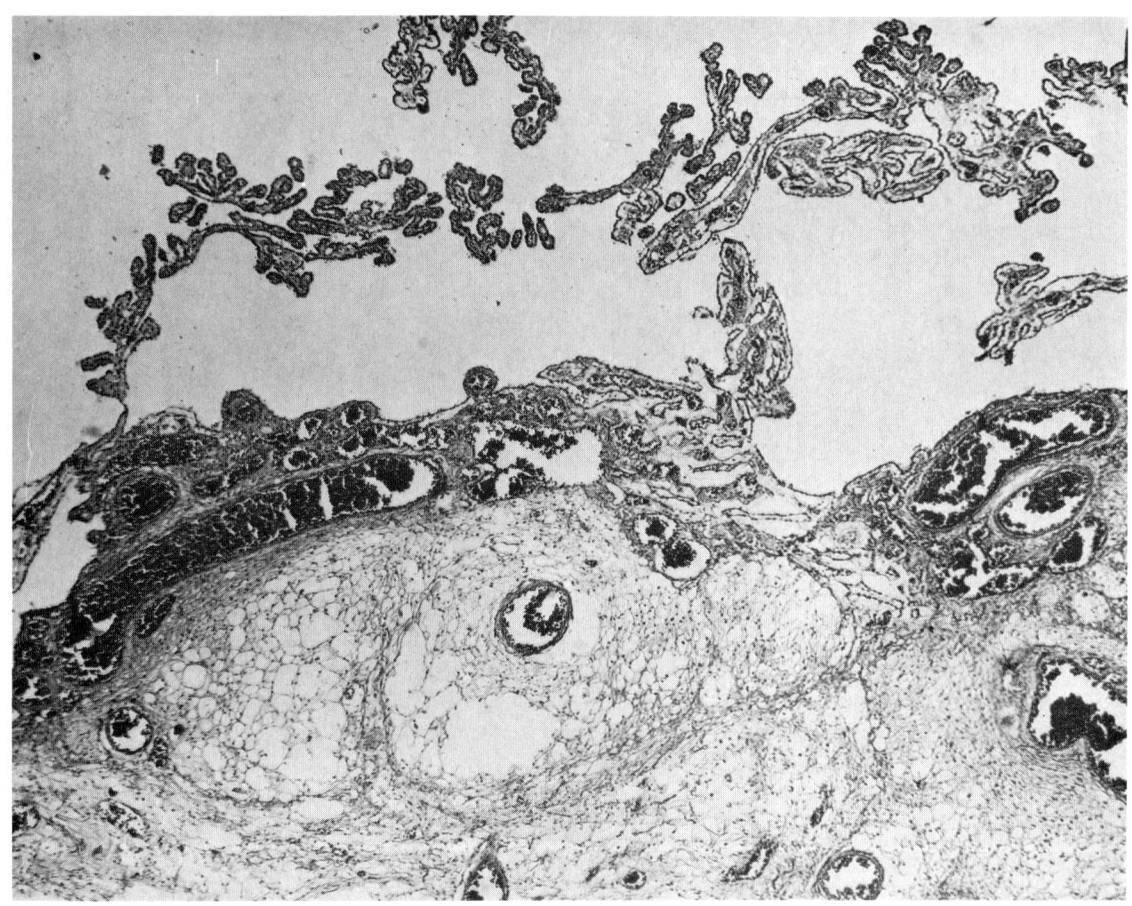

Figure 31–25

Figures 31–25 to 31–27. This set of three photomicrographs illustrates the histologic appearance of the choroid plexus in infants near term.

Figure 31–25. Black male, 5 days old; 43 weeks of gestation; 3,460 grams. Mag. 45×.

Figure 31–26. Male, stillborn; term delivery; 3,250 grams. Mag. 60×.

Figure 31–27. Same infant as Fig. 31–26. Mag. 471×.
Hematoxylin and eosin stain.

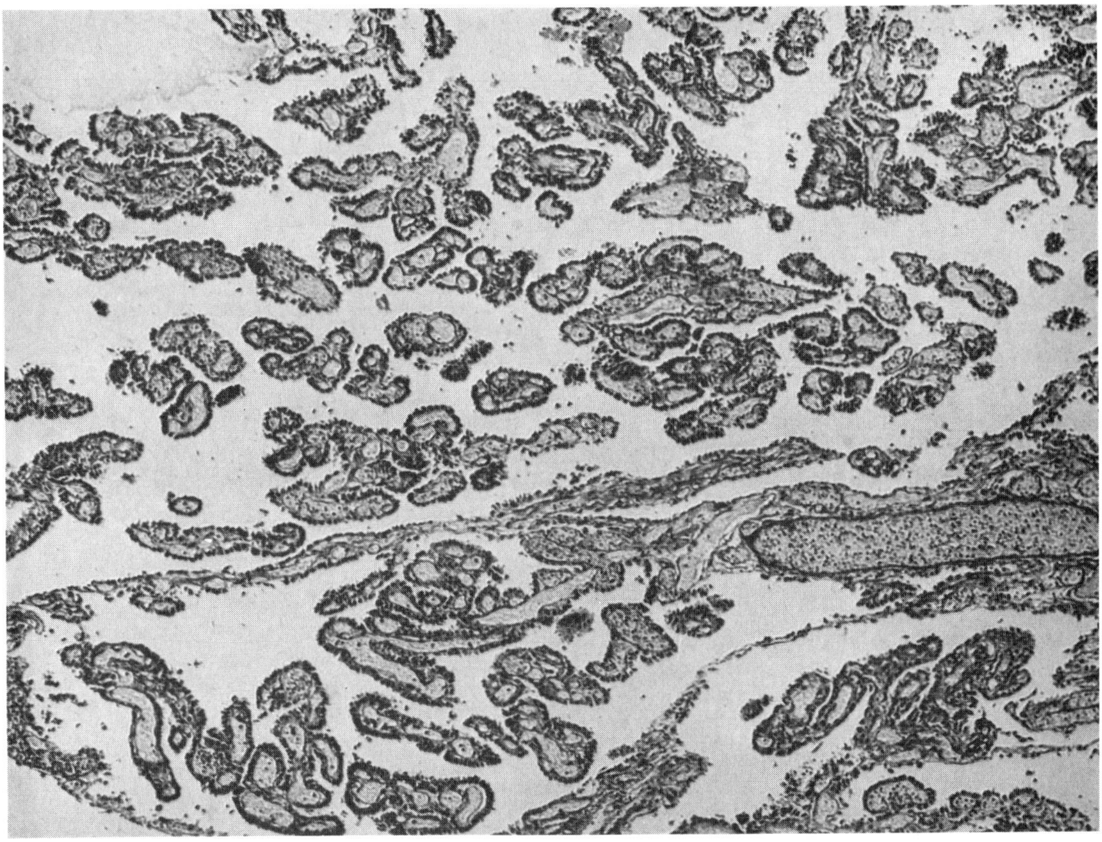

Figure 31-26

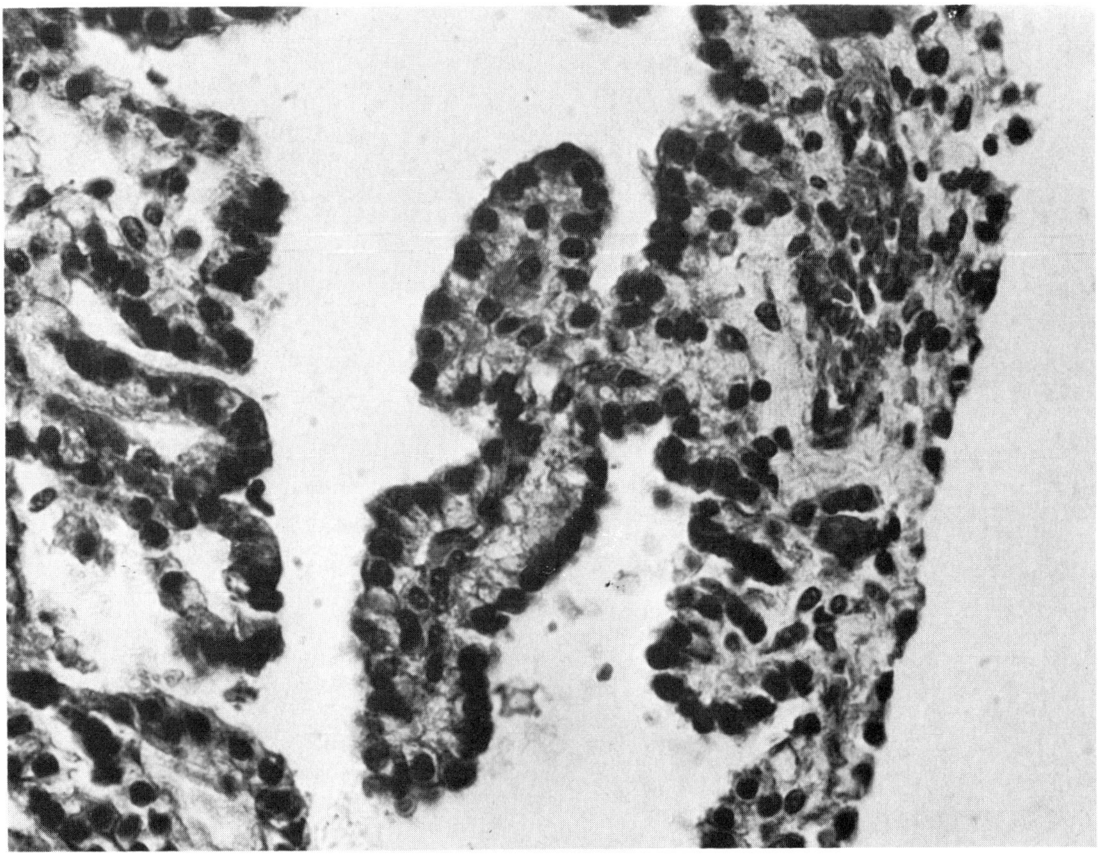

Figure 31-27

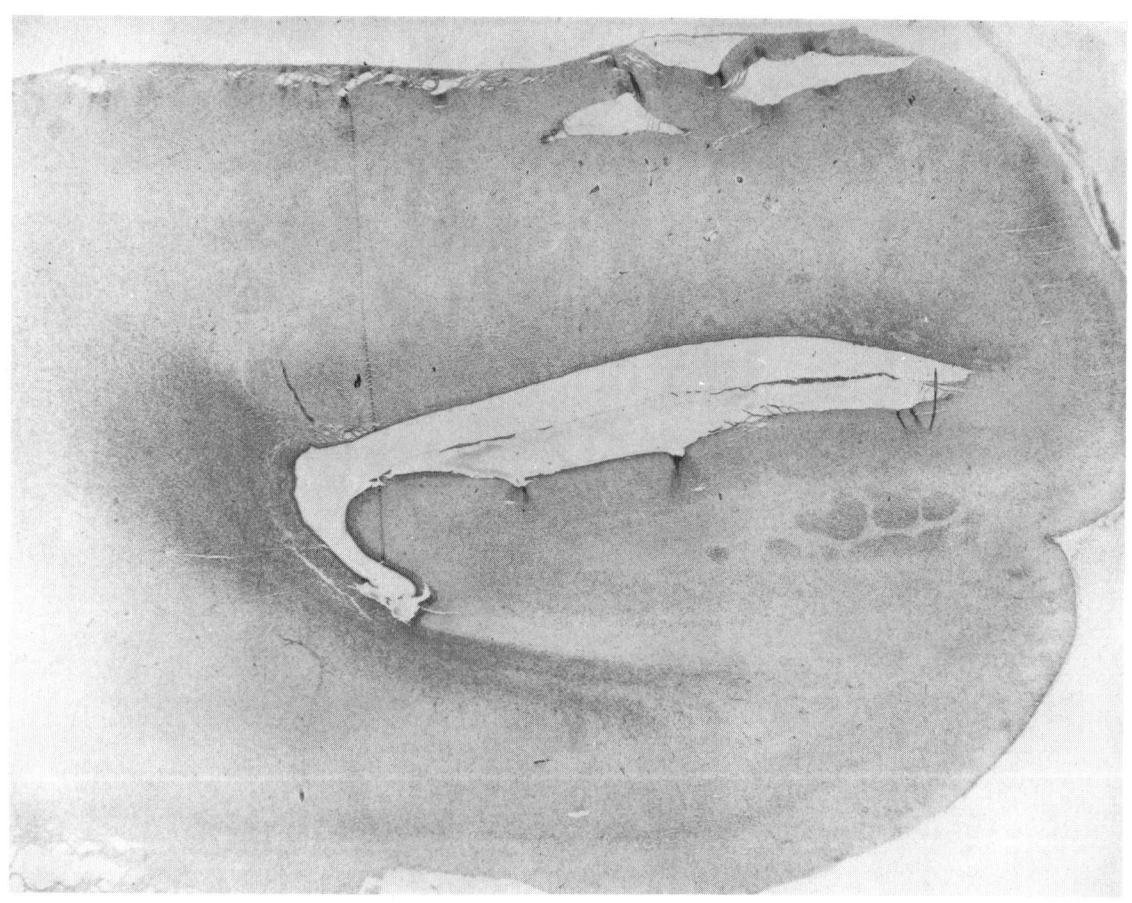

Figure 31–28

Figures 31–28 and 31–29. This pair of photographs, taken from the same section at different degrees of magnification, illustrate the hippocampus of an infant born prematurely in the 30th week of gestation. The section is taken in the coronal plane.

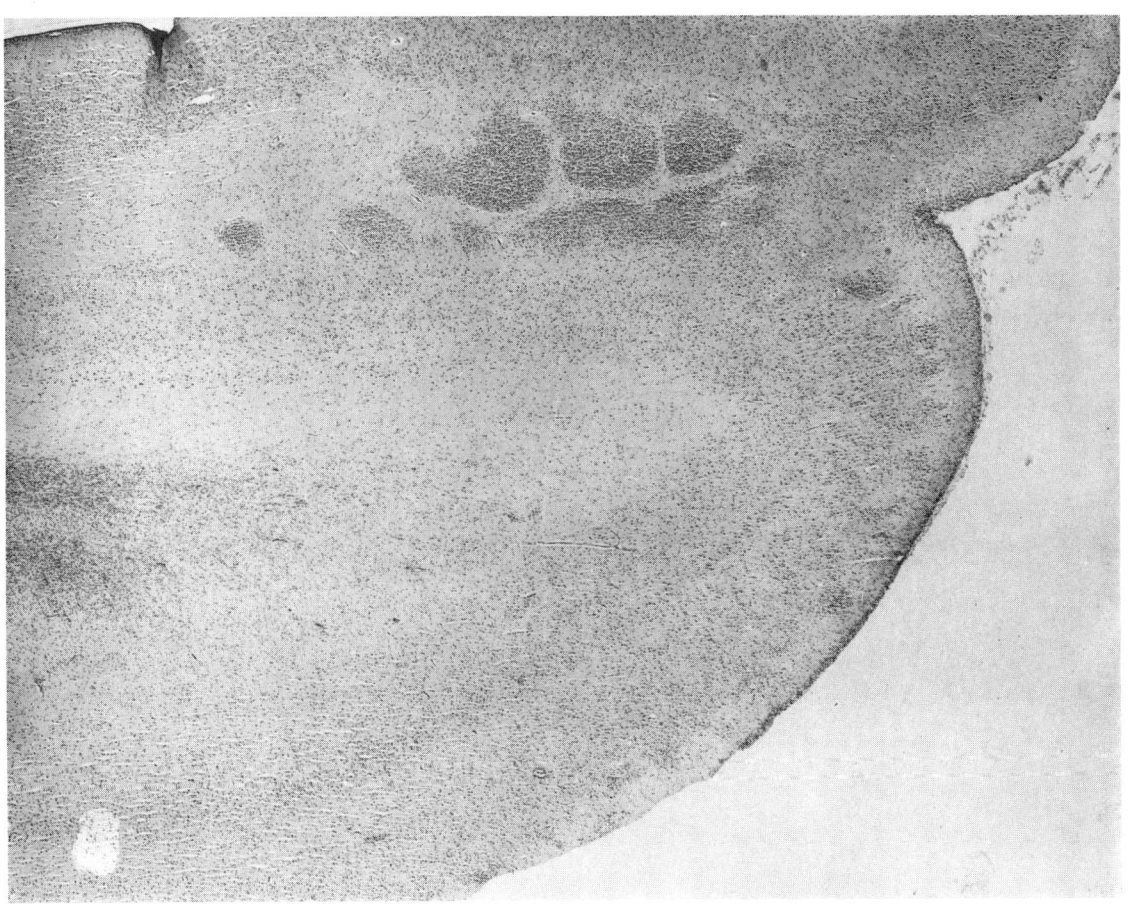

Figure 31–29

The baby was a black male, of 30 weeks gestation, whose body weighed 1,070 grams at autopsy. The infant lived for 4 hours.
Hematoxylin and eosin stain.
Fig. 31–28: Mag. 20.8×.
Fig. 31–29: Mag. 45×.

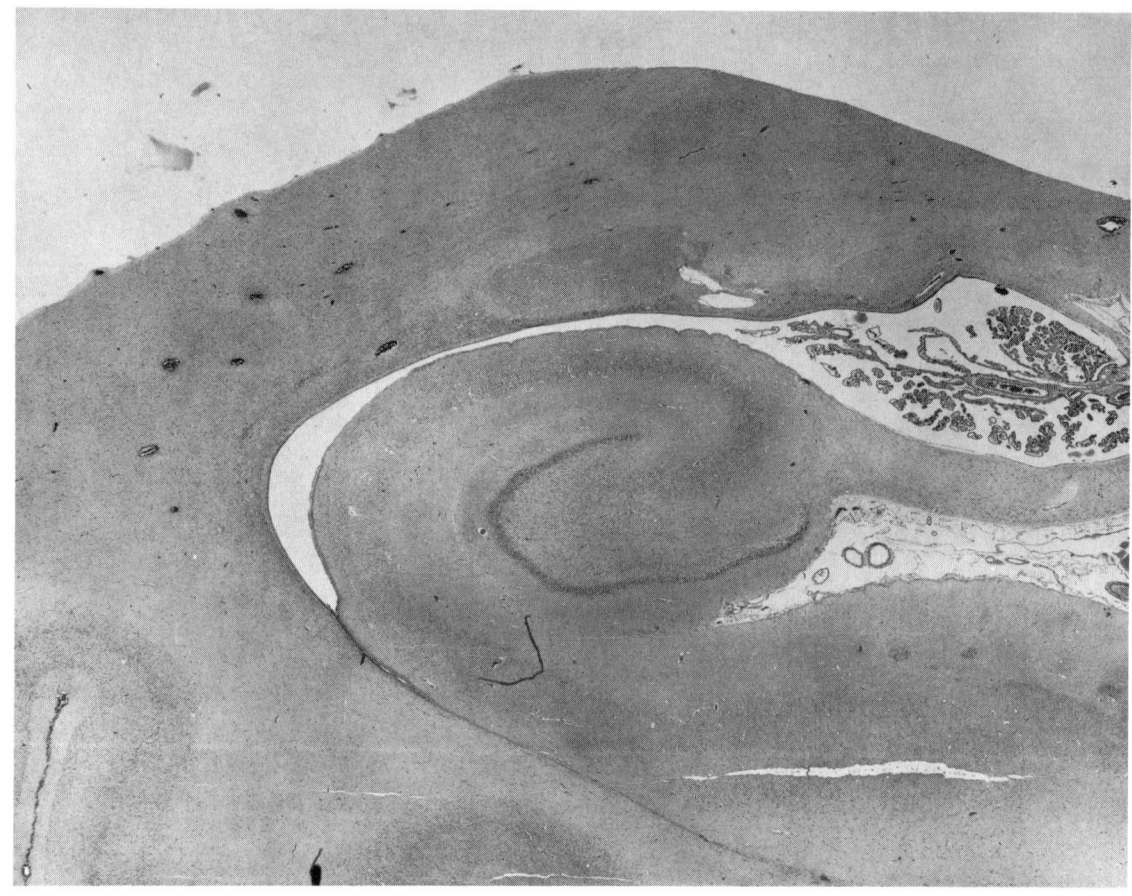

Figure 31–30

Figures 31–30 and 31–31. By contrast with the two preceding photographs, these two depict the hippocampus of an infant born at term. The structure has clearly evolved through time.

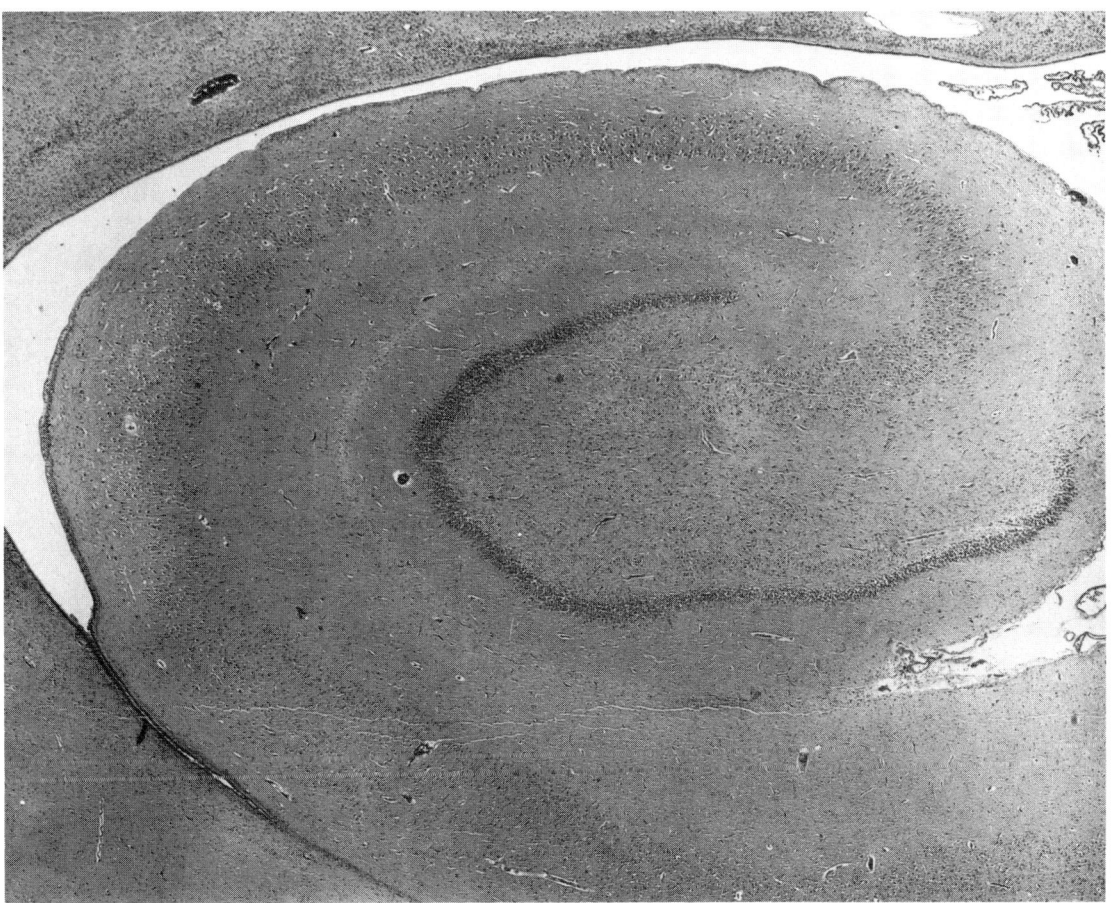

Figure 31–31

This infant was a black female of 40 weeks gestation who lived for one hour and 12 minutes. At postmortem examination, the body weighed 3,200 grams.

Hematoxylin and eosin stain.
Fig. 31–30: Mag. 20.8×.
Fig. 31–31: Mag. 45×.

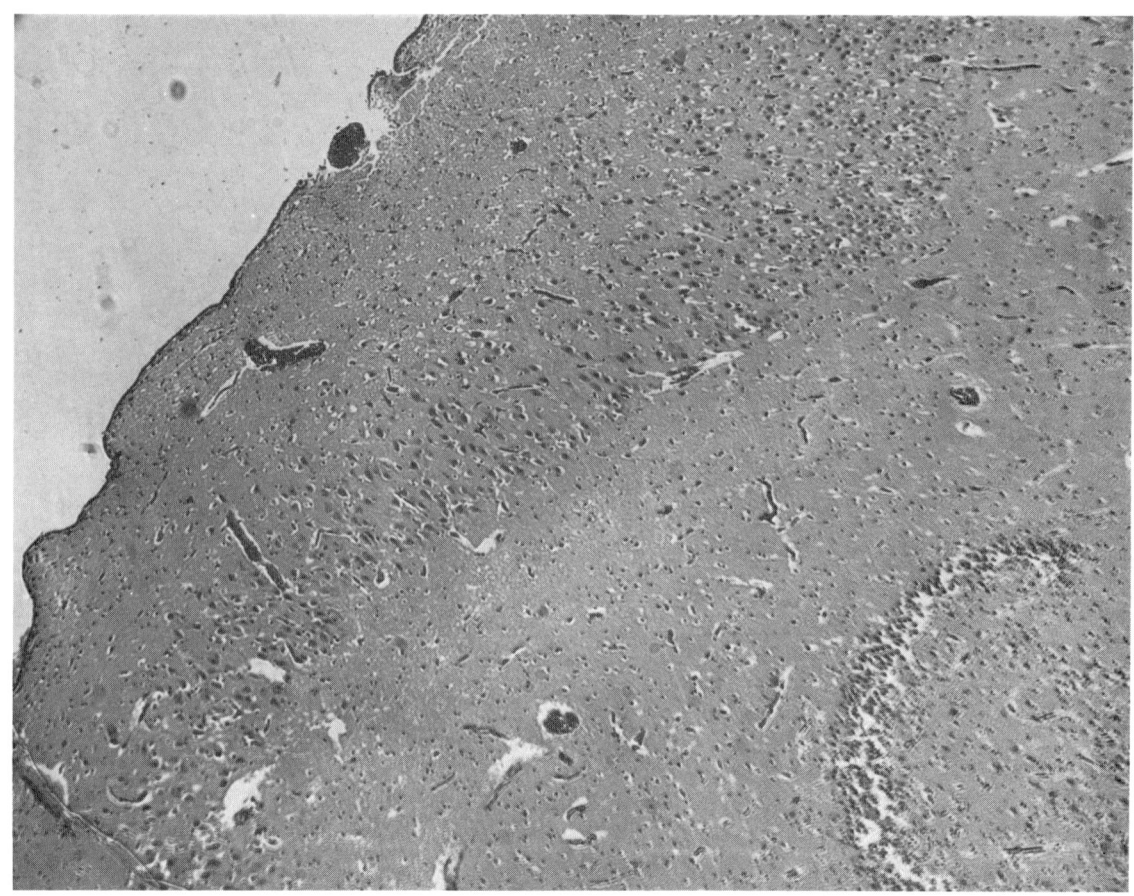

Figure 31–32

Figures 31–32 to 31–34. Taken at progressively higher magnification, these three illustrations show the cells of the hippocampus.

The first and the third sections (Figs. 31–32 and 31–34) are from the same infant, a stillborn black male weighing 2,100 grams, born in about the eighth month of gestation.

Fig. 31–33 is from a 3,470 gram stillborn black male, delivered at term.

Hematoxylin and eosin stain.

Fig. 31–32: Mag. 60×.
Fig. 31–33: Mag. 100×.
Fig. 31–34: Mag. 250×.

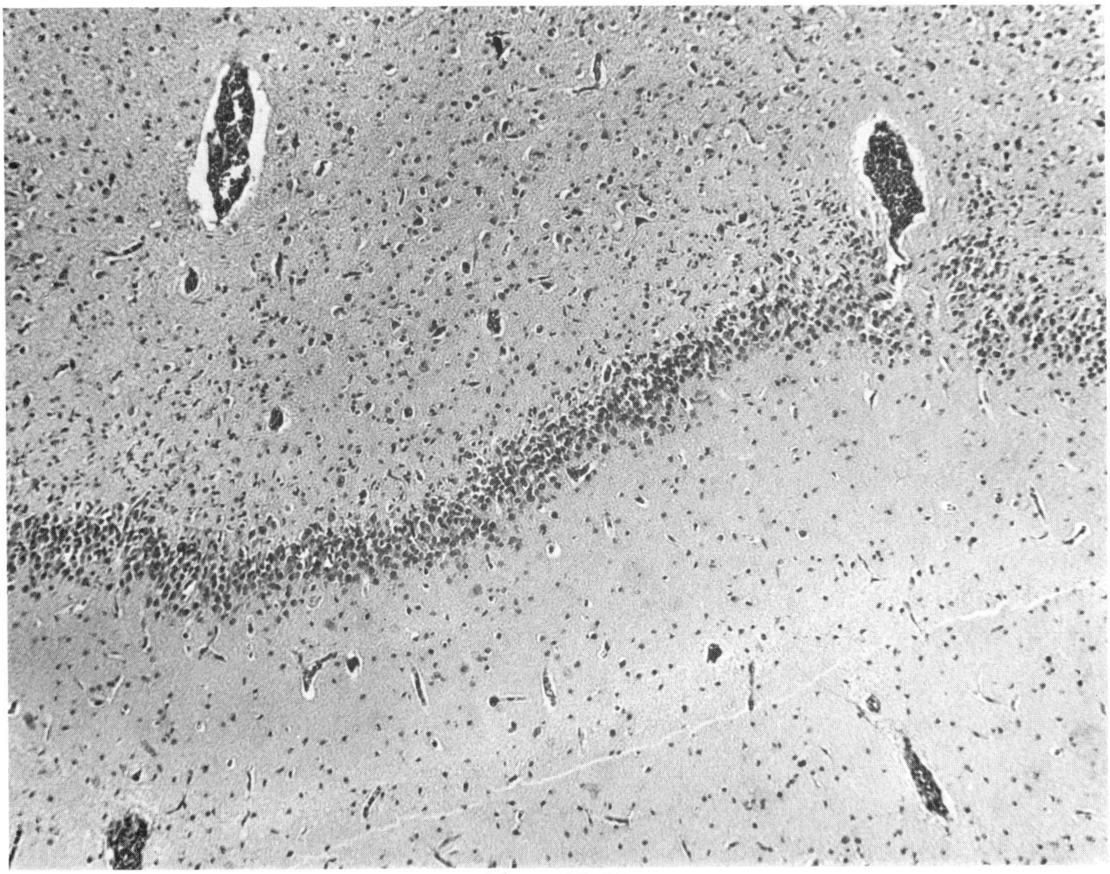

Figure 31–33

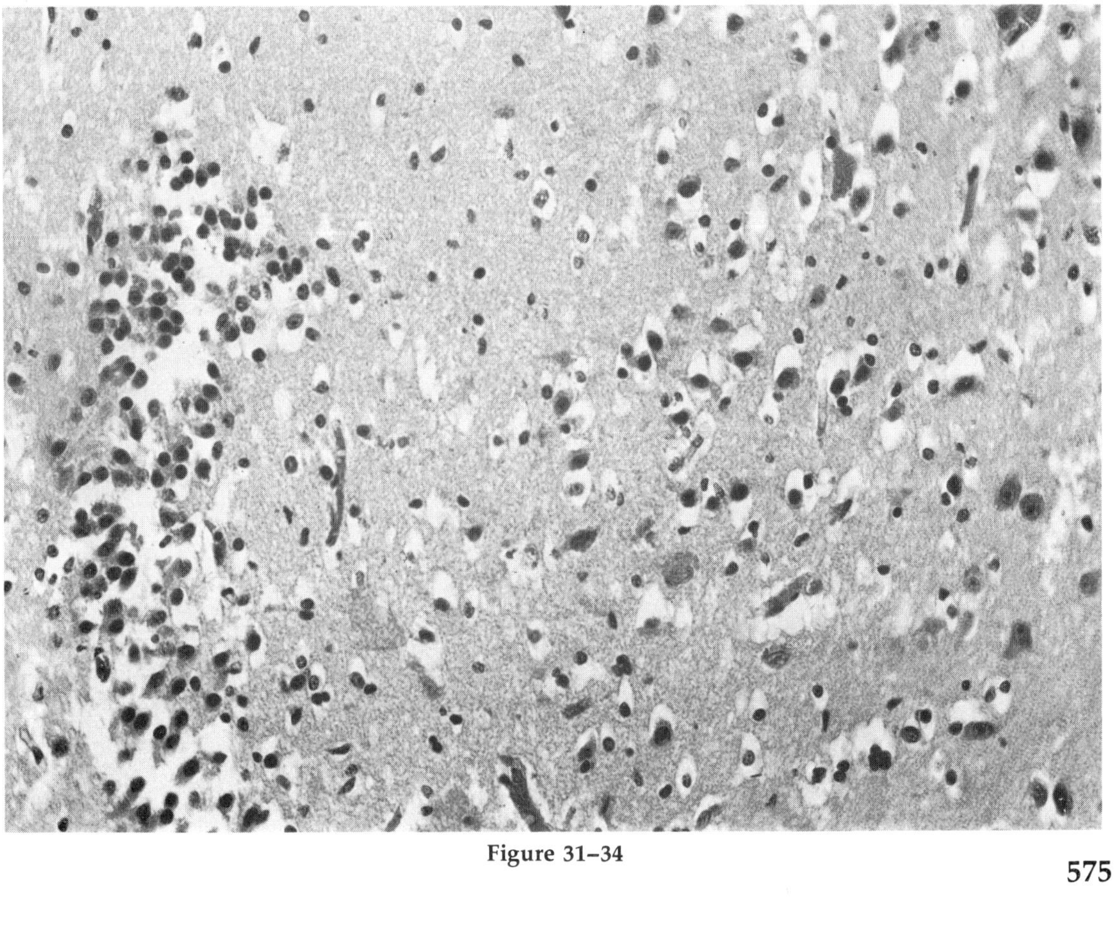

Figure 31–34

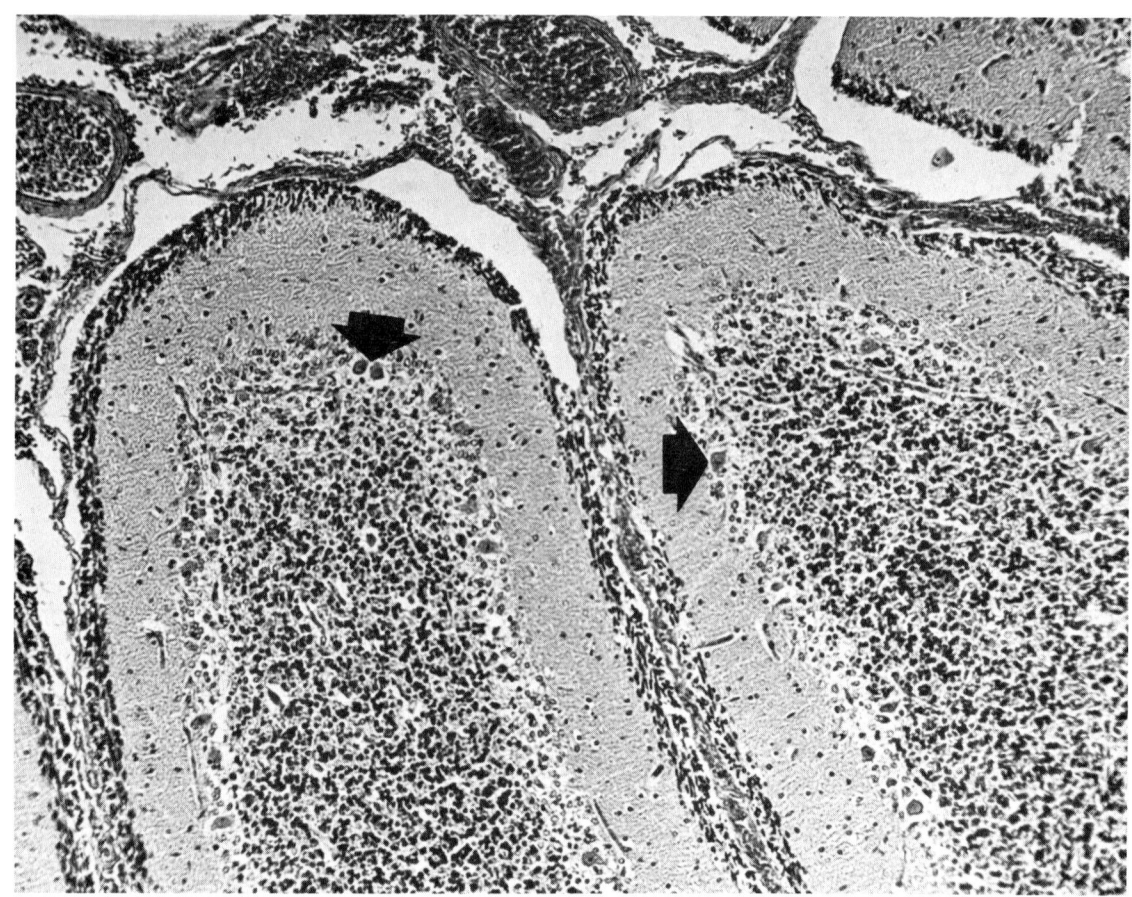

Figure 31–35

Figure 31–35. Two cerebellar folia are depicted here. These are from an infant born in approximately the 33rd week of gestation. This infant lived for 7½ hours.

Marked with arrows are two of the Purkinje cells in these folia, situated at the junction of the pale-staining molecular layer and the more darkly stained granular layer, internally.

Hematoxylin and eosin stain. Mag. 132×.

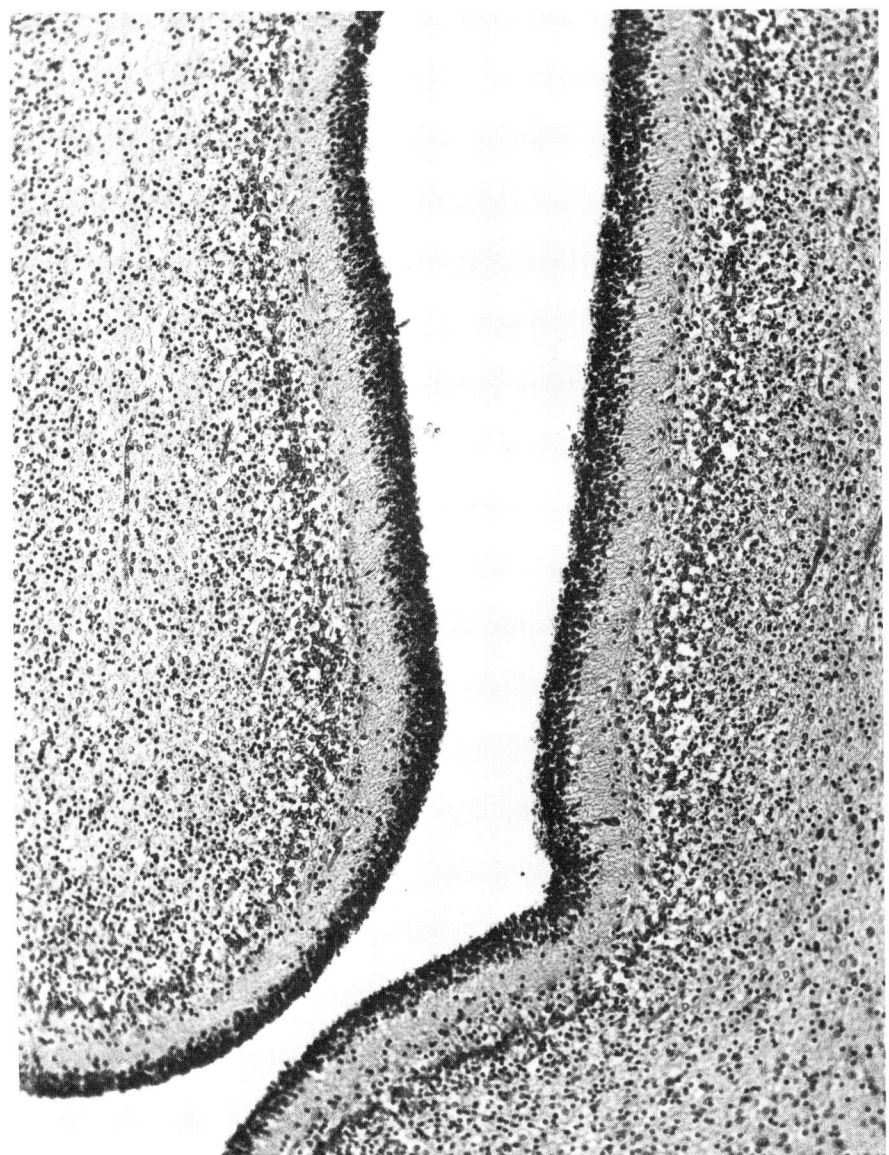

Figure 31–36

Figure 31–36. This is a section of parts of two adjacent cerebellar folia from an infant born in approximately the seventh month of gestation.

In the folium on the left, white matter is seen at the edge of the photograph; the grey ribbon of cells to its right represents the granular layer and the pale, relatively non-cellular layer to the right of that, the molecular layer. Purkinje cells are located between those two.

This infant's body weighed 1,505 grams at autopsy.

Hematoxylin and eosin stain. Mag. 164×.

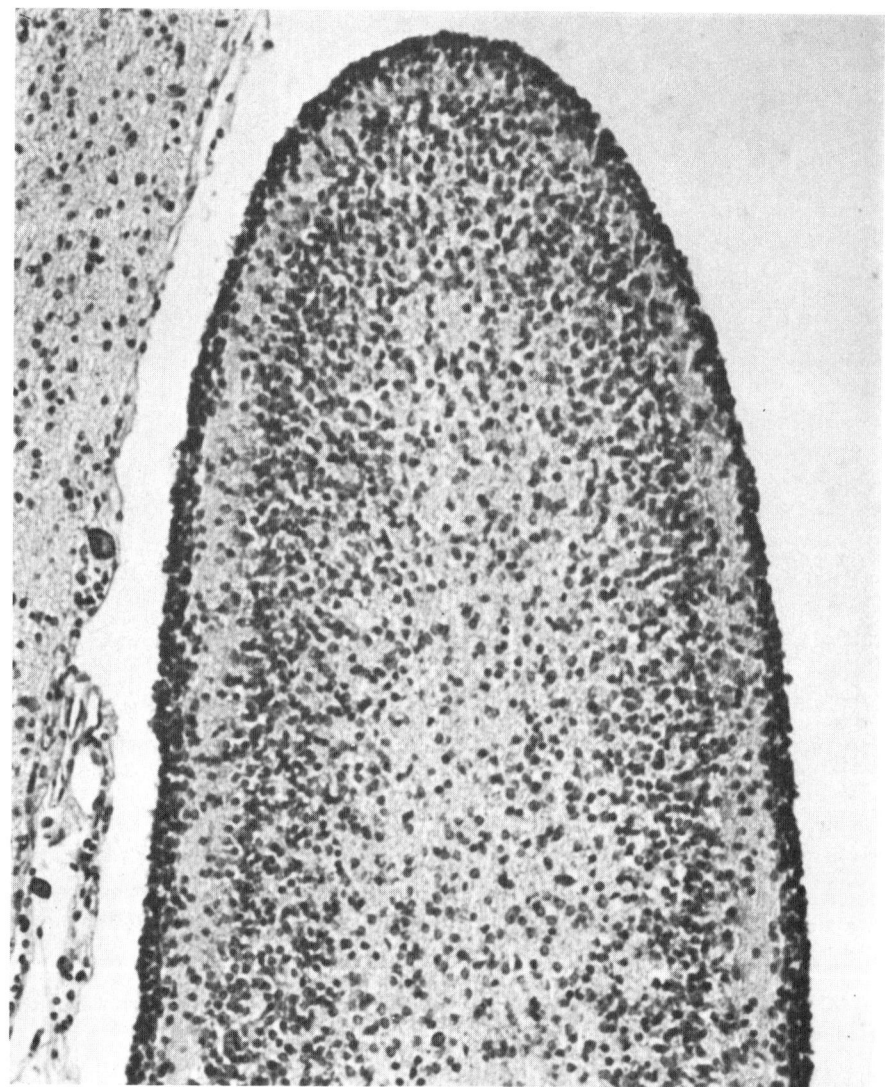

Figure 31-37

Figures 31-37 to 31-39. These three photographs show folia in three different infants in different stages of perinatal development.

Figure 31-37. This is from an infant weighing only 512 grams, a black female who lived for 27 hours. She was born in the 16th week of gestation. Mag. 132×.

Figure 31-38. This infant was a black male weighing 2,460 grams who lived for seven hours and 30 minutes. Gestational age was probably near term. Mag. 267×.

Figure 31-39. This black female infant weighed 4,815 grams at autopsy. She lived for two hours and 35 minutes. Her gestational age is unknown but was probably near term. Mag. 45×. Hematoxylin and eosin stain.

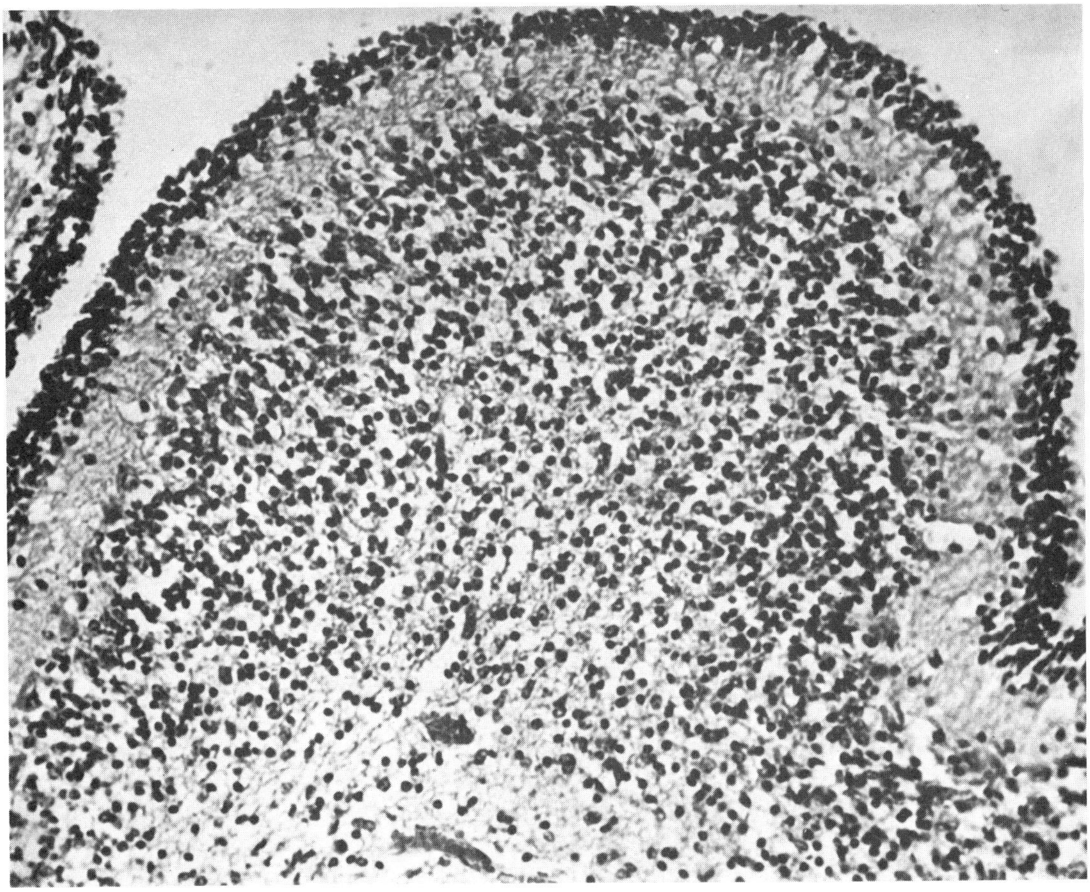

Figure 31–38

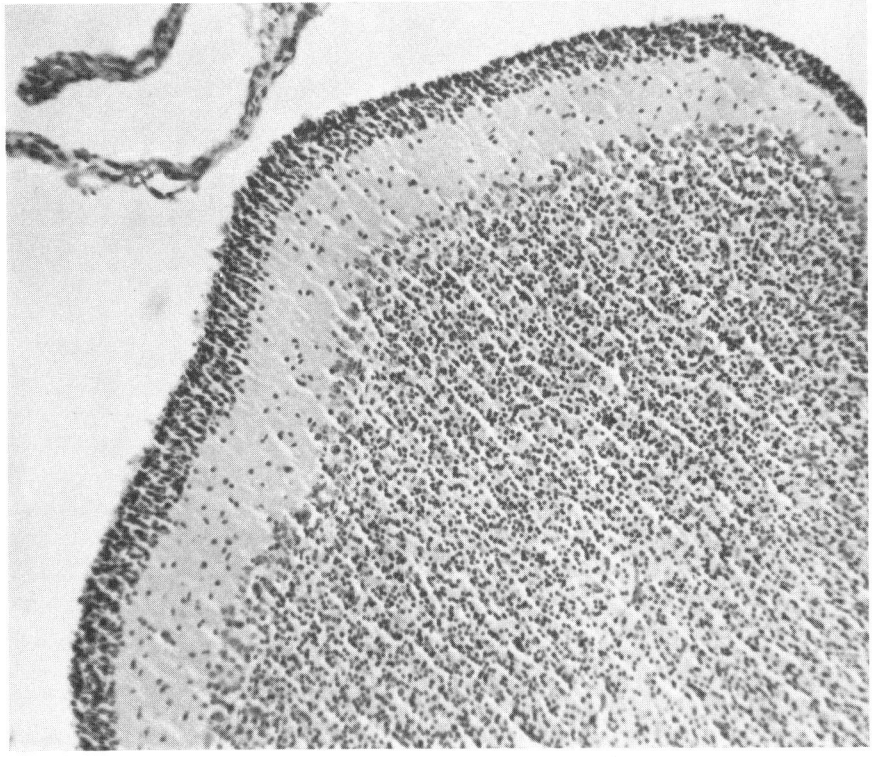

Figure 31–39

580 CENTRAL NERVOUS SYSTEM

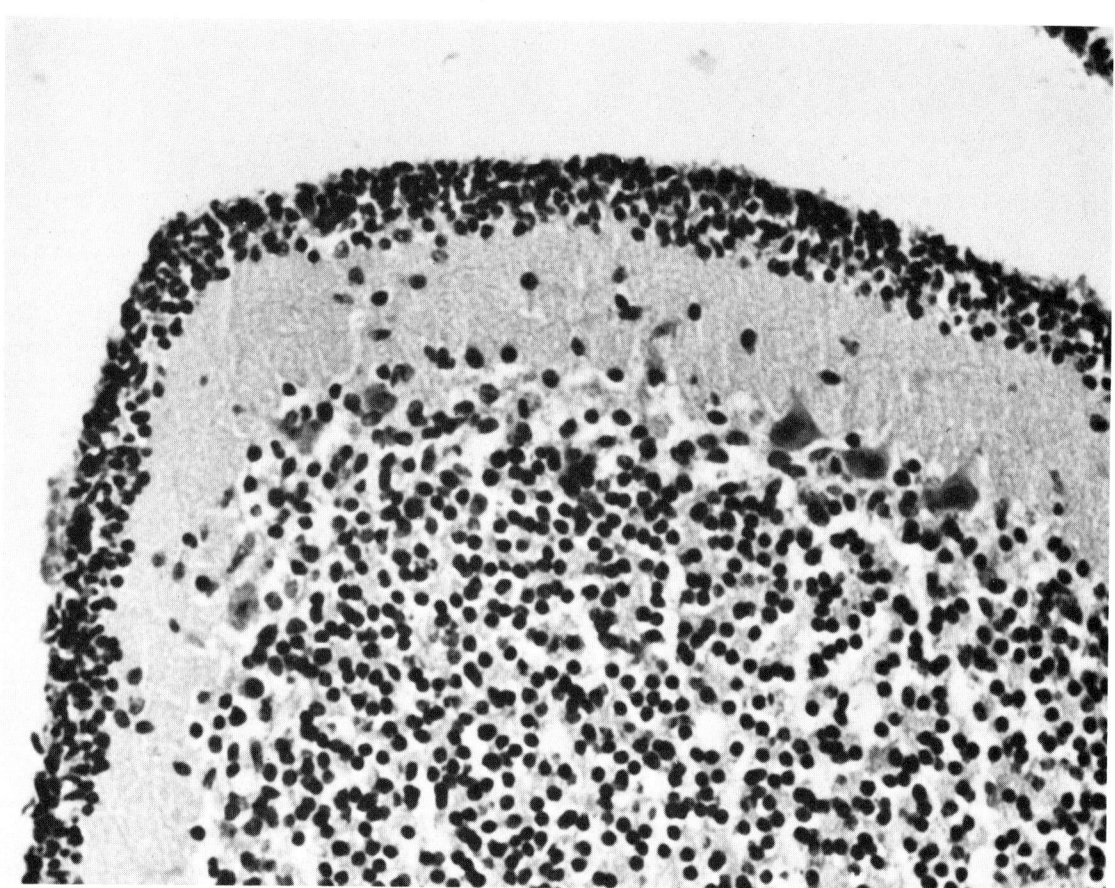

Figure 31-40

Figure 31-40. This photomicrograph shows, at very high magnification, the nature of the cells in the superficial portion of a single cerebellar folium of an infant.

Three prominent Purkinje cells appear on the right between the pale molecular layer above and the darker, more cellular granular layer below.

This patient was a stillborn black male, whose body weighed 2,100 grams at postmortem examination.

Hematoxylin and eosin stain. Mag. 392×.

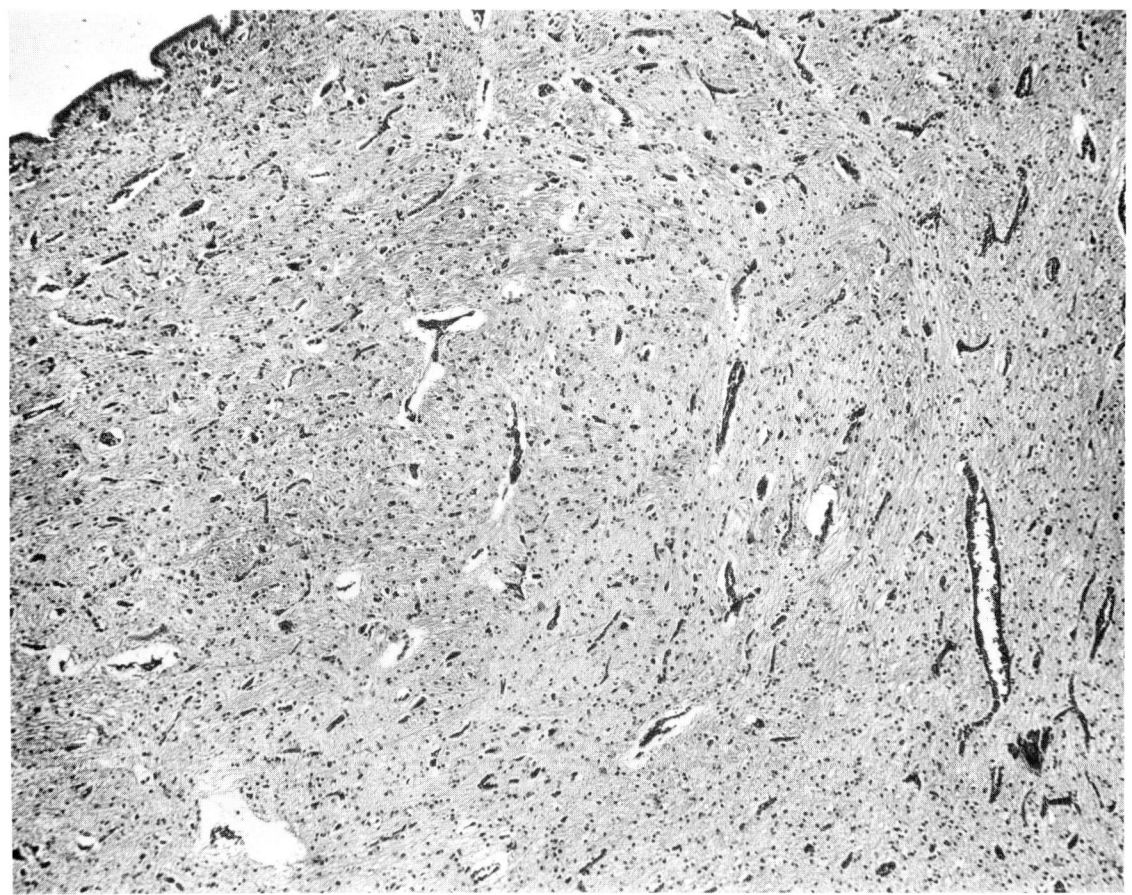

Figure 31–41

Figure 31–41. This is an illustration of the white matter of the cerebellum in an infant in the perinatal period.

This patient was a black male weighing 1,780 grams. He lived for one day and 3 hours. Gestational age was given as eight to eight and a half months.

Hematoxylin and eosin stain. Mag. 72×.

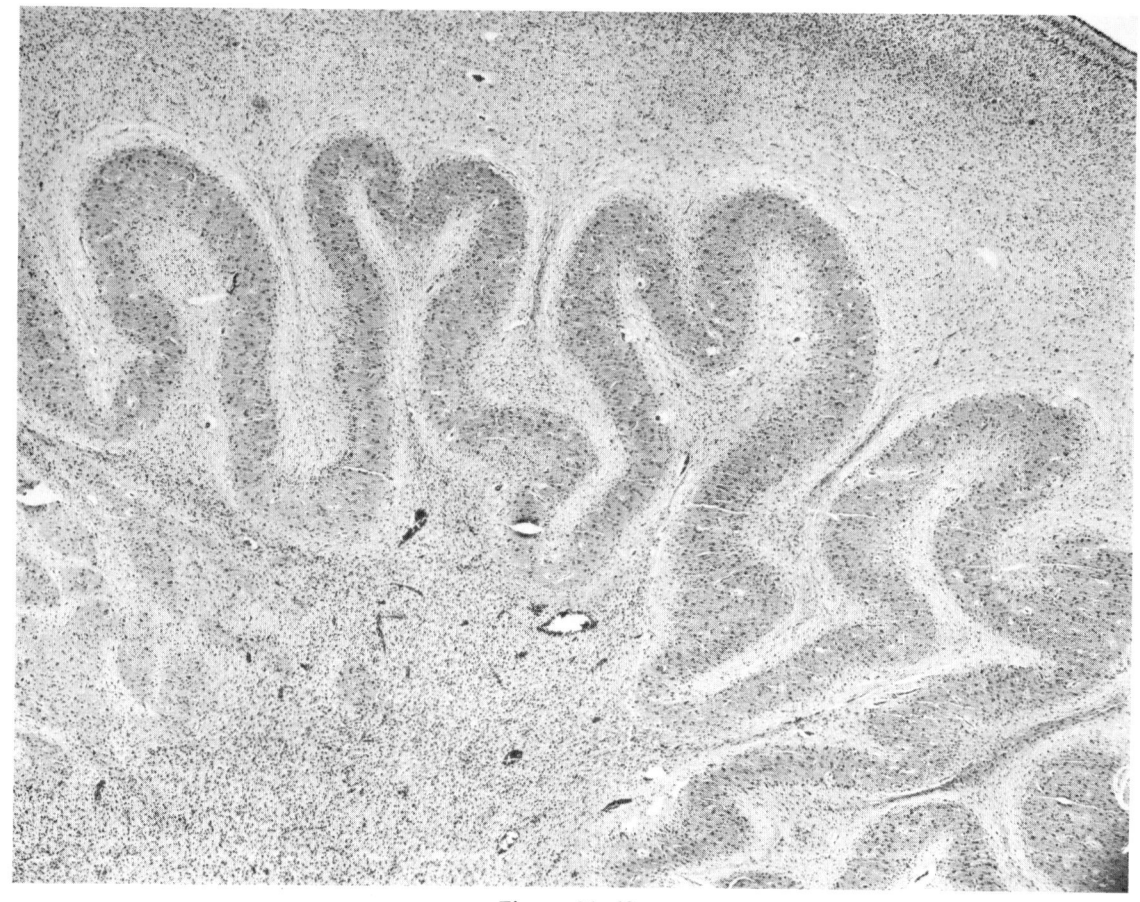

Figure 31–42

Figures 31–42 to 31–44. Taken at the same low magnification, these three photographs depict the dentate nucleus of the cerebellum, a characteristically undulating or crumpled structure.

Figure 31–42. This infant weighed 720 grams at autopsy. He was a black male who lived for three and a half hours. Gestational age was said to be 24 weeks.

Figure 31–43. This baby was a black female whose body weighed 925 grams at postmortem examination. She was stillborn.

Figure 31–44. This patient was a 1,050 gram liveborn who survived for 10½ hours after birth. Estimated gestational age is 24 weeks.

Hematoxylin and eosin stain. Mag. 45×.

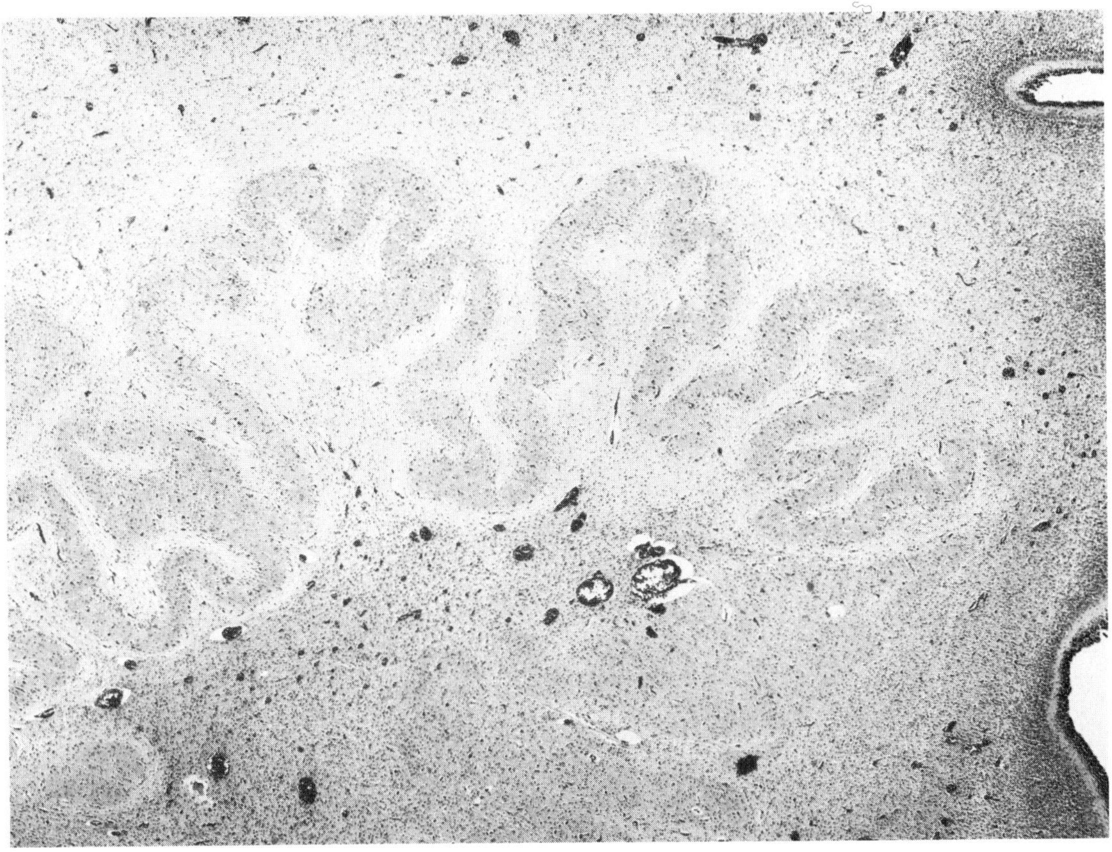

Figure 31-43

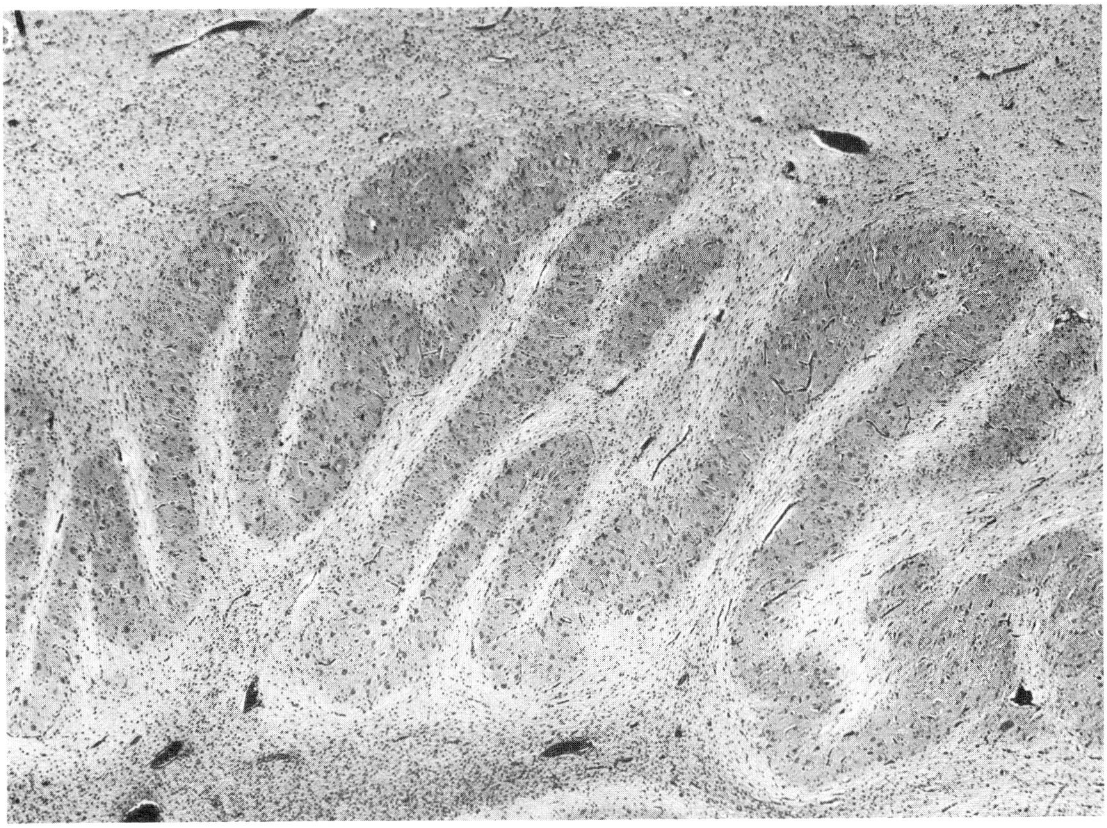

Figure 31-44

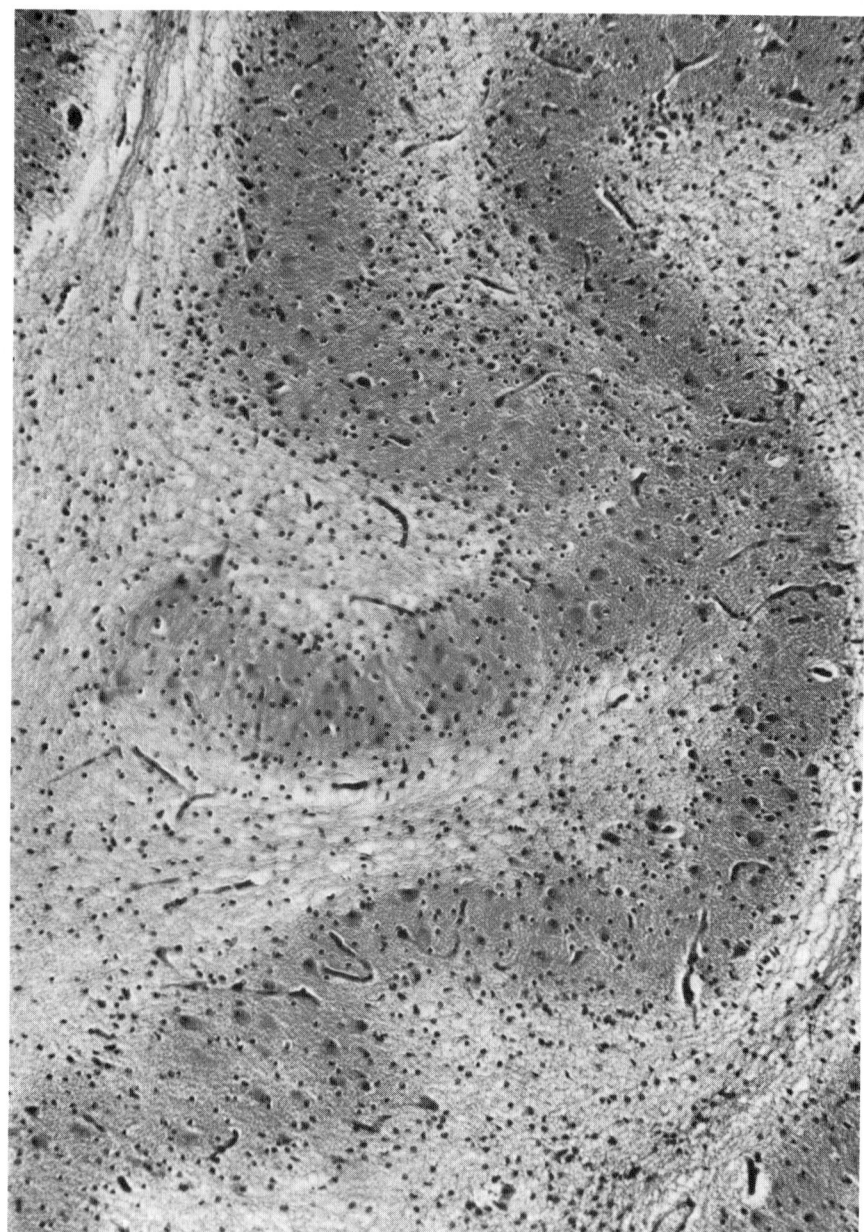

Figure 31–45

Figure 31–45. This photomicrograph illustrates the cells of the dentate nucleus at moderately high magnification.

The patient was a black male infant who lived for two hours and three minutes. His body weight at postmortem examination was 1165 grams. Estimated gestational age is 27 weeks.

Hematoxylin and eosin stain. Mag. 124×.

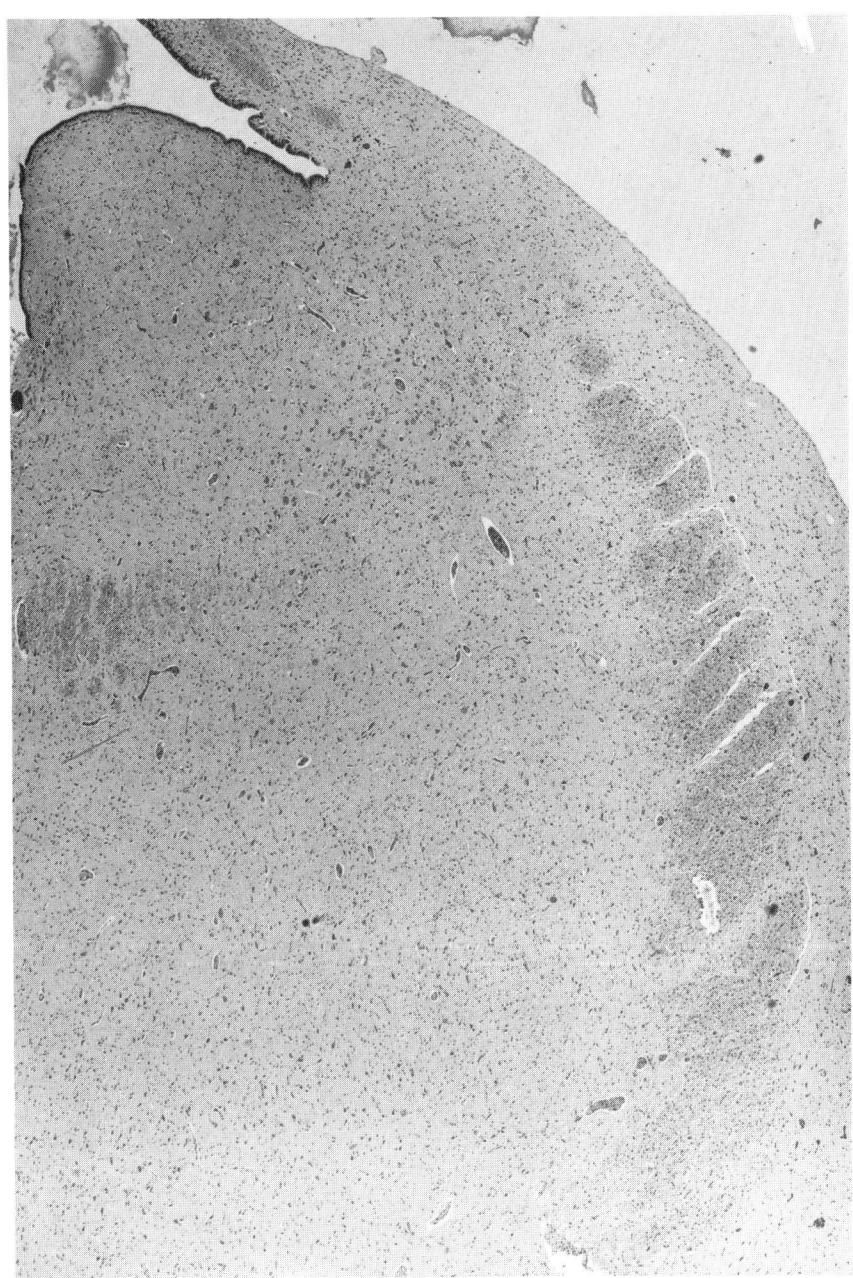

Figure 31–46

Figure 31–46. This is a section of the upper portion of the pons. The aqueduct of Sylvius with its ependymal lining is seen at the top on the left.

This infant was a stillborn white female, who weighed 3,120 grams at autopsy. She was born at term.

Hematoxylin and eosin stain. Mag. 31×.

Figure 31–47. This, too, is a section of the upper portion of the pons immediately adjacent to the midline, which is located on the right-hand margin. The ependymal lining appears as a dark slender line along the upper borders of the section.

The patient was a stillborn black male baby, delivered at term. His body weight at autopsy was 3,775 grams.

Hematoxylin and eosin stain. Mag. 45×.

See illustration on the opposite page

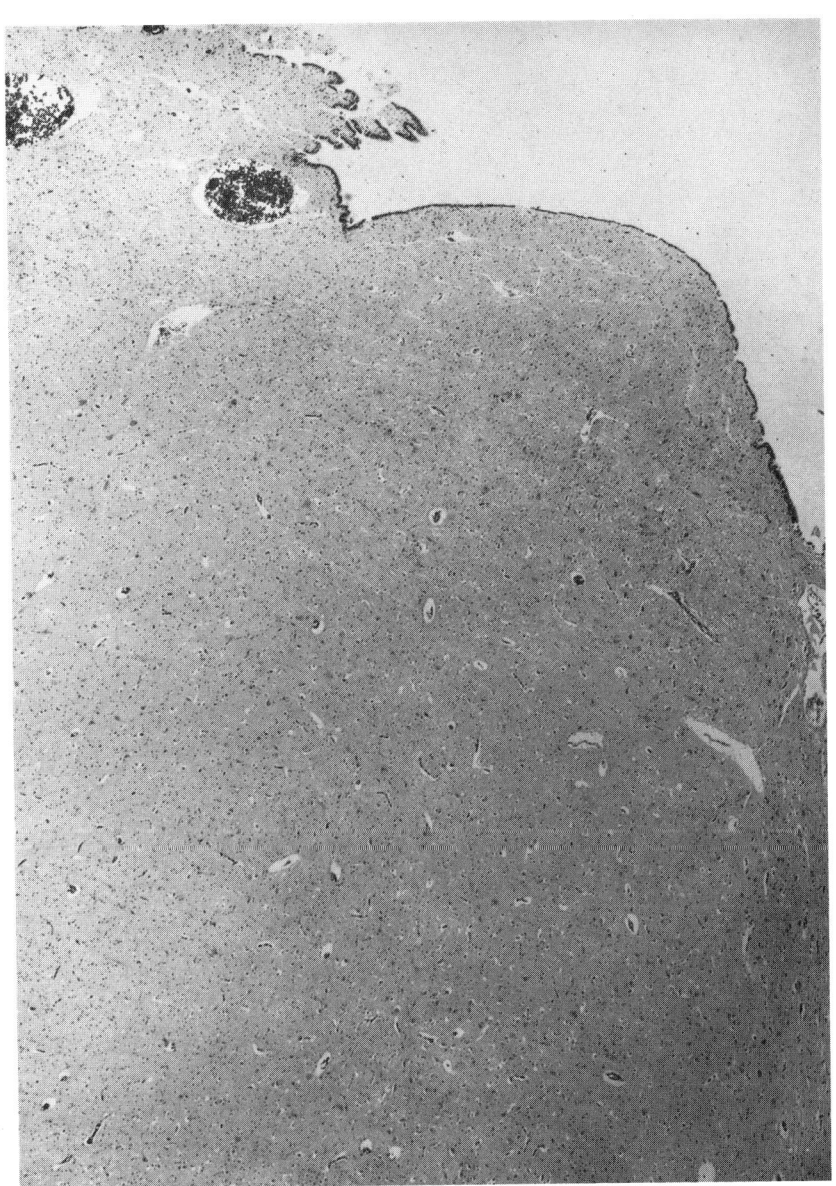
Figure 31-47

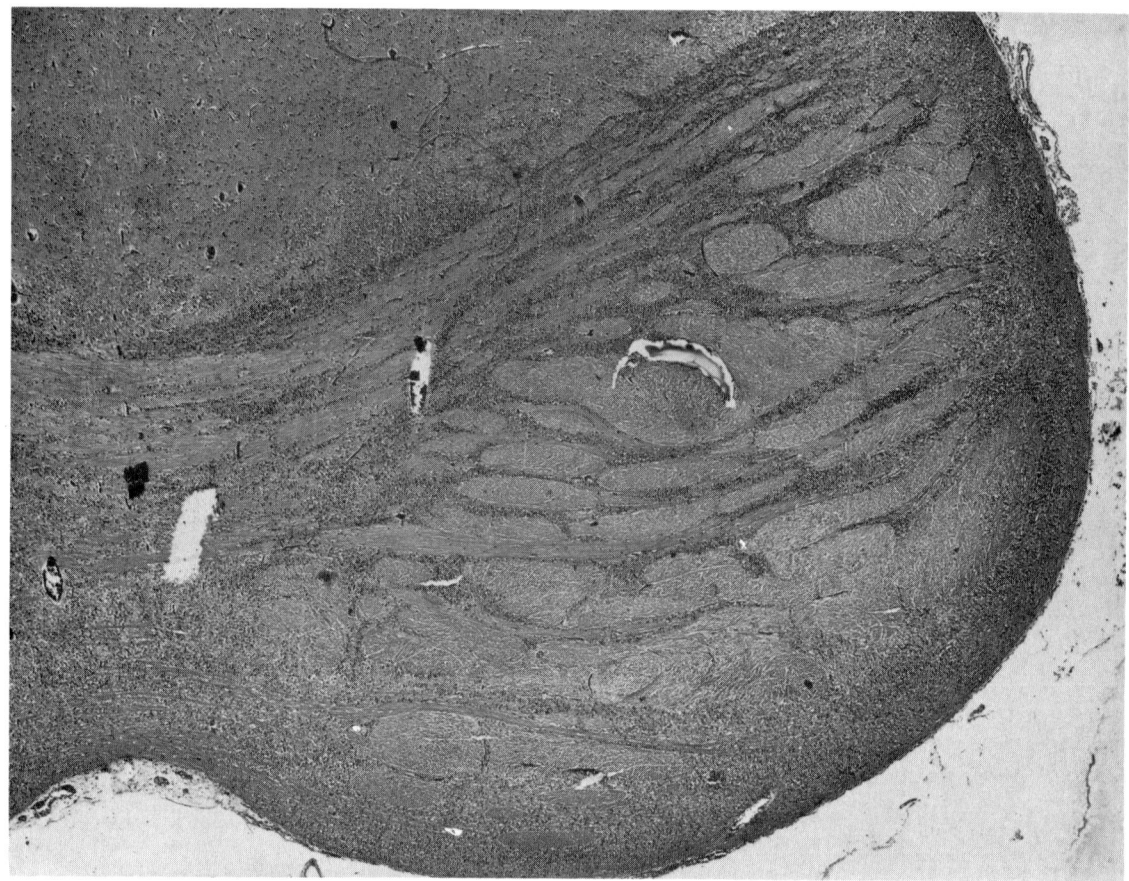

Figure 31–48

Figure 31–48. This is the basis pontis of a very tiny infant, seen at low magnification. The midline is located at the indentation on the inferior margin. The basis pontis contains cortico-pontocerebellar fibers (running horizontally) and corticospinal fibers (running vertically).
The patient was stillborn after 18 weeks of gestation and weighed 370 grams.
Hematoxylin and eosin stain. Mag. 31×.

Figures 31–49 and 31–50. The two figures on the opposite page show, at somewhat higher magnification, the alternating orientation of groups of fibers in horizontal and vertical groups.

Figure 31–49. A 3,775 gram stillborn white female, born after 41 weeks gestation.

Figure 31–50. A 3,120 gram stillborn white female, born at term.
Hematoxylin and eosin stain. Mag. 45×.

See illustration on the opposite page

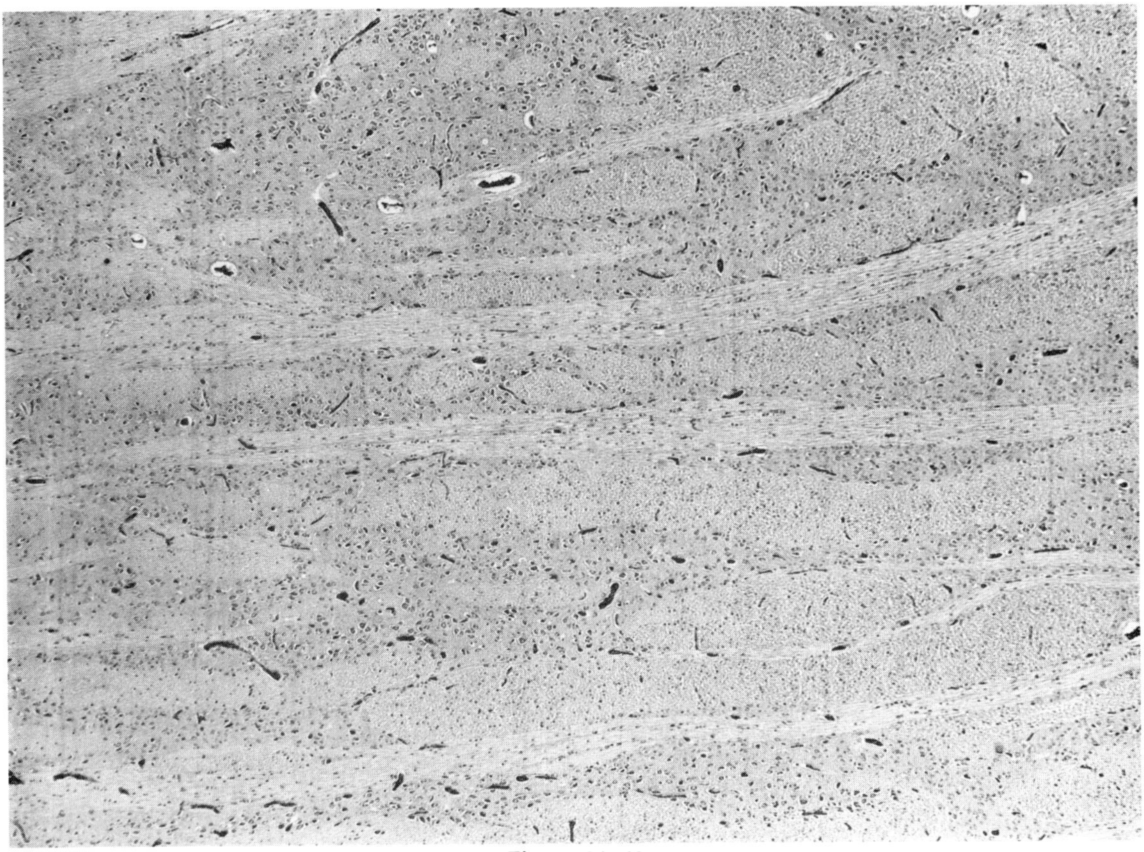

Figure 31-49

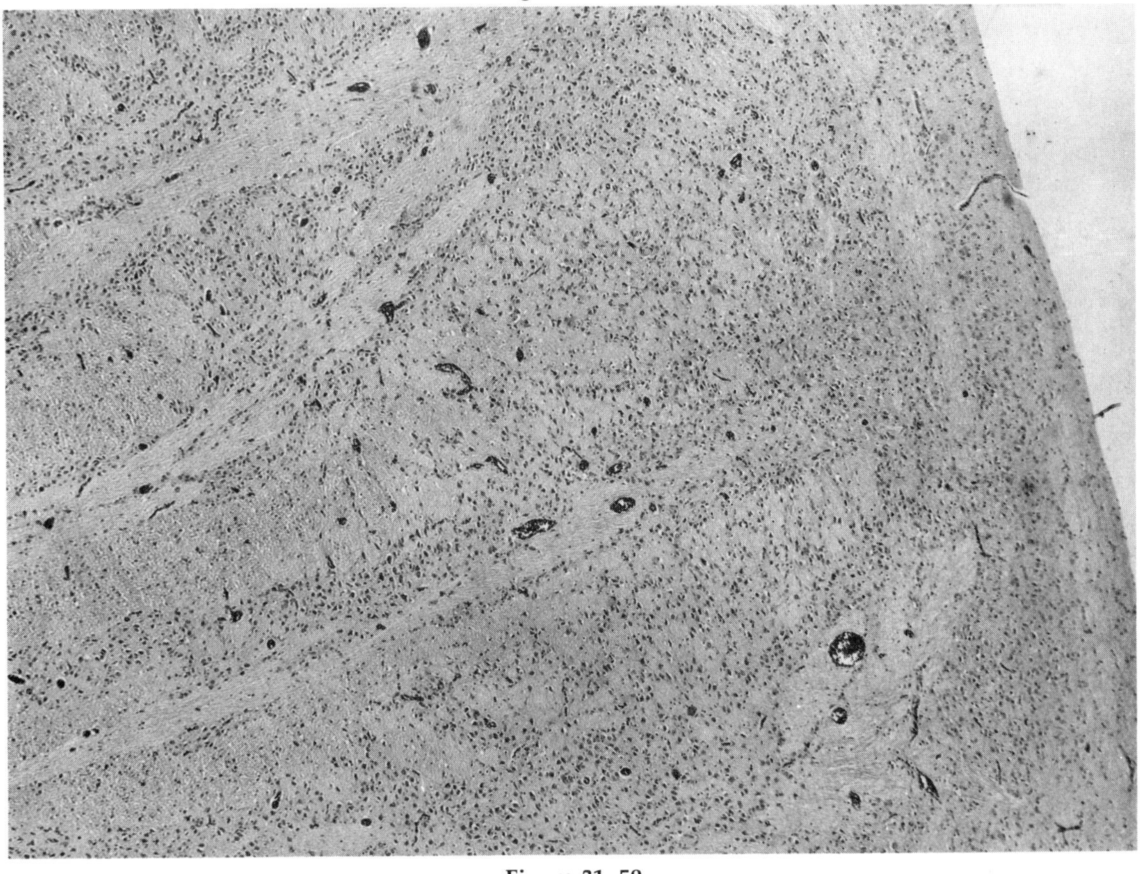

Figure 31-50

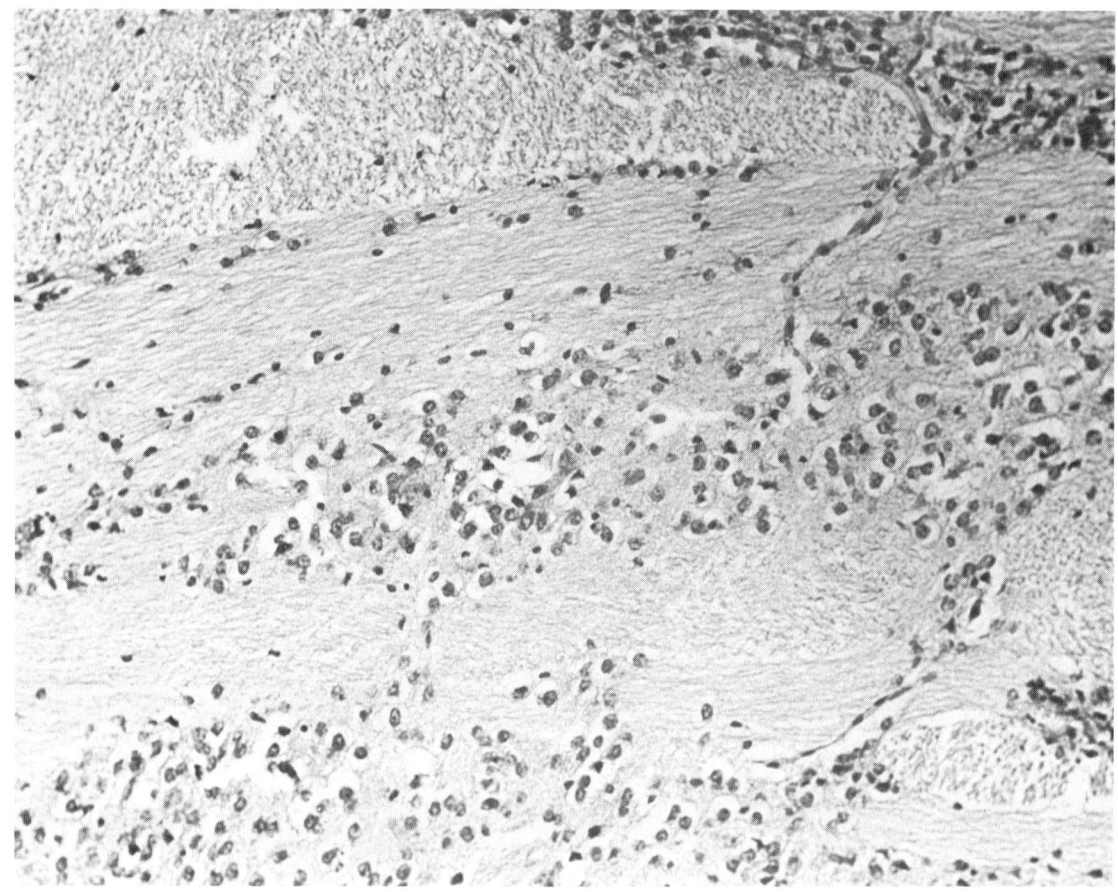

Figure 31–51

Figures 31–51 to 31–53. These are photographs, at intermediate magnification, of the cell population of the basis pontis in three infants spanning a little more than the last trimester of pregnancy. (The succeeding three illustrations are from the same set of three infants.)

Figure 31–51. This is a portion of the basis pontis from a black male infant born in approximately the sixth month of gestation, who lived for 3 hours and 30 minutes. Body weight at autopsy was 720 grams.
Hematoxylin and eosin stain. Mag. 186×.

Figure 31–52. This is roughly the same type of section. It is from an infant who lived for two hours and three minutes. He was a black male whose body, at postmortem examination, weighed 1,165 grams.
Hematoxylin and eosin stain. Mag. 124×.

Figure 31–53. This is a section from the basis pontis of an infant stillborn at 41 weeks of gestation, a white female weighing 3,775 grams.
Hematoxylin and eosin stain. Mag. 124×.

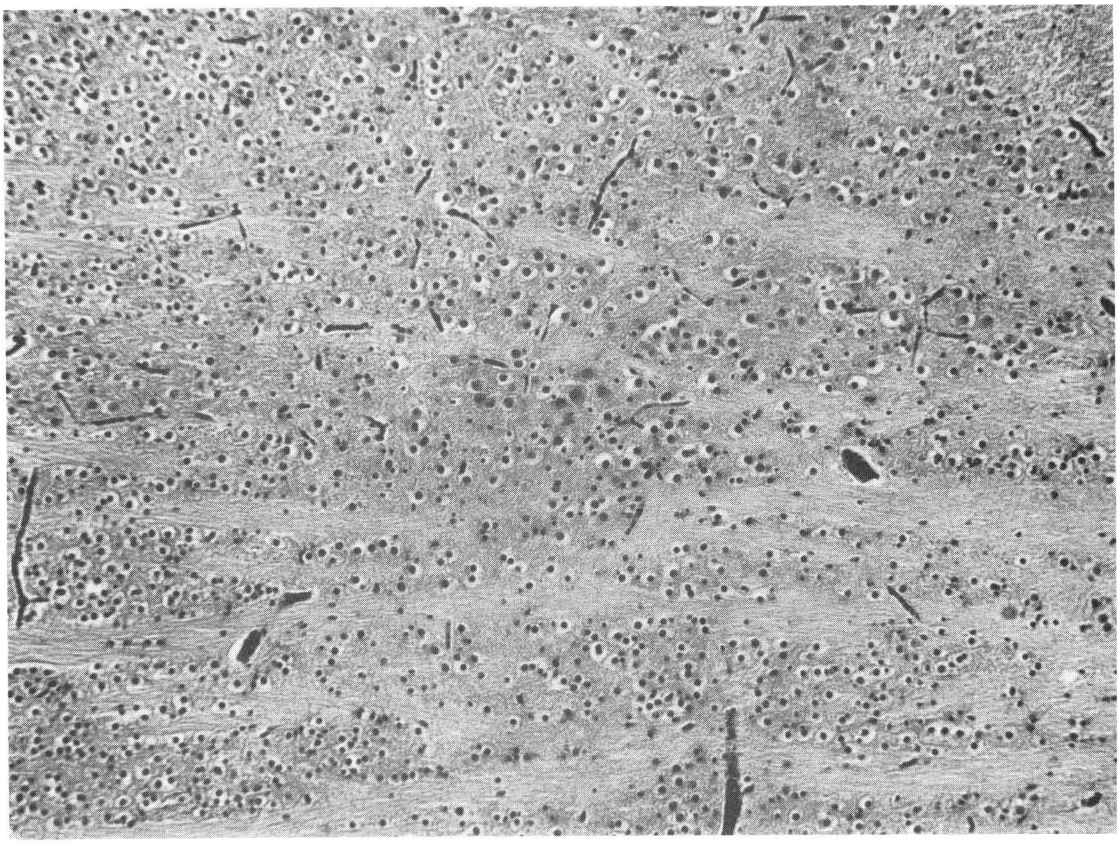

Figure 31-52

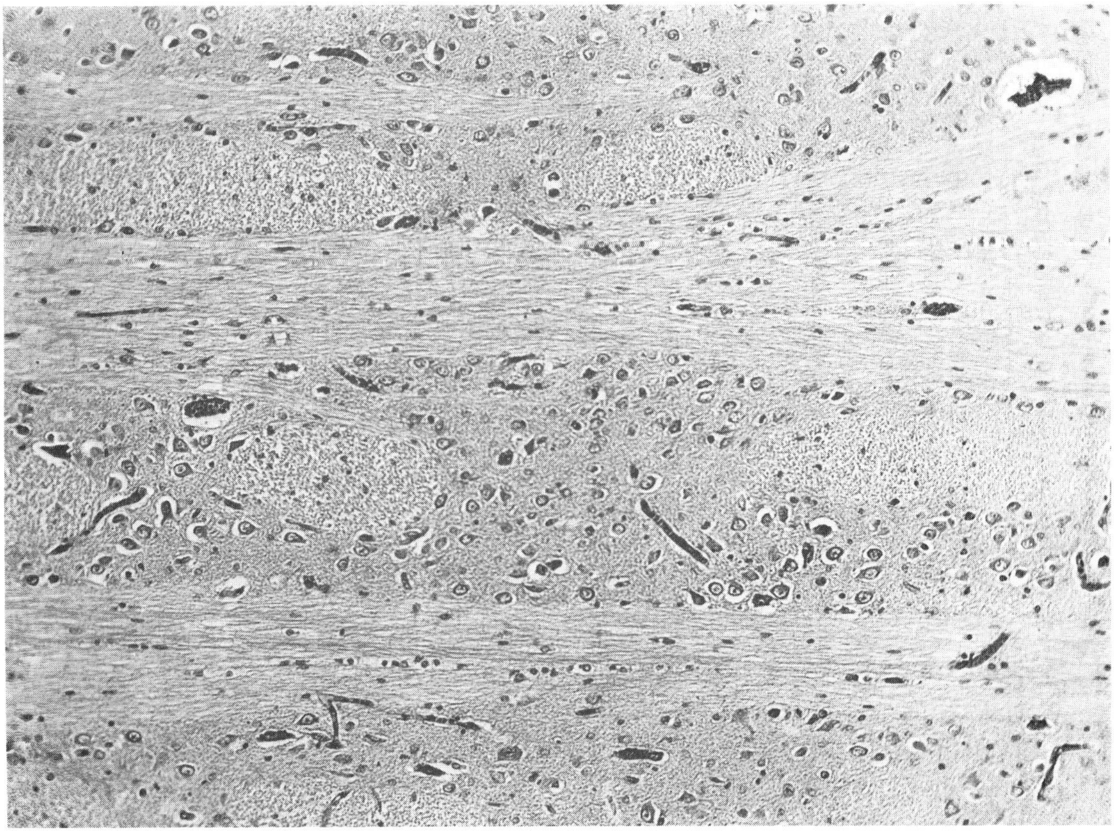

Figure 31-53

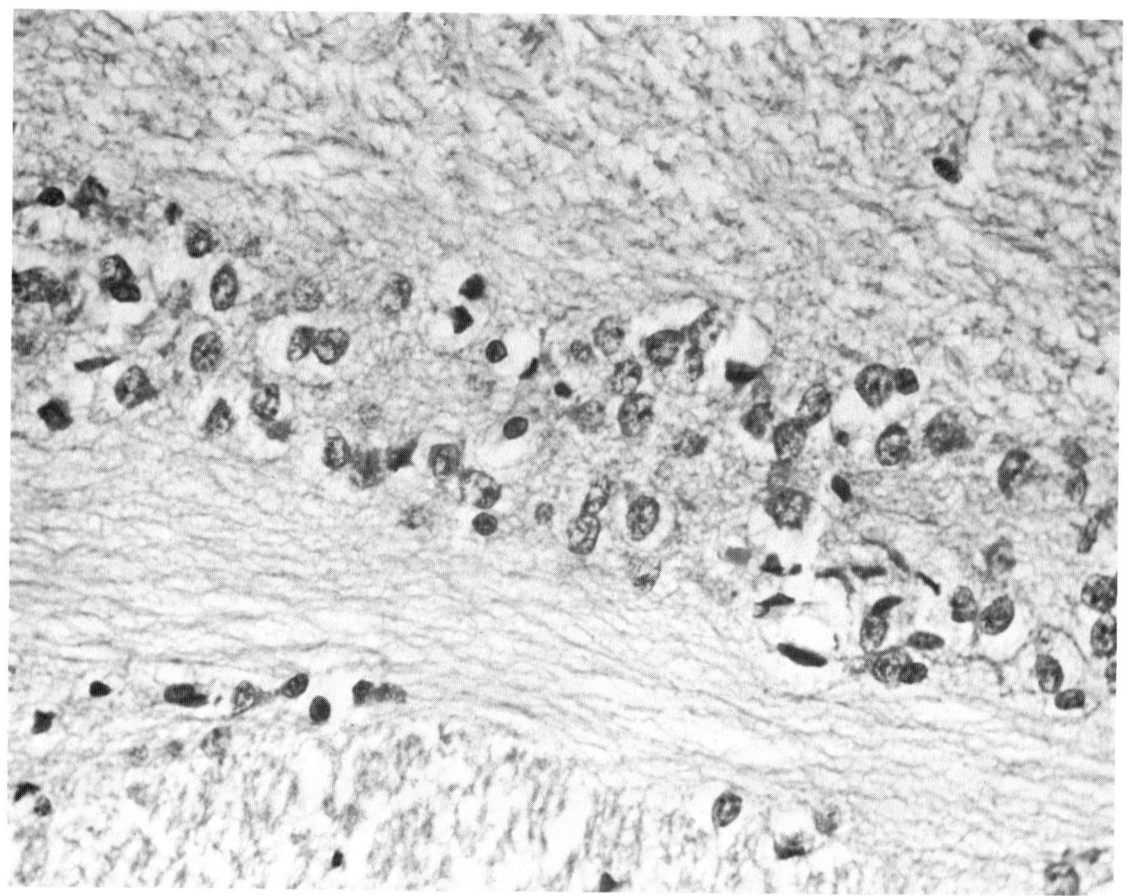

Figure 31-54

Figures 31-54 to 31-56. Seen here at very high magnification are the cells of the basis pontis in three infants who are representative of three different stages of intra-uterine development.

Figure 31-54. This illustration depicts the cells of the basis pontis from the infant described in the legend of Fig. 31-51.
Hematoxylin and eosin stain. Mag. 500×.

Figure 31-55. Taken at the same magnification as the preceding, this photomicrograph shows the same cell population from a somewhat more developed infant, the same one described in the legend of Fig. 31-52.
Hematoxylin and eosin stain. Mag. 500×.

Figure 31-56. At very slightly higher magnification, this is the same view from the infant described in the legend of Fig. 31-53.
Hematoxylin and eosin stain. Mag. 513×.

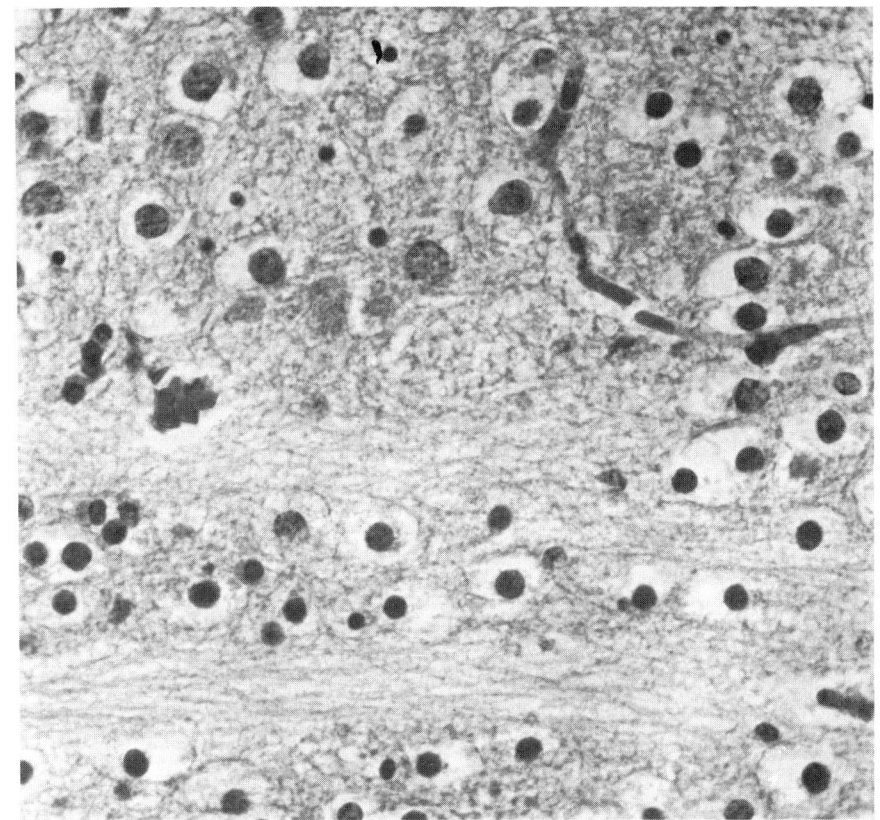

Figure 31–55

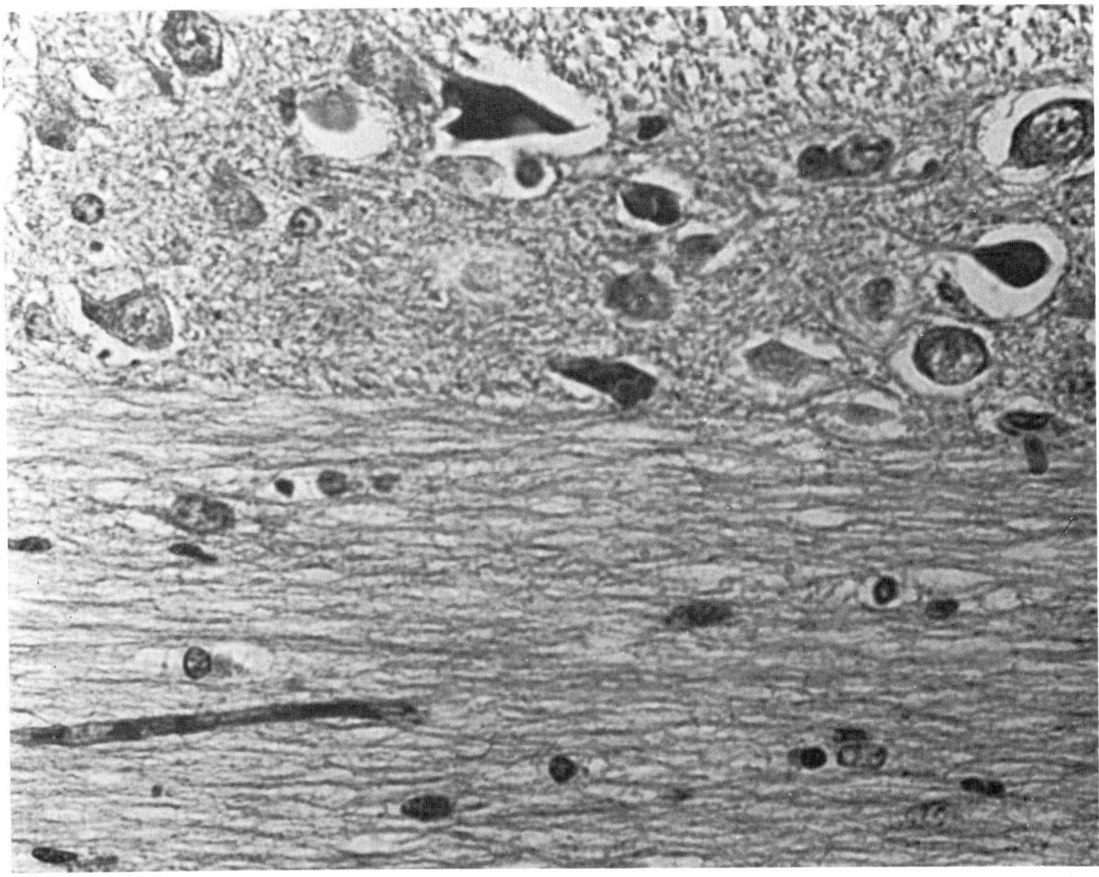

Figure 31–56

594 CENTRAL NERVOUS SYSTEM

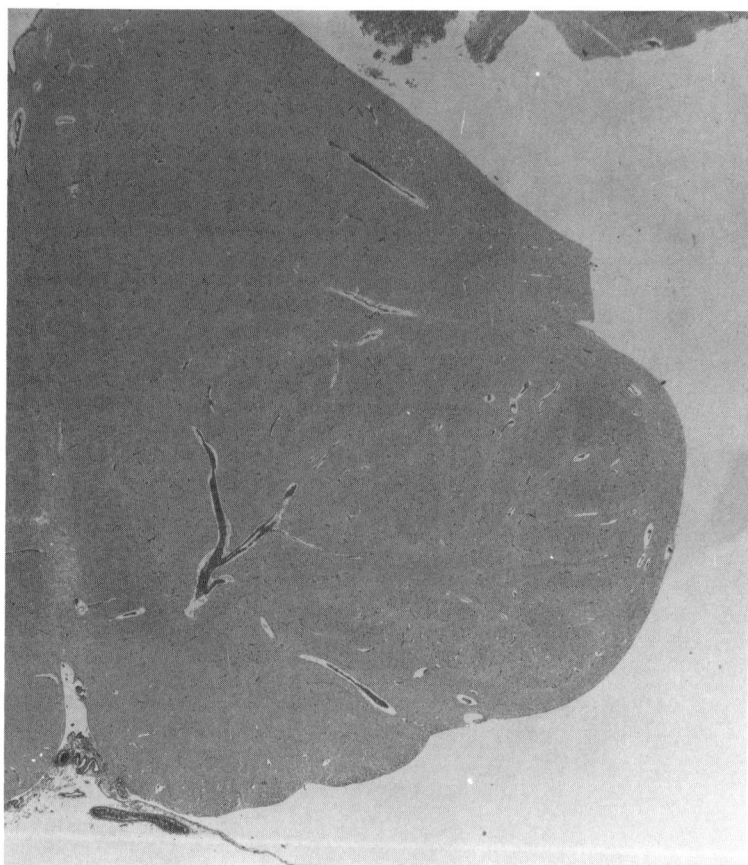

Figure 31–57

Figure 3–57. This is a coronal section of the medulla oblongata from an infant; half is seen here. The cerebral peduncle has been cut away from the upper right margin. Below that, on the right, is the olive appearing as a dark undulating line.

The ependymal lining of this portion of the ventricular system appears in the upper left corner.

The pale triangular body representing the pyramid is just to the right of the cleft in the lower border, the midline of medulla.

This infant was born at term, 41 weeks of gestation. She was a stillborn white female and weighed 3,775 grams at autopsy.

Hematoxylin and eosin stain. Mag. 15×.

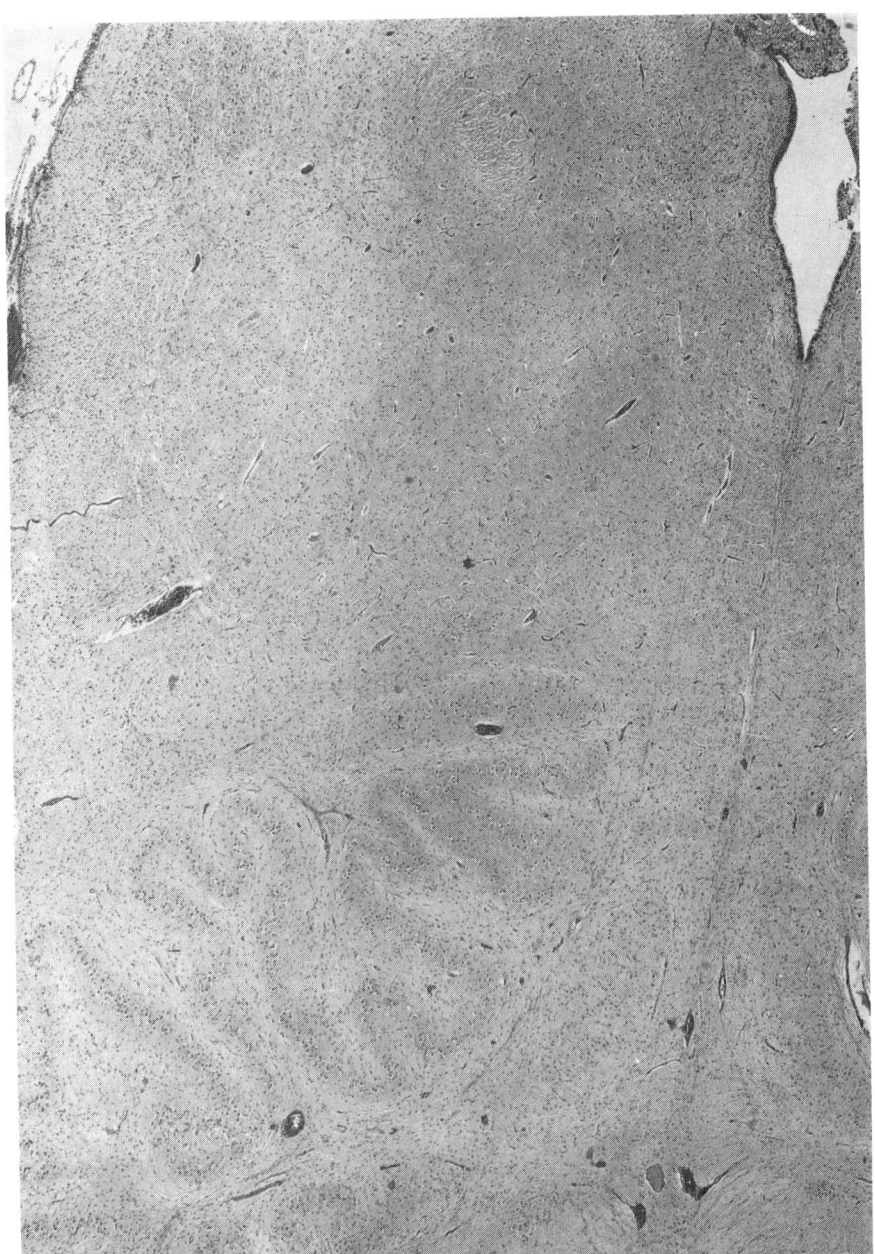

Figure 31–58

Figure 31–58. Taken in the same plane as the preceding, this also is a coronal section of the medulla oblongata. The dark line bordering the space at upper right is the ependymal lining. The olive appears as an undulating delicate dark line in the lower left.

This infant was a pre-term male; he lived for two days and 17 hours, even though his body weight was only 710 grams.

Hematoxylin and eosin stain. Mag. 31×.

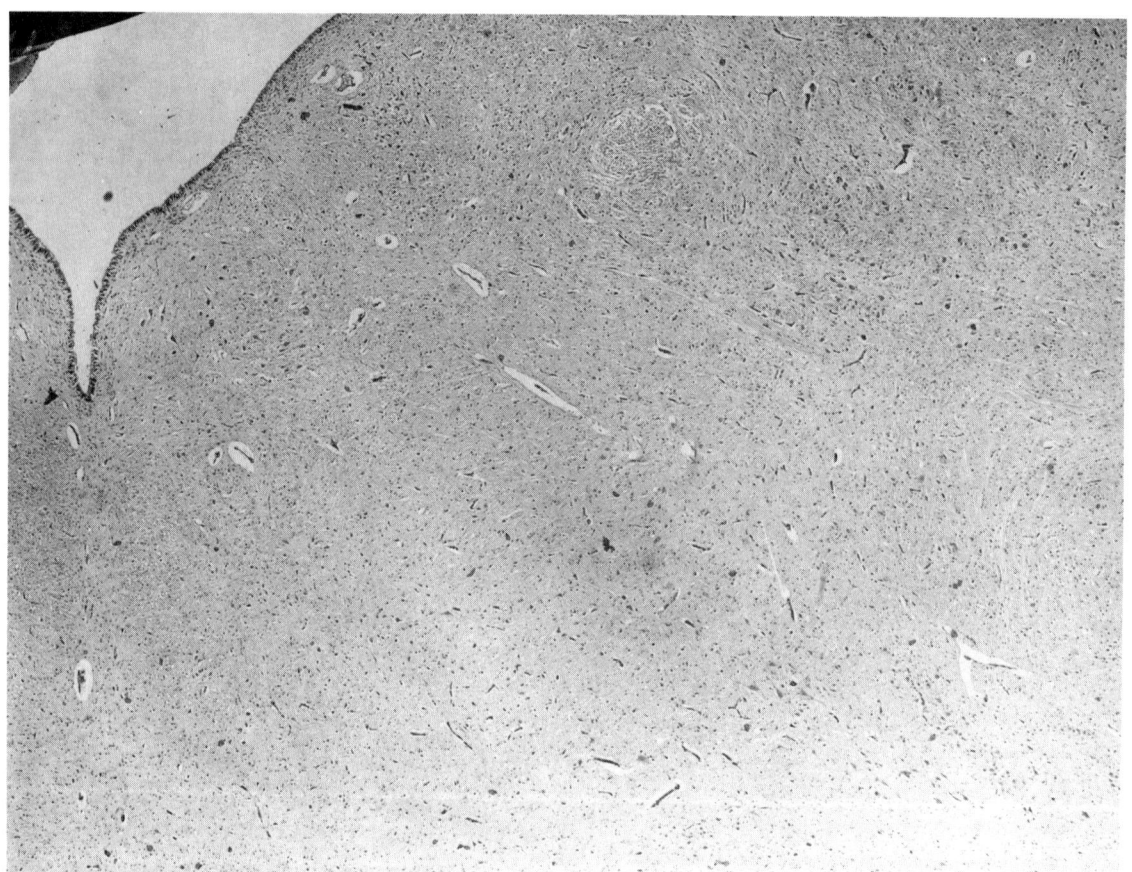

Figure 31–59

Figure 31–59. This photograph depicts, at somewhat higher magnification than the preceding, the upper portion of the medulla oblongata, again in the coronal plane. A portion of the fourth ventricle, upper left, is lined by a single layer of ependymal cells.

The infant from whom this section was taken was a three day old white female who, at postmortem examination, weighed 1,630 grams.

Hematoxylin and eosin stain. Mag. 45×.

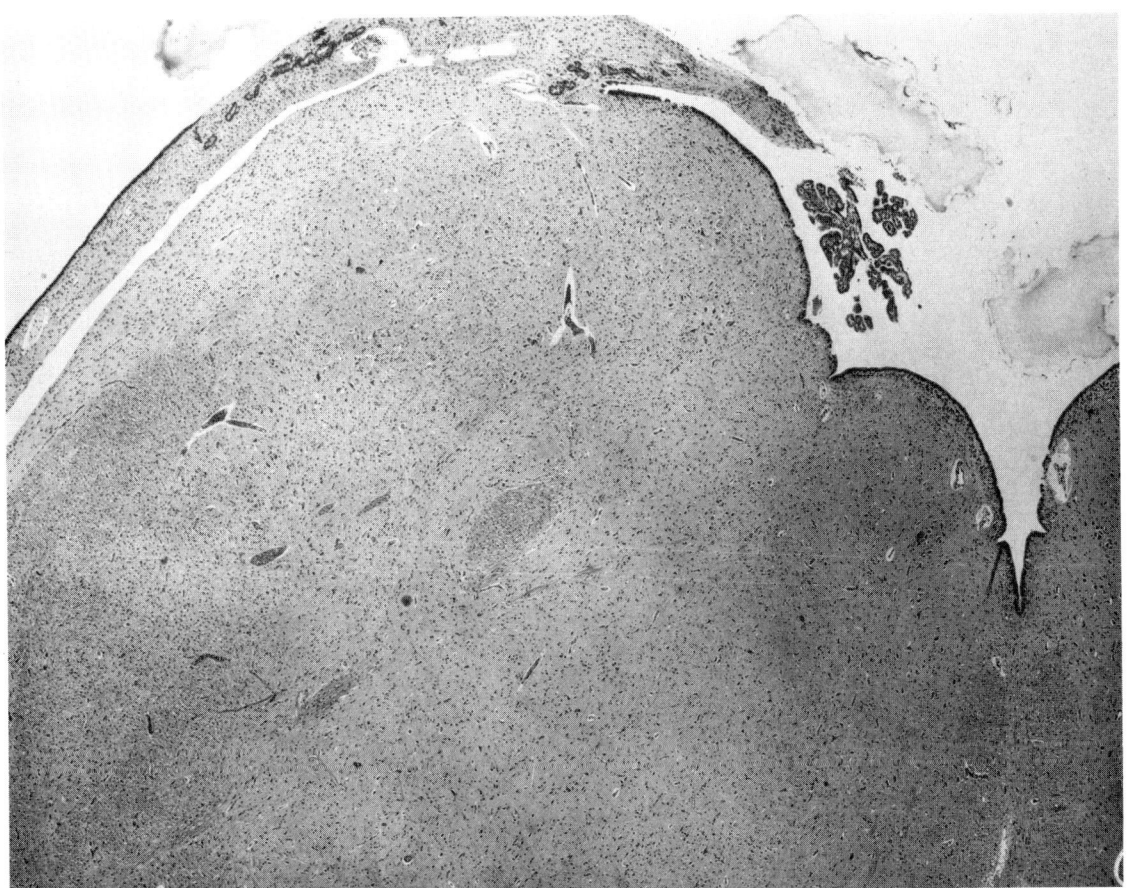

Figure 31-60

Figure 31-60. This photomicrograph depicts a part of the medulla at a slightly different level from that shown in the preceding illustration, but still in the upper portion. A bit of choroid plexus is suspended in the lumen of the fourth ventricle, at the upper right.

This infant was stillborn, delivered at term, a white female weighing 3,120 grams.

Hematoxylin and eosin stain. Mag. 41×.

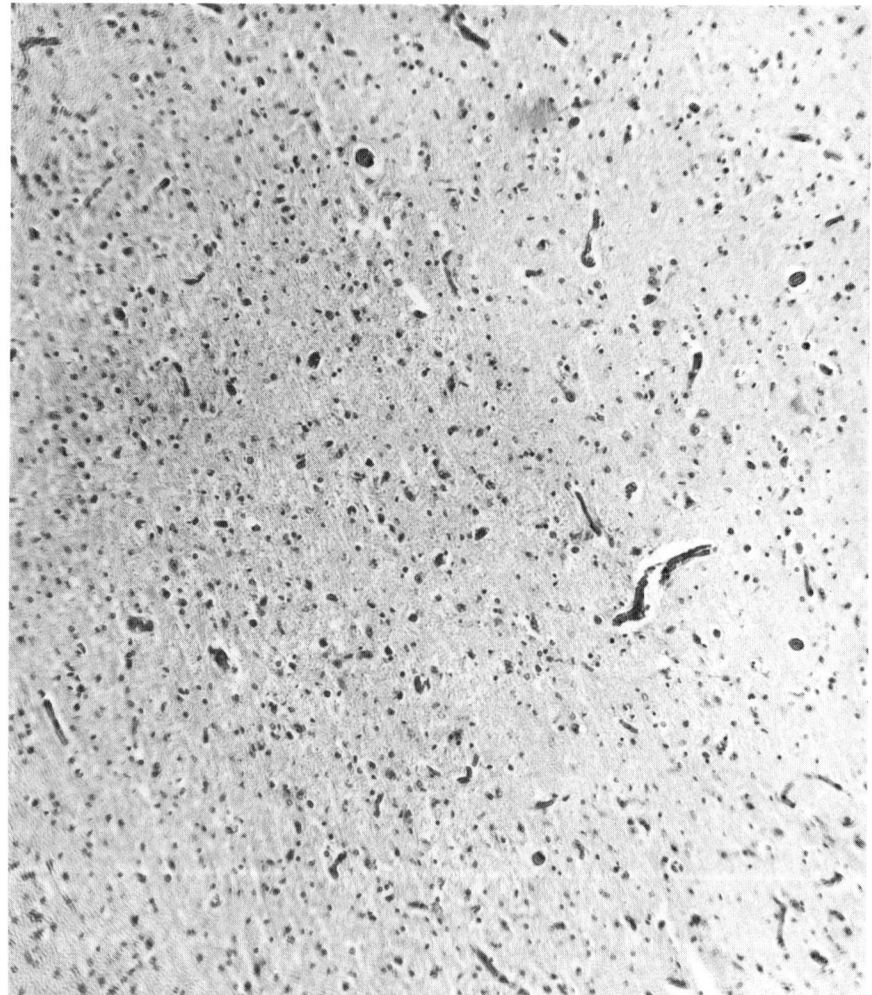

Figure 31-61

Figures 31-61 and 31-62. These two illustrations are taken from the upper portion of the medulla, both at relatively high magnification. The first depicts a single nucleus, while the second shows the ependymal lining of the canal at this level.

Figure 31-61. This photograph shows the nature of the population of cells in this segment of the upper portion of the medulla. The infant was born preterm (in about the 30th week of gestation). Body weight at necropsy was 1,630 grams. The baby, a white female, lived for three days.
Hematoxylin and eosin stain. Mag. 124×.

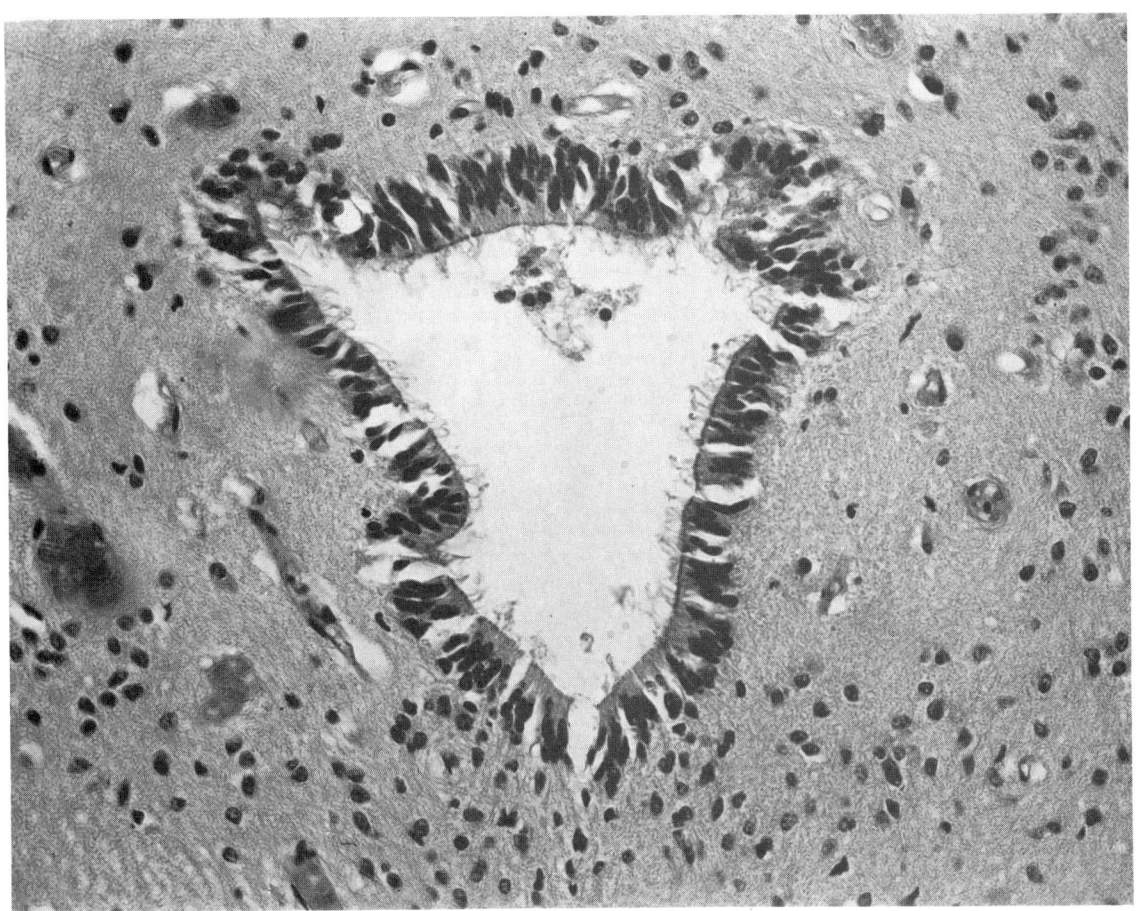

Figure 31-62

Figure 31-62. The ependymal cells that line the canal are very clearly depicted here. This infant was stillborn, a male weighing 3,250 grams.
Hematoxylin and eosin stain. Mag. 290×.

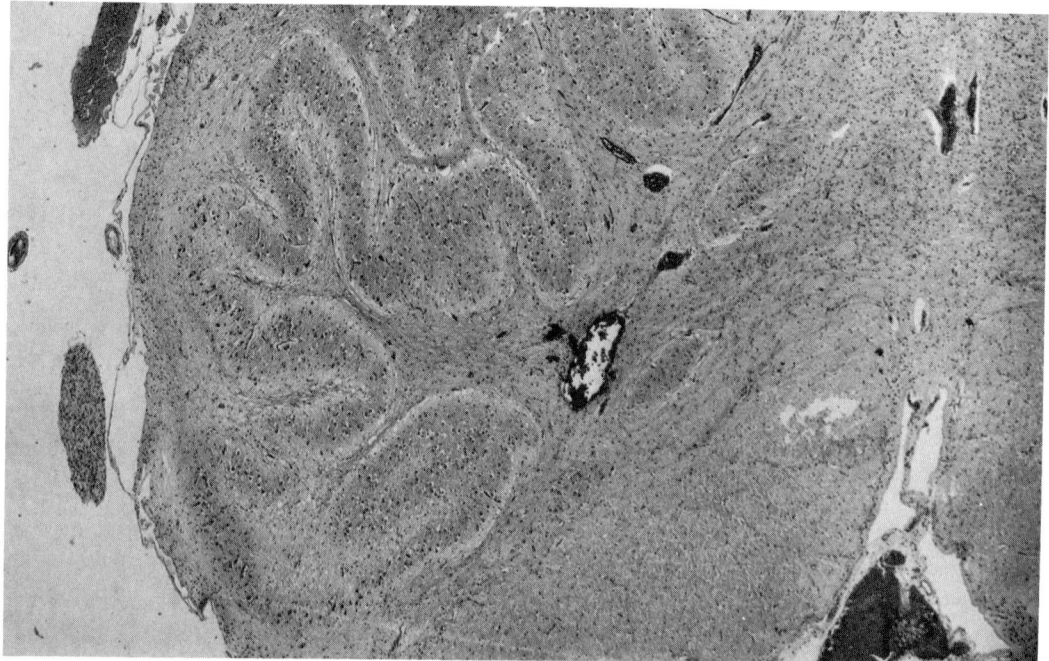

Figure 31–63

Figures 31–63 and 31–64. Taken at roughly the same magnification, these two illustrations depict the appearance of the olive in the infant born prematurely or preterm.

Figure 31–63. This infant was a black male who lived for two hours and three minutes. His body weight at necropsy was 1,165 grams. His gestation is estimated to be about 27 weeks.
Hematoxylin and eosin stain. Mag. 38×.

CENTRAL NERVOUS SYSTEM 601

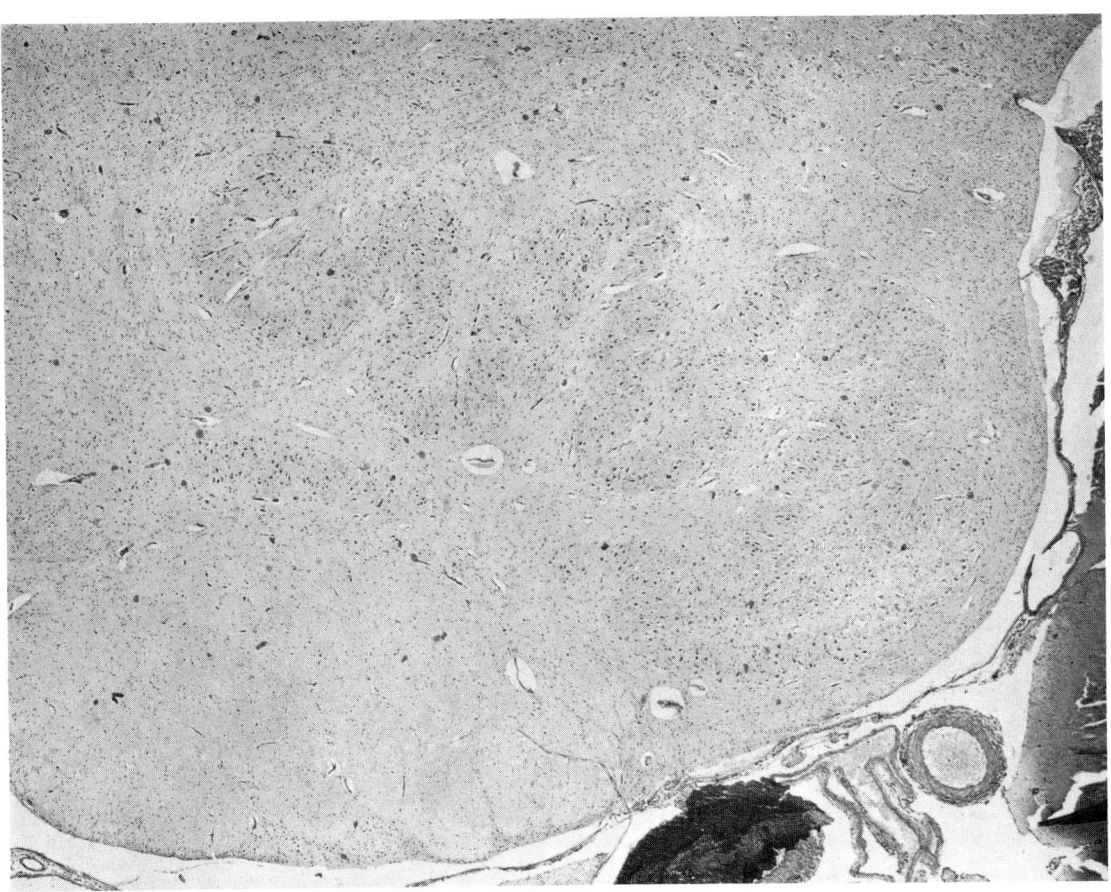

Figure 31-64

Figure 31-64. This is the olive of the medulla oblongata of a three day old white female infant whose body, at autopsy, weighed 1,630 grams. (Estimated gestational age: 30 weeks.) Hematoxylin and eosin stain. Mag. 45×.

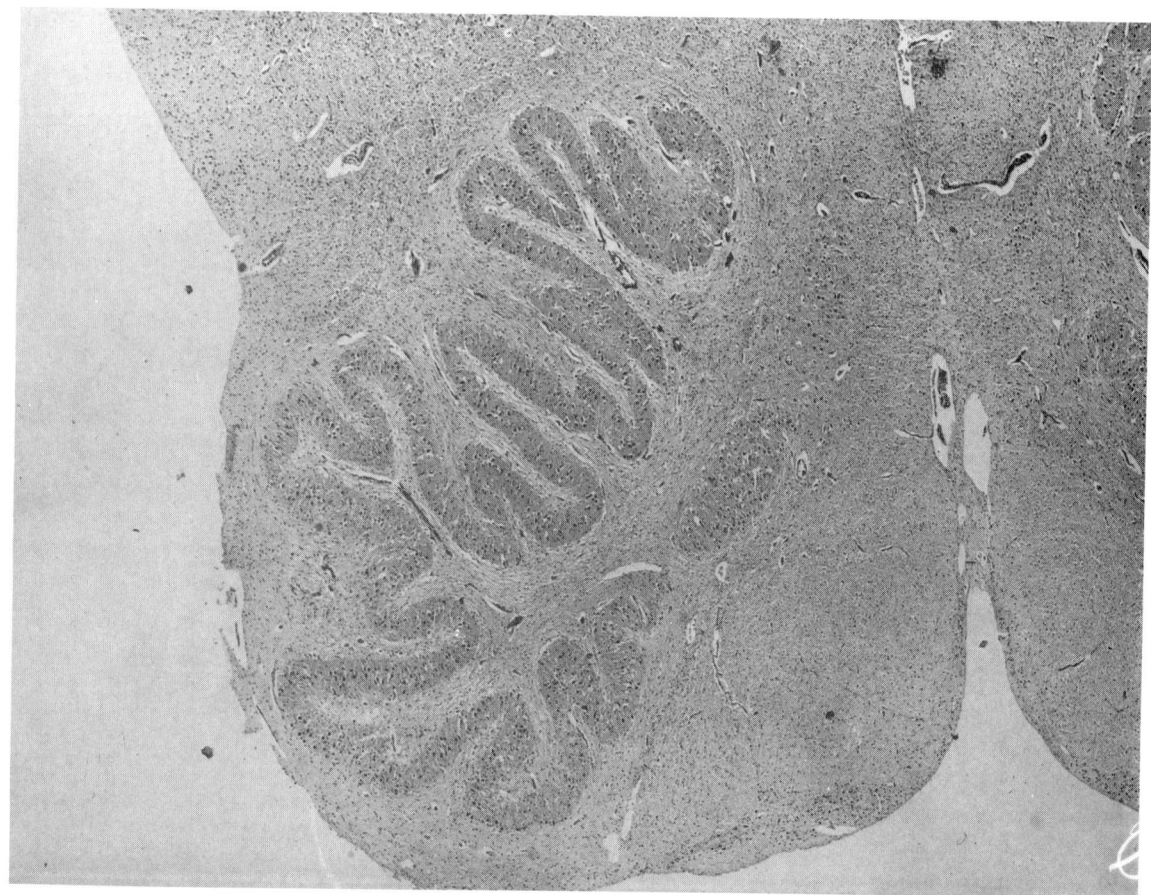

Figure 31–65

Figures 31–65 to 31–67. This set of three photographs depicts the nature of the olive in the infant born at term.
Hematoxylin and eosin stain.

Figure 31–65. This infant, a black male, lived for seven hours and 30 minutes. His body weight at autopsy was 2,460 grams. Gestational age is unknown. Mag. 45×.

Figure 31–66. This baby was a stillborn white female delivered at term, weighing 3,120 grams. Mag. 41×.

Figure 31–67. This infant, also stillborn, was a black male delivered at 8½ months of gestation. His body weight was 3,210 grams. Mag. 38×.

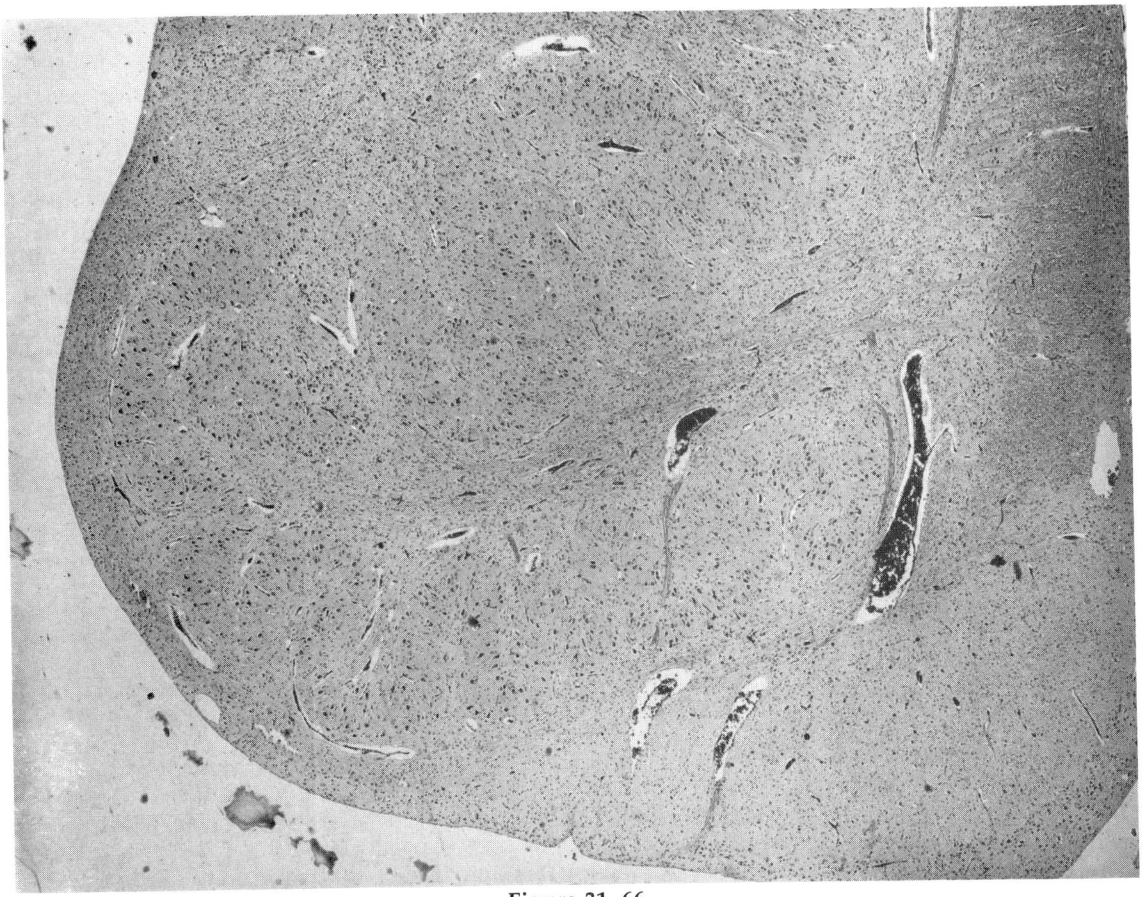

Figure 31–66

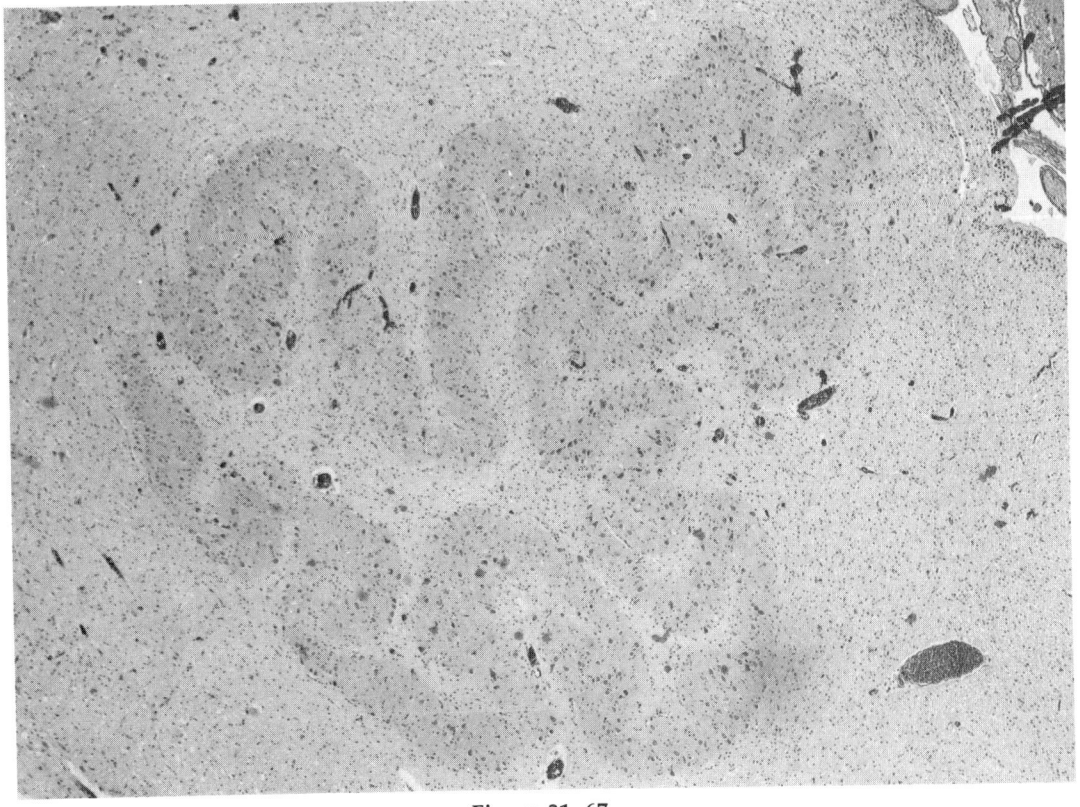

Figure 31–67

603

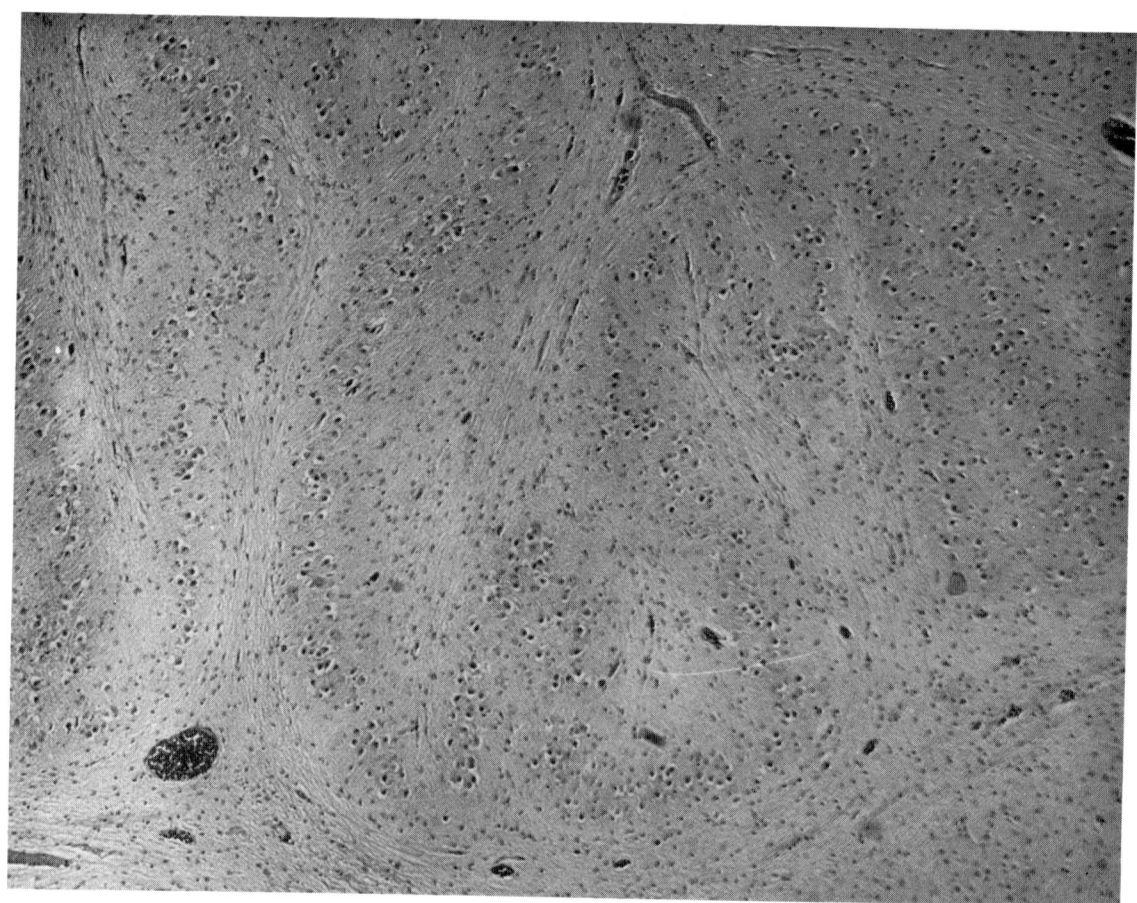

Figure 31-68

Figure 31-68. This picture shows in somewhat greater detail the nature of the cell population in the olive of the medulla oblongata in a neonate.

This male infant weighing 710 grams at autopsy, survived for two days and 17 hours. His estimated gestational age is 23 weeks.

Hematoxylin and eosin stain. Mag. 45×.

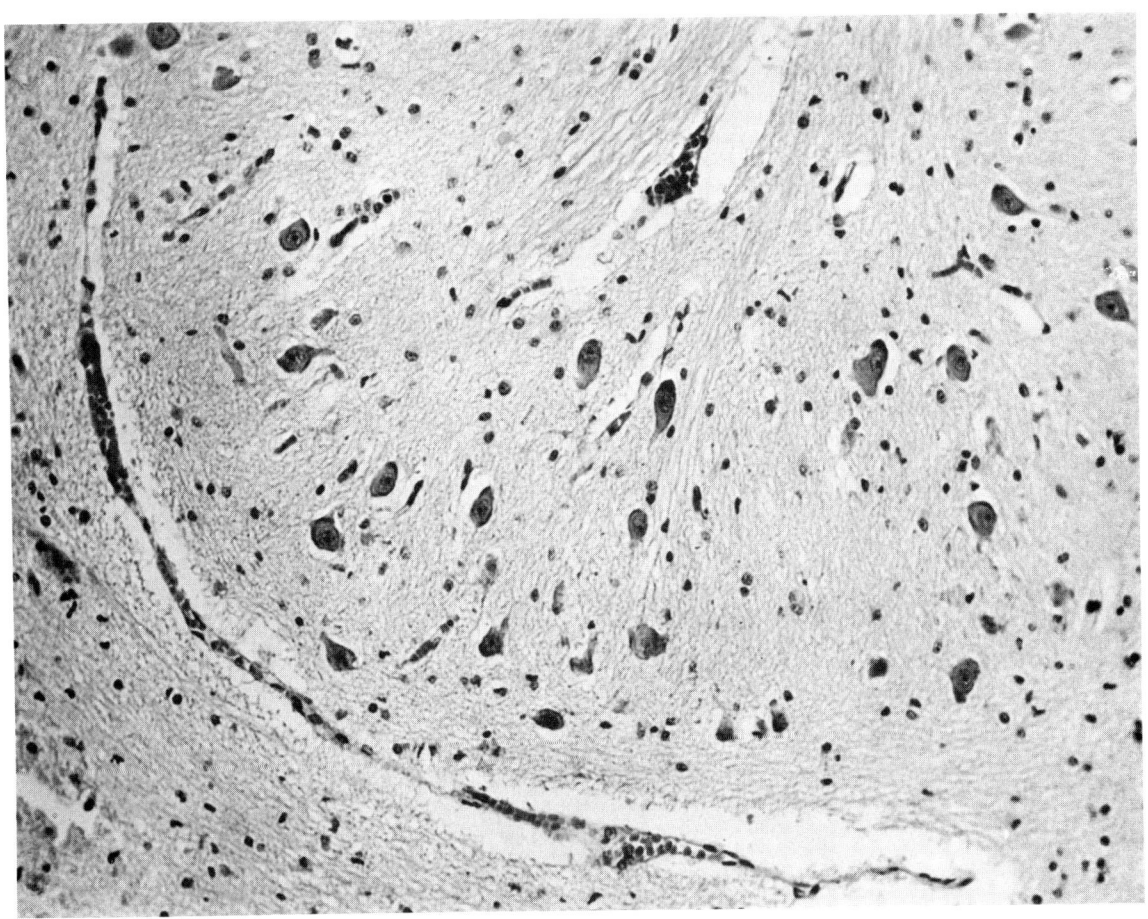

Figure 31–69

Figure 31–69. These are the cells of the olive of medulla oblongata in a newborn. This infant was a stillborn white female weighing 3,120 grams, delivered at term. Hematoxylin and eosin stain. Mag. 208×.

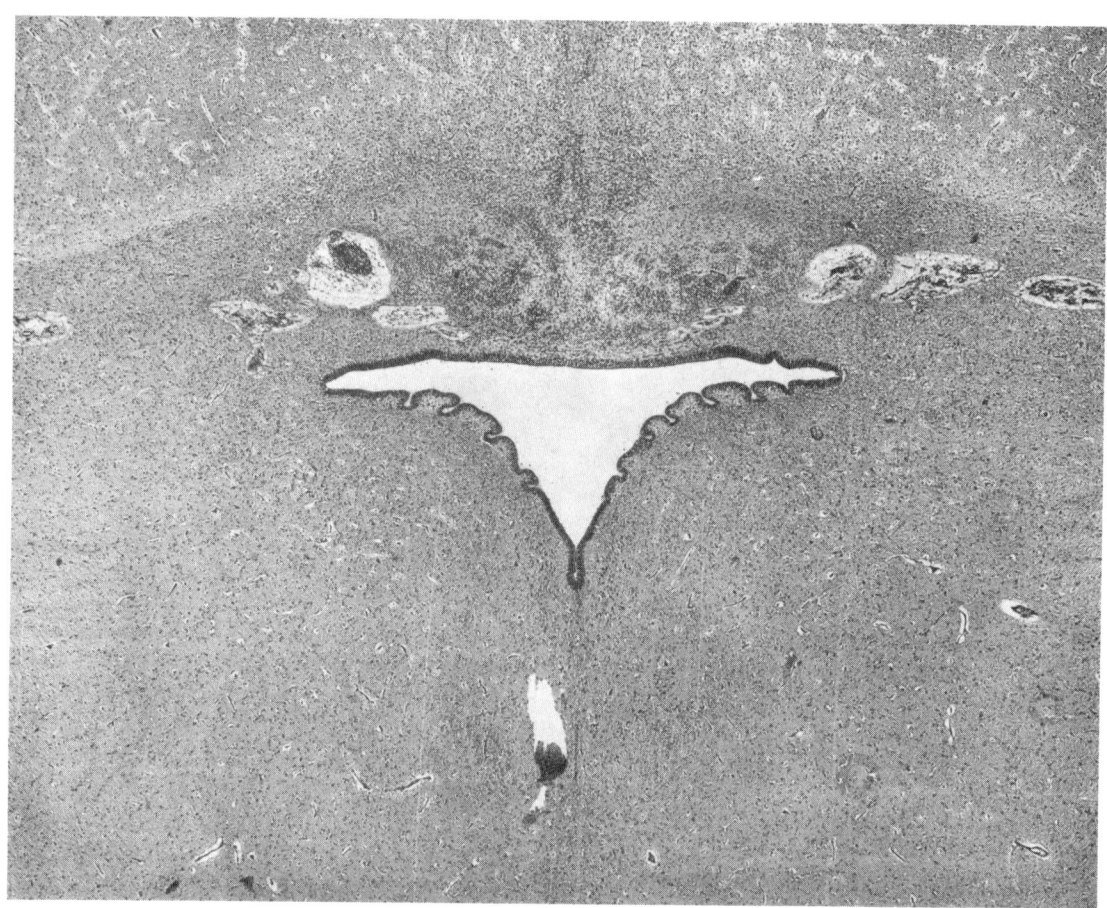

Figure 31–70

Figure 31–70. This is a photograph of the fourth ventricle in a 370 gram stillborn infant who was delivered in the eighteenth week of gestation.
Hematoxylin and eosin stain. Mag. 31×.

CENTRAL NERVOUS SYSTEM 607

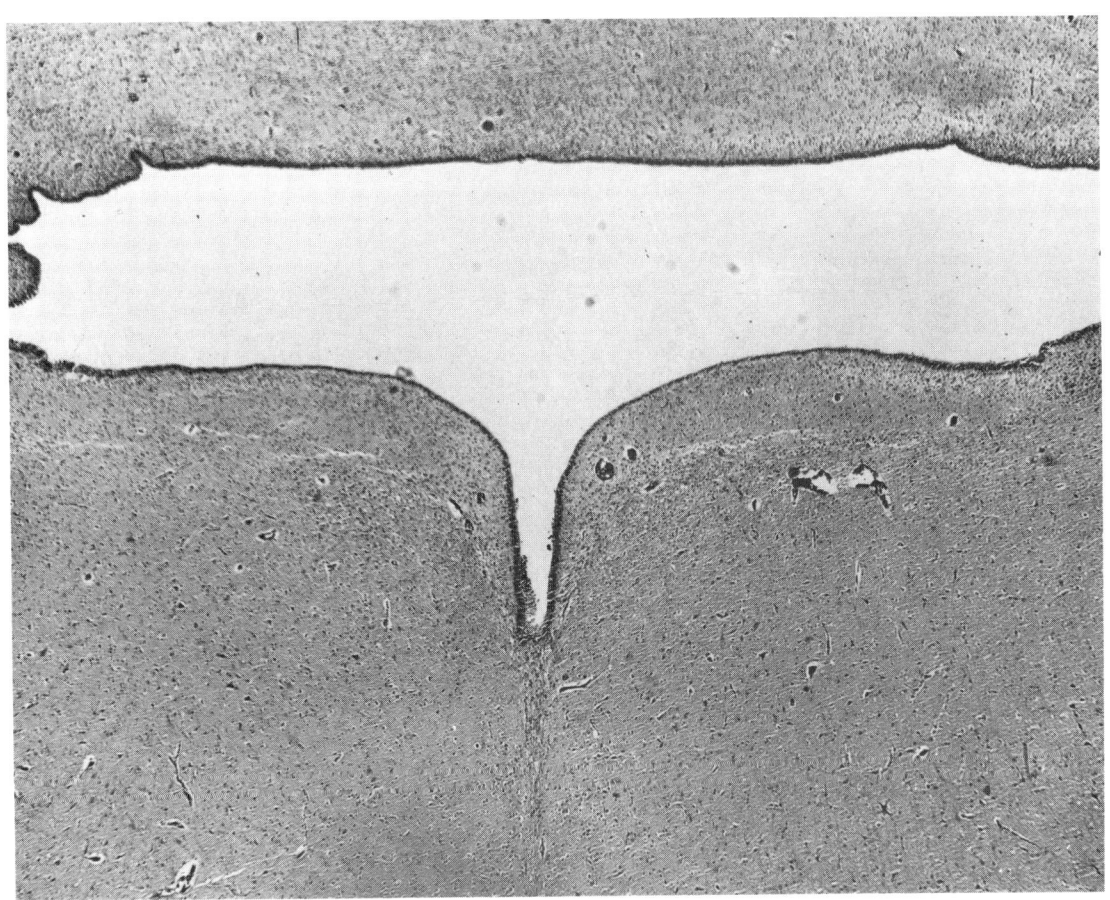

Figure 31–71

Figure 31–71. Depicted here is a coronal section of the superior portion of the pons with the fourth ventricle.

The patient was a black male immature infant born in the 24th week of gestation. The body weight at autopsy was 650 grams.

Hematoxylin and eosin stain. Mag. 35×.

608 CENTRAL NERVOUS SYSTEM

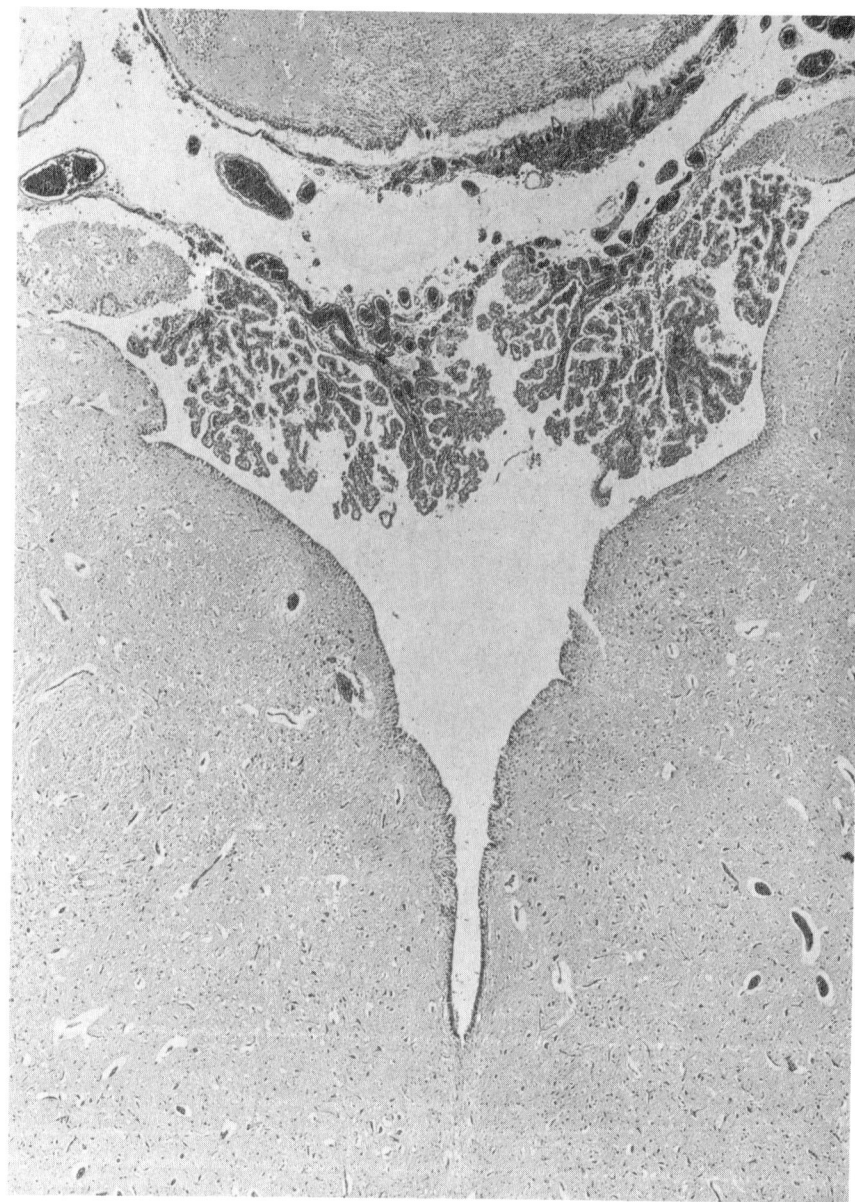

Figure 31–72

Figures 31–72 to 31–74. These are three views of the fourth ventricle, sectioned in the coronal plane, illustrating its unique shape. Suspended from the roof of the fourth ventricle is the tela choroidea or choroid plexus of the fourth ventricle.

Figure 31–72. This black male infant, weighing 2,200 grams, lived for one minute. Mag. 43.5×.

Figure 31–73. This white male infant lived for one month and five days. His body weight was 1,350 grams. Mag. 37×.

Figure 31–74. This one hour and 25 minute old black male weighed 2,960 grams at autopsy. Mag. 37×.

Hematoxylin and eosin stain.

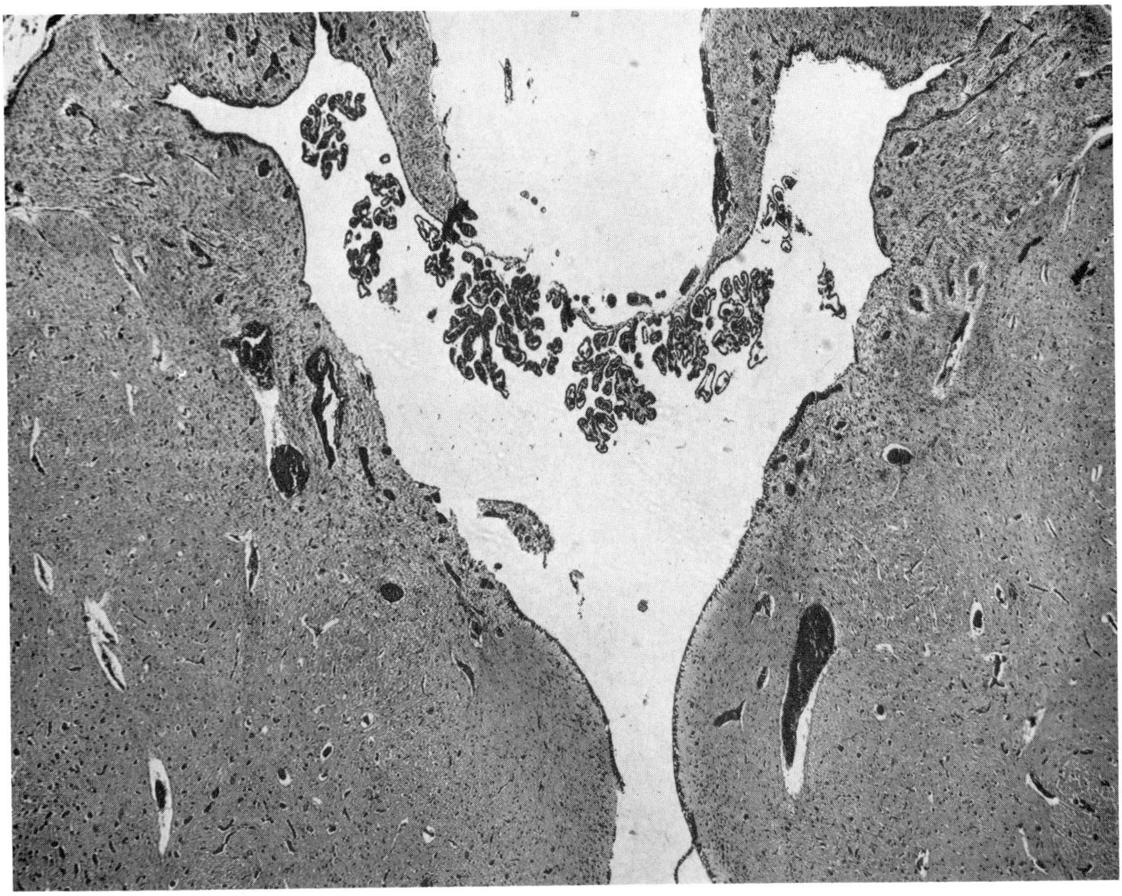

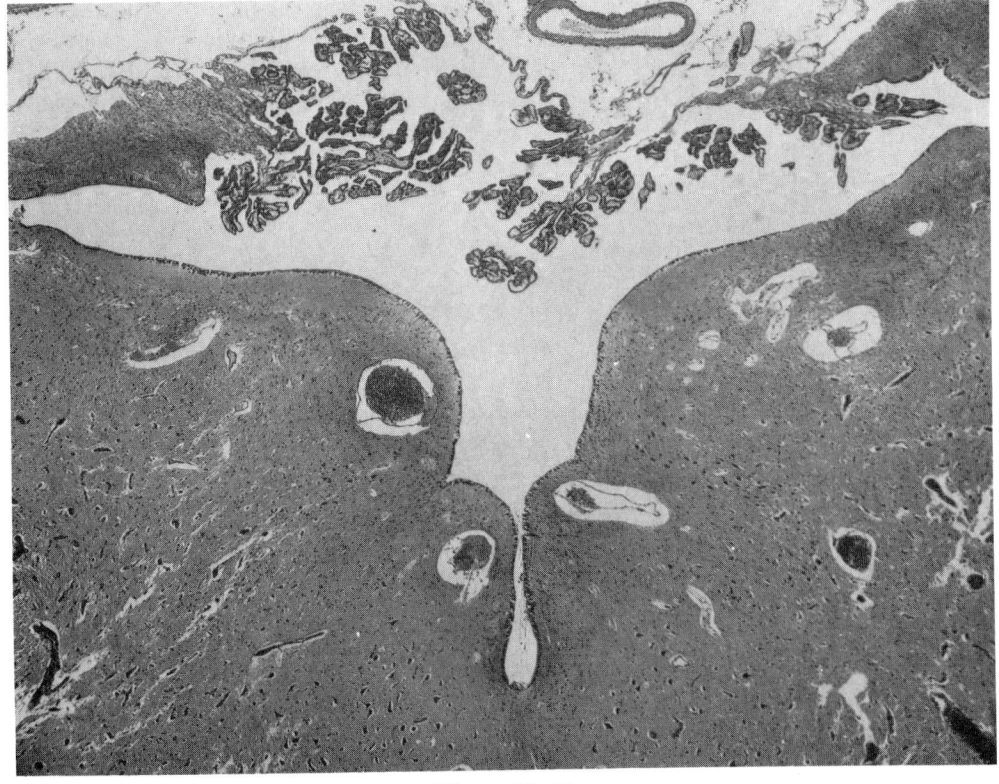

Figure 31–73

Figure 31–74

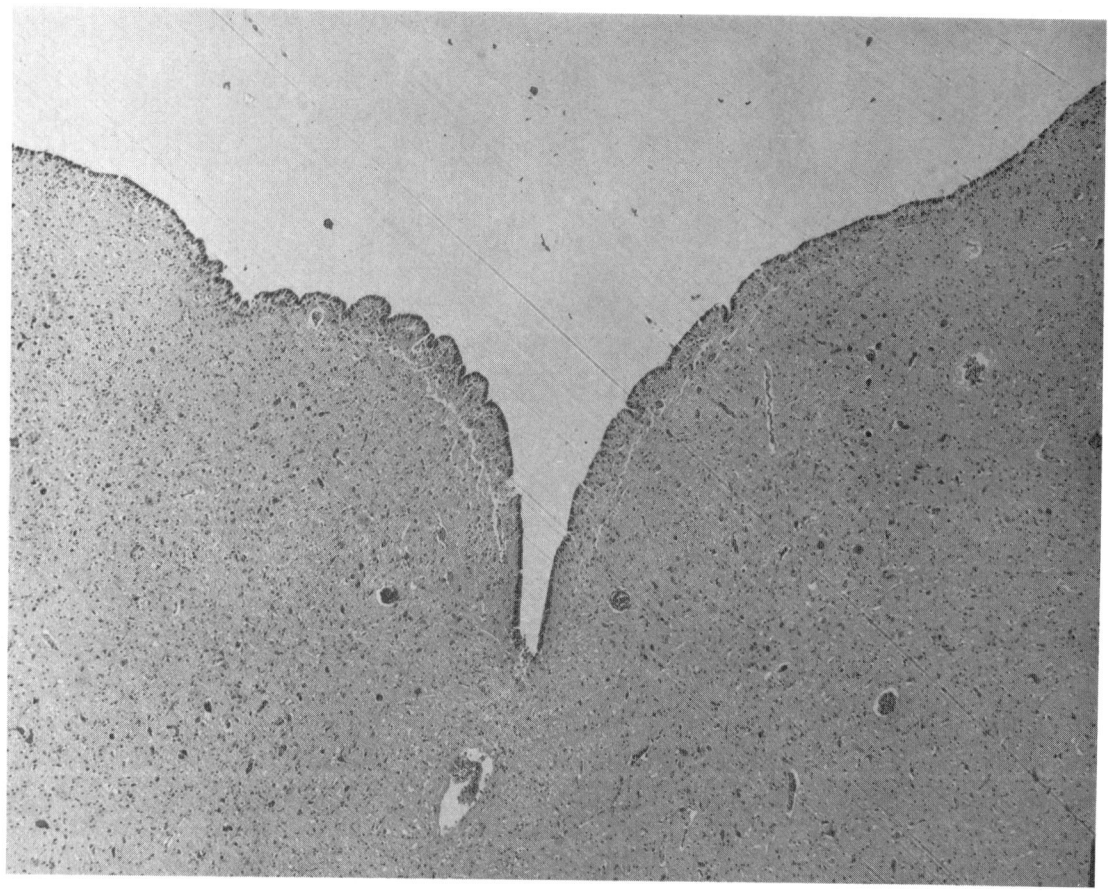

Figure 31-75

Figure 31-75. This is an illustration of the floor of the fourth ventricle from a much more mature infant, a stillborn black male whose weight at autopsy was 3,210 grams.
Hematoxylin and eosin stain. Mag. 45×.

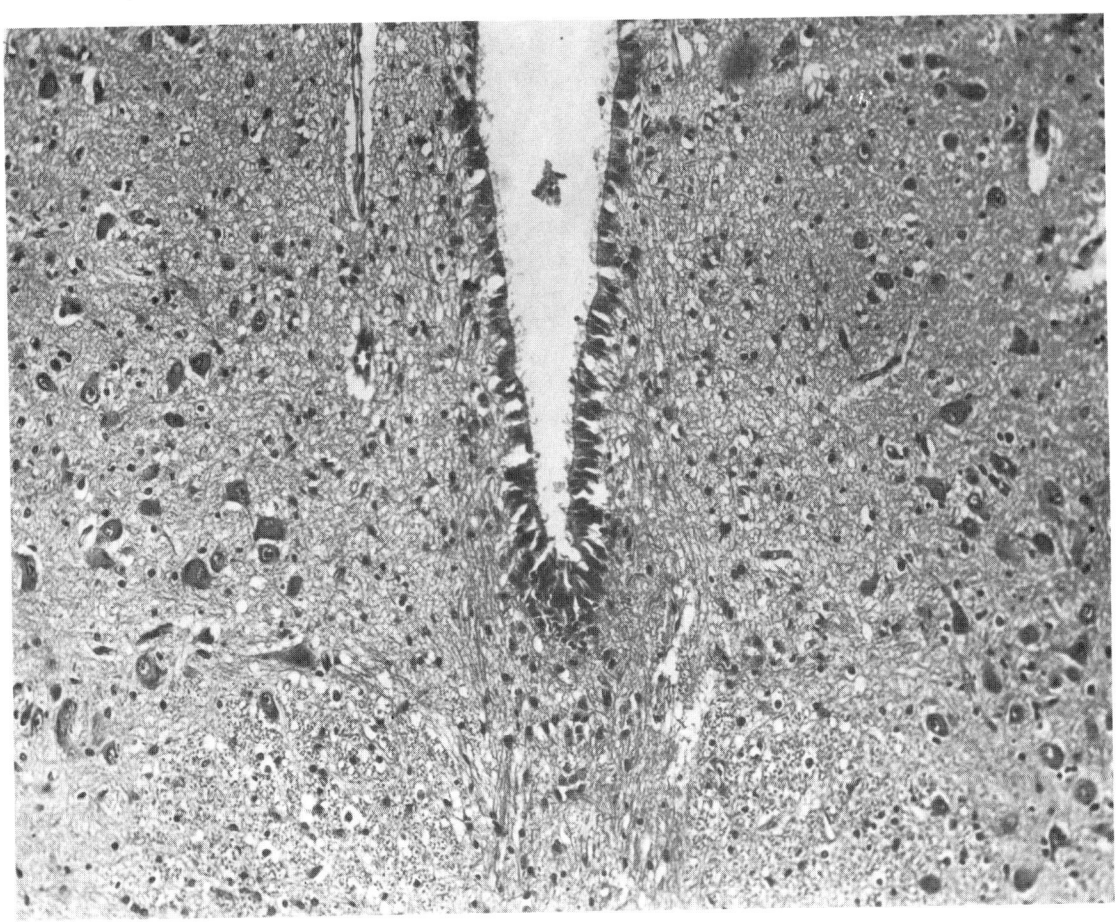

Figure 31–76

Figure 31–76. Seen here at higher magnification is the ependymal lining of the floor of the fourth ventricle, again from an infant born at term. This was a 3,100 gram female who lived for one hour and 32 minutes after birth.
Hematoxylin and eosin stain. Mag. 153×.

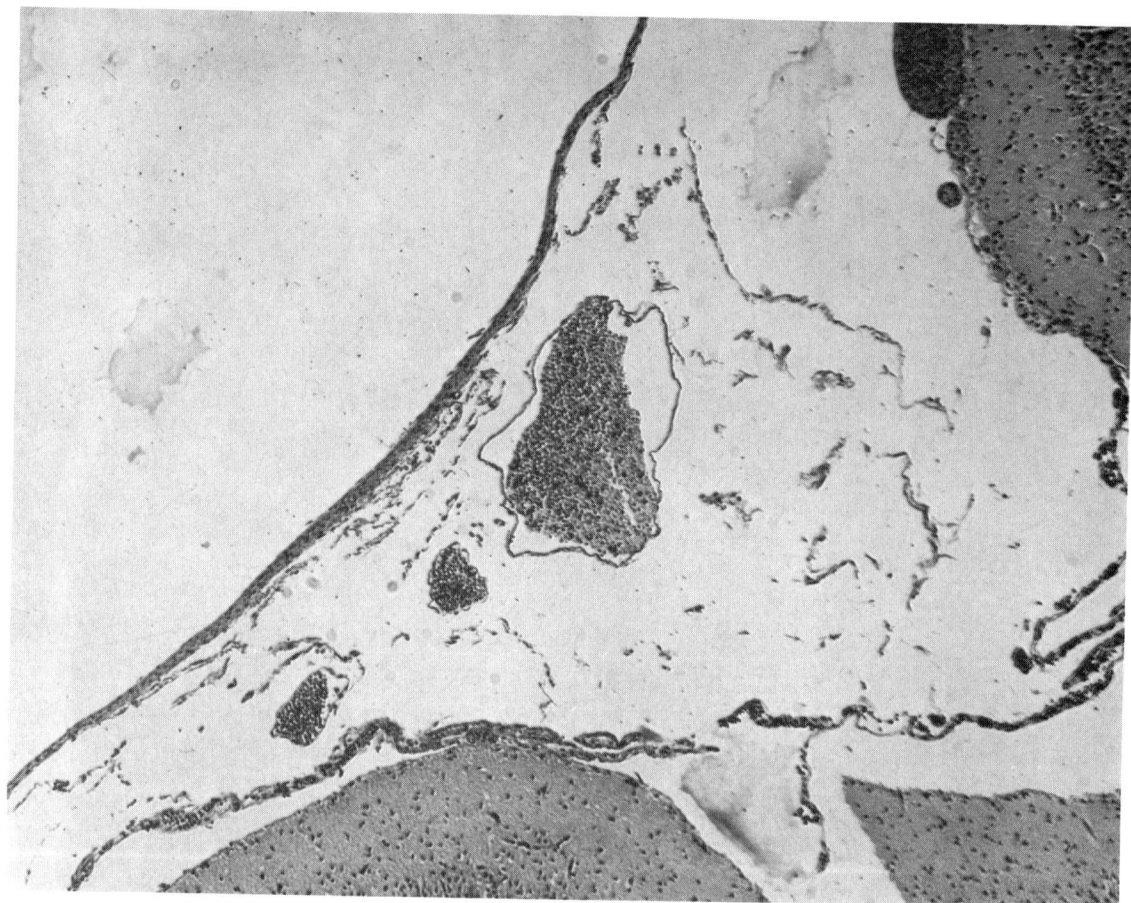

Figure 31-77

Figure 31-77. This is a photomicrograph of the pia arachnoid, covering the cerebral hemisphere. The arachnoid appears as a delicate arc sweeping from the left margin upward to the center of the top. The pia is separated from it and rather intimately applied to the surface of the cortex. Between the two there is loosely woven connective tissue in which are suspended several thin-walled blood vessels.

This infant was a white female, stillborn at term, whose body weight at postmortem examination was 3,120 grams.

Hematoxylin and eosin stain. Mag. 45×.

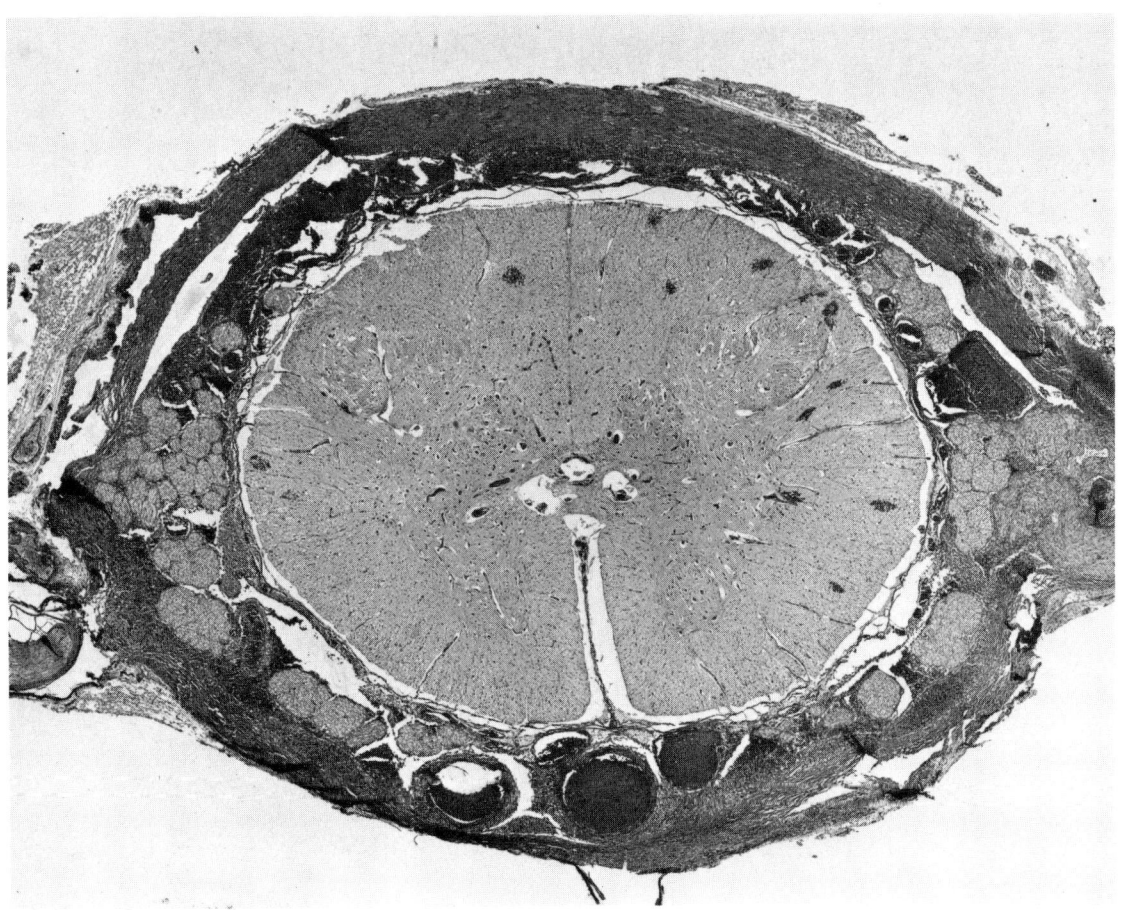

Figure 31–78

Figure 31–78. This is a cross section of the thoracic portion of the spinal cord from a newborn. At this level the cord is surrounded by a moderate number of nerves. The pia arachnoid and the dura are also included in this section.

The infant was a 3,250 gram stillborn delivered at term.

Hematoxylin and eosin stain. Mag. 20.8×.

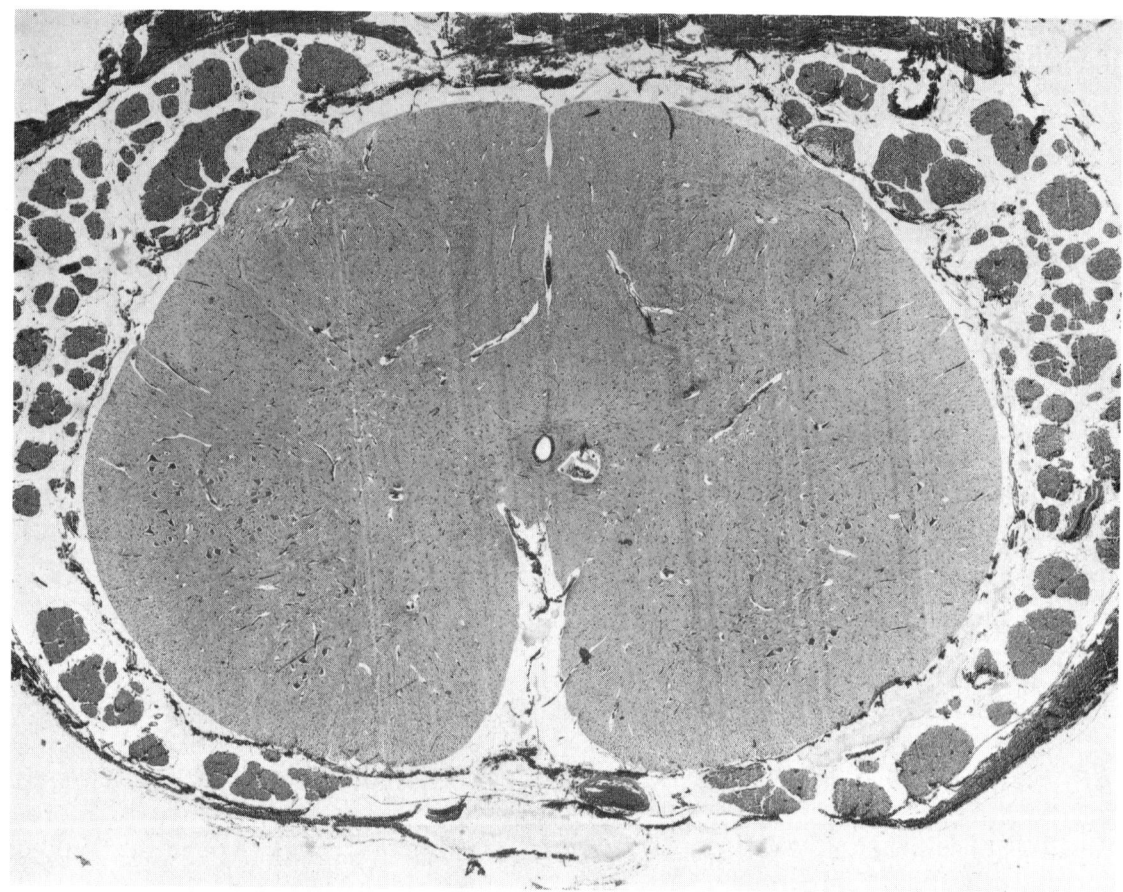

Figure 31-79

Figure 31-79. This is a cross section of the lumbar portion of the spinal cord from a newborn.
Note the large number of nerves surrounding the spinal cord. The delicate pia arachnoid immediately encircles the cord, while the dura embraces the nerves as well as the cord.

This patient was a three month old black female whose body weight at autopsy was 4,610 grams.

Hematoxylin and eosin stain. Mag. 15×.

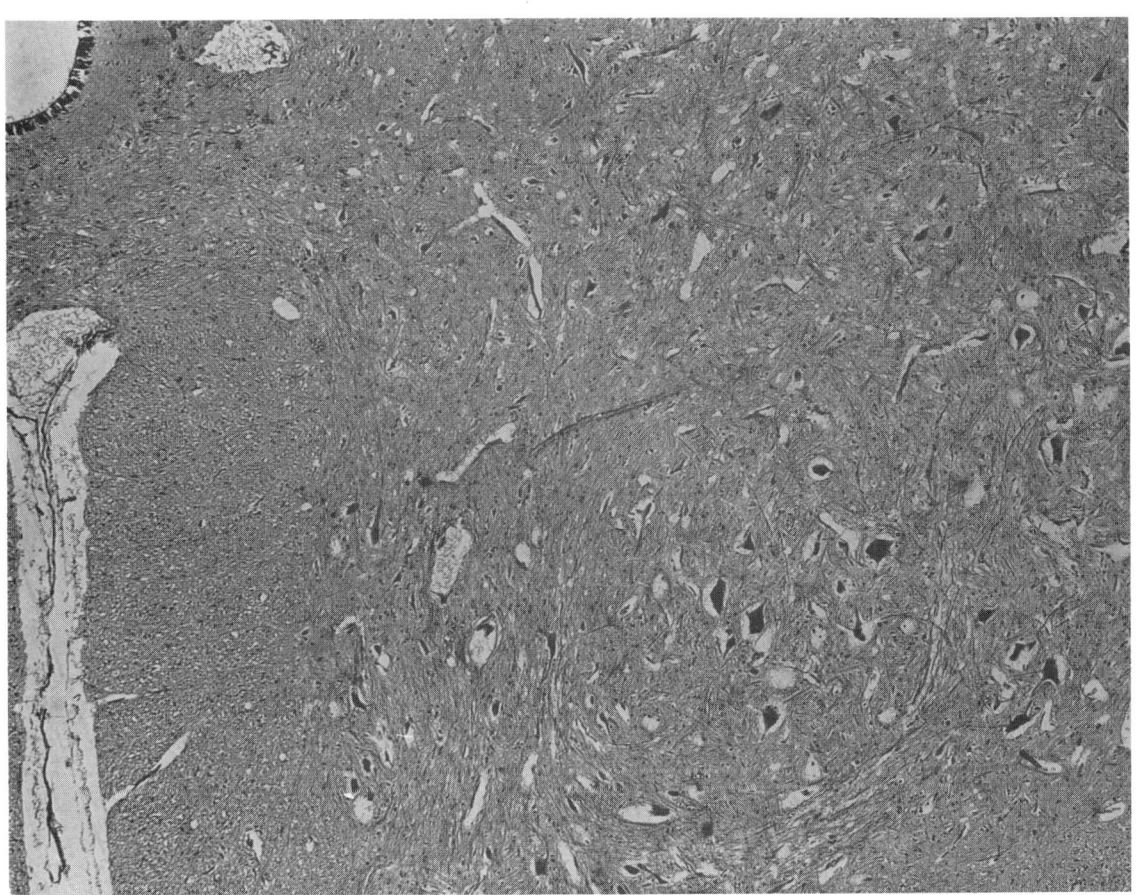

Figure 31-80

Figure 31-80. This photograph depicts the anterior horn of the spinal cord of an infant beyond the newborn period. The anterior horn cells appear as large black irregular forms near the right lower corner of the picture. The central canal is in the upper left.

This infant was nine months old at death. She died of a mediastinal tumor.

Hematoxylin and eosin stain. Mag. 20×.

Figure 31–81. This photograph serves to illustrate the nature of the central canal—not only its shape, but also the nature of the lining ependymal cells.

This baby was a black male who lived for nine hours and 47 minutes. His body weight at autopsy was 1,010 grams.

Hematoxylin and eosin stain. Mag. 267×.

See illustration on the opposite page

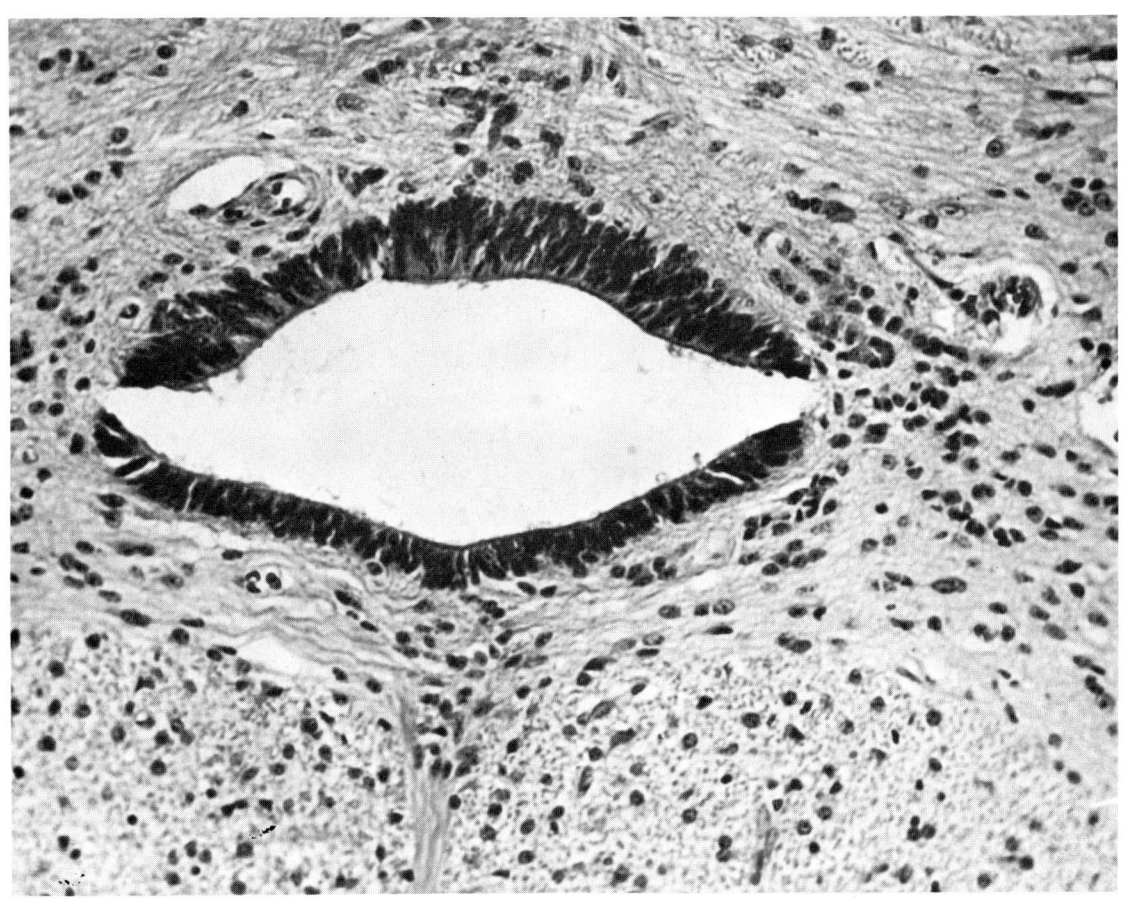

Figure 31–81

618 CENTRAL NERVOUS SYSTEM

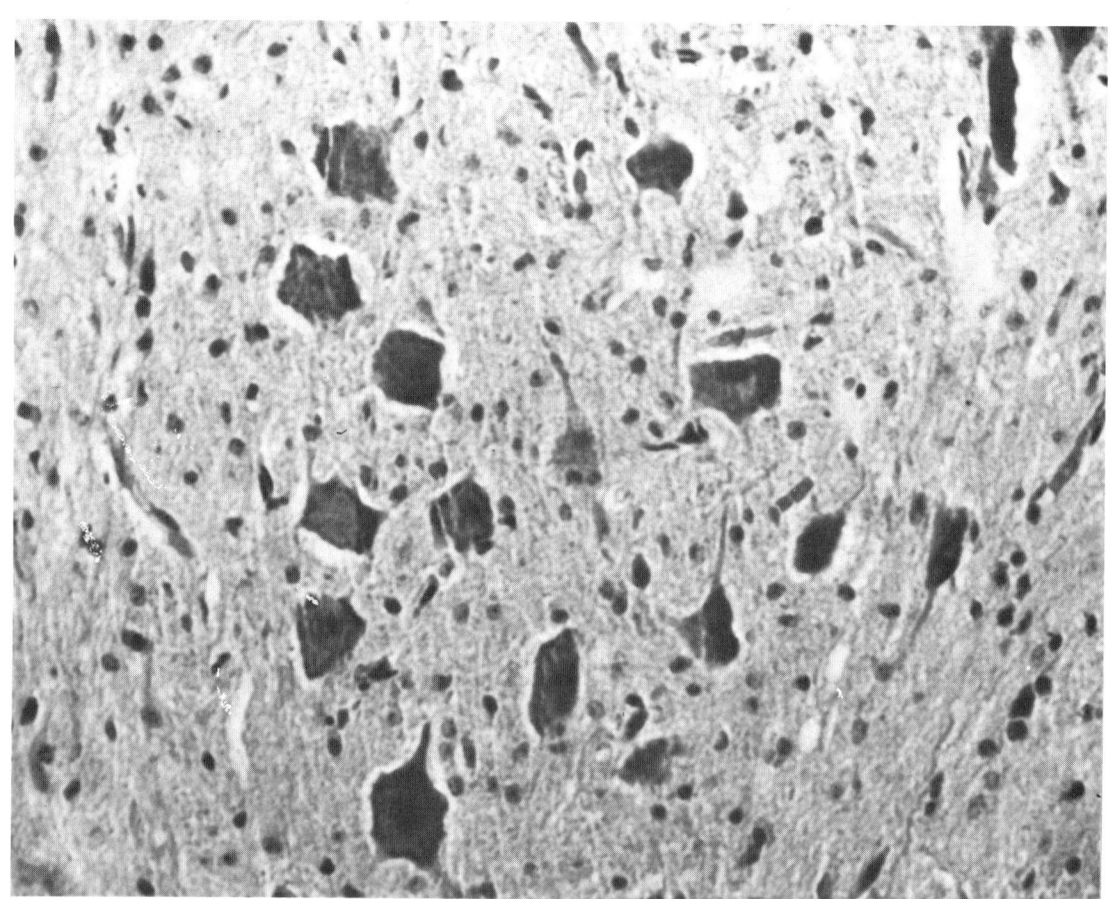

Figure 31–82

Figures 31–82 to 31–84. This set of three photomicrographs shows, at progressively higher magnification, the anterior horn cells of the spinal cord.

Figure 31–82. This baby was a white male weighing 1,030 grams, born at 26 weeks of gestation. Mag. 382×.

Figure 31–83. This was a black male infant weighing 4,225 grams, born at term. He survived for 27 hours. Mag. 513×.

Figure 31–84. This was a black male infant weighing 1,100 grams, who lived for 20 hours. Estimated gestational age is 27 weeks. Mag. 660×.

Hematoxylin and eosin stain.

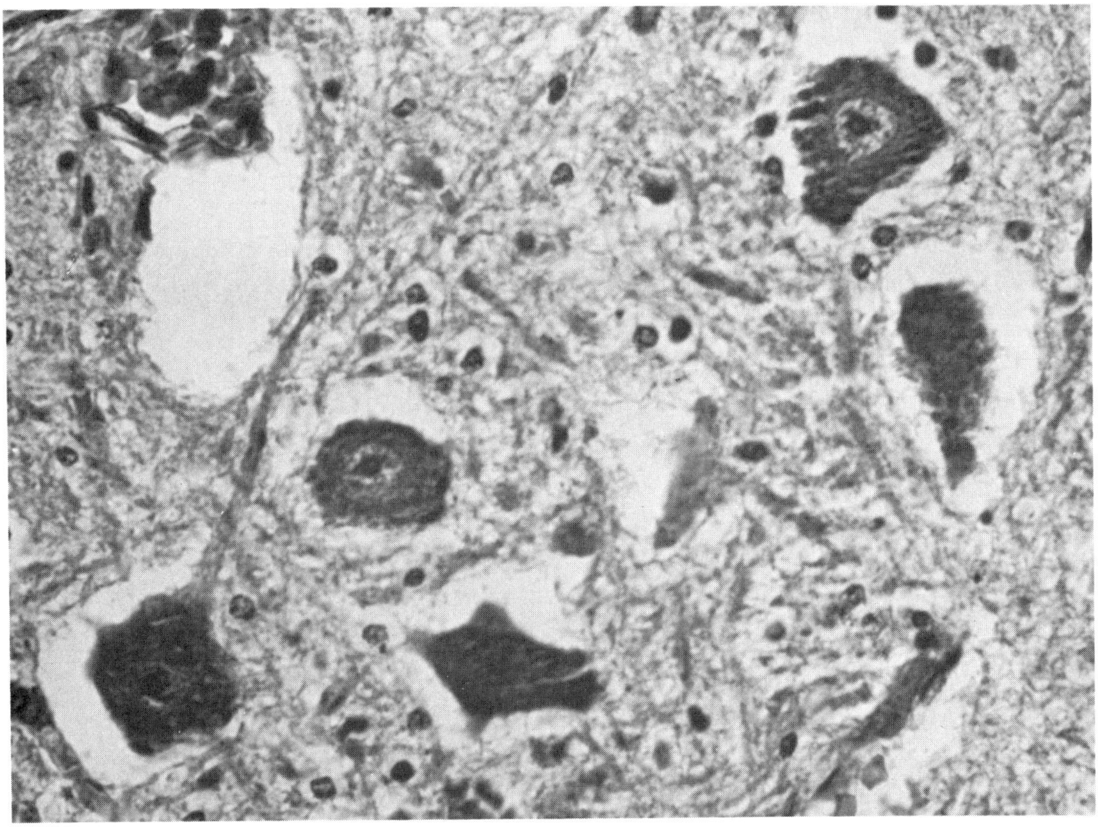

Figure 31-83

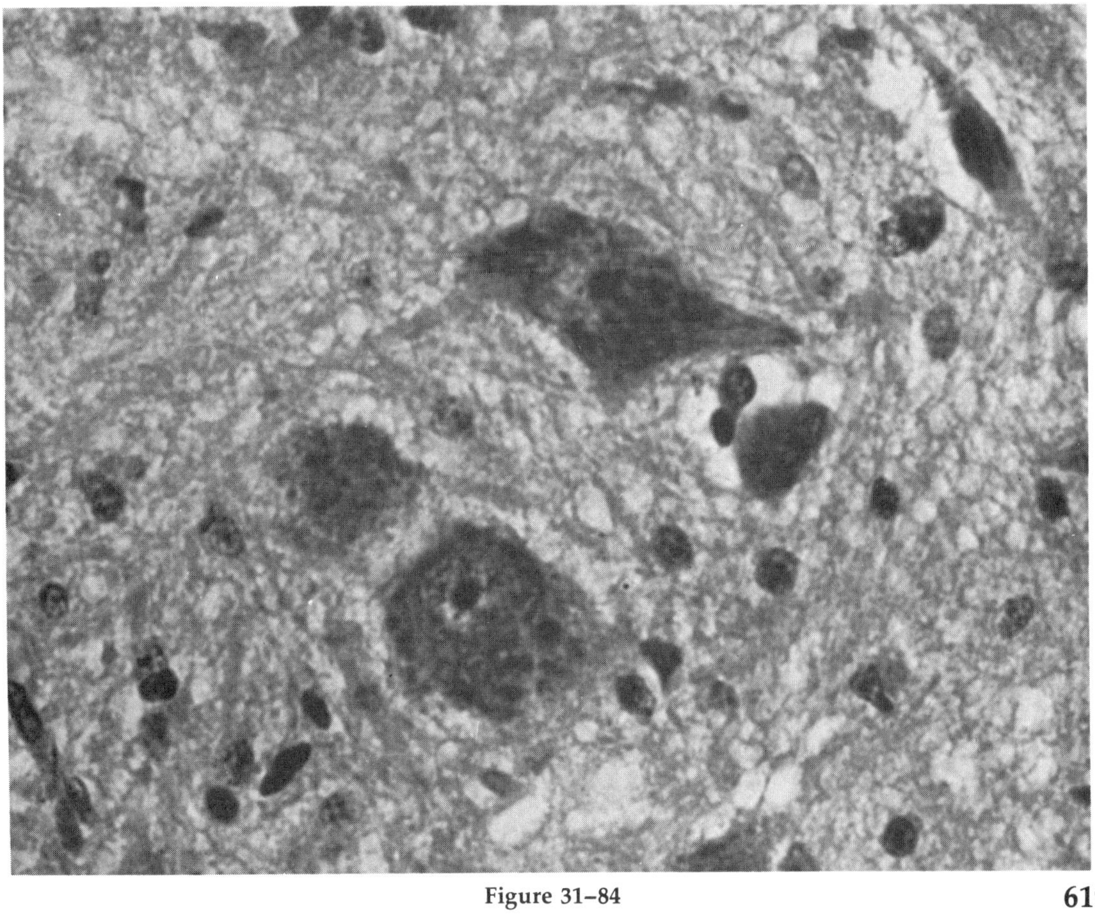

Figure 31-84

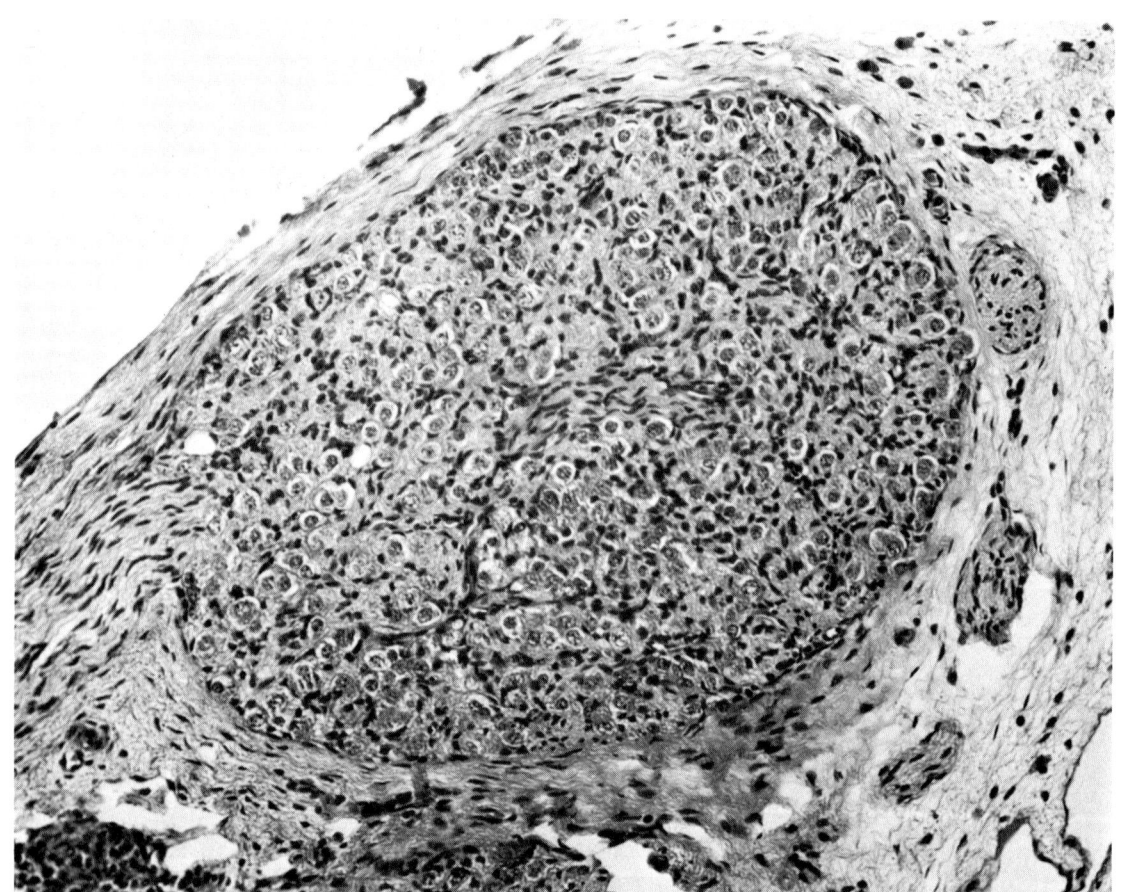

Figure 31–85

Figure 31–85. This is a ganglion from an infant born quite prematurely. A nerve related to this ganglion can be seen on the left.

The infant, who lived for five days, was born in the sixth month of gestation. Her body weight was 568 grams.

Hematoxylin and eosin stain. Mag. 45×.

Part 14

SUPPORTING STRUCTURES

Chapter 32

MUSCULAR SYSTEM

EMBRYOLOGY

The muscular system evolves almost entirely from mesoderm. Muscle tissue develops from primitive cells called myoblasts, which are derived from mesenchyme.[1] The myoblasts that form the skeletal musculature are derived from the mesenchyme of (1) the myotome regions of the somites, (2) the branchial arches, and (3) the somatic mesoderm.

The individual myoblasts, early on, have rather finely granular cytoplasm. They tend to be elongate. Initially the young muscle fiber has a single, large, centrally placed nucleus; soon, however, as it elongates it becomes multinucleated and the nuclei move to the periphery of the cells. During early fetal life, myofibrils appear in the cytoplasm and, by the end of the third month, they show the characteristic cross striations of skeletal muscle fibers.

The musculature of the limbs is developed in situ from mesenchyme surrounding the developing bones. That mesenchyme, in turn, is derived from the somatic layer of the lateral plate mesoderm.[1]

In a fetus at term, the skeletal muscle fibers have all the essential histological characteristics of adult skeletal muscle (Fig. 32–1). However, the fibers are much more slender than those of the adult, and the nuclei are more rounded and less intensely crowded against the sarcolemma.[2]

The first somites to be formed are the most cephalic ones in the series; they appear close behind the auditory placode during the third week of development. They increase rapidly in number until, by the sixth week, their total has reached 39 pairs. Surprisingly constant are the eight cervical, twelve thoracic, five lumbar, and five sacral somites. Added to these are four occipital and five caudal somites, giving 39 pairs.[2]

The developing fibers in the myotomes originally run in a craniocaudal direction. In certain areas the fiber direction changes; but many trunk muscles, especially the intercostal and those associated with the vertebral column, retain their original segmental relations.[2]

As the muscle system differentiates, there are certain commonly repeated types of changes that occur as the adult plan of arrangement is established. These are: (1) the above-mentioned changes in the original direction, (2) longitudinal splitting into two or more portions, (3) tangential splitting into two or more layers, (4) fusion of portions of successive myotomes to form a single muscle mass, (5) migration of muscle primordia to segmental levels different from those of their origin, and (6) degeneration of portions or of the whole of a muscle segment; when it degenerates it tends to become converted into connective tissue, such as an aponeurosis.[2]

ANATOMY

The individual units of skeletal muscle are the muscle fibers, each of which is a single cell with many hundreds of nuclei. The fibers are arranged in bundles of various sizes within the muscle. Connective tissue fills the spaces between the muscle fibers within a bundle, where it is known as the endomysium (Fig. 32–1); each bundle is also surrounded by a stronger connective tissue sheath or perimysium (Fig. 32–2). Surrounding the whole muscle is a stout epimysium, which is continuous with both the perimyseal septa and the connective tissues of surrounding structures.[3]

HISTOLOGY

With the light microscope, skeletal muscle fibers appear as closely packed cylinders in longitudinal section (Fig. 32–1), but they may have circular, elliptical, or polygonal profiles in cross section (Fig. 32–2). Each fiber is elongate and may stretch from one end of the muscle to the other; elsewhere they may extend only part of the length of the muscle and end in some connective tissue intersection that penetrates the body of the muscle.

Their flattened nuclei lie peripherally in a zone immediately beneath the cell membrane or sarcolemma, while their cytoplasm, known as the sarcoplasm, is divided into longitudinal threads or myofibrils. In transverse sections, routinely prepared, the myofibrils often appear aggregated in small groups called the fields of Cohnheim, but this is probably an artifact because better methods of preservation show the myofibrils to be uniformly distributed.

In longitudinal sections or on surface view, the myofibrils are seen to be traversed by striations, which are apparently continuous across the fiber. They vary in staining reaction and optical properties. In the most commonly used terminology, the two principal bands are named the A band and the I band according to their appearance in polarized light. Polarization microscopy reverses the appearance noted by light microscopy so that the dark band becomes bright and the light band dark. The dark band of routine light microscopy, which exhibits birefringence with polarized light, is *anisotropic* and is called the A band. The light band of routine light microscopy is poorly refractile and relatively *isotropic*, and is called the I band.[4]

Both in stained preparations and in living muscle viewed with phase contrast microscopy, a dark transverse line, the Z line, bisects each I band. In exceptional preparations a paler zone, called the H band, may be seen traversing the center of the A band.[5]

The repeating structural unit is the sarcomere, which is defined as the segment between two successive Z lines and therefore includes an A band and half of the two contiguous I bands. In histological sections of skeletal muscle the A bands, the I bands, and the Z lines are usually the only cross striations that are discernible. (Ordinarily not visible in routine preparations, in the very center of the H band as it traverses the A band, is a narrow dark line called the M band or M line.) All of these features are much more readily appreciated in electron micrographs.

Fibers making up a single muscle are not uniform in size or cytological characteristics. Three categories are recognizable: small red fibers (rich in mitochondria), large white fibers (with relatively few mitochondria), and fibers with intermediate characteristics. Variations in the gross color of different muscles, red to white, reflect differing proportions of the three fiber types. Proportions within a given muscle are fairly constant.[5]

References

All references for Part Fourteen are on p. 642.

626 MUSCULAR SYSTEM

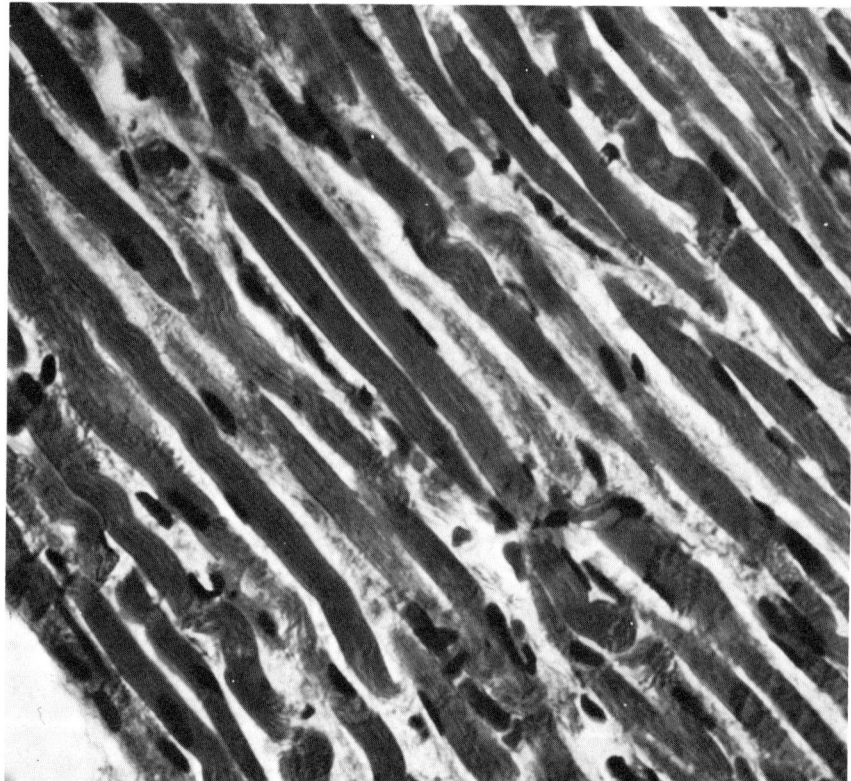

Figure 32–1

Figure 32–1. Depicted here is the skeletal muscle of the diaphragm in longitudinal section. The infant was a 2,080 gram male delivered in the thirty-fourth week of gestation. He survived for 57 hours.

Hematoxylin and eosin stain. Mag. 492×.

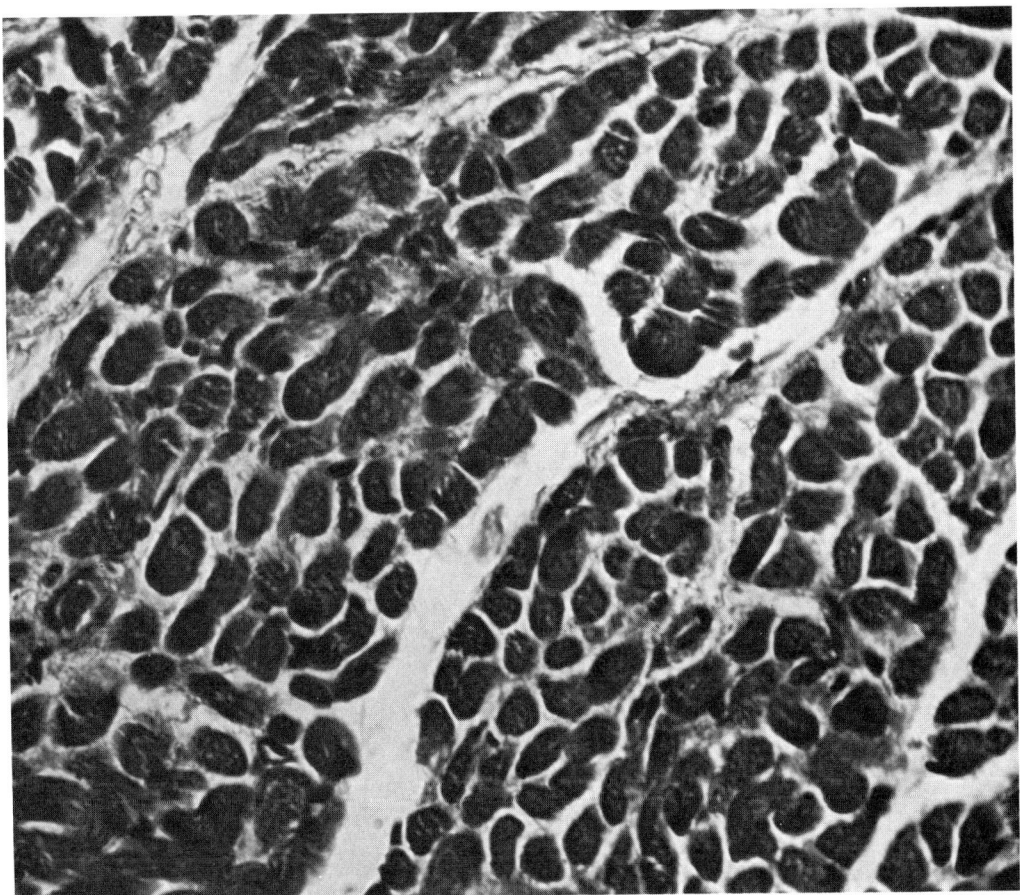

Figure 32–2

Figure 32–2. This is a cross section of the same muscle as is illustrated in Fig. 32–1. The patient is the same.

Note that the muscle fibers are arranged in discrete bundles and that each such bundle is sheathed in a delicate layer of collagenous connective tissue.

One can observe that the muscle nuclei are located along the edges of the fibers, as is characteristic for skeletal muscle.

Hematoxylin and eosin stain. Mag. 492×.

Chapter 33

SKELETAL SYSTEM

EMBRYOLOGY

The skeletal system develops from mesoderm. Most bones of the skeleton first appear as mesenchymal condensations, and then as hyaline cartilage models that become ossified by enchondral ossification. Some bones develop in mesenchyme by intramembranous bone formation.[1]

Cartilage develops from mesenchyme and first appears in embryos of about five weeks. In areas where cartilage is to develop, the mesenchyme condenses and the cells proliferate and become rounded. Subsequently, collagenous fibers or elastic fibers, or both, are deposited in the intercellular substance or matrix. Three types of cartilage (hyaline, fibrocartilage, and elastic) are distinguished, depending upon the nature of the matrix.[1]

Bone always develops by transformation of pre-existing connective tissue; it develops in two types of connective tissue, mesenchyme and cartilage. Intramembranous ossification occurs in mesenchyme. The mesenchyme condenses and becomes very vascular; some cells differentiate into osteoblasts and begin to deposit intercellular substance. That matrix subsequently becomes calcified to form spicules of spongy bone. Some osteoblasts remain trapped in the matrix to become osteocytes as successive layers of lamellae are deposited by other osteoblasts. As the spicules thicken and fuse, plates of compact bone form; haversian systems develop by later internal reorganization. Between the plates the intervening bone remains spongy, and the mesenchyme differentiates to become bone marrow. Remodeling continues by the action of osteoblasts and osteoclasts.

Enchondral or intracartilaginous ossification takes place in pre-existing cartilaginous models. For example, in a long bone the primary ossification center appears in the diaphysis or shaft. Here the cartilage cells increase in size, the matrix becomes calcified, and the cells die. Concurrently, a thin layer of bone is deposited under the perichondrium surrounding the shaft; thus the perichondrium becomes the periosteum. Invasion of vascular connective tissue from the periosteum breaks up the cartilage. Some mesenchymal cells differentiate into hematopoietic cells of the bone marrow, while others differentiate into osteoblasts that deposit bone matrix on the spicules of calcified cartilage. This process continues toward the epiphyses or ends of the bones. The spicules of bone are remodeled by the action of osteoblasts and osteoclasts.[1]

Growth in the length of long bones takes place at the junction of the shaft and the epiphysis, the epiphyseal line (Figs. 33-2, 33-3, and 33-6). The cartilage cells in that region proliferate by mitosis. In the vicinity of the shaft they hypertrophy, and the matrix becomes calcified and broken up into spicules by vessels from the marrow or medullary cavity. Bone is deposited on these spicules. Resorption of the bone keeps the spongy bone masses relatively constant in length and enlarges the marrow cavity. At birth the shaft is largely ossified (Figs. 33-4 to 33-6), but most epiphyses are still cartilaginous (Figs. 33-2 and 33-3).

Secondary ossification centers appear in the epiphyses during the postnatal period. The epiphyseal cartilage cells hypertrophy, and there is invasion of vascular connective tissue. Ossification, as described above, spreads out in all directions from the center; only the articular cartilage and a transverse plate of cartilage called the epiphyseal plate remain cartilaginous. After the epiphyses are well established, growth occurs on the shaft side of the plate only. Growth in the diameter of the bone results from the deposition of bone beneath the periosteum and its resorption on the medullary surface. The rates of deposition and resorption are balanced to regulate the thickness of the compact bone and the size of the marrow cavity.

Irregular bones develop in a way similar to that of the epiphyses of long bones. Ossification begins centrally and spreads in all directions.

ANATOMY

The skeletal tissues, cartilage and bone, are essentially specialized connective tissues and consist of the same three elements: cells, embedded in an intercellular matrix, permeated by a system of fibers. These sclerous tissues are different from generalized connective tissues because their matrix is solidified. Yet cartilage and bone are distinct, structurally and physically, and in their patterns of growth and regeneration.[3]

The matrix of cartilage varies in its gross appearance when freshly cut and in the nature of its fibers. Hence it is classified as either (1) hyaline cartilage, (2) white fibrocartilage, or (3) yellow elastic fibrocartilage. Cartilage is relatively avascular, the majority of cartilage cells being at a considerable distance from the nearest exchange vessels.

Bone, by contrast, is a highly vascular, living, constantly changing mineralized connective tissue, remarkable for its hardness, resilience, growth mechanisms, and regenerative capacities.

A long bone such as the tibia typically has become, at birth, ossified throughout its shaft or diaphysis by the activity of the primary center, which appears in the seventh week of gestation. Its two extremities, the epiphyses (Figs. 33-2 and 33-3), are subsequently transformed into osseous tissue by secondary centers there.[3] The actively growing part of the diaphysis, adjacent to the epiphyseal cartilage, is known as the metaphysis (Fig. 33-6).

Macroscopically, the cut surface of bone may be either compact in the ivory-like surface layers of mature bone or spongy in the interior of mature bones (this is also called cancellous or trabecular bone). Early embryonic bone is also spongy.

The inorganic matrix of bone may exist as irregular dense masses with bone cells scattered through it, or it may be arranged in series of thin sheets or lamellae with intervening rows of bone cells; both types develop as roughly cylindrical masses known as osteons, each having a central vascular canal. Almost all mature bone is of the lamellar type.[3]

HISTOLOGY

Cartilage cells occupy small spaces or lacunae in the matrix, which conform to the shape of the cell. Young cells or chondroblasts are small, irregular, and often flattened. Mature cells or chondrocytes are more rounded.

The intercellular components predominate over the cells; the matrix appears homogeneous in part because the ground substance and the collagen embedded within it have approximately the same refractive index and in part because of the small size of the collagen fibrils. The principal constituent of the ground substance is chondromucoprotein.

In a section of the shaft of a long bone such as is illustrated in Figure 33–4, the cortical portion, which is very slender in a newborn, is composed of compact bone while the medullary cavity is so-called spongy bone.

Compact bone consists largely of matrix, a mineralized interstitial substance, deposited in layers or lamellae. Uniformly spaced throughout it are tiny spaces or lacunae, each filled by an osteocyte. Radiating in all directions from each lacuna are tubular passages, the canaliculi anastomosing with canaliculi of neighboring lacunae. Thus there is a continuous system of cavities interconnected by minute canals. These provide for the nutrition of the bone cells.

The lamellae of compact bone are arranged in three patterns. (1) The most regular are the haversian systems or osteons, each of which is a cylindrical structural unit with a central, longitudinally oriented vessel. In cross section the osteon looks like a series of concentric rings around a central circular opening. (2) Between the osteons are irregular fragments of lamellar bone known as the interstitial systems. The limits between the haversian and interstitial systems are demarcated by prominent refractile lines called cement lines, so that a cross section of compact bone resembles a mosaic of round and angular pieces cemented together. (3) Along the external and internal surfaces of compact bone are several "boundary lamellae" that continue uninterruptedly around much of the circumference of the shaft. These are the outer and inner circumferential lamellae.[5]

In the perinatal period (Figs. 33–2 and 33–3), the cortex of long bones such as the ribs appears to be extremely delicate and discontinuous.

Cancellous or spongy bone is also composed of lamellae (Figs. 33–4 and 33–5), but the trabeculae are thin and not usually penetrated by blood vessels; therefore, they do not usually contain haversian systems but are merely a mosaic of angular pieces of lamellar bone. The bone cells here are nourished by diffusion from the endosteal surface via minute canaliculi.

The periosteum, during the embryonic and postnatal period, presents an inner layer of bone-forming cells, the osteoblasts (Fig. 33–4). The outer layer is relatively acellular dense connective tissue containing blood vessels.

The endosteum (Fig. 33-4) is a thin layer of squamous cells lining the walls of the marrow cavities; it is the peripheral layer of the stroma of the bone marrow where it is in contact with bone. It resembles the periosteum in its osteogenic potential, but it is much thinner. All of the cavities of bone, including the haversian canals, are lined by endosteum that is said to have the capacity to make bone.[5]

The interstitial substance of bone is composed of two major components, an organic matrix and inorganic salts. The organic matrix consists of collagenous fibers embedded in an amorphous ground substance. The inorganic matter consists of submicroscopic deposits of a form of calcium phosphate.[5]

Growth in Length of Long Bones (Figs. 33-2, 33-3, and 33-6). In the continuing growth in length of the cartilage model, after the appearance of the diaphyseal center of ossification, the chondrocytes in the adjacent regions of the epiphyses become arranged in longitudinal columns. The cells within the columns are separated by thin transverse septa, while adjacent columns are separated by wider longitudinal bars of hyaline matrix (Fig. 33-6). The most distal cells proliferate; those in the next group mature and enlarge and become provisionally calcified; and finally the chondrocytes degenerate. The open ends of their enlarged lacunae become invaded by capillary loops from the marrow and by primitive osteogenic cells from the diaphysis. As the spaces are invaded, osteoblasts congregate on the surfaces of the longitudinal bars of persisting calcified cartilage; a thin new layer of bone matrix is deposited on the surface, which begins to calcify and become bone. This transitional zone where cartilage is being replaced by bone is called the metaphysis (Fig. 33-6). The primary spongy bone in this zone undergoes extensive reorganization as the growth passes it by. As the bone grows longer, the diaphyseal ends of the trabeculae are continually being eroded by osteoclasts at about the same rate that additions are made at the epiphyseal end, with the result that the metaphysis tends to remain relatively constant in length.[5]

Growth in Diameter of Long Bones. As mentioned previously, growth in the diameter of the shaft is the result of deposition of new membranous bone beneath the periosteum. Deposition on the outside is accompanied by the appearance of osteoclasts that erode the inner aspect of subperiosteal trabeculae to enlarge the marrow cavity. The two processes are so balanced that the shaft expands rapidly while the thickness of its wall increases more slowly.

References

All references for Part Fourteen are on p. 642.

SKELETAL SYSTEM 633

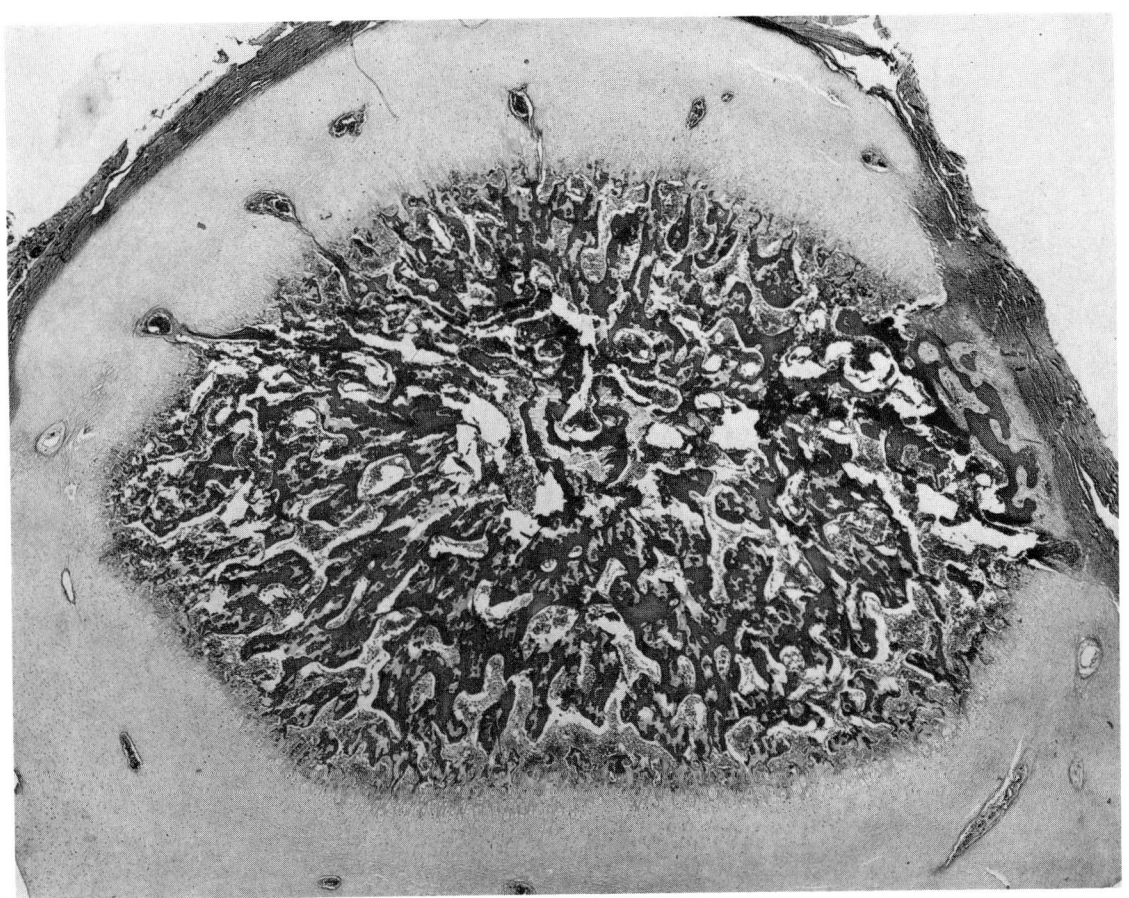

Figure 33–1

Figure 33–1. This is a cross section of a vertebral body of a very small and prematurely born baby. The period of gestation was probably late in the fourth month; body weight at autopsy was only 251 grams. The infant was a female and lived for one hour and eight minutes.

Note the pale-staining band of cartilage about the perimeter and the transition to bone centrally.

Hematoxylin and eosin stain. Mag. 20.8×.

634   SKELETAL SYSTEM

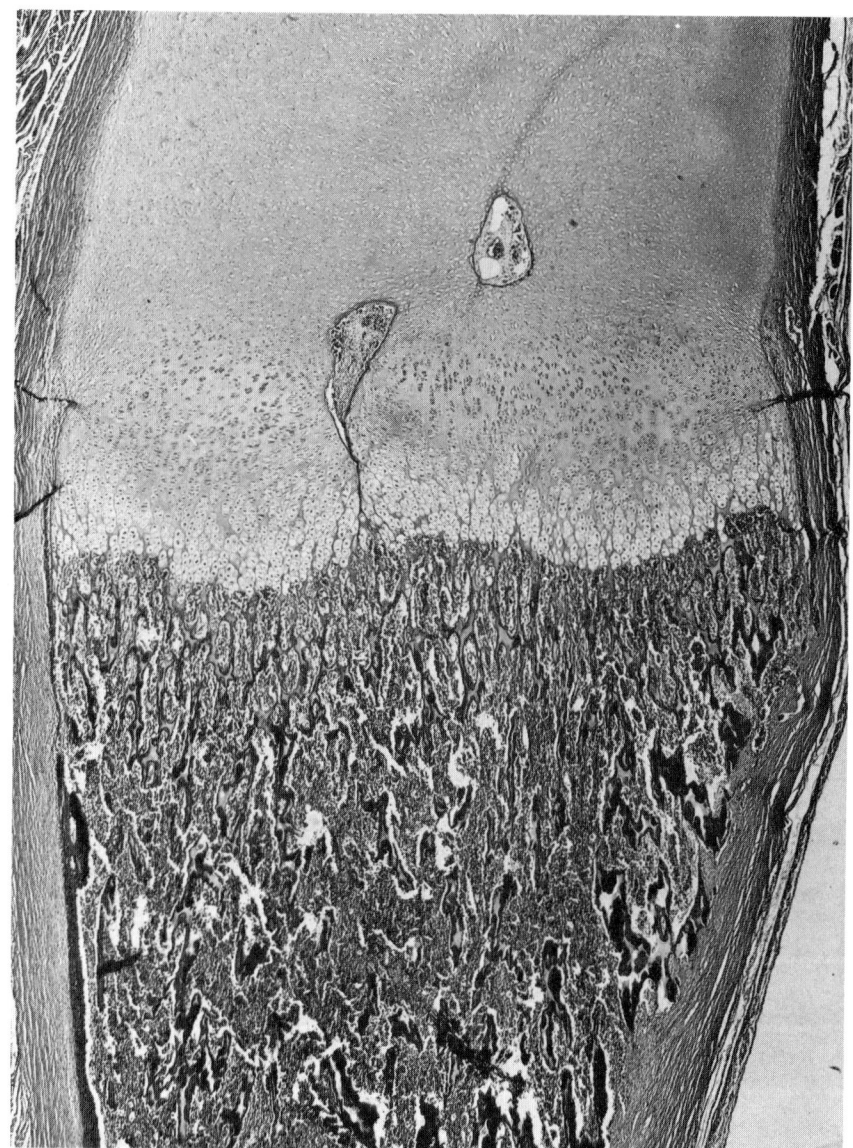

Figure 33-2

Figure 33-2. Pictured here is a longitudinal section of the epiphyseal line in a rib at the costochondral junction.

This infant was a black female who lived for 11 hours. At postmortem examination her body weighed 2,125 grams, even though delivery was said to have been accomplished several weeks past the due date. Mother was a 17 year old girl.

The rather sharply delineated epiphyseal line shows particularly well here. The columns of cartilage cells are nicely longitudinally oriented. The bony trabeculae are delicate, as is the cortex.

Hematoxylin and eosin stain. Mag. 28.5×.

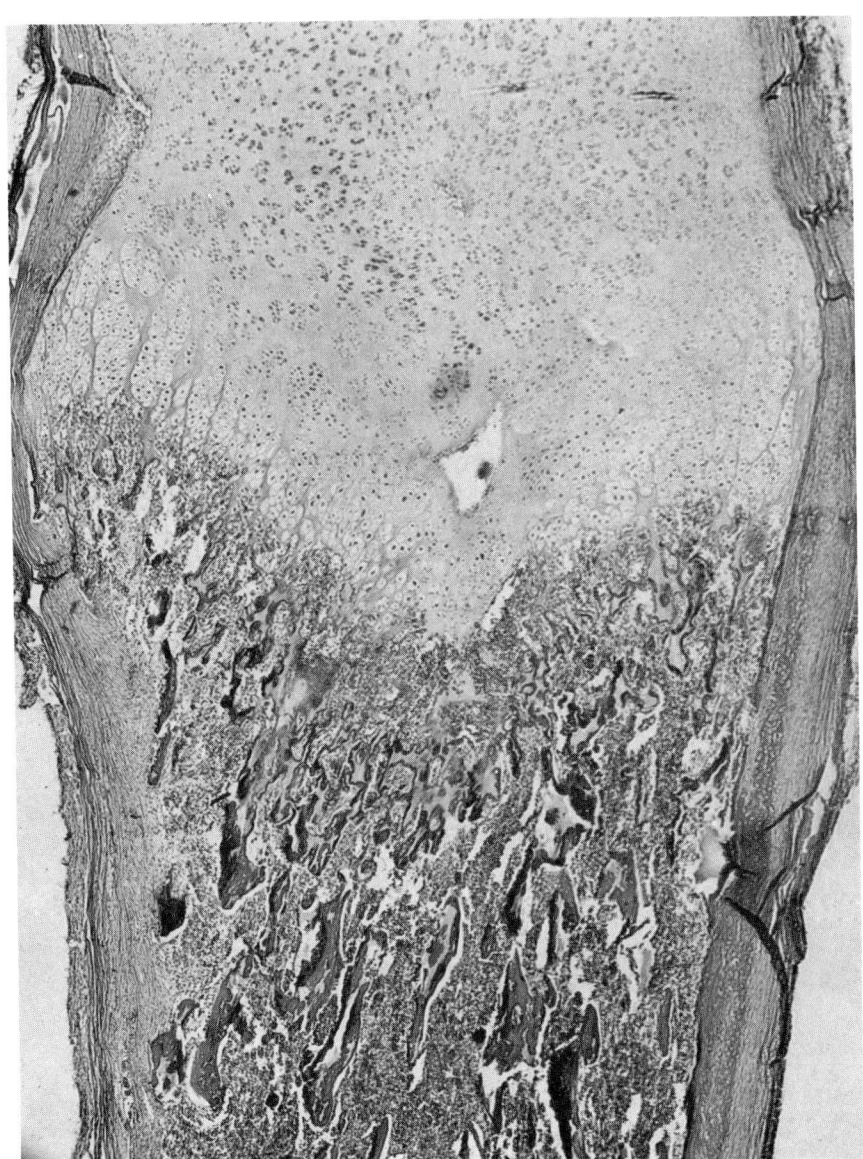

Figure 33–3

Figure 33–3. This V-shaped configuration of the epiphyseal line is also seen at times, in longitudinal sections of the costochondral junction.

This baby was a 2,280 gram black female, born at term, who lived for five hours and nine minutes.

Hematoxylin and eosin stain. Mag. 38×.

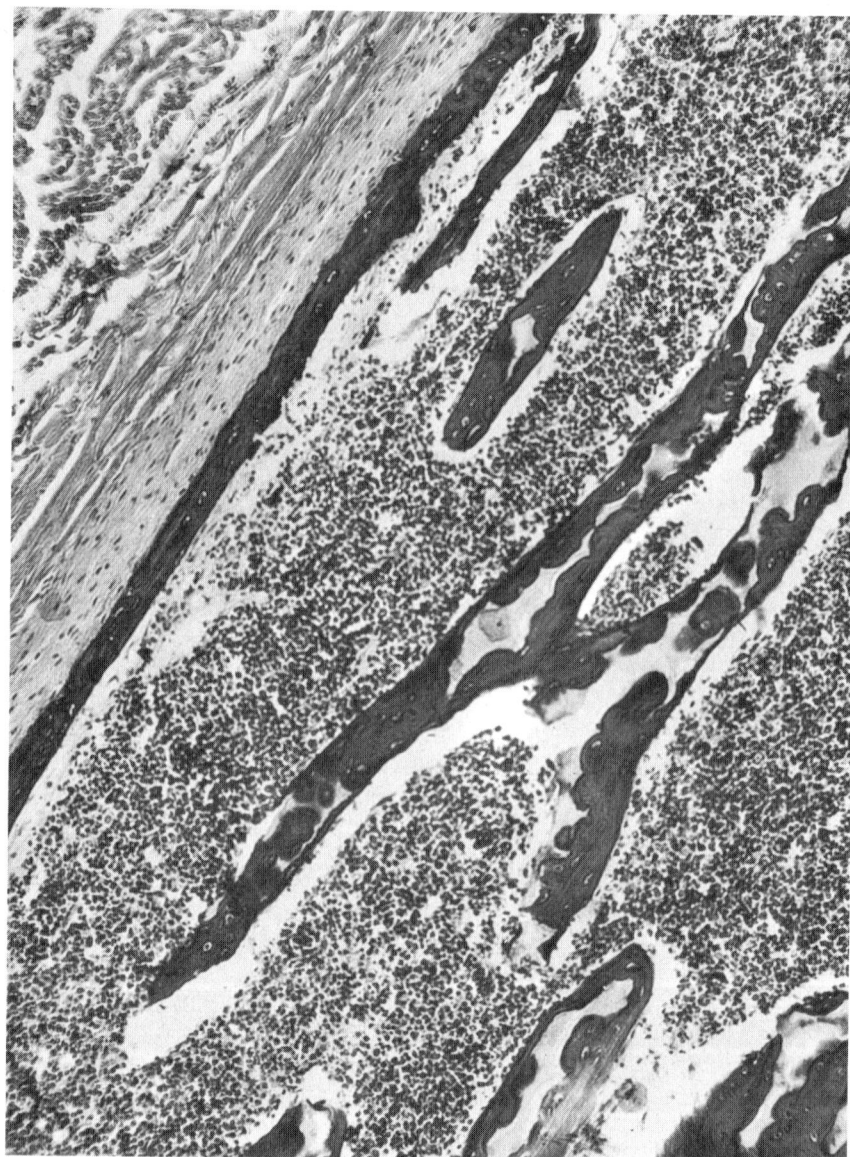

Figure 33-4

Figure 33-4. Seen here at higher magnification is the shaft of the rib to illustrate the nature of the bony trabeculae; the cellularity of the marrow, which at this age is completely hematopoietic with no adipose tissue elements; and the delicate quality of the cortex. Note just beyond the cortex the densely cellular fibrous periosteum.

Within the trabeculae, the pale-staining material in the central portion represents the osteoid and the darker-staining exterior is mineralized bone. Osteocytes can be seen within the tiny lacunae there.

This section was taken from a stillborn baby weighing 1,325 grams, delivered after 20 to 24 weeks of gestation.

Hematoxylin and eosin stain. Mag. 132×.

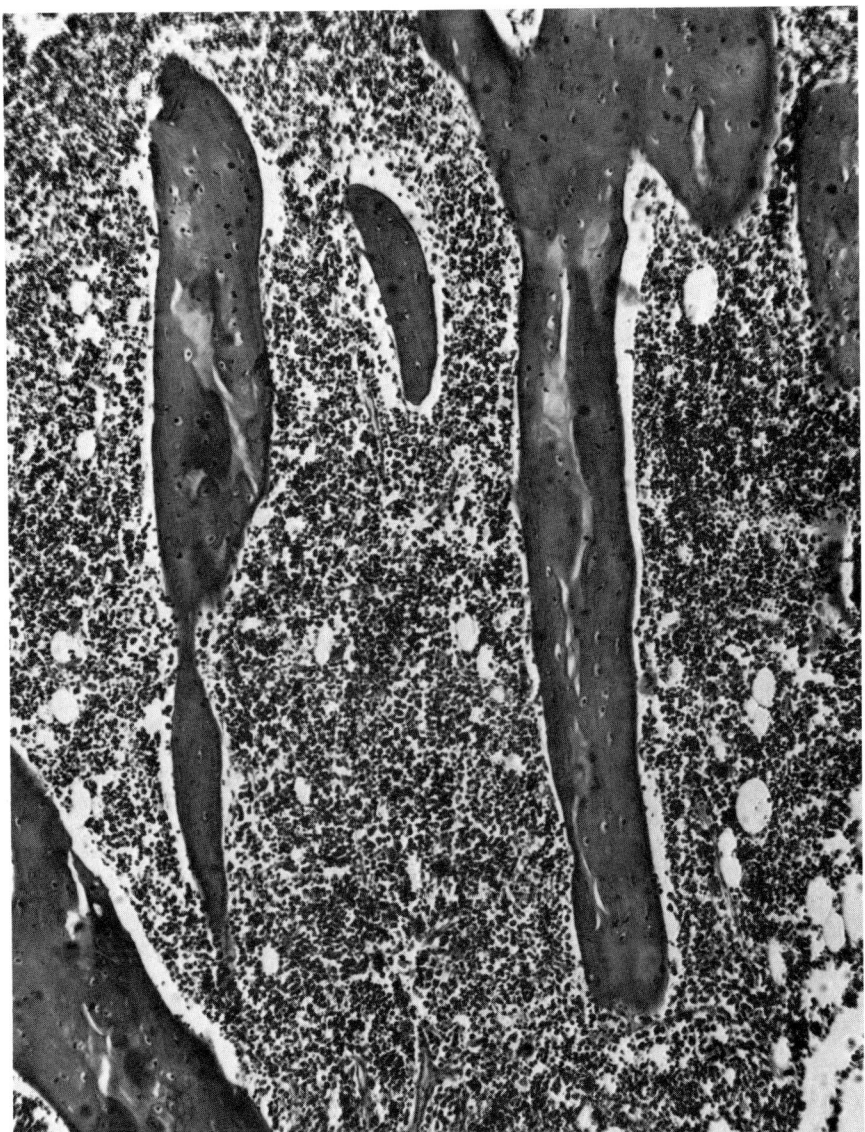

Figure 33–5

Figure 33–5. Like Fig. 33–4, this represents a longitudinal section of the shaft of a rib. The infant was a little more developed than that shown in the preceding figure. The trabeculae contain less osteoid and they are stouter. There are a few adipose tissue cells within the bone marrow, but they are certainly not many.

This infant, a female weighing 2,575 grams, was born at term and lived for one day.

Hematoxylin and eosin stain. Mag. 132×.

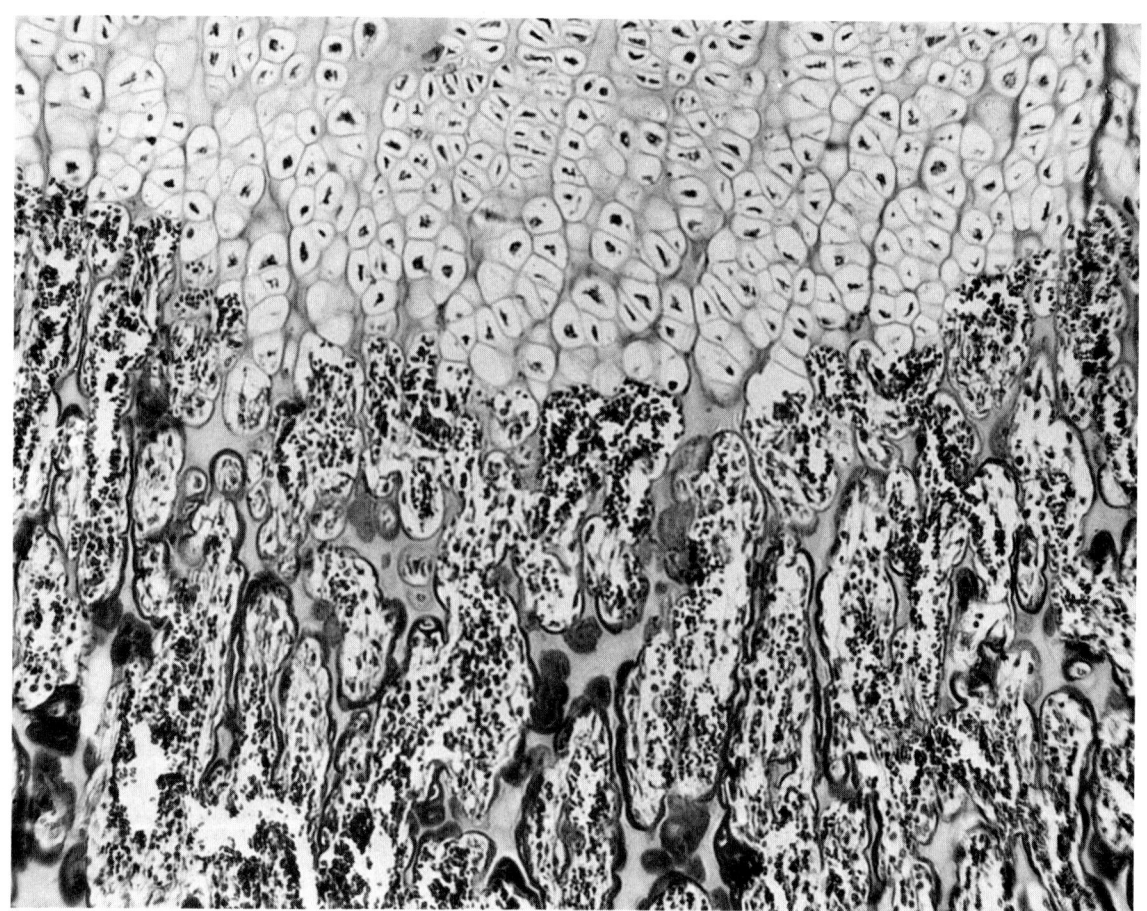

Figure 33–6

Figure 33–6. This photograph was taken, at rather high magnification, to illustrate in some detail the intimate morphology of the epiphyseal line.

Note the columns of cartilage cells directed downward from above and the abundant osteoid in the not yet very well developed trabeculae below. The marrow is very cellular.

This infant, a 2,125 gram female, was born to a 17 year old mother some weeks after the expected date of confinement. The baby lived for 11 hours.

Hematoxylin and eosin stain. Mag. 132×.

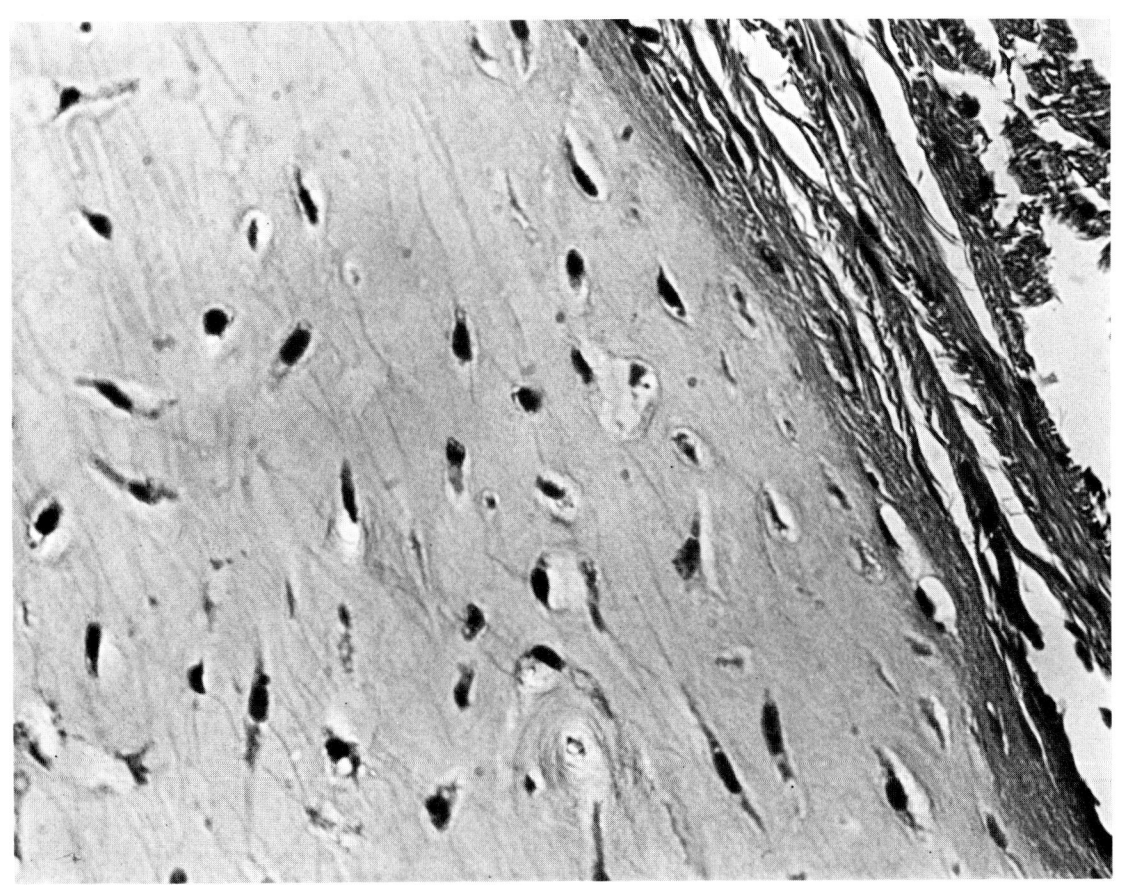

Figure 33–7

Figure 33–7. This photomicrograph was taken to illustrate the fine features of hyaline cartilage in infants during the perinatal period.

This particle of tissue comprised a portion of the sella turcica. The fibrous sheath of perichondrium appears in the upper right corner.

The baby was a 3,290 gram male born at 41 weeks of gestation, who lived for 12¼ hours.

Hematoxylin and eosin stain. Mag. 471×.

Chapter 34

ADIPOSE TISSUE

EMBRYOLOGY

From the seventeenth to the twentieth week of intrauterine life, deposits of fat form. At first the fat accumulates in the form of many small droplets within the cytoplasm of the cells (Fig. 34–1). These droplets later tend to increase in size and coalesce, causing the cell to round out and enlarge and crowding the nucleus toward the periphery (Fig. 34–3). Extensive accumulations of subcutaneous fat do not begin to be laid down in the fetus until the last two months of gestation; the wizened appearance of the prematurely born infant is due in large part to the lack of subcutaneous adipose tissue.

At various special locations in the fetus, especially along the dorsal body wall, certain groups of fat cells tend to retain their multiple small lipid droplets long after such droplets have coalesced in fat cells in other parts of the body. These are the so-called brown fat cells. In the human their relative numbers diminish steadily during the first year of extrauterine life.[6, 7]

ANATOMY

During the seventh month of gestation the body of the fetus becomes more plump and rounded in its contours and the skin loses its wrinkled appearance because of increased deposition of subcutaneous adipose tissue.

The special paired deposits of brown fat, such as appear in envelopes around the developing adrenal glands, are particularly prominent along the coelomic side of the dorsal body wall. Sizeable masses of brown fat can be seen in the newborn infant in the axillae as well as at the nape of the neck and in the posterior triangles of the neck. Smaller lobules are found near the thyroid, along the carotid sheaths, and in the hilus of each kidney. From the beginning these clusters of fat cells are divided into distinct lobules.

HISTOLOGY

It is thought that fixed undifferentiated mesenchymal cells give rise to the so-called lipoblasts. The lipoblasts take up lipid in a soluble form and store it within their cytoplasm as droplets. In the beginning, the nuclei of these cells are centrally located. Later, as the droplets become larger and coalesce, the nuclei are pushed to the perimeter of the cells (Fig. 34–2 and 34–3). By the end of the first month of life, many adipose tissue cells, such as those in the subcutaneous tissues, are large and unilocular; these are the so-called white fat cells or adult fat cells.

References

1. Moore, K. L.: The Developing Human: Clinically Oriented Embryology. Philadelphia, W. B. Saunders Co., 1973, pp. 218–297.
2. Patten, B. M.: Human Embryology, 2nd ed. New York, McGraw-Hill Book Co., Inc., 1953, pp. 295–302 and 250.
3. Warwick, R., and Williams, P. L.: Gray's Anatomy, 35th British ed. Philadelphia, W. B. Saunders Co., 1973, pp. 210–220 and 474–475.
4. Bergman, R. A., and Afifi, A. K.: Atlas of Microscopic Anatomy. Philadelphia, W. B. Saunders Co., 1974, pp. 85–94.
5. Bloom, W., and Fawcett, D. W.: A Textbook of Histology. Philadelphia, W. B. Saunders Co., 1975, pp. 244–285 and 296–308.
6. Hull, D: Brown adipose tissue in the newborn; in E. E. Philipp, J. Barnes, and M. Newton (Eds.): Scientific Foundations of Obstetrics & Gynecology. London, William Heinemann, Ltd., 1970, pp. 407–411.
7. Valdés-Dapena, M. A., Gillane, M. M., and Catherman, R.: Brown fat retention in the Sudden Infant Death Syndrome. Arch. Pathol. Lab. Med., *100*:547–549, 1976.

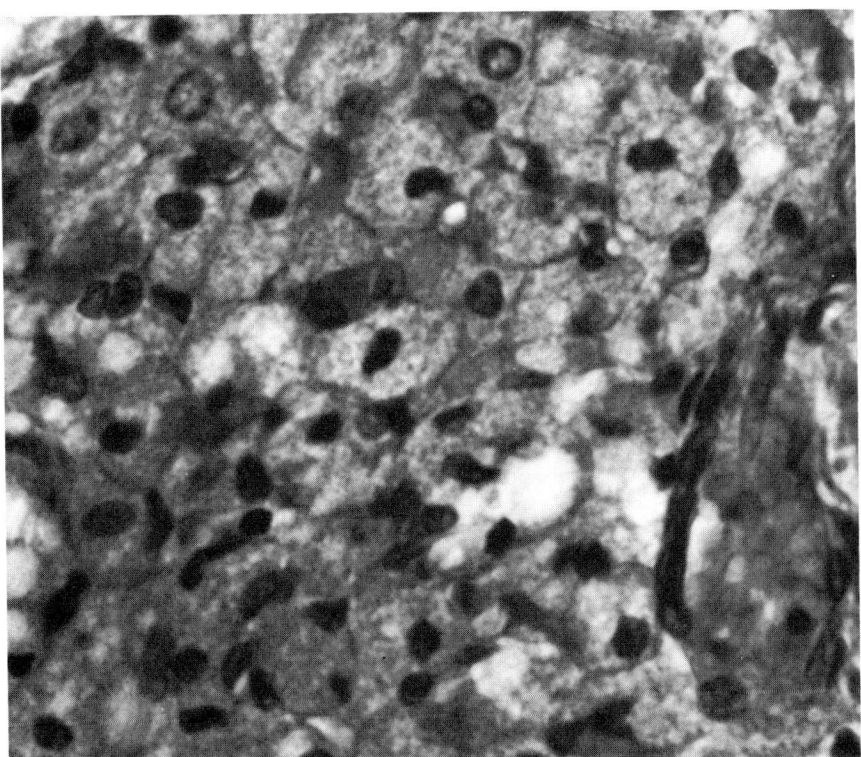

Figure 34–1

Figure 34–1. This is a section of brown fat from a six day old white female infant. The gestational age is unknown. The baby's body at autopsy weighed 2,800 grams.

Note that the nuclei of most of these cells are still centrally located. Although most of the vacuoles are extremely fine, a few are several times larger than the nuclei.

Hematoxylin and eosin stain. Mag. 660×.

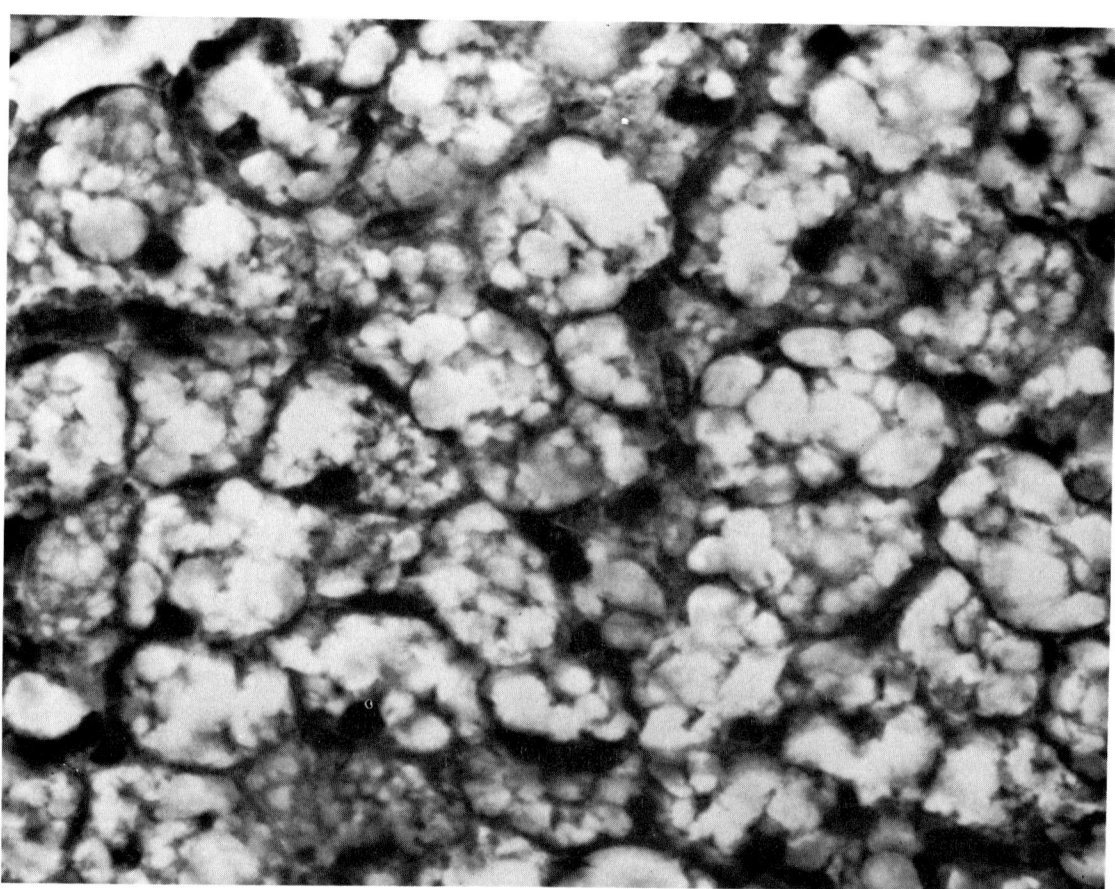

Figure 34–2

Figure 34–2. This is a section of so-called brown fat. It may or may not represent that. At least by light microscopy, these are multiloculated adipose tissue cells such as comprise the envelope of fat surrounding the adrenals. Each cell is as large as a white fat cell and its nucleus is pushed to the perimeter, as in a white fat cell, but its cytoplasm seems to contain many vacuoles separated from one another by extremely delicate walls.

This type of adipose tissue makes up most of the periadrenal envelope in newborns less than one month of age, and diminishes relative to the white fat, thereafter, throughout the first year.

Hematoxylin and eosin stain. Mag. 660×.

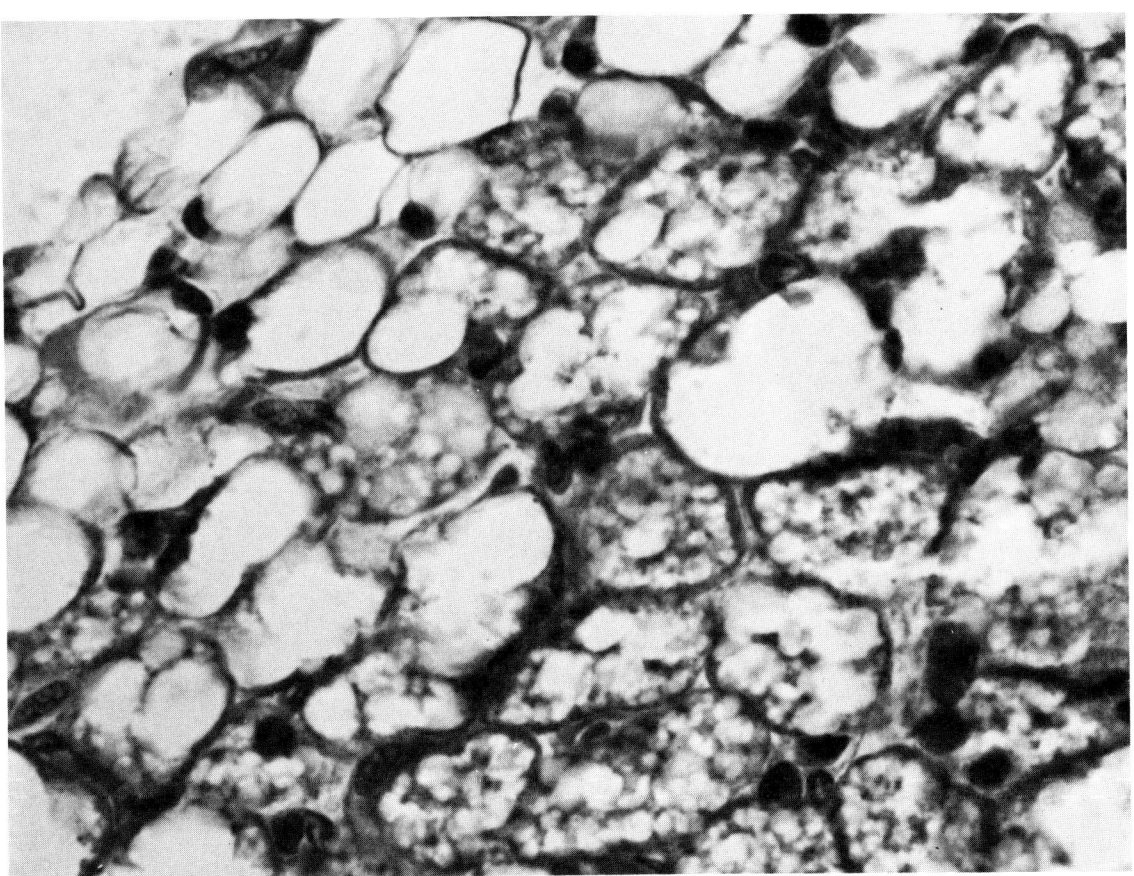

Figure 34–3

Figure 34–3. We no longer have any record of the infants from whom this section and that in Fig. 34–2 were taken.

Nevertheless, this picture illustrates a mixture of uni- and multilocular fat cells—which may or may not correspond to white and brown fat cells. (There is disagreement among authorities as to whether or not that judgment can be made on the basis of light microscopy alone.) The white or adult fat cells are the unilocular ones appearing in the left upper corner.

Hematoxylin and eosin stain. Mag. 660×.

Index

Page numbers in *italics* indicate illustrations.

A band, of myofibrils, 624–625
Acinus(i), pancreatic, 278–279
   thyroid, 117–118, *124–125*
Adenohypophysis, 104–105, *106, 108–109.*
   See also *Pituitary gland.*
Adipose tissue, 641–642, *643–645*
   anatomy of, 641
   cells of, *644–645*
   embryology of, 641
   histology of, 642
   of adrenal gland, *152–153*
   of epicardium, *22*
Adrenal gland, 131–134, *135–153*
   adipose tissue of, *152–153*
   anatomy of, 132
   cells around, brown fat, *152–153*
      giant, 133, *144–145*
      sympathochromaffin, *151*
   cortex of, 131–133, *135–145*
      "adenoid change" in, 133, *135, 146–147*
      adult, 131–132, *135, 138–141*
      cells of, 133, *145*
      embryology of, 131, *138–139*
      fetal, 131–133, *135, 138–139, 142–145*
      nodules of, 133, *149*
   embryology of, 131–132
   glomerular zone of, 131–133
   hematopoiesis in, extramedullary, *148*
   histology of, 132–134, *135–139*
   medulla of, 132–134, *150*
      embryology of, 132
      vein of, central, *138, 150*
Aganglionosis, 235, *240*
Airway, *301*
Alpha cells, of pituitary gland, 104, *108–109*
Alveolus, of lung, 309–313, *328–333, 336–337*
      after artificial respiration, *337*
      development of, 310
      duct(s) of, 311–312, *322–323, 337*
      histology of, *332–333*
      lumen of, *338–339*
      sac(s) of, 311–312, *322*
Ampulla of Vater, 265, *268*
Anitschkow myocyte, 4–5, *14–15*
Annulus fibrosus, 5
Anorectal canal, *242–244*
Aorta, 32, *34–38*
Apocrine gland, 160–161

Appendix, vermiform, 234
Appendix epididymis, 398, 400, *407–409, 414*
   anatomy of, 398
   embryology of, 398
   histology of, 400
Appendix testis, anatomy of, 398
   embryology of, 398
   histology of, 400
Aqueduct, of Sylvius, 585
Aqueous fluid, 517
Arachnoid, 542
Arrectores pilorum, 160, *163*
Artery(ies), coronary, *24*
   pulmonary, 310, 313
   splenic, *40,* 83, *98–99*
Arytenoid swelling, 287–288
Atrium, cardiac, 3–4
Auerbach, plexus of, *236–239*

Basis pontis, 544–545, *588–593*
Bellini, papillary ducts of, 348
Beta cells, of pituitary gland, 104–105, *108–109, 112*
Bile duct, 245–246, *258–259*
Bladder, urinary. See *Urinary bladder.*
Blood vessel(s), 31–33, *34–41*
   anatomy of, 32
   coronary, *24–25*
   embryology of, 31–32
   histology of, 32–33
   umbilical, 33, *41*
Bone, cancellous, 630–631
   compact, 631
   development of, 629–630
   interstitial substance of, 632
   lamellar, 631
   long, growth of, 632
   trabecular, 630, *636–637*
Bowman's capsule, 346, *371*
   urinary pole of, 347
Brain, 533–546. See also *Forebrain, Hindbrain,* and *Midbrain.*
   capsule of, internal, 539–540, 543, *554–555*
   embryology of, 533–537
   meninges of, 542
   nucleus of, caudate, 543, *556–557*
      lenticular, 543

Brain stem, 537
Breast, 501-505, 506-511. See also *Mammary glands.*
  anatomy of, 504
  development of, at term, 510
  embryology of, 503-504
  histology of, 504
  supportive tissue of, 508-509
Bronchiole(s), respiratory, 311-312, 320-323
  epithelial lining of, 319
Bronchus(i), 288-289, 291, 307, 309-313, 314-317
  anatomy of, 289
  embryology of, 288
  epithelial lining of, 318
  histology of, 291, 311-312
  stem, 288
Brown fat cell(s), 641, 643-644
  around adrenal gland, 152-153
Brunner's glands, 225, 226-227
Bulbus cordis, 4

C cells, of pituitary gland, 104-105, 108-109
Call-Exner bodies, 452
Calyx, of kidney, 380
Capsule, Glisson's, 247, 264
  hepatic, 264
  internal, of brain, 539-540, 543, 554-555
  of lymph nodes, 66-67
  of spleen, 83, 91
Cardiac atrium, 3-4
Cardiac glands, 208
Cardiac orifice, 207
Cardiac septum, 3-5, 16, 26-28
Cardiac valves, 5, 18-19
Cardiovascular system, 1-41. See also *Blood vessels* and *Heart.*
Cartilage, of skeletal system, elastic, 629-630
  hyaline, 629-630, 639
Cecum, 233-234
Cell(s), acidophilic, of pituitary gland, 104, 108-109
  alveolar, 338-339
  basophilic, of pituitary gland, 104-105, 108-109, 112
  chromophobe, of pituitary gland, 104-105, 108-109
  ependymal, of brain, 544, 546-565, 598-599
  epithelial, of pituitary gland, 104-105, 108-109
  fat, 641-642, 643-645
  ganglion, of large intestine, 235, 238-241
  giant, of adrenal gland, 133, 144-145
  glial, 558-559, 562-563
  hematopoietic, of pancreas, 281
  hilus, of ovary, 436, 458-459
  Kupffer, 246-247, 253
  Leydig, 399, 404
  Paneth, 230-231
  Purkinje, 576-577, 580
  Sertoli, 397
  stave, of spleen, 83
  sympathochromaffin, of adrenal gland, 151
Central nervous system, 533-546, 547-620. See also *Brain* and *Spinal cord.*
  anatomy of, 537-542
  embryology of, 533-537
  fourth ventricle of, 545-546, 596-597, 606-611

Central nervous system (*Continued*)
  histology of, 542-546
  lateral ventricle of, 533, 543-544, 560-565
Cerebellum, 540-541
  folia of, 576-580
  formation of, 536
  histology of, 544
  nucleus of, dentate, 544, 582-584
  white matter of, 581
Cerebral cortex, 534-535, 542-543, 547-553
  histology of, 542-543
  layers of, 542-543
  superficial, 552-553
Cerebral dura, 542
Cerebrum, 534-535, 537-540
  cortex of. See *Cerebral cortex.*
Cervical canal, 492-493
"Cervical erosion," 481
Cervix, 479-481, 489-491, 497-499
  glands of, 481, 491, 494-496
Choroid, 516, 518
Choroid plexus, 544, 597, 608-609
  histology of, 568-569
  morphology of, 566-567
Cloaca, 233
Cohnheim, fields of, 624
Collagen, of myocardium, 30
Colon, histology of, 236-237
Conduction system, myocardial, 5, 26-30
Copula, of tongue, 168
Cord(s), ovigerous, 442-444
Corium. See *Dermis.*
Cornea, 516-518, 523
Coronary blood vessels, 24-25
Coronary sinus, 23
Corpus atreticum, of ovary, 435-436, 453
Corpus callosum, 535
Corpus fibrosum, 435
Corpus striatum, 535
Corpuscle(s), Hassall's, 46-47, 52, 54-56
  Malpighian, of spleen, 86-87
Cortex, cerebral, 534-535, 542-543, 547-553
  histology of, 542-543
  superficial, 552-553
  ovarian, 433-434, 443, 453
  renal, 346-347, 350-354
   morphology of, 349-353, 356-359
  thymic, 46, 52-53
Cricoid, 301
Crypt(s), of Lieberkühn, 234-235, 236-237
  tonsillar, 59, 62-63
Cumulus oophorus, 449
Cyst(s), follicular, 437
  of pars intermedia, 105, 114

Dermis, 157-161
  papillary layer of, 160-161
  reticular layer of, 160-161
Diaphragm, skeletal muscle of, 626-627
Diaphysis, 632, 636-637
Diencephalon, 533-534
Disse, space of, 247
Duct(s), alveolar, 311-312, 322-323, 337
  bile, 245-246, 258-259
  ejaculatory, 416, 425
  esophageal, 194, 200-203
  genital. See *Genital ducts.*
  mesonephric, 345

Duct(s) (*Continued*)
  Müllerian, 397, 415, 479
  of Bellini, 348
  of Santorini, 269
  of Wirsung, 269
  pancreatic, 269–270, *274–277*
  paraurethral, 384
  prostatic, 416, *423–427*
  Stensen's, 184
  thyroglossal, 117
  ureteric, 346
  Wharton's, 184
  Wolffian, 345, 397, *456–457*
Ductus arteriosus, 32, *37, 39*
Ductus deferens, 399, *411*
Duodenum, 223–224, *226–227*
Dura mater, 542

Eccrine glands, 160–161
Ejaculatory ducts, 416, *425*
Elastic fiber(s), of myocardium, *30*
Endocardium, 4, *20–21*
Endocrine glands, 101–153. See also *Adrenal gland, Parathyroid glands, Pituitary gland,* and *Thyroid gland.*
Endometrium, 480–481, *485–486*
  glands of, 481, *485, 487*
    morphology of, *487*
  stroma of, *488*
Endomysium, 624
Endosteum, 632
Epicardium, 5, *22–23*
  adipose tissue of, *22*
Epidermis, 157–159, *166*
Epididymis, 398–399, *407–408*
  ductules of, *409–410*
Epiglottis, 287–290, *293–296*
  anatomy of, 288
  embryology of, 287
  histology of, 289–290
Epimysium, 624
Epiphysis(es), 630, *634–635, 638*
Epithelium, germinal, of ovary, 436, *454–455*
  of testis, 399, *403*
Esophagus, 193–195, *196–206*
  anatomy of, 193–194
  embryology of, 193
  epithelial lining of, *198–200*
  gland of, 194–195, *200–201*
    duct of, *200–203*
  histology of, 194–195, *196–197*
  muscle of, 194, *204–205*
Eye, 513–519, *520–529*
  anatomy of, 516–517
  choroid of, 516, 518
  ciliary body of, 516–518
  cornea of, 516–518, *523*
  embryology of, 515–516
  fetal, *529*
  histology of, 517–519
  iris of, 515, 517–518, *522*
  lens of, 516–518
  nerves of, 518–519, *526–529*
  retina of, 515–518, *524–527*
  sclera of, 516–517
  tunic of, fibrous, 516–518
    vascular, 518
  vitreous body of, 518

Fallopian tubes, 469–470, *471–477*
  anatomy of, 469
  embryology of, 469
  histology of, 469–470
  mucosa of, 469–470, *476–477*
  muscular coat of, 470
  serosa of, 470
Fat cell(s), 641–642, *643–645*
Fiber, elastic, of myocardium, *30*
  muscle, 624
  Purkinje, 5
Fibrocartilage, skeletal, 629–630
Fibrous trigone, of heart, 5
Fingerprint(s), patterns of, 159
Follicle, Graafian, *448–451*
  hair, 159, *164–165*
  ovarian. See *Ovary, follicle of.*
Foramen, of Luschka, 533
  of Magendie, 545
Foramen cecum, 117, 170
Forebrain, anatomy of, 537–540
  embryology of, 533–535
  gyrus(i) of, 538
  hippocampus of, 540, 544, *574–575*
    immature, *570–571*
    mature, *572–573*
  lobes of, 538–539
  sulcus(i) of, 538
Fourth ventricle, of central nervous system, 536, 540–541, 545–546, 596, *606–611*
  choroid plexus of, 544, *566–569, 608–609*
  ependymal lining of, *611*
Frenulum linguae, 169

Gallbladder, 265–266, *267–268*
  anatomy of, 265
  embryology of, 265
  histology of, 265–266
  wall of, *267*
Ganglion, neural, 546, *620*
Gastric glands, 207–208, *214–219*
Gastric mucosa, *214–215*
Gastric perforation, spontaneous, *220*
Gastrointestinal tract, 167–283. See also *Esophagus, Gallbladder, Large intestine, Liver, Pancreas, Salivary glands, Small intestine, Stomach,* and *Tongue.*
Genital ducts, 397–400, *409–411*
  anatomy of, 398
  embryology of, 397–398
  histology of, 399–400
Gland(s), adrenal. See *Adrenal gland.*
  apocrine, 160–161
  Brunner's, 225, *226–227*
  cardiac, 208
  cervical, 481, *491, 494–495*
    squamous epithelium of, *496*
  eccrine, 160–161
  endocrine, 101–153. See also *Adrenal gland, Parathyroid gland, Pituitary gland,* and *Thyroid gland.*
  endometrial, 481, *485, 487*
  esophageal, 194–195, *200–201*
    duct of, *200–203*
  gastric, 207–208, *214–219*
  lingual, 170–171, *179–181*
  mammary. See *Mammary glands.*
  parathyroid. See *Parathyroid glands.*
  parotid, 183–184

Gland (*Continued*)
  periurethral, 392
  pituitary. See *Pituitary gland.*
  prostatic. See *Prostate.*
  pyloric, 208, *211, 214–217*
  salivary. See *Salivary glands.*
  sebaceous, 160–161, *164*
  seminal, 393, 399–400, *412–413*
  sublingual, 183–184
  submandibular, 183–184, *185–190*
  thymus. See *Thymus.*
  thyroid. See *Thyroid gland.*
  tubuloalveolar, of prostate, *428–429*
  urethral, 384, 392
Glial cells, 558–559, *562–563*
Glisson's capsule, 247, *264*
Glomerular zone, adrenal, 131–133
Glomerulosclerosis, 368
Glomerulus, renal, 347, *366–367*
Glottis, primitive, 287–288
Graafian follicle, *448–451*

H band, of myofibrils, *624–625*
Hair, 159–160
Hair follicle, 159, *164–165*
Hassall's corpuscles, 46–47, *52, 54–56*
Haversian system(s), 631
Heart, 3–5, *6–30.* See also *Cardiac.*
  conduction system of, 5
  embryology of, 3–5
  morphology of, 4–5
Heister, spiral valve of, 265
Hematopoiesis, extramedullary, adrenal, *148*
  hepatic, 260–263
  mammary, 508–509
  pancreatic, 270
  thymic, 57
Henle, loop of, 346
Hepatic. See *Liver.*
Hepatocyte(s), 246–247, *252*
Hilus cell(s), of ovary, 436, *458–459*
Hindbrain, anatomy of, 540–542
  embryology of, 535–536
Hippocampus, 540, 544, *574–575*
  immature, *570–571*
  mature, *572–573*
Hormone(s), testicular, 397–398
Hypophysis. See *Pituitary gland.*

I band, of myofibrils, *624–625*
Ileum, 224, *228*
Infundibulum, pituitary, 103
  uterine, *475*
Interstitial system(s), 631
Intestine. See *Large intestine* and *Small intestine.*
Iris, 515, 517–518, *522*

Jejunum, 224

Kidney, 345–348, *349–381*
  anatomy of, 346–347
  calyx of, *380*

Kidney (*Continued*)
  cortex of, 346–347, *350–354*
    morphology of, *349–353, 356–359*
  embryology of, 345–346
  glomerulus of, 347, *366–367*
    sclerotic, 368
  histology of, 347–348
  juxtaglomerular apparatus of, *369*
  medulla of, 347, *355*
  nephrogenic zone of, *357–358, 360–365*
  pelvis of, 379
  pyramid of, *350–353, 376–378*
  tubules of, 347–348
    collecting, *370–375*
    cortical, *366–367*
    secretory, 346
Kupffer cells, 246–247, *253*

Langerhans, islets of, 270, *280*
Lanugo hair, 159
Large intestine, 233–235, *236–244*
  anatomy of, 234
  embryology of, 233–234
  histology of, 235
Larynx, 287–290, *297–298*
  anatomy of, 288–289
  embryology of, 287–288
  histology of, 290
  lumen of, *299–300*
  sinus of, 289
  ventricle of, 289, *292, 300*
  vestibule of, 289
Lens, optic, 516–518
Leptomeninges, 542
  histology of, 546
Leydig cells, 399, *404*
Lieberkühn, crypts of, 234–235, *236–237*
Lingual gland(s), 170–171, *179–180*
Lipoblast(s), 642
Liver, 245–247, *248–264*
  anatomy of, 246
  capsule of, *264*
  embryology of, 245–246
  hematopoiesis in, extramedullary, 260–263, 270
  histology of, 246–247, *248–249*
  lobule of, 246, *250–251*
  parenchyma of, *260*
  portal areas of, *256–257*
  sinusoids of, 246–247
  vein of, *254–255*
Lobule, hepatic, 246, *250–251*
  of lung, 311
  pancreatic, *272, 279*
  thymic, *50–51*
Loop of Henle, 346, 347
Lower respiratory tract, 309–313, *314–341.*
  See also *Bronchiole(s), Bronchus(i),* and *Lung(s).*
  anatomy of, 310–311
  embryology of, 309–310
  histology of, 311–313
Lung(s), 309–313, *314–341*
  alveolus of. See *Alveolus.*
  anatomy of, 310–311
  embryology of, 309–310
  histology of, 311–313, *324–327, 334–335*
  lobules of, 311
  visceral pleura of, 313, *340*

INDEX

"Lung bud," 288
Luschka, foramen of, 533
Lymph node(s), 65–67, 68–77
  anatomy of, 66
  capsule of, 66–67
  cortex of, 66–67
    nodules of, 74–75, 77
  embryology of, 65, 68–73, 76
  histology of, 66–67
  mesenteric, 73–75
  medulla of, 66–67
  sinuses of, 66–67
Lymphatic aggregates, of spleen, 94–96
Lymphatic channels, 76
Lymphatic sinus, 66–67
Lymphocyte(s), pancreatic, 282
  thymic, 46
Lymphoid tissue, 43–77. See also *Lymph node(s)*, *Thymus*, and *Tonsils, palatine.*

M band, of myofibrils, 625
Magendie, foramen of, 545
Mall, space of, 247
Malpighian corpuscles, of spleen, 86–87
Mammary glands, 501–511. See also *Breast*.
  ducts of, 504, 508–511
  milk channels of, 503
  nipple of, 503–504, 506–507
Meconium, 234
Medulla, of lymph nodes, 66–67
  renal, 347, 355
  thymic, 52–53, 56
Medulla oblongata, 536, 541, 594–597
  cells of, 598–599
  histology of, 545
  olive of, 541, 594–595, 600–603
    cells of, 604–605
Membranous septum, of heart, 5
Meninges, 542
Mesencephalon. See *Midbrain*.
Mesoderm, 623, 629
Metanephros, 345–346
Metaphysis, 632
Metencephalon, 536
Midbrain, anatomy of, 540
  embryology of, 535
Milk channels, 503
Mitral valve, of heart, 18–19
"Mongolian spots," 158
Müllerian ducts, 397, 415, 479
Muscle, skeletal, 626–627
Muscle fibers, 623–625, 626–627
  of heart. See *Myocardium*.
Muscular system, 623–625, 626–627
  anatomy of, 624
  embryology of, 623–624
  histology of, 624–625
Myelencephalon, 536
Myocardium, 4–5, 6–17, 26–30
  conduction system of, 5, 26–30
  ventricular, 10–12, 14–15
Myocyte, Antischkow, 4–5, 14–15
Myofibril(s), 624–625
  cardiac, 5
Myometrium, 481, 488

Nephrogenic zone, 357–358
  morphology of, 360–365

Nerve(s), of eye, 518–519, 526–529
Nerve plexus, autonomic, 283
Neural tissues, 531–620. See also *Brain* and *Spinal cord*.
Neurohypophysis, 104–105, 106, 115
Nipple, 503–504, 506–508
Nucleus, of brain, caudate, 543, 556–557
    dentate, 582–584
    lenticular, 543

Olive, of medulla oblongata, 541, 594–595, 600–603
  cells of, 604–605
Oocyte(s), binuclear, 464–465
  development of, 434–435, 445–448
    Class A, 434, 445–446
    Class B, 434, 445–446
    Class BC, 445–446
    Class C, 445–446
  disappearance of, in infancy, 435–436
  multinuclear, 437
Optic lens, 516–518
Optic nerve, 518–519, 526–529
Ossification, 629–630
  secondary centers of, 630
Osteon(s), 631
Ovary, 433–437, 438–467
  adrenal cortical rests in, 436, 460
  anatomy of, 434
  cortex of, 433–434, 443, 453
    superficial, 440–441
  embryology of, 433–434
  epithelium of, germinal, 436, 454–455
  follicle of, 434–435, 445–448
    Class BC, 434
    Class C, 434–435
    Class CD, 435
    Class D1, 435, 445–446
    Class D2, 435, 445, 447, 452
    Class E, 435, 445, 447
    Class F, 435, 448–449, 450–451
  cysts in, 437, 466–467
  disappearance of, in infancy, 435–436
  multiovular, 436, 462–463
  hilus cells of, 436, 458–459
  histology of, 434
    aberrations in, 436–437
  hyperplasia in, 436, 461
  para-ovarian remnants of, 436, 456–457
  sex cords of, 442–444
    cells of, 444
  stroma of, 455

Palatine tonsils. See *Tonsils, palatine*.
Pancreas, 269–271, 272–283
  acinus of, 278–279
  anatomy of, 269
  ducts of, 269–270, 274–277
  embryology of, 269
  exocrine, 278
  hematopoietic cells of, 281
  histology of, 270, 272–274, 281
  islet of, 269, 280
  lobule of, 272, 279
  lymphocytic infiltration of, 282
  neural elements in, 283

Pancreatic impression, of spleen, 90
Paneth cell, 230–231
Papilla(e), of tongue, filiform, 169–170, 174–175
    foliate, 170
    fungiform, 169–170
    vallate, 169–170, 176–177
Parathyroid glands, 126–127, 128–130
    anatomy of, 126–127
    cells of, 129
    embedded, 130
    embryology of, 126
    histology of, 127, 128
    petechiae in, 126, 130
Parenchyma, hepatic, 260
Parotid gland, 183–184
Periderm, 157
Perimysium, 624
Periosteum, 631
Petechia(e), of parathyroid, 126, 130
Peyer's patches, 224–225, 228
Pharynx, posterior, 297, 301
Pia arachnoid, 612–613
Pia mater, 526, 528, 534, 542
Pituicyte, 103, 105, 115
Pituitary gland, 103–105, 106–115
    cells of, 104–105, 108–109
    embryology of, 103
    histology of, 104–105
    lobes of, 107, 115
    morphology of, 104
    pars distalis of, 104, 107–109
    pars intermedia of, 104, 105, 107, 110–113
        cysts of, 105, 114
    pars nervosa of, 103
    pars tuberalis of, 103–104
Pleura, visceral, 313, 340–341
Plexus, choroid. See *Choroid plexus*.
    of Auerbach, 236–239
Pons, of hindbrain, 541, 544–545, 585–589, 607
    cells of, 592–593
    formation of, 536
    histology of, 544–545
Pouch, of Rathke, 103, 114
    pharyngeal, 126
Pronephros, 345
Prosencephalon. See *Forebrain*.
Prostate, 415–416, 417–429
    anatomy of, 415
    ducts of, 416, 423–427
    embryology of, 415
    histology of, 415–416
    sinus of, 415, 418
    stroma of, 419
    tubuloalveolar glands of, 416, 428–429
    utricle of, 420–422
Pulmonary artery, 310
Pulmonary system. See *Lung(s)*.
Pulp, splenic, 82, 92–93, 97
Purkinje cells, 576–577, 580
Purkinje fibers, 5
Pylorus, 208, 211, 214–217

Rathke's pouch, 103, 114
Renal cortex, 346–347, 350–354
    morphology of, 349–353, 356–359

Reproductive system, female, 431–477. See also *Fallopian tubes, Ovary, Uterus,* and *Vagina*.
    male, 395–429. See also *Prostate* and *Testis*.
Respiratory system, 285–341
Respiratory tract, lower, 309–313, 314–341. See also *Bronchiole(s), Bronchus(i),* and *Lung(s)*.
    upper, 287–291, 292–307. See also *Bronchus(i), Epiglottis, Larynx,* and *Trachea*.
Rete testis, 397, 401
Retina, 515–518, 524–527
    histology of, 518
Rhombencephalon. See *Hindbrain*.

Sac(s), alveolar, 311–312, 322
Salivary glands, 183–185, 186–191
    anatomy of, 183–184
    embryology of, 183
    histology of, 184–185
    minor, 171, 182
    parotid, 183
    sublingual, 183–185
    submandibular, 183–184, 186–191
Santorini, duct of, 269
Sarcolemma, 624
Sarcomere, 624
Sarcoplasm, 624
Sclera, of eye, 516–517
Sebaceous glands, 160–161, 164
Sella turcica, 106, 639
Seminal gland(s), 393, 399–400, 412–413
Seminiferous tubules, 399, 402, 404–405
    histology of, 399
Septum(a), cardiac, 3–5, 16, 26–28
    interalveolar, 312
    urorectal, 233
Sertoli, cells of, 397
Sex cords, 442–444
Sinus, coronary, 23
    laryngeal, 289
    lymphatic, 66–67
    prostatic, 415
Sinusoid(s), hepatic, 246–247
Skeletal muscle, 626–627
Skeletal system, 629–632, 633–639
    anatomy of, 630–631
    embryology of, 629–630
    histology of, 631–632
Skin, 155–161, 162–166
    anatomy of, 158–160
    appendages of, 158–159
    embryology of, 157–158
    hair-bearing, 163
    hair follicle of, 164–165
    histology of, 160–161, 162
    layers of, 160–161
Small bowel. See *Small intestine*.
Small intestine, 223–225, 226–231
    anatomy of, 224
    embryology of, 223
    histology of, 224–225, 230–231
    lamina propria of, 225
    mucosa of, 224–225
Somite(s), 623
Space, of Disse, 247
    of Mall, 247

INDEX 653

Spermatogonia, 397
Spinal canal, *616–617*
Spinal cord, anatomy of, 541–542
   anterior horn of, *615, 618–619*
   embryology of, 536–537
   histology of, 546
   lumbar, *614*
   meninges of, 542
   thoracic, *613*
Spinal dura, 542
Spleen, 79–83, *84–99*
   anatomy of, 81–82
   arteries of, *40*, 83, *98–99*
   capsule of, 83, *91*
   cells of, 83
   clefts of, *89*
   embryology of, 81
   hilus of, 88
   histology of, 82, *84–87*
   lymphatic aggregates of, *94–96*
   Malpighian corpuscles of, *86–87*
   pancreatic impression of, *90*
   pulp of, red, 82, *92–93*
      white, 82, *97*
   veins of, 83
Stem bronchus, 288
Stensen's duct, 184
Stomach, 207–209, *210–221*
   anatomy of, 207–208
   corpus of, 208
   embryology of, 207
   fundus of, 207–208, *218–219*
   glands of, 207–208, *214–219*
   greater curvature of, 207
   histology of, 208–209
   lesser curvature of, 207–208
   mucosa of, 208–209, *214–215*
   muscular coat of, 209, *220–221*
   pylorus of, 208, *211, 214–217*
   wall of, *210, 212–213*
Stratum basale, 160
Stratum corneum, 160
Stratum germinativum, 157, 160
Stratum granulosum, 160
Stratum lucidum, 160
Stratum malpighii, 160
Stratum spinosum, 160
Stroma, endometrial, *488*
   ovarian, *455*
   prostatic, *419*
Sublingual gland, 183–184
Submandibular gland, 183–184, *185–190*
Supporting structures, 621–645
Sweat gland, 160–161
Sylvius, aqueduct of, 585

Taste buds, 168–169, 171, *178*
   development of, 168–169
Telencephalon, 533–534. See also *Cerebrum.*
Testis, 397–400, *401–414*
   anatomy of, 398
   cells of, 397, 399, *404, 406*
   ducts of, 397–400, *410–411*
   embryology of, 397–398
   epididymis of, 398, *407–409, 414*
   histology of, 398–400, *406*
   hormones of, 397–398
   seminal gland of, 398, *412–413*

Testis (*Continued*)
   tubules of, 397, 399, *402, 404–405*
   tunica albuginea of, 398, *401, 403*
Theca interna, ovarian, hyperplasia of, 436, *461*
Thymus, 45–47, *48–58*
   anatomy of, 46–47, *48–49*
   cortex of, 46, *52–53*
   embryology of, 45–46
   epithelial tissue of, 58
   hematopoiesis in, extramedullary, 57
   lobules of, *50–51*
   medulla of, *52–53, 56*
Thyroid gland, 117–118, *119–125*
   acinus of, 117–118, *124–125*
   anatomy of, 118
   embryology of, 117–118
   histology of, 118, *119–123*
   lobes of, *302*
Tissue, adipose. See *Adipose tissue.*
   epithelial, thymic, 58
   lymphoid, 43–77. See also *Lymph node(s), Thymus,* and *Tonsils, palatine.*
   neural, 531–620. See also *Brain* and *Spinal cord.*
Tongue, 168–171, *172–182*, 293–295
   anatomy of, 169–170
   base of, *293, 295*
   embryology of, 168–169
   foramen cecum of, 168–169
   histology of, 170–171
   lingual glands of, 170–171, *179–181*
   mucous membrane of, 170
   oral part of, *172–177*
   papillae of, 169–170, *173–177*
   salivary glands of, 171, *182*
   terminal sulcus of, 168–169
Tonsils, palatine, 59–60, *61–63*
   anatomy of, 59
   crypts of, 59, *62–63*
   embryology of, 59, *61–63*
   histology of, 60
Trabecula(e), bony, 636–637
Trachea, 288–290, *302–306*
   anatomy of, 289
   embryology of, 288
   histology of, 290
   mucosa of, *303, 305–306*
   wall of, *304*
Truncus arteriosus, 4
Tube, fallopian. See *Fallopian tubes.*
Tuberculum impar, 168
Tubule(s), seminiferous, 399, *402, 404–405*
   histology of, 399
Tunica adventitia, of blood vessels, 31–32, *36–37*
Tunica albuginea, of testis, 397–398, *401, 403*
Tunica intima, of blood vessels, 31–32, *36–37, 39*
Tunica media, of blood vessels, 31–32, *36–37, 39*
Tunica vaginalis, of testis, 398

Umbilicus, vasculature of, 33, *41*
Upper respiratory tract, 287–291, *292–307*. See also *Bronchus(i), Epiglottis, Larynx,* and *Trachea.*
   anatomy of, 288–289

Upper respiratory tract (*Continued*)
  embryology of, 287–288
  histology of, 289–291
Urachus, 383
  histology of, 385
  remnants of, *391*
Ureter, *381*, 384–385
Urethra, 383–385, *386–393*
  anatomy of, 384
  ducts of, 384
  glands of, 384, *392*
  embryology of, 383
  epithelial lining of, *392*
  histology of, 384–385
  seminal vesicle in, *393*
Urethral crest, *420–421*
Urinary bladder, 383–385, *386–393*
  anatomy of, 384
  embryology of, 383
  epithelial lining of, *389*
  fundus of, *390*
  histology of, 384
  wall of, *386–388*
Urinary system, 343–393
Uterine tube. See *Fallopian tubes.*
Uterus, 479–482, *483–499*
  anatomy of, 479–480
  embryology of, 479
  histology of, 480–481
Utricle, prostatic, *420–422*

Vagina, 479–482, *483–499*
  anatomy of, 479–480
  embryology of, 479
  histology of, 480–481
Valves, cardiac, 5, *18–19*
  spiral, of Heister, 265

Vas deferens, 398
Vein, adrenal, central, 138, *150*
  coronary, 24
  hepatic, central, *254–255*
  umbilical, *41*
Vellus hair, 159–160
Ventricle, cardiac, 4
  fourth, of central nervous system, 545–546, 596–597, *606–611*
    choroid plexus of, 544, *566–569*, 597, *608–609*
    ependymal lining of, *585–587*, *595*, *599*, *611*
  laryngeal, 289, *292*, *300*
  lateral, of central nervous system, 533, 543–544, *560–565*
    ependymal cells of, 544, *564–565*, *598–599*
    morphologic changes in, *560–563*
Vernix caseosa, 158
Vertebral body, *633*
Verumontanum, *418*
Vessel(s), blood, 31–33, *34–41*
Vitreous body, of eye, 516
Vocal cords, histology of, 290

Wharton's duct, 184
White fat cell(s), 642, *645*
Wirsung, duct of, 269
"Witch's milk," 504, *510*
Wolffian duct, 345, 397, *456–457*

Z line, of myofibrils, 624–625